Colposcopy

Ralph J. Lellé • Volkmar Küppers

Colposcopy

Comprehensive Textbook and Atlas

With contributions by Widyorini Hanafy and John France Rwegoshora

Springer

Ralph J. Lellé
Department of Obstetrics & Gynaecology
University of Münster
Münster, Germany

Volkmar Küppers
Düsseldorf, Germany

Translation from the German language edition: Kolposkopie in der Praxis by Ralph J. Lellé, and Volkmar Küppers, © Springer-Verlag Berlin Heidelberg 2014. Published by Springer-Verlag Berlin Heidelberg. All Rights Reserved.

ISBN 978-3-030-85386-0 ISBN 978-3-030-85388-4 (eBook)
https://doi.org/10.1007/978-3-030-85388-4

This Springer imprint is published by the registered company Springer Nature Switzerland AG
The registered company address is: Gewerbestrasse 11, 6330 Cham, Switzerland

We dedicate this book to our patients as well as our fellow health care providers around the world who work hard to care for the health of women, sometimes under difficult circumstances.

May our efforts be another step forward towards the ultimate goal: eliminating cancer of the cervix!

Preface

Cancer of the cervix uteri is a unique type of malignancy. On one hand, it is the second most common cancer of women worldwide. On the other hand, it is amenable to a broad range of preventive measures through secondary screening. By identifying and removing precancerous lesions, incidence rates of invasive cervical cancer have declined dramatically within the last 50 years. Unfortunately, this is only true in so-called developed countries where people possess the considerable financial and structural means to establish and maintain a screening program based on cytopathology and HPV testing.

With the introduction of HPV vaccination in 2006, worldwide elimination of cervical cancer is on the horizon. However, for years to come, vaccination efforts need to be complemented by effective secondary screening programs which are to be adapted to local resources.

This book is intended to provide a comprehensive review of available strategies for screening, triage, and treatment of cervical cancer and its precursors as well as other neoplastic and preneoplastic diseases of the lower genital tract.

As visual diagnosis of many of these diseases is feasible, a comprehensive collection of color illustrations is included. Furthermore, individual clinical scenarios are discussed, including the management of patients within a low resource environment.

May this publication be a contribution to the World Health Organization's global strategy for elimination of cervical cancer!

Münster, Germany — Ralph J. Lellé
Düsseldorf, Germany — Volkmar Küppers
November 2022

Acknowledgements

We thank the numerous people who have contributed to this book.

Special thanks go to

- Ms. Alexandra Woltering for her invaluable assistance with the manuscript's creation
- Willi Kramer and Christiane Schliemann, Media Center of Münster University, Germany, for the illustrations
- Rita Ruland, RN
- the entire team of Dr. Küppers, Düsseldorf, Germany
- Univ.-Prof. Dr. med. Gabriele Köhler, the former Director of the Gerhard Domagk Institute of Pathology, Münster University, Germany
- Birgit Konert and Magdalena Marciniak, Cytological laboratory of the Gerhard Domagk Institute for Pathology of Münster University, Germany
- Dr. Supriyatiningsih, M.Kes.,Sp.OG, Obstetrics and Gynecology Department, PKU Muhammadiyah Gamping UMY Teaching Hospital, Faculty of Medicine and Health Sciences, Universitas Muhammadiyah Yogyakarta, Indonesia
- Heinke Schimanowski-Thomsen, M.D., Matema Lutheran Hospital, Tukuyu, Tanzania, East Africa

and of course our wives, children, and grandchildren.

Contents

Abbreviations

ACIS	Adenocarcinoma in situ
ACOG	American College of Obstetrics and Gynecology
ACS	American Cancer Society
AGC	Atypical glandular cells
AGCPC	Arbeitsgemeinschaft für Zervixpathologie und Kolposkopie (= German Federation of Cervical Pathology and Colposcopy)
AIN	Anal intraepithelial neoplasia
AIS	Adenocarcinoma in situ
ASCCP	American Society of Colposcopy and Cervical Pathology
ASC-H	Atypical squamous cells favor high grade
ASC-US	Atypical squamous cells of undetermined significance
CI	Confidence interval
CIN1	Cervical intraepithelial neoplasia grade 1
CIN2	Cervical intraepithelial neoplasia grade 2
CIN3	Cervical intraepithelial neoplasia grade 3
CIS	Carcinoma in situ
CVLP	Chimeric virus-like particle
DIMDI	Deutsches Institut für Medizinische Dokumentation und Information
ECC	endocervical curettage
EFC	European Federation of Colposcopy
FDA	Food and Drug Administration
FIGO	Federation Internationale de Gynécologie et Obstétrique
GTN	Gestational trophoplastic neoplasia
HC2	Hybrid Capture 2 test
HGCGIN	High-grade cervical glandular intraepithelial neoplasia
HLA	Human leukocyte antigens
HPV	Human papillomavirus
HSIL	High-grade squamous intraepithelial lesion
IACR	International Agency for Research on Cancer
ICSI	Intracytoplasmic sperm injection
IFCPC	International Federation of Cervical Pathology and Colposcopy
ISSVD	International Society for the Study of Vulvovaginal Diseases
JHPIEGO	Johns Hopkins Program for International Education in Gynecology and Obstetrics
LBC	Liquid-based cytology
LEEP	Loop electrosurgical excision procedure

LLETZ	Large loop excision of the transformation zone
LSIL	Low-grade squamous intraepithelial lesion
MN III	Münchner Nomenklatur III
N/C ratio	Nuclear to cytoplasmic ratio
NILM	Negative for intraepithelial lesion or malignancy
PCR	Polymerase chain reaction
SGO	Society of Gynecologic Oncology
SIL	Squamous intraepithelial lesion
STD	Sexually transmitted disease
STIKO	Ständige Impfkommission
TCA	Trichloroacetic acid
VAIN	Vaginal intraepithelial neoplasia
VAIN 1	Vaginal intraepithelial neoplasia grade 1
VAIN 2	Vaginal intraepithelial neoplasia grade 2
VAIN 3	Vaginal intraepithelial neoplasia grade 3
VIA	Visual inspection (of the cervix) with acetic acid
VIAM	VIA with magnification
VILI	Visual inspection with Lugol's iodine
VIN	Vulvar intraepithelial neoplasia
VLP	Virus-like particle

1 Introduction

Contents

Colposcopy as a method of optically magnifying the inspection of the external and internal genitalia was first described by Hans Hinselmann from Bonn University, Germany, in 1925. While cytopathology and, more recently, HPV testing have become the methods of choice for many screening programs, colposcopy is the universally recognized procedure and gold standard for triage of abnormal Pap smears and/or positive HPV test results.

1.1 The Origin of Colposcopy

In 1925, the journal "Münchner Medizinische Wochenschrift" (Munich Medical Weekly) published the article "Verbesserung der Inspektionsmöglichkeiten von Vulva, Vagina und Portio" ("Improving the possibilities of the inspection of vulva, vagina, and cervix") by Prof. Dr. Hans Hinselmann (1884–1959), then a senior physician at the Department of Gynecology of Bonn University, Germany (Hinselmann 1925).

In his introduction, Hinselmann wrote[1]:

> **Based on the needs for early diagnosis and the etiology of cervical carcinoma, I was striving to improve the inspection of the cervix. (...) For this purpose, I have equipped the Leitz binocular magnifying device for dissection with a light source. Thus magnifications of 3.5 and more can be achieved with a long distance to the object and intense illumination of vagina and cervix. [...] It allows us to study all diseases of the vulva, the vestibulum, the vagina and the cervix in a way which previously has not been possible.**

Hinselmann called this device "colposcope" (Fig. 1.1). With the colposcope, it became possible for the first time to study the early stages of cervical cancer and the characteristics of intraepithelial changes. The colposcope also offered an opportunity to diagnose and treat preinvasive cervical disease.

[1] Authors' translation.

R. J. Lellé, V. Küppers, *Colposcopy*, https://doi.org/10.1007/978-3-030-85388-4_1

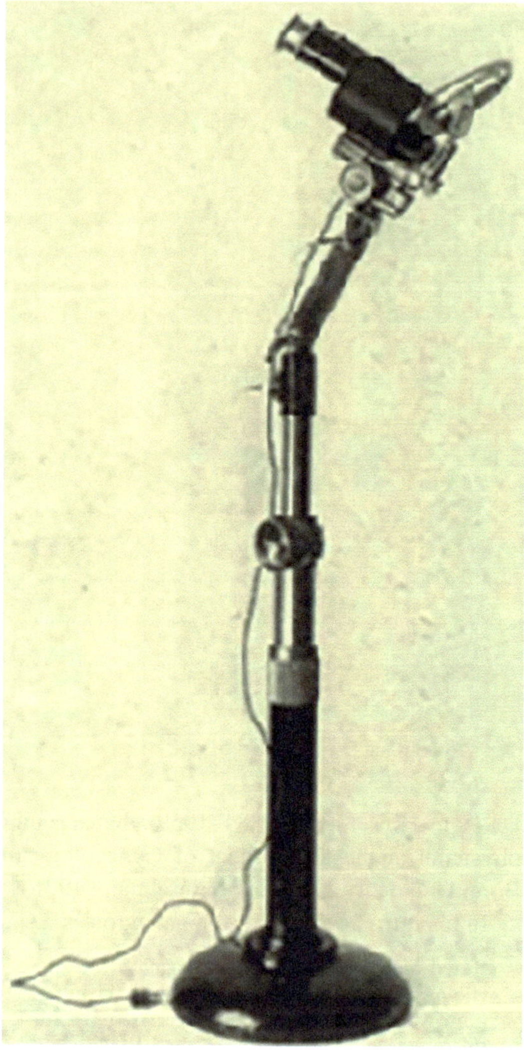

Fig. 1.1 The first colposcope as described by Hinselmann in 1925 (Hinselmann 1925)

Hinselmann could not foresee that "colposcopy" as conceived by him would become an internationally recognized and practiced method as well as a synonym for any kind of cervical diagnosis.

Hans Hinselmann left the University of Bonn in 1933 and went to Hamburg, Germany, where he became head of the Altona Women's Hospital. Only recently, Hinselmann's massive ethical misdemeanors during Nazi rule have been documented.

In a 2007 article for the American journal "The Forward" titled "*The deadly origins of a life-saving procedure*,""[2] the author Ruth Jolanda Weinberger, a scientific researcher at the "Ludwig Boltzmann Institute for Historical Social Science" based in Vienna, Austria, states: "*… inasmuch as it is possible to reconstruct events more than six decades after the fact, there appears to be enough circumstantial evidence to charge Hinselmann with at least passive knowledge of the horrifically cruel medical experiments conducted in Auschwitz.*"

The connection between Hinselmann and Auschwitz is based on the fact that one of his residents at Hamburg Altona, Helmut Wirths, had been a brother to Eduard Wirths, also a gynecologist by training and then the commanding physician at the Auschwitz concentration camp. Most likely, a colposcope had been provided to Auschwitz by Hinselmann to study the cervix of female prisoners that were photographed and subsequently removed completely. Those samples were sent to Hamburg to be studied by Hinselmann and Helmut Wirths.

Weinberger states, "*Following the fall of the Third Reich, Hinselmann was found guilty by the Allies of having conducted forced sterilizations of Gypsy women at his gynecological clinic in Hamburg. But what about his knowledge of the medical experiments performed on Jewish women in Auschwitz's Block 10, perhaps the greatest violation of the Hippocratic Oath in modern history? Should judgment not also be passed on his at least passive complicity in this most heinous of crimes?*"

Thanks to the research conducted by Bruno Halioua from France (Halioua 2010) and based on testimony from Adélaide Hautval (1906–1988), a French physician who had been imprisoned in Auschwitz (Halioua and Hauptmann 2015) and became a witness to crimes committed on women under the pretext of medical research,

[2] http://forward.com/opinion/9946/the-deadly-origins-of-a-life-saving-procedure/.

the dubious nature of Hinselmann's actions are now well known to the medical community.

Subsequently, the historical circumstances have also been documented in Germany (Ebert and David 2014), and further studies are under way (Hübner 2016). In the meantime, the "Deutsche Gesellschaft für Gynäkologie und Geburtshilfe" (German Society of Gynecology and Obstetrics) has officially distanced itself from its honorary member Hans Hinselmann.

The discussions and the competition between supporters of colposcopy as a primary screening tool and supporters of cytopathology as established by Papanicolaou had lasted for decades and are settled now. Cytopathology and colposcopy do not compete but rather complement each other.

Cytopathological examination is a simple and fast procedure and has become the screening method of choice in most Western countries. In fact, it can be regarded as the gold standard of cervical screening at which all other methods need to be measured such as HPV screening, either alone or in combination with cytopathology.

On the other hand, colposcopic examination is the crucial method for further triage of abnormal cytopathological findings. Thus, colposcopy is the most important requisite to decide whether to observe or to treat cervical precancer. If the decision to treat has been made, the colposcope guides the surgeon in order to ensure small volume resections, especially in younger women.

1.2 Acetic Acid Test

Inspection of the cervix with or without magnification may identify cervical cancer. However, identification of very early stage disease or the differential diagnosis of precancerous lesions is not possible, as the normal cervix is covered by mucus. Furthermore, epithelial changes due to high-grade squamous intraepithelial lesions are not readily visible under colposcopic magnification. Therefore, the realization that application of a 3–5% solution of acetic acid applied to the cervix will cause "acetowhite" staining together with a whole range of other diagnostic clues has revolutionized the visual diagnosis of dysplasia.

As the acetic acid reaction of squamous epithelium with HSIL changes will lead to a clearly visible "acetowhite" reaction, identification of some of these characteristic changes is feasible even without the colposcope. This is the basis for VIA (visual inspection (of the cervix) with acetic acid), thus providing an effective screening tool that can be used within a low-resource environment.

It is unclear by whom and when acetic acid application as an adjunct to colposcopy was conceived. Initially, Hans Hinselmann, who introduced colposcopy and the colposcope in 1925, did not use acetic acid. Instead, he and his German colleagues focused on "leukoplakia" (Hinselmann 1927b; Hinselmann 1927a; von Franqué 1927), which is caused by hyperkeratinization and is sometimes, but not always, associated with cervical dysplasia or cancer (Fig. 1.2). Subsequently, Hinselmann described the phenomenon of mosaic formation as a colposcopic sign of precancerous lesions, again without the use of acetic acid (Hinselmann 1928a).

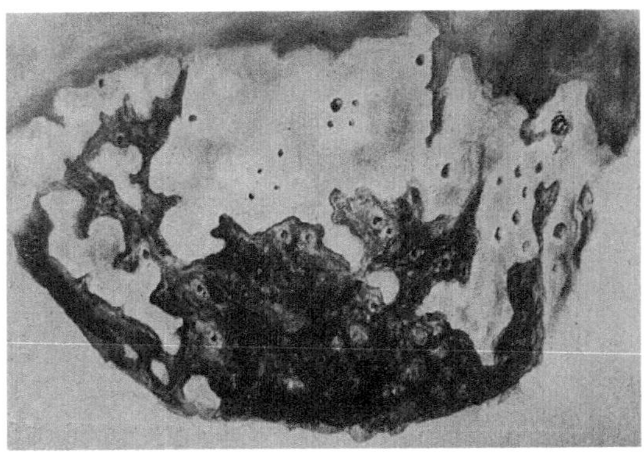

Fig. 1.2 Colposcopic drawing of the cervix from a 24-year-old prostitute with a precancerous lesion. Large areas of leukoplakia are seen, which Hinselmann in 1927 interpreted as the most significant colposcopic sign of a precancerous condition (Hinselmann 1927b)

1.3 Schiller's Iodine Test

Walter Schiller (1987–1960) from Vienna, Austria, who later became Director of Laboratories in New York and Chicago, used iodine solution to perform an in vivo stain of the cervical epithelium (Schiller 1928). He called this test, which would later carry his name, "Jodpinselung" or "brushing with iodine" (Schiller 1929). Right from the beginning, he recognized that abnormal epithelial cells do not store a sufficient amount of glycogen and do not react with the iodine. On the other hand, a positive stain can be used to rule out cancer or precancer. In 1929, Schiller used his test as a guide from where on the cervix to obtain cervical biopsies or rather scrapings from the surface epithelium ("Abschabung des Portioepithel"). Initially, Schiller did not make use of Hinselmann's colposcope. However, as early as 1928, Hinselmann suggested to combine all of these methods (Hans Hinselmann 1928b).

Today, Schiller's test is an integral part of colposcopic inspection and may even be used without colposcopic magnification as a screening tool within a low-resource environment.

References

Ebert A, David M (2014) Historische Behandlungsmethode. Die Erfindung der Kolposkopie. Geburtshilfe Frauenheilkd 74(07):631–633. https://doi.org/10.1055/s-0034-1368424

Halioua B (2010) The participation of Hans Hinselmann in medical experiments at Auschwitz. J Low Genit Tract Dis 14(1):1–4. https://doi.org/10.1097/LGT.0b013e3181af30ef

Halioua B, Hauptmann G (2015) Adélaïde Hautval (1906–1988): une personnalité médicale exemplaire. Presse Med 44(12):1290–1296. https://doi.org/10.1016/j.lpm.2015.05.012

Hinselmann H (1925) Verbesserung der Inspektionsmöglichkeiten von Vulva, Vagina und Portio. Mmw 72:1733

Hinselmann H (1927a) Über die Methodik der Diagnose der Portioleukoplakien. Zentralbl Gynaecol 51(50):3162–3163

Hinselmann H (1927b) Zur Kenntnis der präcancerösen Veränderungen der Portio. Zentralbl Gynaecol 51:901–903

Hinselmann H (1928a) Schichtungskugeln in dem Epithel der weißlichen Felder der Umwandlungszone der Portio. Zentralbl Gynaecol 52(20):1244–1247

Hinselmann H (1928b) Zur Frage der Frühdiagnose des Portiokarzioms anläßlich der Ausführungen von Kermauner im Halban-Seitz Bd. IV, 1927. Zentralbl Gynaecol 52(3):168–169

Hübner J (2016) Kolposkopie ohne Menschlichkeit?! Hinselmann und die Versuche an Frauen in Auschwitz. Geburtshilfe Frauenheilkd 76(03):A11. https://doi.org/10.1055/s-0036-1571408

Schiller W (1928) Zur klinischen Frühdiagnose des Portiokarzinoms. Zentralbl Gynaecol 52(30):1886–1892

Schiller W (1929) Jodpinselung und Abschabung des Portioepithels. Zentralbl Gynaecol 53(17):1056–1064

von Franqué O (1927) Leukoplakie und präcanceröse Veränderung des Plattenepithels. Zentralbl Gynaecol 51(15):898–899

2 Normal Anatomy of the Cervix

Contents

Understanding the transformations zone, where squamous and glandular epithelium meet, is the basis for understanding colposcopic diagnosis. Squamous cell carcinoma and its predecessors develop within the transformation zone on the basis of human papillomavirus infection. Transformation and metaplasia cause a variety of physiologic phenomena, which need to be recognized by the colposcopists and distinguished from pathologic findings.

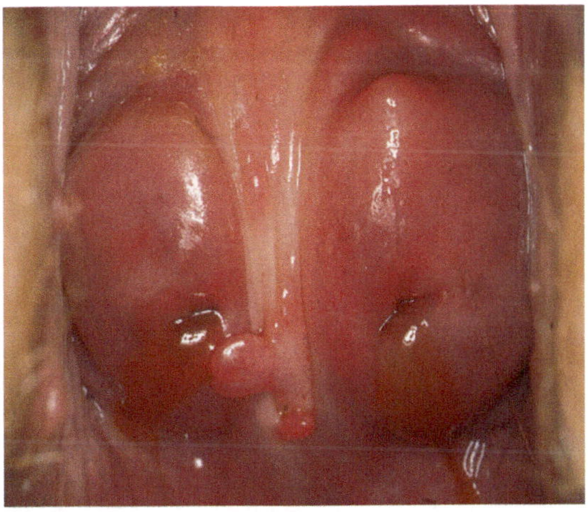

Fig. 2.1 Uterus bicollis

2.1 General Principles of Cervical Anatomy

The cervix develops through fusion of the distal part of the Müllerian ducts. If this fusion is incomplete, various malformations of the genital tract may result (Fig. 2.1). The Müllerian ducts are lined by glandular epithelium. The vagina is derived from the urogenital plate and is covered by squamous epithelium. Eventually, these two types of epithelium meet and will later form the so-called original squamocolumnar junction. At the time the embryo is fully developed and the child is born, this junction is located within the cervical canal.

Through colposcopy, only part of the cervix can be visualized. This part or portion ("portio") of the cervix extends into the vagina and is called

R. J. Lellé, V. Küppers, *Colposcopy*, https://doi.org/10.1007/978-3-030-85388-4_2

the "portio vaginalis uteri" (Figs. 2.2 and 2.3). The portio vaginalis comprises only about 30–50% of the entire length of the cervix, which is approximately 3 cm long. The length and size as well as the overall anatomy of the cervix are quite variable.

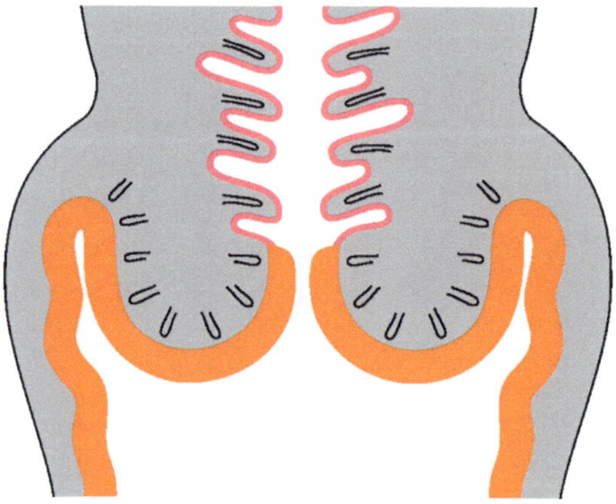

Fig. 2.2 Schematic drawing of vaginal and cervical epithelium. Vagina and cervix are both lined by multilayer squamous epithelium (yellow), which becomes a single-layered columnar epithelium within the endocervix (red)

The glandular epithelium of the cervix forms invaginations and crypts up to a depth of about 7 mm. This increases the surface of the secreting epithelium. In a strict sense, the term "endocervical gland," which is frequently used for histopathological descriptions, does not apply, since the so-called glands are merely a part of these invaginations.

The location of the squamocolumnar junction is variable. If this junction between glandular and squamous epithelium is located in the periphery of the outer cervix, and the process of transformation or metaplasia (see below) is still incomplete, the thin monolayer of columnar cells has a bloodred appearance due to blood vessels within the underlying stroma. This phenomenon is called "ectopy" (Figs. 2.4, 2.5, and 2.6). The term "erosion" is misleading and should be considered obsolete.

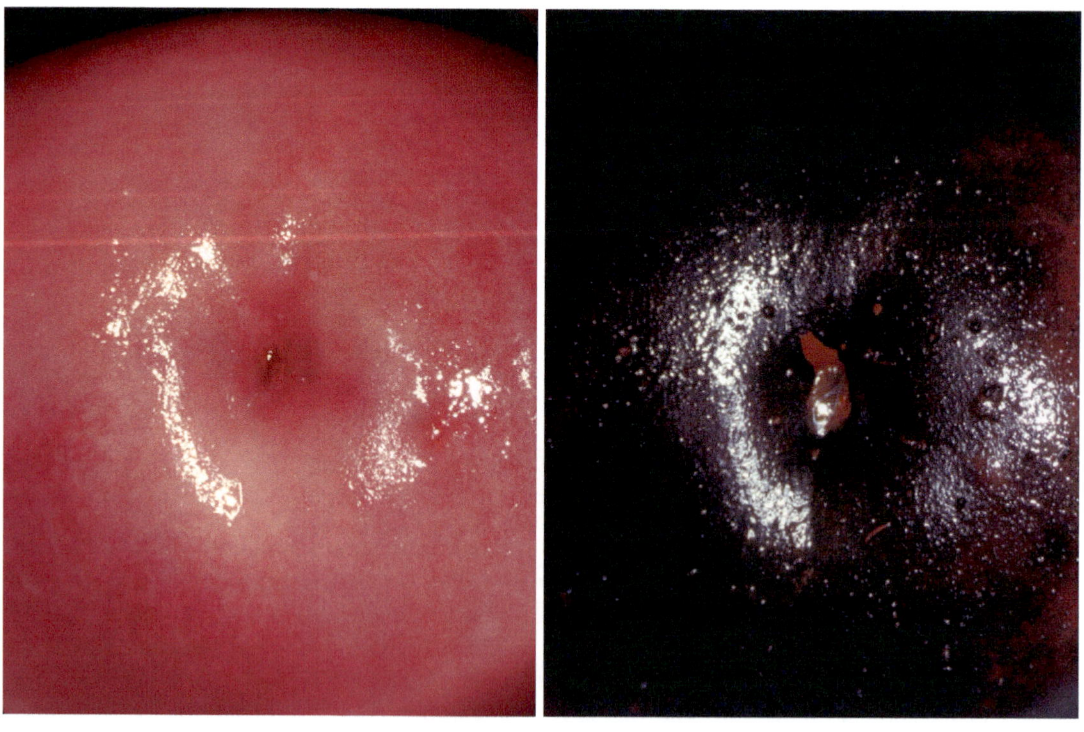

Fig. 2.3 Colposcopic image of a cervix covered by squamous epithelium (left: acetic acid test, right: Schiller's test). The squamocolumnar junction is not visible. Close to the opening of the cervical canal, a tiny area of immature metaplasia can be seen, which is Lugol (iodine)-negative

Squamous metaplasia is the decisive physiological mechanism and a basic prerequisite for the development of cervical intraepithelial neoplasia or CIN.

Metaplasia means that one type of cells/epithelium is transformed into another type of cells/epithelium. This mechanism occurs in several sites of the human body, for example, salivary glands, bronchi, stomach, or anus. In the case of cervical metaplasia, transformation of mature glandular epithelium into mature squamous cell epithelium can be observed.

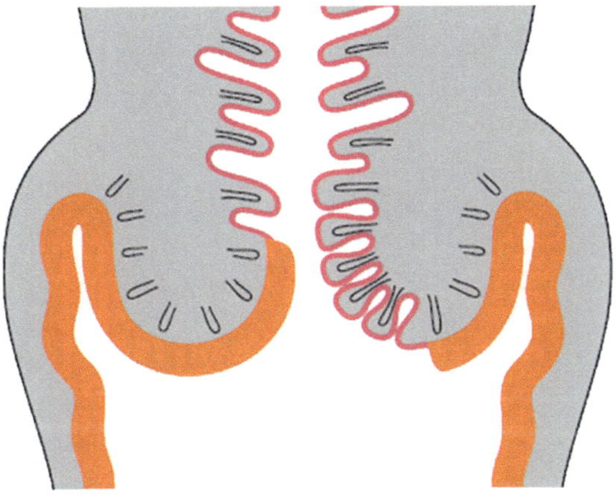

Fig. 2.4 Schematic drawing of ectopy. The glandular epithelium has not yet been modified by metaplasia and is visible on the ectocervix (on the right)

Metaplastic transformation is triggered when the columnar epithelium is situated in the ectocervix, i.e., outside the cervical canal. Obviously, external influences such as mechanical irritation, inflammation, and bacteria, a low pH, or estrogenic stimulation may be triggers for metaplastic transformation.

The process of metaplasia starts at the level of so-called reserve cells. Reserve cells form a single-layer epithelium located between the glandular epithelium and the basement membrane. These undifferentiated cells play a crucial role as they are the primary target of HPV infection.

After transformation is completed, the new metaplastic squamous epithelium is neither colposcopically nor cytologically different from the original squamous epithelium. However, on histopathological tissue sections,

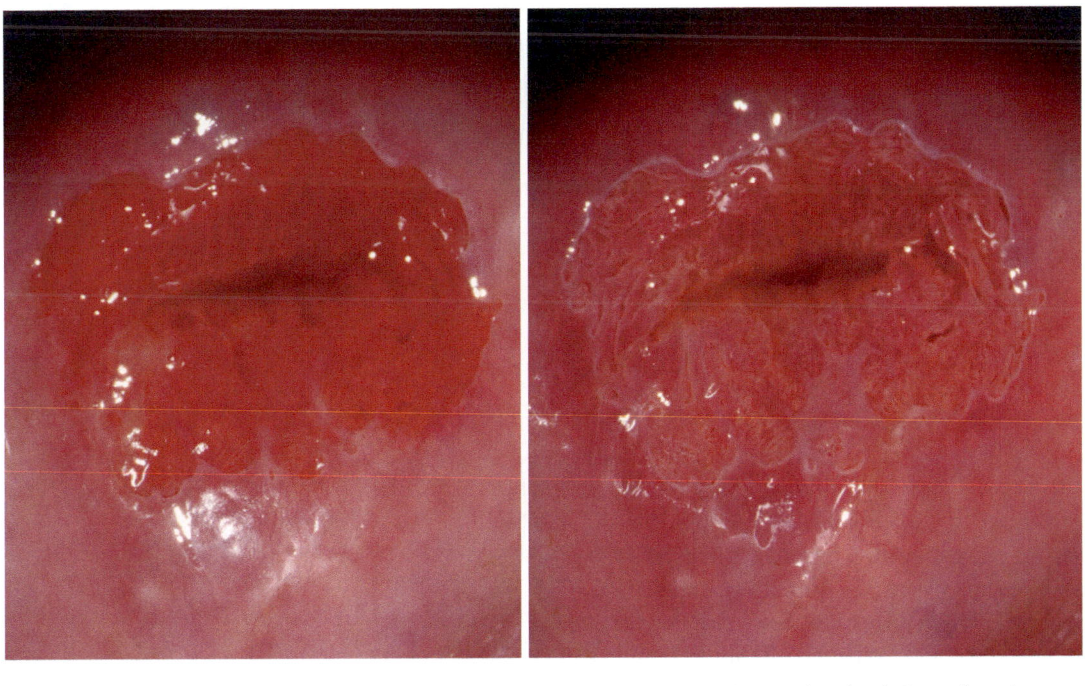

Fig. 2.5 Ectopy before and after the application of acetic acid. The squamocolumnar junction is located on the ectocervix. The glandular epithelium, which has not yet been modified by metaplasia, is bright red. At 6 o'clock, there is a small area of immature metaplasia

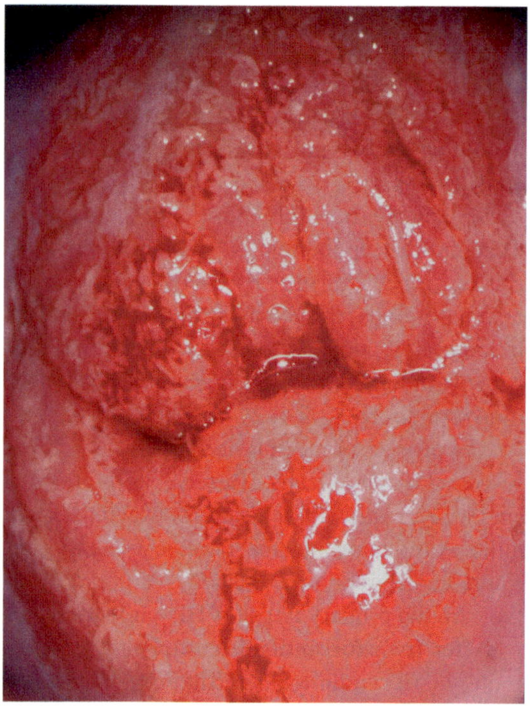

Fig. 2.6 Ectopy without metaplasia that encompasses the entire ectocervix and exhibits a villous morphology

there will be residual glandular cells underneath the new squamous cell layer.

Colposcopically, small round openings of the squamous surface are seen, which can secrete cervical mucus. If the metaplastic squamous epithelium does not leave gland openings, cysts will form through continuous excretions of the glandular epithelium, eventually leading to cysts of variable sizes. These cysts are called "ovula Nabothi" or Nabothian cysts, referring to Martin Naboth (1675–1721), a professor at Leipzig University in Germany (Baskett 2001). Naboth called these cysts "ovula," i.e., eggs, as he imagined that they represent a repository for ova.

The inner border of the transformation zone is the original gland epithelium. This is considered the "new" squamocolumnar junction. The outer border is the transition between the newly formed metaplastic squamous epithelium and the original squamous epithelium (the "old" squamocolumnar junction). Whereas the inner border can be seen clearly unless it is located within the cervical canal, the outer border of the transformation zone may be less well defined, especially when the metaplastic squamous epithelium has reached a high degree of maturity. Only the occasional gland opening and/or Nabothian cyst will indicate the metaplastic nature of the cells.

Identification of the newly formed squamous epithelial border is critical for colposcopy diagnosis (Fig. 2.7). It is recognizable by

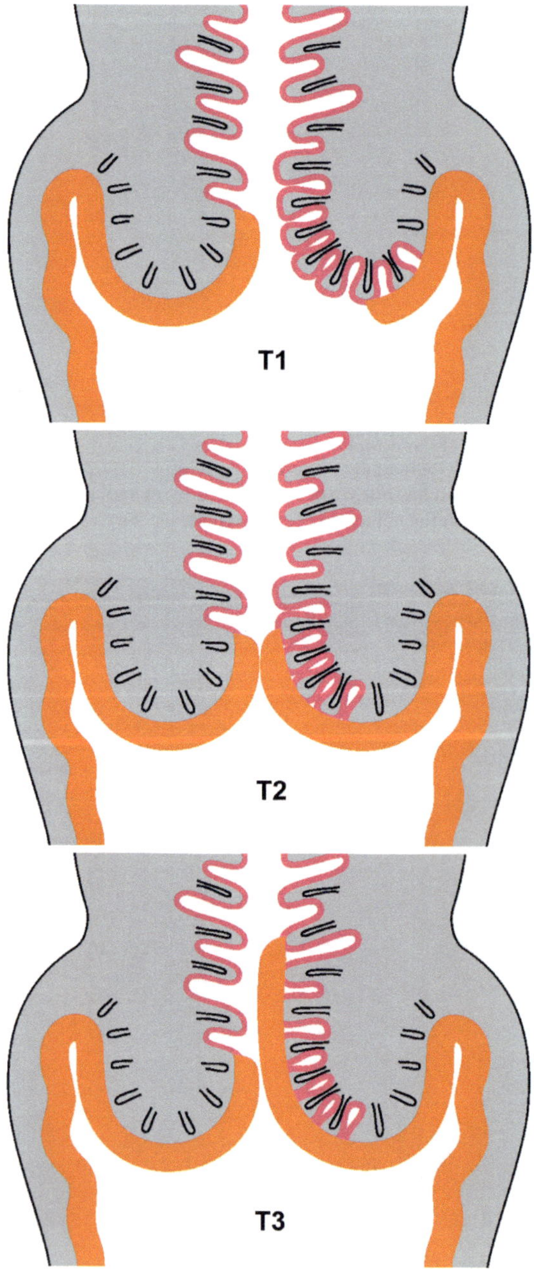

Fig. 2.7 Three different positions of the newly formed squamocolumnar junction (T1, T2, T3) after metaplastic transformation

the sharp contrast between the more or less mature metaplastic epithelium and the deep red original glandular epithelium. If this transition is fully visualized during the colposcopy examination—if necessary by spreading the cervical os—the entire transformation zone can be viewed, and thus the area critical for the development of squamous epithelial neoplasia can be assessed colposcopically.

For every colposcopic examination, this is an important aspect, which needs to be documented. Previous colposcopic nomenclatures have called a colposcopic exam "satisfactory" when the squamocolumnar junction is fully visible (Walker et al. 2003).

2.2 Colposcopic Appearance of the Normal Cervix

The colposcopic appearance of the normal transformation zone is highly variable. Therefore, the basic prerequisite for colposcopic recognition of various dysplastic findings is to familiarize oneself with the different manifestations of normal metaplastic transformation (Fig. 2.8).

In part, the different colors of the cervix can be explained by the different amount of light reflected by the cervical epithelium. The completely matured squamous epithelium consists of several cell layers so that the light from the blood vessels located within the stroma is only partially reflected. Therefore, normal squamous epithelium will appear light red or pink. The original glandular epithelium, on the other hand, will be deep red, because the stromal capillaries shine through the single-layered cylindrical epithelium. The metaplastic tissue of the transformation zone will reflect the white light from the colposcope, depending on its state of maturity.

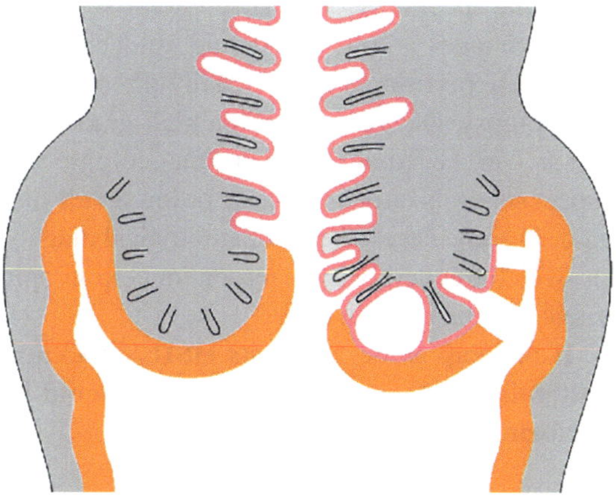

Fig. 2.8 Two characteristic phenomena of metaplastic transformation: gland openings and Nabothian cysts

Nabothian cysts are a characteristic phenomenon of the normal transformation zone. There may be only a discrete elevation of the squamous epithelium with a yellowish hue or there may be multiple cysts, sometimes with a diameter of several centimeters, so that they can be seen well on vaginal ultrasound examination (Figs. 2.9, 2.10, and 2.11).

Frequently, large-caliber vessels are seen on the surface of larger Nabothian cysts. Here, the stromal capillaries are pushed toward the epi-

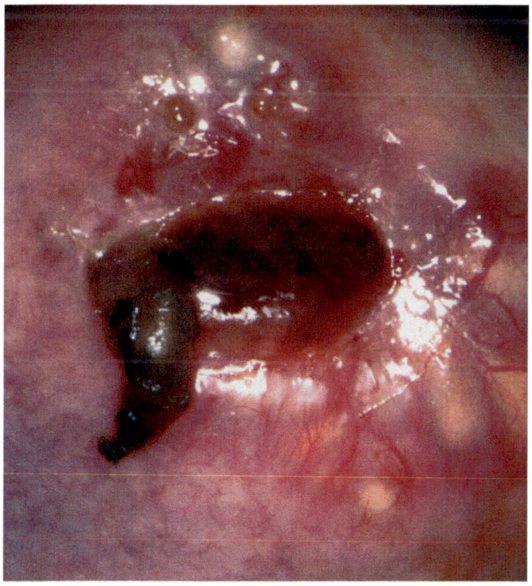

Fig. 2.9 Nabothian cysts. The cysts are of varying size with a yellowish color covered by prominent but regular blood vessels. This particular patient was sent to the colposcopy clinic after multiple cysts had been documented on ultrasound exam

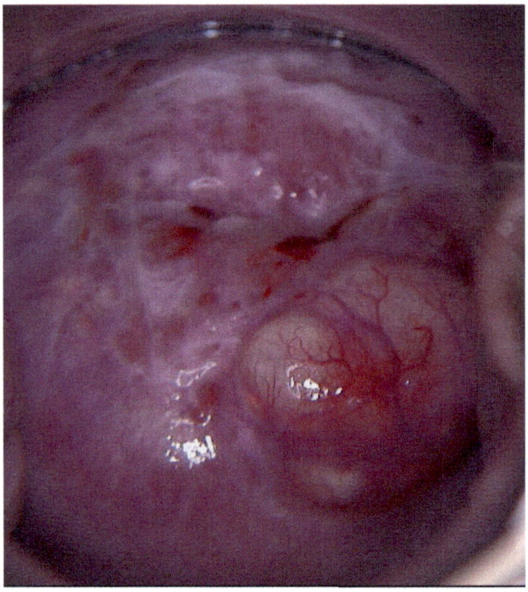

Fig. 2.10 Nabothian cysts. The 50-year-old patient was referred for further diagnosis of a "large exophytic tumor"

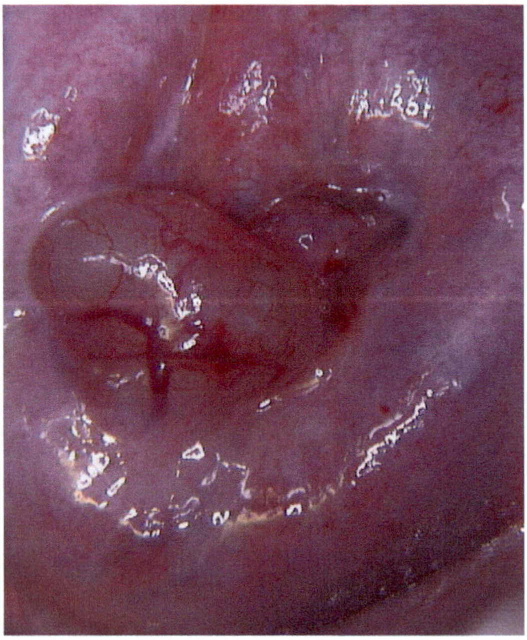

Fig. 2.11 Large Nabothian cyst from a 34-year-old patient

thelial surface by the accumulated secretion. The differential diagnosis of atypical vessels is not difficult, since there are no fluctuations in the caliber of the vessels; rather, the vessel diameter tapers toward the periphery.

When 3–5% acetic acid solution is applied to the normal cervix, it has little effect on squamous cell or glandular epithelium. However, metaplastic tissue sometimes produces a white ("acetowhite") staining. This is due to the fact that the nuclei within the metaplastic tissue are enlarged in relation to the cytoplasm. Acetic acid leads to dehydration of the cytoplasm. Thus, the metaplastic nuclei are more densely packed resulting in increased light reflection. After a few seconds or a few minutes, this effect decreases, as the cell cytoplasm is slowly rehydrated (Figs. 2.12 and 2.13).

Through colposcopy, the positive acetic acid reaction of immature metaplasia—when the nuclear/cytoplasmic (N/C) ratio is high—cannot be reliably distinguished from low-grade squamous intraepithelial dysplasia.

In addition, stromal capillaries may become more prominent during the process of metaplasia. On colposcopic examination, after the application of acetic acid, a fine mosaic pattern and/or punctation are seen. These vascular phenomena of metaplasia may complicate the colposcopic diagnosis of intraepithelial neoplasia.

As the specificity of colposcopy for so-called minor changes is low, one should not hesitate to frequently perform colposcopically directed cervical biopsy. Occasionally, even high-grade dysplasia can be found whereas the colposcopic aspect suggests only metaplasia or low-grade disease. In some cases, the cytopathological diagnosis, which frequently is the reason for colposcopic triage, can be helpful.

If the Pap smear suggests HSIL/CIN3 and only minor lesions are seen, biopsy should be performed.

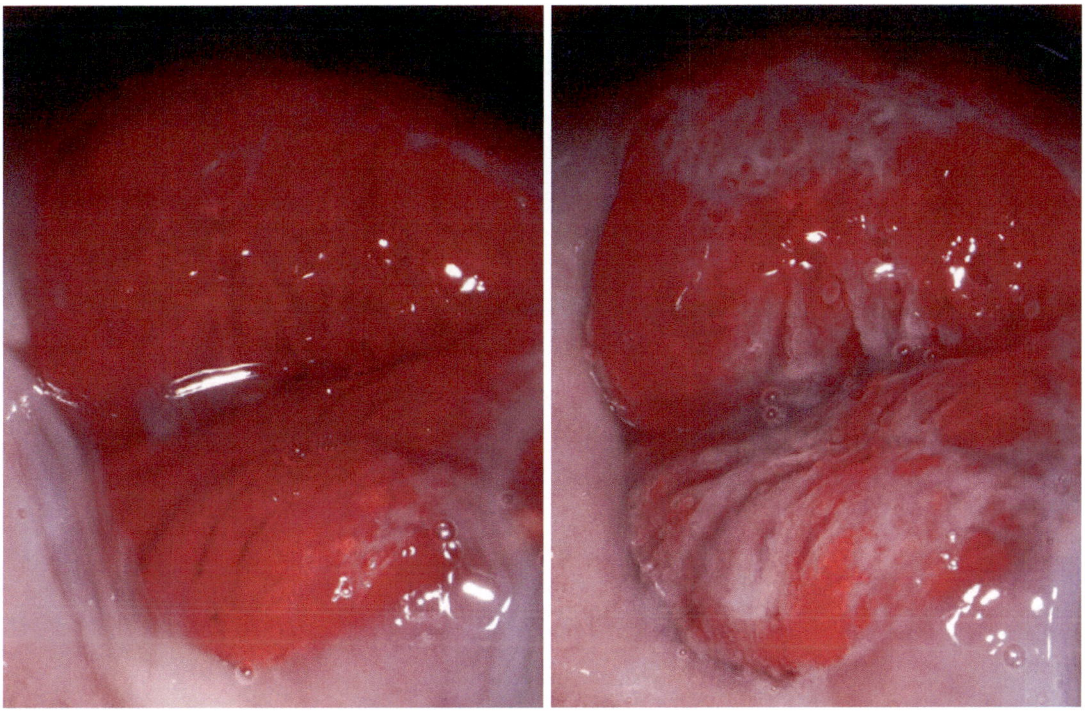

Fig. 2.12 Metaplasia before and after the application of acetic acid

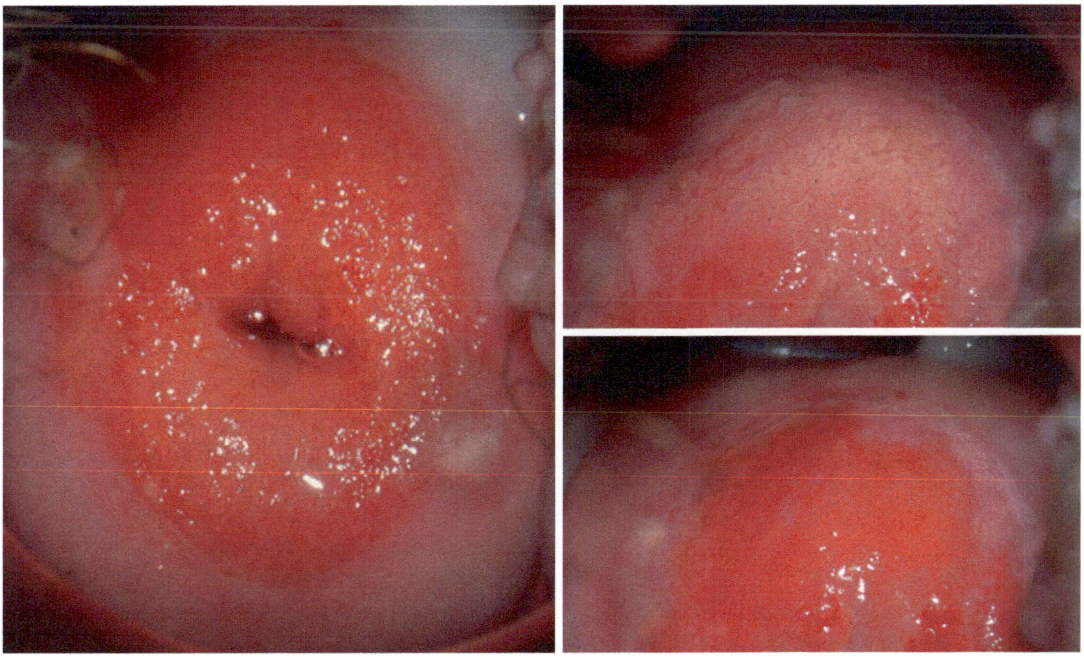

Fig. 2.13 Dynamics of the acetic acid reaction. The large image on the left shows the cervix before application of acetic acid. Thirty seconds later, metaplasia with acetowhite squamous epithelium is visible at the ventral aspect of the cervix. After 60 seconds, the epithelium still remains acetowhite in the periphery

References

Baskett TF (2001) On the shoulders of giants: eponyms and names in obstetrics and gynaecology. RCOG Press, London

Walker P, Dexeus S, De Palo G, Barrasso R, Campion M, Girardi F et al (2003) International terminology of colposcopy: an updated report from the International Federation for Cervical Pathology and Colposcopy. Obstet Gynecol 101:175–177

3 Abnormal Findings of the Cervix

Contents

After applying 4–5% acetic acid solution, vascular phenomena of the cervix can be visualized, which, for example, are described as punctation or mosaic. When learning colposcopy, the criteria for low- and high-grade changes and, most importantly, for invasive disease need to be practiced. This chapter describes in detail the relationship between precancerous and invasive processes with human papillomavirus (HPV).

3.1 Introduction

Essentially, the main scope of colposcopy is the recognition of precancerous changes. These changes are also referred to as dysplasia and are classified into three grades: mild, moderate, and severe dysplasia or "carcinoma in situ." Moderate and severe changes are often summarized as high-grade lesions. The term "cervical intraepithelial neoplasia" or "CIN" is just as commonly used as the term "dysplasia." Mild, moderate, and severe dysplasia are called CIN1, CIN2, and CIN3, respectively.

The following criteria are helpful in order to distinguish between normal and abnormal colposcopic findings:

- The color of the epithelium before and after application of acetic acid ("acetowhite")
- The type of delineation of acetowhite areas: indistinct versus sharp borders
- The presence and appearance of capillary vessels
- The tissue reaction to Schiller's test (Lugol's iodine solution)

Before describing and illustrating the typical colposcopic phenomena, an important aid for colposcopic evaluation, i.e., Schiller's iodine test, will be addressed in more detail.

Schiller used an iodine solution originally developed by Jean Guillaume Auguste Lugol

R. J. Lellé, V. Küppers, *Colposcopy*, https://doi.org/10.1007/978-3-030-85388-4_3

(1788–1851) for the treatment of skin tuberculosis, in order to identify the glycogen-containing epithelium of cervix and vagina. Therefore, Schiller's iodine is also called Lugol's iodine solution (Table 3.1).

Table 3.1 Preparation of Lugol's solution for Schiller's test (Sankaranarayanan and Wesley 2003)

Ingredients	Quantity
1. Potassium iodide	10 g
2. Distilled water	100 mL
3. Iodine crystals	5 g
Preparation	
(a) Dissolve 10 g potassium iodide in 100 ml of distilled water.	
(b) Slowly add 5 g iodine crystals, while shaking.	
(c) Filter and store in a tightly stoppered brown bottle.	

Schiller's test is carried out after acetic acid application and is the final step of the colposcopic examination procedure. Whenever possible, an image of Schiller's iodine test has been added to the illustrations below.

The presence of iodine-negative epithelium is not always to be regarded as pathological. Normal glandular epithelium, an immature transformation zone, or atrophic/inflammatory squamous epithelium do not contain glycogen and thus are iodine-negative.

If an area with a usually dysplasia-related phenomenon such as punctation or mosaic turns out to be iodine-positive, dysplasia can be reliably ruled out. Thus, the patient can be spared unnecessary biopsies (Fig. 3.1).

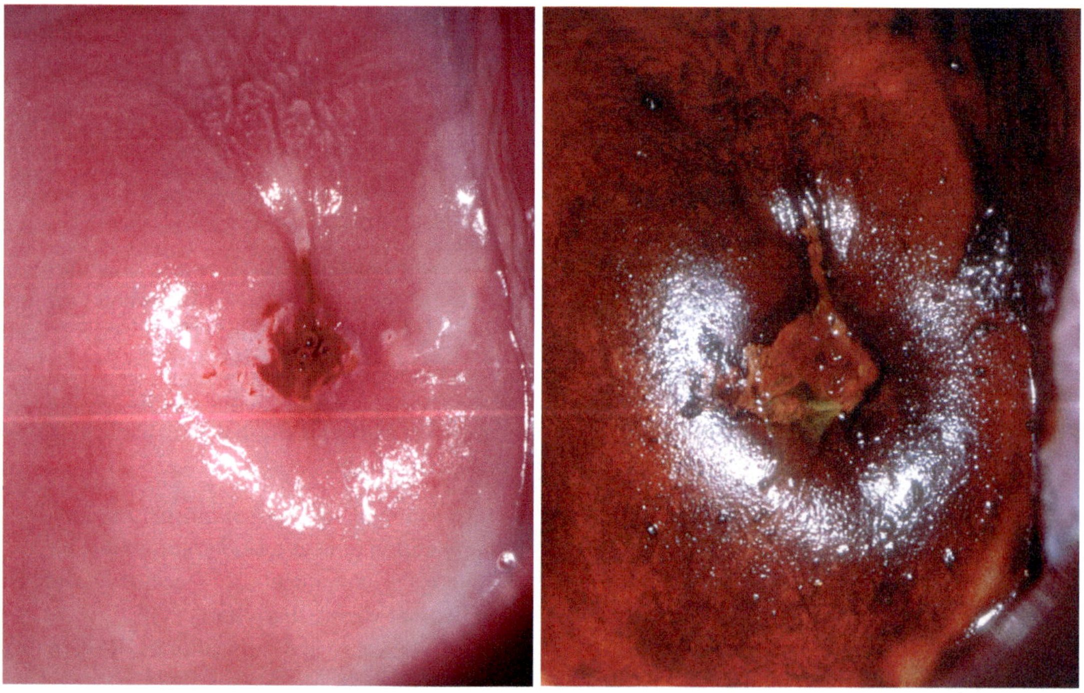

Fig. 3.1 Iodine-positive "pseudo-mosaic" in a 19-year-old patient with no further evidence of cervical dysplasia. A slightly raised gyrated pattern is seen on the ventral cervix that may be misinterpreted as dysplasia-associated mosaic. However, the entire lesion is Lugol-positive, thus ruling out dysplasia

3.1.1 Leukoplakia

Leukoplakia presents as a white area that is visible before acetic acid is applied. Leukoplakia may be located both inside and outside the transformation zone. Histologically, thickened keratinized squamous epithelium is seen. Keratinized tissue areas will reflect the light completely and therefore appear white on colposcopic inspection (Fig. 3.2).

Leukoplakia may be caused by local irritation of the epithelium, for example, by trauma or chronic infection (Fig. 3.3). Leukoplakia is particularly pronounced when cervical condyloma is present (Fig. 3.4).

Although the underlying causes of leukoplakia are usually benign, both cervical intraepithelial neoplasia as well as keratinizing squamous cell carcinoma need to be ruled out.

In many cases of leukoplakia, tissue biopsy is necessary in order to distinguish between benign and neoplastic squamous cell epithelium.

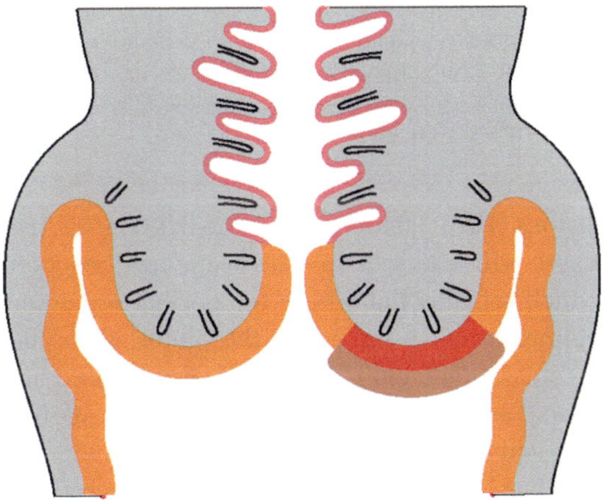

Fig. 3.2 Leukoplakia. A thick keratinizing layer covers the squamous epithelium. This layer is opaque and appears white when viewed from above

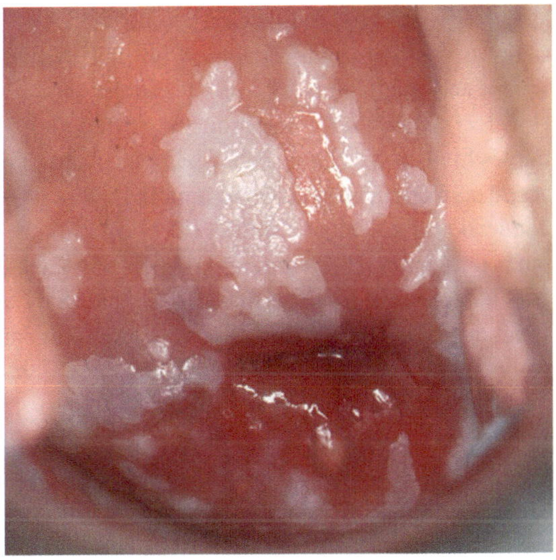

Fig. 3.3 Leukoplakia without dysplasia. The Pap smear is normal, and the HPV test (Hybrid Capture 2) is negative

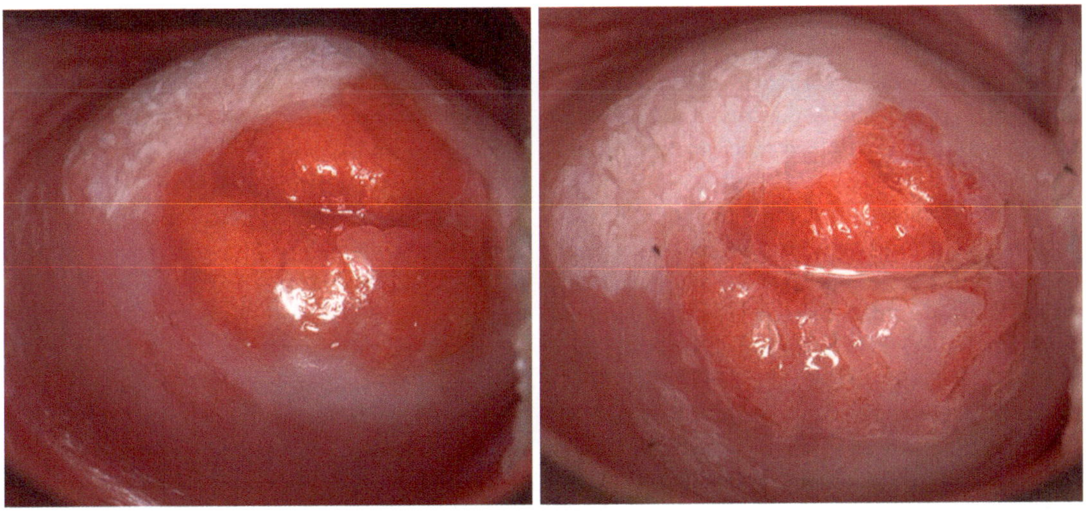

Fig. 3.4 Typical cervical condyloma before and after application of acetic acid

3.1.2 Acetowhite Epithelium

The acetic acid test is the most important part of the colposcopic examination. Assessment of the acetic acid reaction without the colposcope is more meaningful than colposcopic examination without the application of acetic acid, as demonstrated by VIA-based screening programs.

A 4–5% acetic acid solution is applied to the cervix. As a result, the cervical mucus coagulates and can be removed mechanically. The acetic acid solution has no visible effect on normal mature squamous epithelium or on glandular tissue. However, when the protein content of the epithelium is high, as it is the case in squamous dysplasia, acetic acid application leads to a more or less pronounced white color change. High-grade squamous intraepithelial lesions, and particularly CIN3, are characterized by large nuclei surrounded by a small amount of cytoplasm. Thus, protein content within the epithelium layer is high, as there is an increase of the nuclear/cytoplasmic ratio.

The hyperosmolar acetic acid causes the cells to shrink by dehydration of the cytoplasm and coagulates the nuclear proteins. The cell nuclei move closer together and render the epithelium opaque. As a result, it loses its pink color and appears to be white, as it reflects the incoming light beams (Fig. 3.5).

The nuclear/cytoplasmic ratio is high in precancerous lesions, especially in high-grade squamous intraepithelial lesions (CIN2 and CIN3). However, immature metaplastic cells will also have a higher nuclear/cytoplasmic ratio and thus, to a certain extent, will also react positive to the acetic acid test.

If, however, the cells contain abundant glycogen, the acetic acid solution can only penetrate into the superficial cell layers. The epithelium will retain its normal color. Normal squamous cell epithelium will therefore not change its color. The most pronounced acetowhite reaction will be triggered in the presence of severe dysplasia, as the dysplastic tissue is characterized by large nuclei with abundant protein.

Histologically and cytologically, the nuclear/cytoplasmic ratio is higher in CIN2 and CIN3 lesions (HSIL) than in CIN1 (LSIL). Thus, CIN1 tissue will lead to a delicate acetic acid reaction, which remains flat within the normal squamous epithelium that surrounds the abnormal tissue, whereas CIN2 and CIN3 lead to pronounced and coarse acetowhite discolorization with a slightly elevated tissue surface.

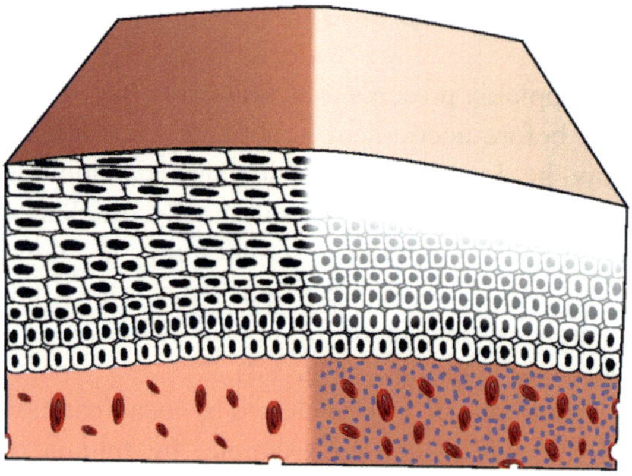

Fig. 3.5 Acetic acid effect on normal epithelium (left) in contrast to dysplasia (right). Dysplastic epithelium has a higher protein content. Acid leads to dehydration of the cytoplasm. Subsequently, crowding of the abnormal nuclei makes the tissue opaque or white ("acetowhite") when viewed from above

Thus, acetowhite epithelium is not necessarily dysplastic, especially when there is still only a delicate hue of acetowhite. Metaplastically developed, not yet mature squamous epithelium also consists of cells with a high nuclear/cytoplasmic ratio and thus have a high protein content. It is not possible to distinguish immature metaplasia from mild dysplasia by acetic acid reaction alone. In addition, dysplastic epithelium and immature metaplastic epithelium may share other features such as a sharp delineation.

In summary, the following findings may be associated with enlarged nuclei and/or a high nuclear/cytoplasmic ratio and thus lead to a positive acetic acid reaction:

- Immature metaplasia
- Squamous intraepithelial neoplasia (CIN2 and CIN3 more pronounced than CIN1)
- Invasive carcinoma
- Cell trauma and repair after infection or mechanical stress (pessary)

3.1.3 Punctation and Mosaic

Punctation and mosaic are vascular phenomena, which can be visualized by the application of acetic acid.

Occasionally, punctation and mosaic may be visible without the acetic acid, when the green filter is used, as the vessels can be seen more clearly.

The effect of punctation is caused by vessels (Fig. 3.6), which are located in the dermal papillae reaching close to the epithelial surface. Punctation may be described as "fine" versus "coarse" and "regular" as opposed to "irregular" (Figs. 3.7 and 3.8).

Fine regular punctation is a frequent sign of mild dysplasia as well as immature metaplasia, as these two diagnostic entities cannot be distinguished colposcopically. On the other hand, coarse and irregular punctation is seen in the presence of high-grade precancerous lesions.

Just like punctation, mosaic—originally described by Hinselmann as "Felderung"—is also a vascular phenomenon. Proliferating capillary structures surround these polygonal or round areas of dysplastic epithelial cells, resulting in a mosaic-like appearance (Fig. 3.9).

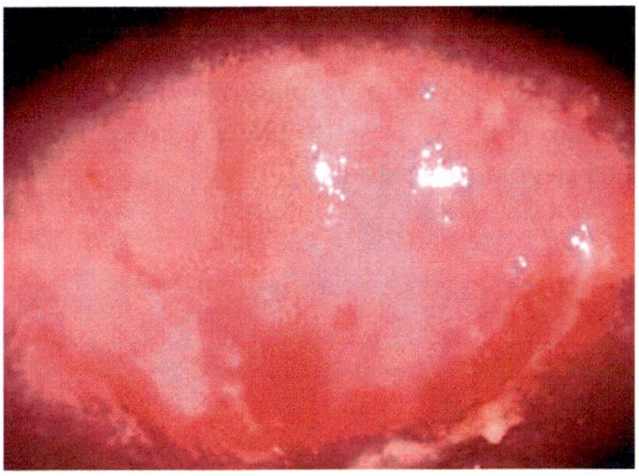

Fig. 3.7 Fine punctation on the anterior (ventral) cervix

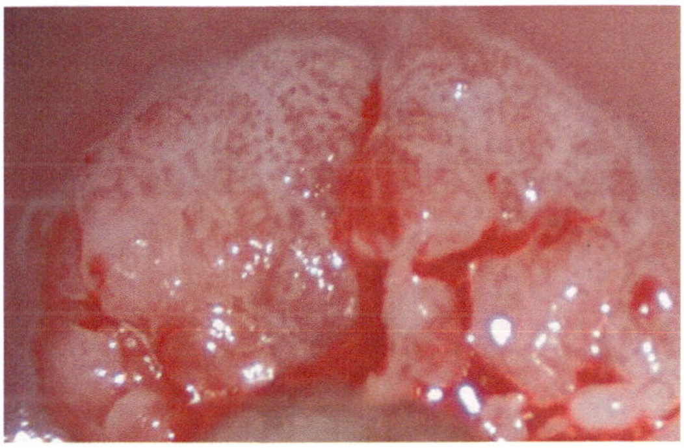

Fig. 3.8 Coarse and irregular punctation

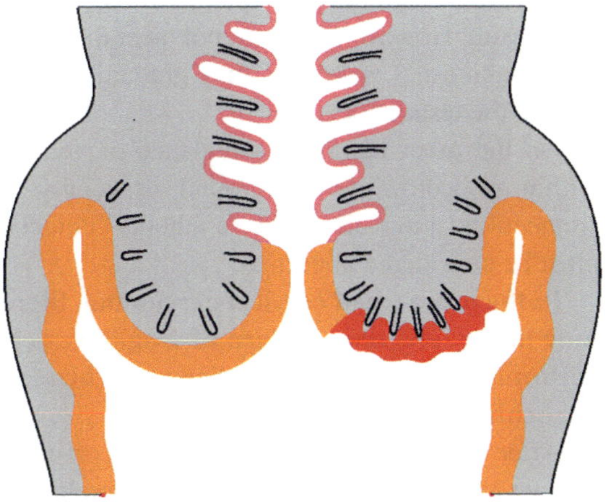

Fig. 3.6 Punctation is caused by single-looped terminal capillaries within stromal papillae of squamous epithelium. As these vessels are situated perpendicular to the epithelial surface, and the atypical epithelium is attenuated after the application of acetic acid, red dots are seen colposcopically. These dots may be regular or irregular, fine or coarse

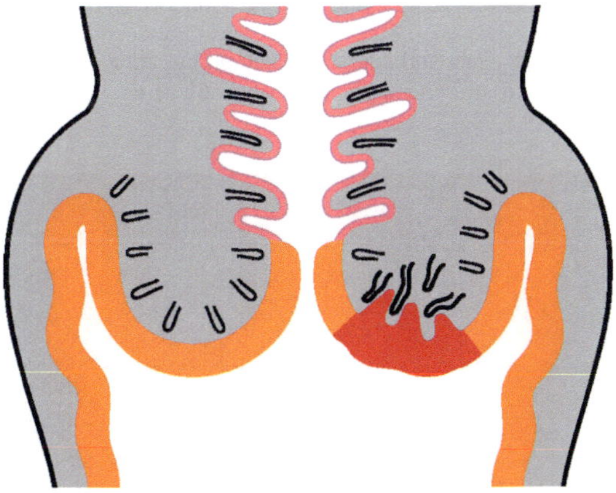

Fig. 3.9 Mosaic-like punctation is a vascular phenomenon, i.e., capillaries in stromal papillae perpendicular to the epithelial surface forming a honeycomb or cobblestone-like pattern when viewed through the colposcope

A delicate or fine mosaic (Fig. 3.10) is more likely associated with a low-grade dysplastic lesion (or immature dysplasia), while a coarse mosaic (Fig. 3.11) most likely corresponds to higher-grade dysplasia.

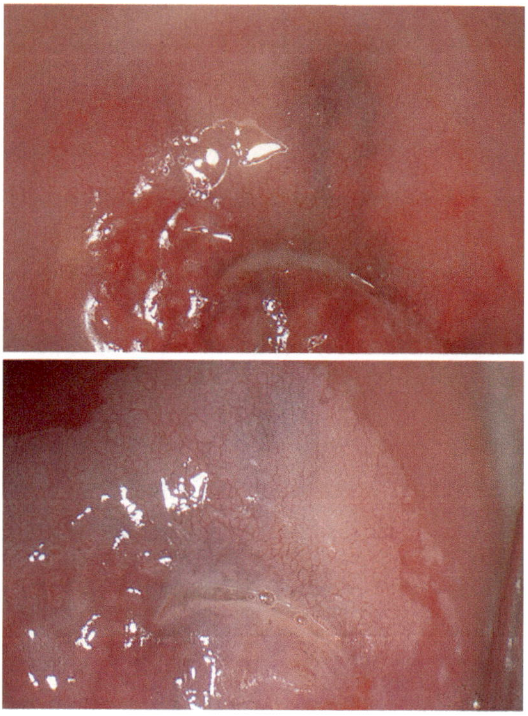

Fig. 3.10 Fine and coarse mosaic on the anterior cervix before and after the application of acetic acid

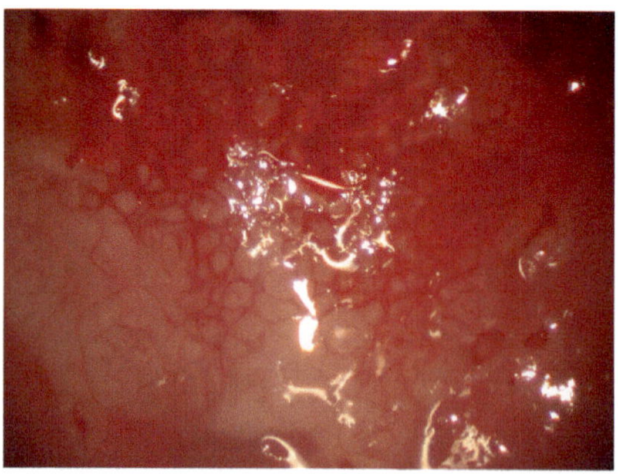

Fig. 3.11 Coarse and irregular mosaic on the posterior cervix

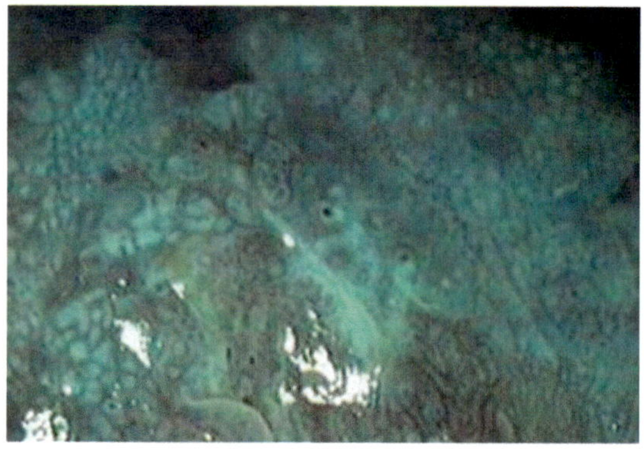

Fig. 3.12 Coarse and irregular mosaic in a patient with high-grade dysplasia. Every colposcope is equipped with a green filter. The filter absorbs red light so that blood vessels appear black and can be seen more clearly against the green background

Since the red color of the blood vessels, which causes the appearance of mosaic and punctation, is more pronounced under green light, every colposcope is equipped with a green filter (Fig. 3.12).

3.1.4 Abnormal Vessels

The mature transformation zone can have numerous prominent blood vessels (Fig. 3.13), especially when a Nabothian cyst bulges the squamous epithelium. However, these do not meet the criteria for abnormal vessels as they gradually taper toward the terminal end.

On the other hand, an abundance of vessels within an acetowhite background, especially in connection with ulcerative epithelial defects, must be considered abnormal.

In the presence of cervical carcinoma, there may be an irregular pattern of fragile vessels with massive caliber fluctuations and bizarre branching.

After introduction of the speculum, or upon contact with a cotton swab, abnormal vessels will bleed easily (Figs. 3.14 and 3.15).

Although abnormal vessels are typical for invasive lesions, they may occasionally occur in benign changes such as granulation tissue, radiation changes, inflammation, or exophytic condylomata acuminata.

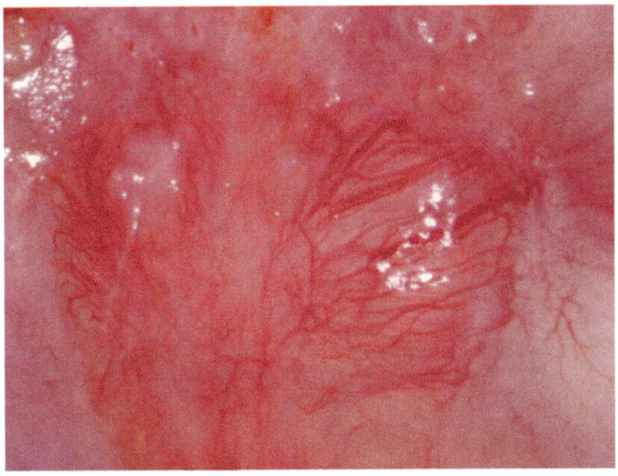

Fig. 3.13 Normal vessels within the transformation zone. The vessels are of regular caliber that gradually constricts toward the periphery

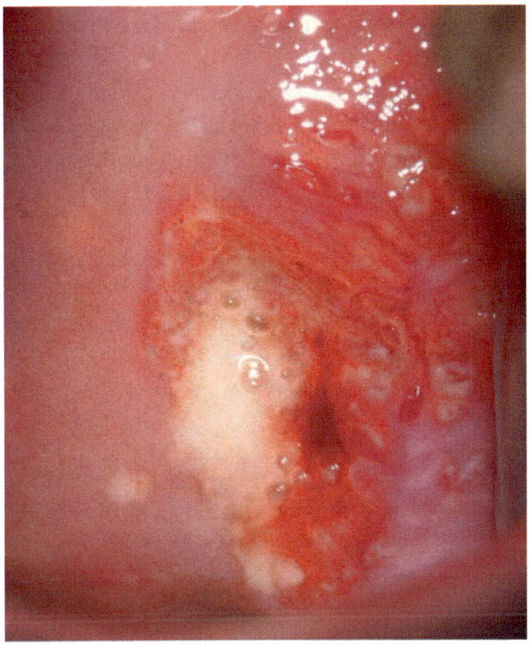

Fig. 3.14 Abnormal vessels in a 29-year-old patient with carcinoma of the cervix

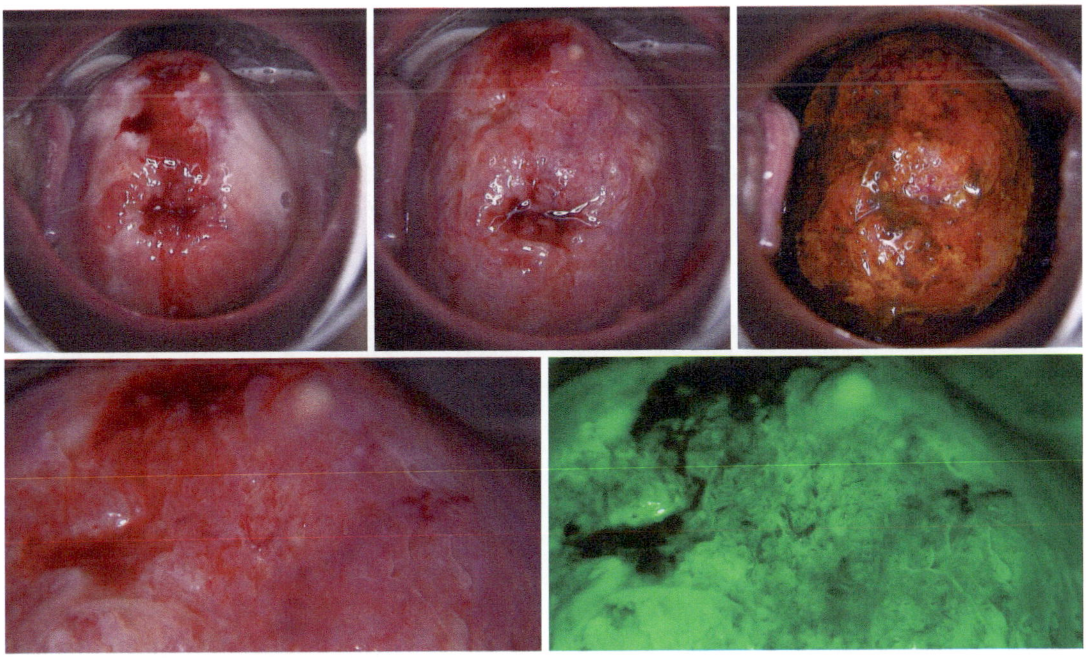

Fig. 3.15 Abnormal vessels in a 30-year-old patient with squamous cell carcinoma of the cervix FIGO stage IB

3.1.5 True Erosion Versus Ulceration

True erosion (Figs. 3.16 and 3.17) is caused by trauma, for example, when a tampon or speculum is inserted into the vagina. If high-grade dysplasia is present, the abnormal epithelium is particularly friable, since the number of desmosomes responsible for cell cohesion is reduced ("peeling edges").

True erosion must be distinguished from ulceration. Ulceration leads to distinct epithelial defects and is always suspicious of invasive carcinoma.

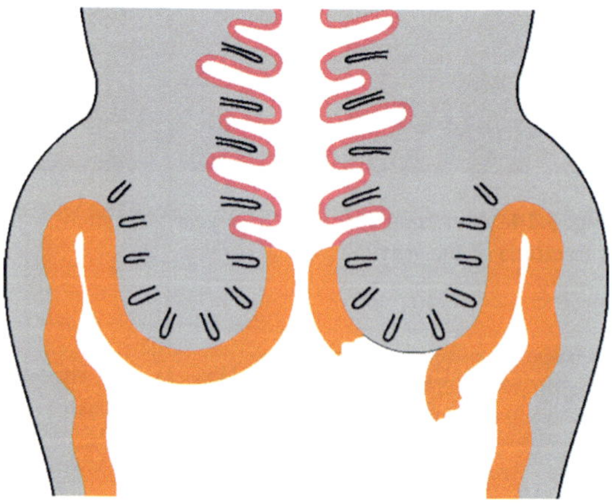

Fig. 3.16 Erosion means sloughing of the squamous epithelium due to a local trauma. Sometimes, the expression "true erosion" is used to distinguish erosion from ulceration or ectopia

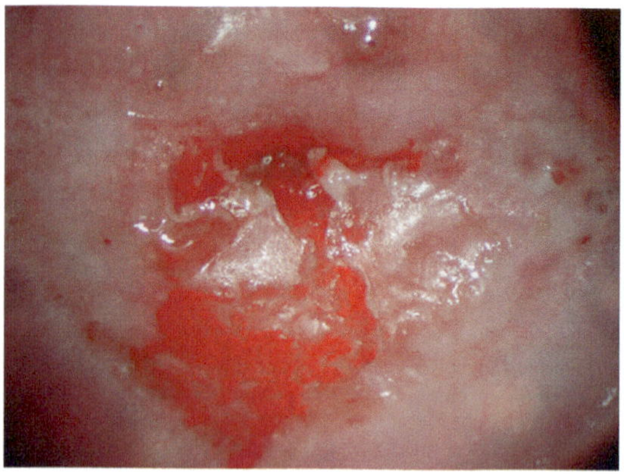

Fig. 3.17 True erosion. The epithelium on the posterior cervix is partially sloughed after inserting the speculum

3.1.6 Atrophy

If there is prominent atrophy of the squamous epithelium, characteristic petechial bleeding occurs when the speculum is inserted, since the atrophic epithelium is quite vulnerable (Figs. 3.18, 3.19, 3.20, 3.21, and 3.22).

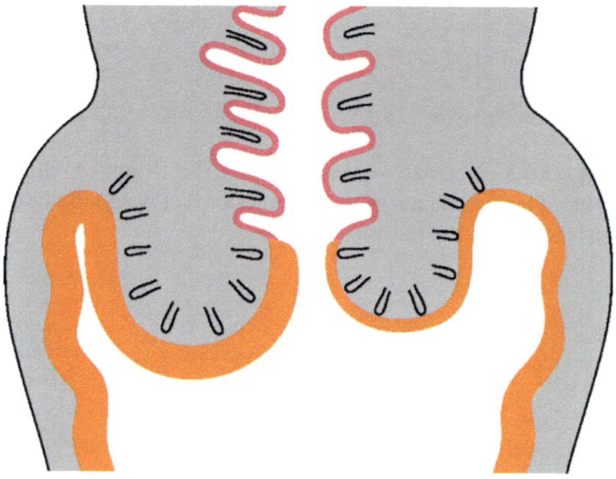

Fig. 3.18 Atrophy. The epithelium is flat and vulnerable

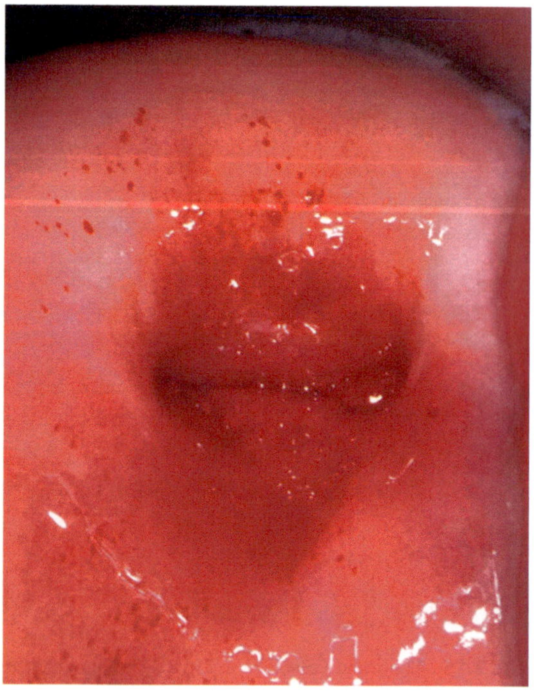

Fig. 3.19 Severe atrophy of the squamous epithelium with petechial hemorrhage

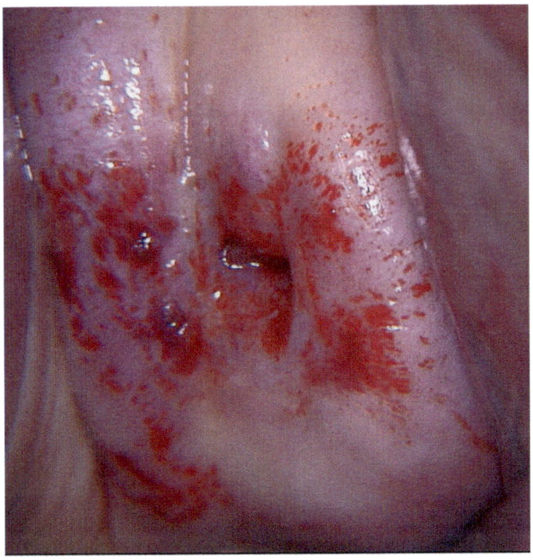

Fig. 3.20 Atrophy of the cervix in a 69-year-old patient

Due to atrophic epithelial changes, both cytological as well as colposcopic assessment can be severely impaired so that satisfactory evaluation is impossible. Usually, atrophy is due to estrogen deficiency and should be treated by local estrogen application for 2–3 weeks. Then the colposcopic examination is repeated.

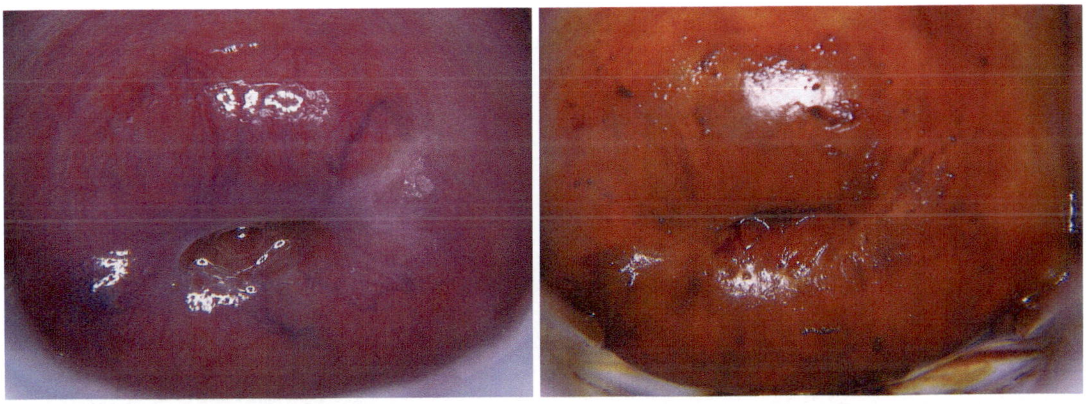

Fig. 3.21 A 59-year-old patient with atrophy. After acetic acid application, blood vessels are visible through the thinned-out epithelium. As no glycogen is present, the ectocervix reacts Lugol-negative

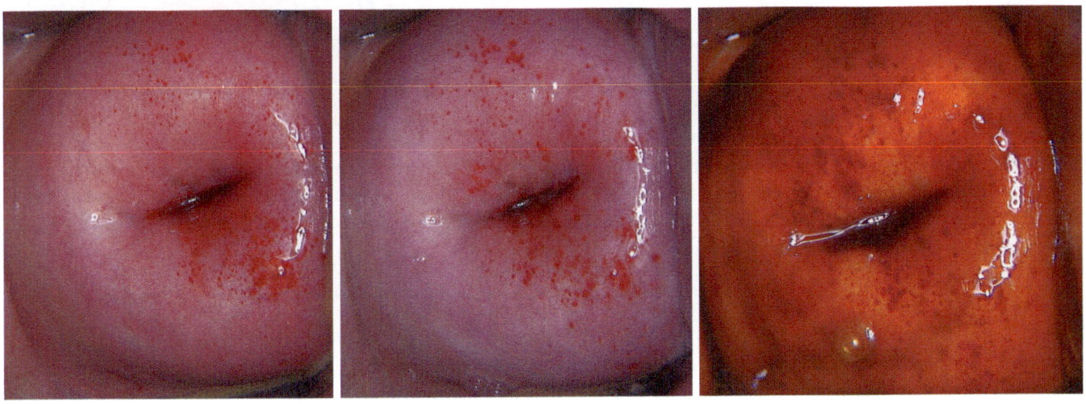

Fig. 3.22 A 70-year-old patient with atrophic cervix and petechial bleeding. There is almost no difference after application of acetic acid (center). The entire cervix is Lugol-negative

3.1.7 Inflammation

Acute inflammatory changes of the vaginal and cervical epithelium are another factor that may severely impair colposcopic evaluation. Topical anti-inflammatory treatment and/or estrogen will be helpful to improve both cytological as well as colposcopic assessment.

During inflammation, the capillary pattern is more pronounced (Fig. 3.23). Colposcopically, a characteristic red discoloration may be seen, which differs from neoplastic punctation (Fig. 3.24). The glycogen storage capacity of the squamous epithelium is also impaired, resulting in a partially negative Schiller's test.

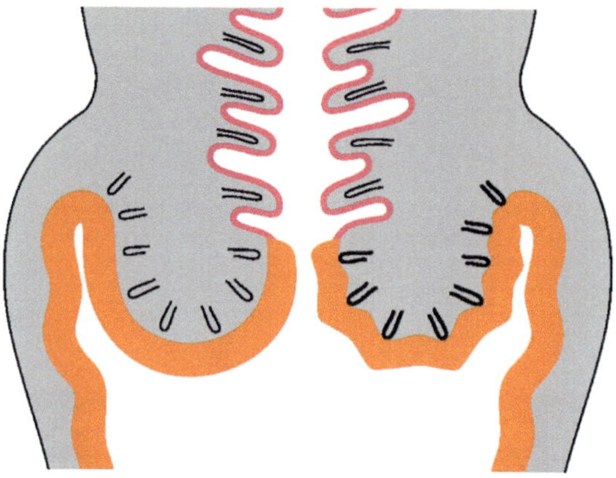

Fig. 3.23 Inflammation. The capillary pattern is more pronounced, giving a typical spotty red color on colposcopic exam

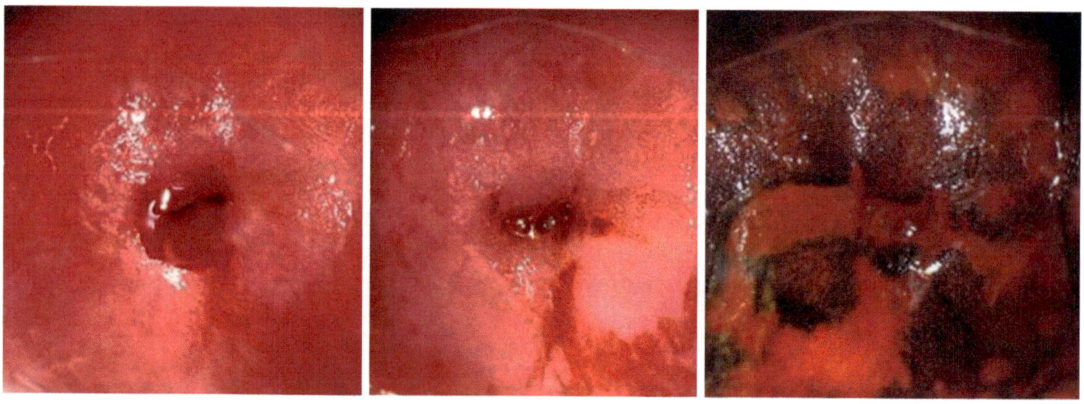

Fig. 3.24 A 34-year-old patient with recurrent fungal infections. The cervix has a patchy red appearance with nonspecific acetowhite staining (center) due to inflammation. At 9 o'clock, there is punctation that is fine and regular, and at 4–5 o'clock, discrete erosion. Only part of the tissue is able to store glycogen and therefore reacts Lugol-positive

3.2 Intraepithelial Neoplasia

The presence of human papillomaviruses (HPV) is a necessary prerequisite for the formation of intraepithelial neoplasia of the cervix as well as various other anogenital lesions.

In 2008, Harald zur Hausen from the German Cancer Research Center in Heidelberg received the Nobel Prize for Medicine for the discovery of the relationship between human papillomavirus infection and cervical carcinoma (zur Hausen 2009). Also, cervical cancer precursors (cervical intraepithelial neoplasia) are also triggered through HPV infection. HP virus DNA alone is sufficient for the development of dysplasia, without the presence of particles capable of replication.

It has been accepted as common knowledge that in the vast majority of cases, human papillomavirus infection is transmitted through sexual intercourse. However, there is a certain percentage of children and adolescents who may be HPV positive prior to sexual activity (Chap. 15).

Only certain HPV types, which are called "high-risk viruses," are involved in the development of dysplasia and ultimately cervical carcinoma, particularly HPV types 16, 18, 31, and 45. Presumably, the gene products of DNA segments E6 and E7 interfere with apoptotic control mechanisms (Fig. 3.25). E6 blocks the tumor suppressor protein p53, E7 the retinoblastoma protein (pRB). Under normal circumstances, damaged cells regularly occur, which are destroyed by apoptosis. Because of the presence of viral E6 and E7, those damaged cells are no longer eliminated so that mutations will accumulate, which may lead to malignant transformation.

The disruption of cell replication caused by human papillomaviruses of the high risk type occurs within the transformation zone, as this area is characterized by increased proliferative activity, that makes it particularly susceptible to HPV.

Obviously, other cofactors are required for preneoplasia or neoplasia development from HPV high-risk infection. The immune system certainly plays an important role. In drug-induced immunosuppression, for example, after organ transplantation or in the case of HIV infection, preneoplasia will develop more frequently. Consequently, the cancer risk is increased. Furthermore, a connection between smoking and dysplasia has been known for a long time. Benzopyrenes in the cigarette smoke can be identified in the cervical mucus. These contaminants are able to raise the titers of HPV high risk types 16, 18, and 31 (Alam et al. 2007).

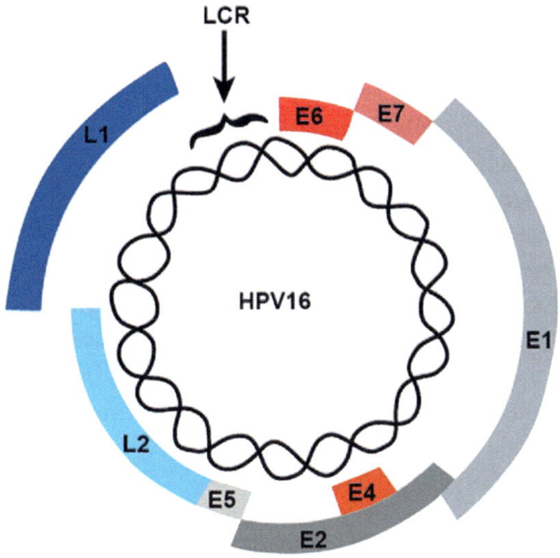

Fig. 3.25 Schematic representation of the HPV 16 genome. Presumably, the gene products of DNA regions E6 and E7 interfere with apoptosis control mechanisms

Although many aspects of cervical cancer development through HPV infection are still unclear, several conclusions can be drawn from epidemiological studies: In sexually active women, HPV high-risk DNA is frequently detected within the cervical region. According to Ho et al. (1998), 43% of college students at one point were HPV positive, when tested at 6 months intervals.

Therefore, women with a positive HPV high-risk test result cannot be regarded as "ill" solely based on the HPV test. HPV positivity, especially in young women and/or after HPV-related disease has been ruled out, is a frequent source of misunderstandings between patients and clinicians that needs to be clarified.

HPV high-risk positivity is not a disease by itself but, depending on the individual circumstances, may indicate a necessity of further

observation or cytopathologic/colposcopic triage.

Only a very small percentage of patients with positive HPV high-risk test result will ever develop cervical dysplasia. Furthermore, it takes at least 3–4 years until preneoplasia of the cervix may develop following HPV infection. Based on the increasing knowledge about the human papillomavirus and its influence on cervical disease, highly effective prevention programs have been established with well-defined screening intervals either in combination with Pap testing (Petry et al. 2003) or as primary HPV screening (Koliopoulos et al. 2007).

In the following section, the two most important clinical manifestations of HPV-related disease are discussed: mild or low-grade dysplasia (cervical intraepithelial neoplasia grade 1, CIN1) and high-grade dysplasia (cervical intraepithelial neoplasia grades 2 and 3, CIN2, and CIN3). The distinction of CIN1 versus CIN2 and CIN3 is of particular importance.

Low-grade cervical intraepithelial neoplasia (CIN1) is an entity that is morphologically, clinically, as well as etiologically distinct from higher-grade precancer (CIN2 and CIN3). Clinical management is also quite different.

Thus, any cyto- or histopathology report has to make a clear distinction between low- and high-grade disease. In Germany, where traditionally a five-class Pap system is used, a basic problem has only been fixed recently. Previously, the "Pap IIID" designation had been used for the cytopathological diagnosis of both mild and moderate dysplasia. With the introduction of the Munich III nomenclature (see below), this has eventually been corrected ("Pap $IIID_1$" versus "Pap $IIID_2$").

The basis for the clinical management of intraepithelial disease is its respective probability for progression and regression.

In principle, all three grades of dysplasia (CIN1 to CIN3) have the potential to regress spontaneously. Understandably, data on the natural history of dysplasia are sparse as observation of untreated cervical intraepithelial neoplasia, possibly until the development of invasive disease, would be highly inappropriate. However, in 1993, Östör (1993) published an extensive literature review on the natural history of precancer that encompasses all pertinent articles published since 1950. Östör concluded that in the vast majority of cases, CIN1 will either regress or persist and that only 10% of CIN1 lesions eventually progress to CIN3 with only a 1% cancer risk. Even in CIN3 disease, one-third of cases may regress. However, both in CIN2 and CIN3, cancer risk is significantly higher (5% and >12%, respectively).

In the case of low-grade dysplasia, a wait-and-see strategy, i.e., expectant management and observation, is acceptable. Based on a longitudinal study on 342 women, Duggan et al. (1998) estimated a likelihood of progression (CIN1 to CIN2/3) of 18.6%. Another 18.6% of patients had persistent disease, and about two-thirds of patients regressed (62.7%).

As shown by a statistical analysis of data obtained from the British National Health Service, 80% of all high-grade lesions (CIN2 and CIN3) will not progress to cancer (Raffle et al. 2003). A meta-analysis by Cantor et al. (2005) came to the conclusion that the average annual transition probability for CIN1 to CIN2 or CIN3 is only 7.20%. On the other hand, regression of CIN1 is much more likely: 14.80% per year.

A British study shows what happens to women who are suspected to have high-grade intracervical disease on cytopathological screening: Those who had to wait for more than 6 months until colposcopic triage was performed were compared to patients who were examined in a more timely manner. Surprisingly, the extended waiting period did not lead to an increase in the development of cancer. Rather, significantly fewer operations were necessary in this group (Fakokunde and Selo-Ojeme 2008).

Moderate and severe dysplasia (CIN2 and CIN3) are best summarized under the term of high-grade dysplasia. In the American Bethesda classification, the term "high-grade squamous intraepithelial lesion" or HSIL is used for both cytological and histopathological nomenclature as is the term "low-grade squamous intraepithelial lesion" (LSIL).

Probability of cancer development in the presence of high-risk HPV:

- Data on the natural history of cervical intraepithelial neoplasia are sparse despite the fact that these data are the basis of clinical decision-making.
- Low-grade dysplasia (CIN1) is much more likely to regress than to progress to CIN2/3 or cancer.
- Even high-grade dysplasia (CIN3) has only a limited potential of malignant progression and may regress spontaneously.

Thus, most cases of higher-grade dysplasia (CIN2/3) are treated surgically (either ablation or destruction), whereas for low-grade disease (CIN1), clinical follow-up exams are preferred, as cell changes are more likely to regress spontaneously.

3.2.1 Low-Grade Dysplasia

3.2.1.1 Pathogenesis

Low-grade squamous intraepithelial lesions (LSIL) or cervical intraepithelial neoplasia grade 1 (CIN1) are the morphological expression of HPV infection. The American ALTS study ("ASC-US/LSIL Triage Study") has shown that in 58.9% of cases, multiple HPV types are present, with 86.1% being of the HPV high-risk variety (ALTS 2000). However, until to date, it has not been shown conclusively that the identification of low- and high-risk virus DNA allows identification of mild dysplasia with a high progression probability.

It is not possible to reliably predict which cases of low-grade dysplasia will regress spontaneously and when the diagnosis of CIN1 must be considered as a first step to the development of high-grade dysplasia or even carcinoma. Thus, the group of low-grade dysplasia consists of two biologically different entities, which cannot be reliably distinguished by today's laboratory tests. However, it is obvious that the risk for progression to invasive cancer is very low (<1%).

Most likely, sexual intercourse is the most frequent mode of HPV infection. However, Doerfler et al. (2009) found that HPV high-risk DNA could be detected in approximately 14% of girls who not yet had had sexual intercourse after sexual abuse had been ruled out. Shew et al. (2013) identified HPV DNA in 10 out of 22 adolescents (14–17 years old), who denied previous vaginal sex. However, 7 of the 10 HPV-positive girls reported noncoital behavior that might have contributed to HPV infection.

The HP virus is thought to penetrate the cervical epithelium during sexual intercourse. The immature metaplastic epithelium of the transformation zone is more susceptible to HPV infection than the original multilayered squamous epithelium. The virus is eventually integrated into the DNA of the basal cells.

However, HPV infection alone does not lead to the morphologically detectable changes that define intraepithelial neoplasia. Most HPV infections do not result in cervical dysplasia. To date, it is not entirely clear which cofactors are required to trigger the activation of viral DNA. Definitely, the immune system plays an important role, which is shown by the frequent occurrence of cervical dysplasia with an increased risk for progression in immunosuppressed patients. Immunosuppression may be due to medication following organ transplantation or by HIV infection. The negative influence of toxins in cigarette smoke has also been documented (Alam et al. 2007).

If the HP virus is activated under the influence of these cofactors, replication of the viruses occurs in the intermediate and superficial cells of the squamous epithelium. The so-called koilocytosis constitutes the morphological expression of HPV infection. The name "koilocyte" is derived from Greek "koilos," which means "hollow" or "hollowed out." The term "koilocyte" or "koilocytotic atypia" was coined in 1956 by Koss and Durfee (1956), who described this cell type as "large cells with relatively small but irregular and

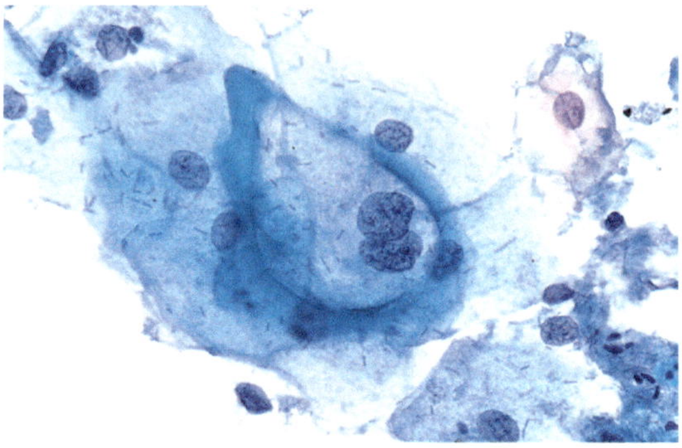

Fig. 3.26 Koilocyte surrounded by normal intermediate squamous cells. Both nuclei are enlarged, slightly irregular, and surrounded by bright cytoplasm

hyperchromatic nuclei surrounded by clear and transparent cytoplasm" (Fig. 3.26). As early as 1960, Ayre expressed the opinion that koilocytes are caused by viral infections. According to Naylor's historical research (Naylor 2000), it was Meisels and Fortin who identified human papillomaviruses as the cause of koilocytic atypia.

In koilocytosis, there is an irregularly shaped nucleus with a distinct perinuclear transparency of the cytoplasm ("halo") and an increased nuclear/cytoplasmic ratio. The cells often have more than one nucleus. Sometimes, the cytoplasm shows signs of disintegration with a patchy eosinophilic pattern ("measle cells").

Low-grade dysplastic changes typically occur in younger women, and the rate of spontaneous regression is high. According to a study on a college population (Ho et al. 1998), 70% of new HPV infections spontaneously regress within 8 months. As already mentioned, the progression probability (low-grade to higher-grade dysplasia) is only 18.6%. A similar percentage of lesions persisted, and 62.7% regressed spontaneously (Duggan et al. 1998).

Only in the case of persistent infection is there a risk for the development of clinically relevant intraepithelial neoplasia. However, HPV persistence, i.e., continuing infection with the same HPV high-risk type, cannot be conclusively diagnosed in individual patients.

According to the present management concept, mild dysplasia (CIN1) is usually not to be treated immediately, as CIN1 lesions are not a significant risk factor for the subsequent development of CIN3 (Castle et al. 2011).

3.2.1.2 Colposcopic Appearance

The most important prerequisite for colposcopic assessment is the acetic test. Application of a 4–5% acetic acid solution to the cervix leads to a whitish stain of the dysplastic epithelium (Fig. 3.27). The acetic acid effect is only temporary. The white color will fade gradually as cells reabsorb fluid from their environment, i.e., they are rehydrated. In the case of low-grade dysplasia, the intensity of the acetowhite reaction can be quite variable. Usually, there is only a faint acetic reaction. The white epithelium remains slightly transparent. The acetowhite tissue stays level with the surrounding squamous epithelium. Compared to high-grade lesions, it usually takes longer for the staining to manifest itself. Furthermore, the acetic acid effect disappears faster in low-grade than in higher-grade dysplasia.

The capillary loops in the epidermis are visible through the epithelium. The capillaries are compressed by the acetic acid effect and will extend toward the epithelial surface. This leads to the appearance of fine punctation and/or mosaic. In contrast to high-grade dysplasia, punctation or mosaic form a regular pattern (Fig. 3.28).

Mild dysplasia usually has well-defined borders toward the surrounding normal squamous epithelium (Fig. 3.29). However, in contrast to high-grade dysplasia, borders may also be less well delineated.

In all dysplastic changes including mild dysplasia, Schiller's iodine test will be negative. However, iodine negativity may be less pronounced in low-grade dysplasia. In the case of condylomatous changes, irregular iodine staining may be observed, sometimes called "tiger skin pattern" (Fig. 3.30).

Hellberg and Nilsson (1990) described the following colposcopic features in 165 women with histologically proven CIN1:

- Acetowhite staining 52.1%
- Punctation 22.4%
- Mosaic 18.2%
- Atypical vessels 12.4%

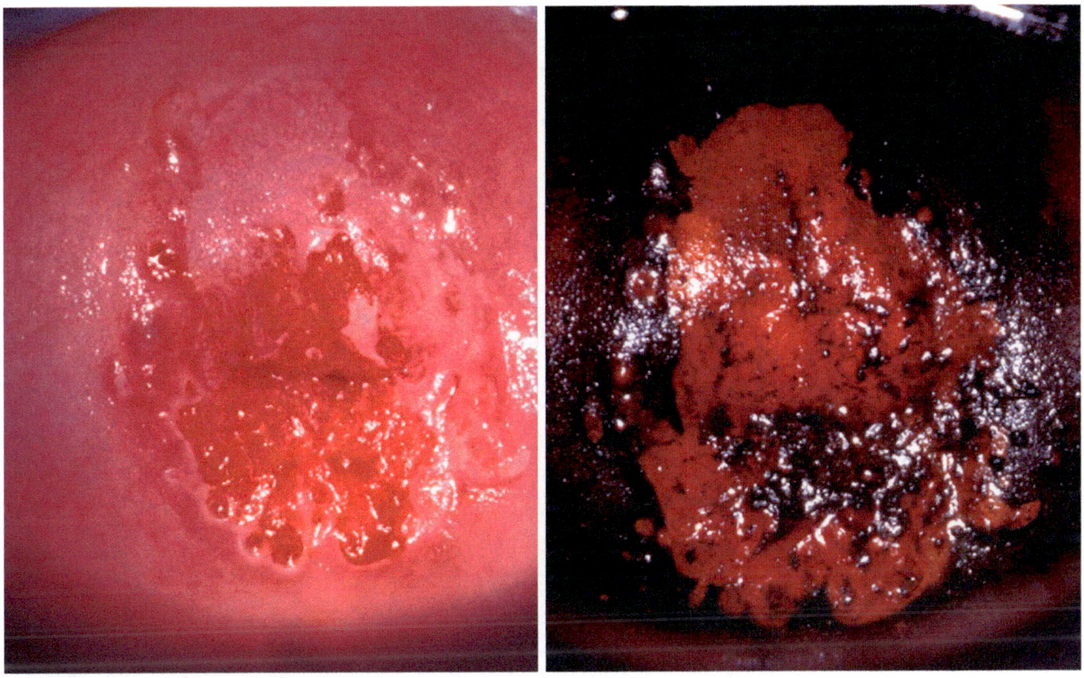

Fig. 3.27 CIN1 in a 20-year-old patient. At 11 and 12 o'clock, there is a thin acetowhite lesion, which is not raised in relation to the surrounding tissue. The abnormal tissue is Lugol-negative

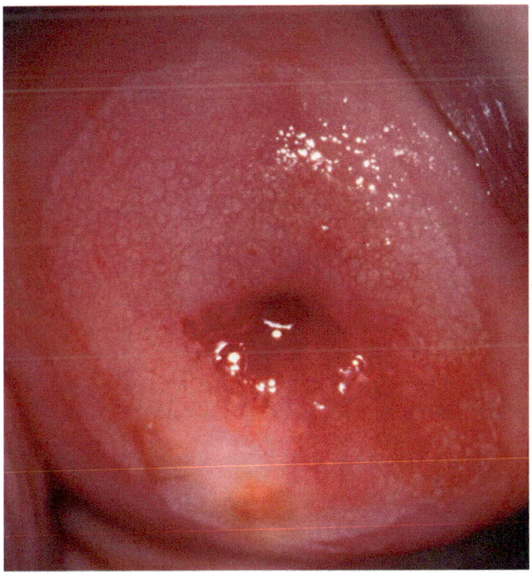

Fig. 3.28 Histologically confirmed CIN1 with fine and regular mosaic

As mentioned earlier, a reliable diagnosis of mild dysplasia based on colposcopy alone is not feasible. According to a literature review by Hopman et al. (1998), only 42.8% of colposcopically diagnosed CIN1 lesions could be confirmed by histopathologic evaluation. When the same investigator was asked to reevaluate the colposcopic images after an interval of 3 months, there was only a 51% intraobserver concordance.

Flat condylomata do not have the characteristic and easily recognizable appearance of condylomata acuminata and may be confused with mild dysplasia. The raised margin and the intense acetowhite staining with sharp borders may even suggest high-grade dysplasia. As shown in Fig. 3.31, flat condylomata are frequently located in the periphery of the cervix rather than near the cervical canal or the squamocolumnar junction.

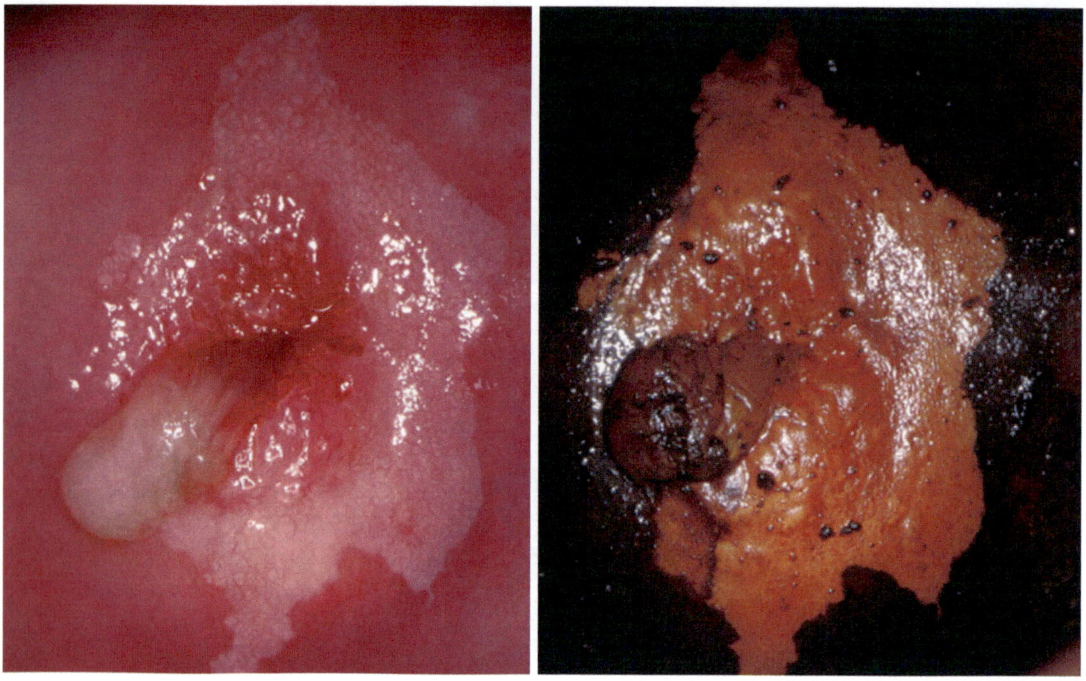

Fig. 3.29 CIN1 in a 25-year-old patient confirmed by biopsy at 6 o'clock. Characteristically, the acetowhite Lugol-negative lesion exhibits sharp borders

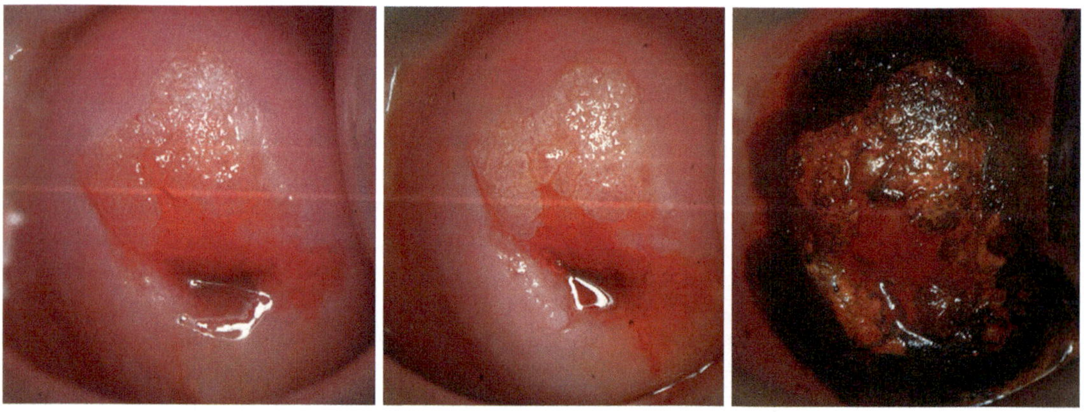

Fig. 3.30 Condyloma as well as CIN2. A large condylomatous slightly raised lesion on the anterior cervix that is acetowhite and partially Lugol-positive ("tiger skin pattern")

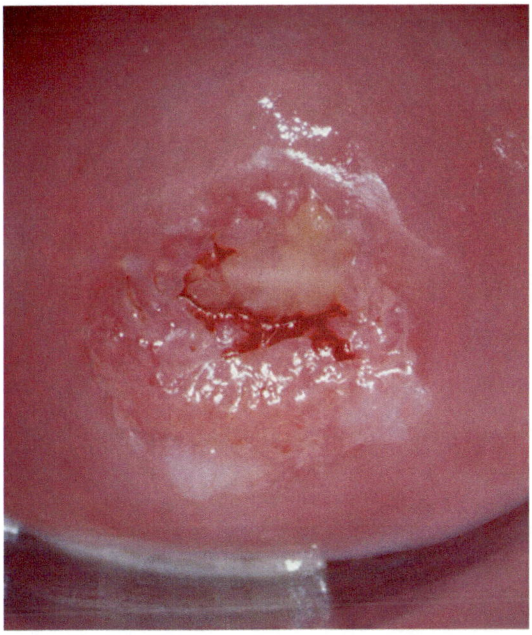

Fig. 3.31 Flat condyloma of the cervix. The 18-year-old patient has already been surgically treated three times for vulvar condylomata acuminata. Now similar condylomata are found on the cervix: at 12 o'clock close to the cervical canal and more peripherally at 4 and 7 o'clock

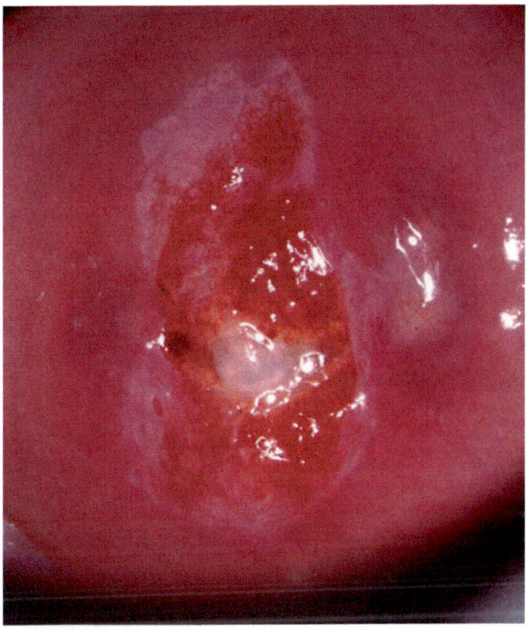

Fig. 3.32 Fine transparent acetowhite areas within the transformation zone. On the anterior (ventral) cervix, there is also a regular mosaic. In a patient like this, it is impossible to distinguish between immature metaplasia and low-grade dysplasia

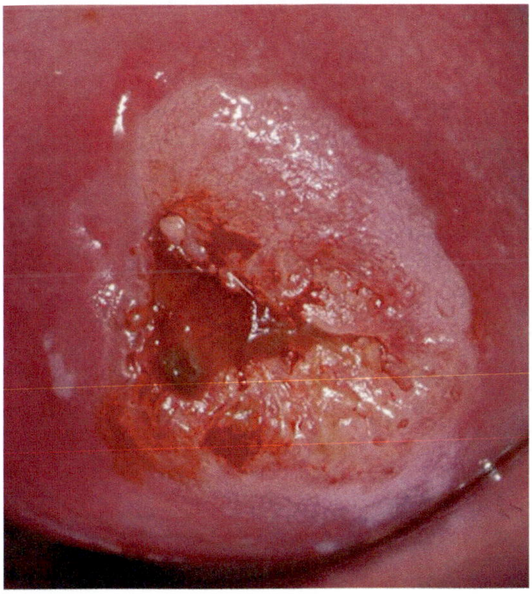

Fig. 3.33 Immature metaplasia with fine mosaic. In this 22-year-old patient, the Pap smear is normal, and the Hybrid Capture 2 test is negative for HPV DNA

However, overinterpretation of metaplastic changes is more likely than confusion of low- and high-grade dysplasia. In particular, immature metaplasia cells have a high protein content and lead to a pale acetowhite reaction. The glycogen content is not yet sufficient for a positive iodine reaction. However, the borders are rather irregular and less well defined than in dysplasia. Sometimes, a fine and regular punctation or mosaic pattern is visible (Figs. 3.32 and 3.33). Thus, colposcopic differentiation between immature metaplasia and low-grade dysplasia is not possible.

In postmenopausal women, the colposcopic diagnosis of low-grade dysplasia should be made with care as in these patients, colposcopic criteria of high-grade dysplasia may be less prominent and resemble those of CIN1 (Figs. 3.34, 3.35, 3.36, 3.37, 3.38, 3.39, 3.40, and 3.41).

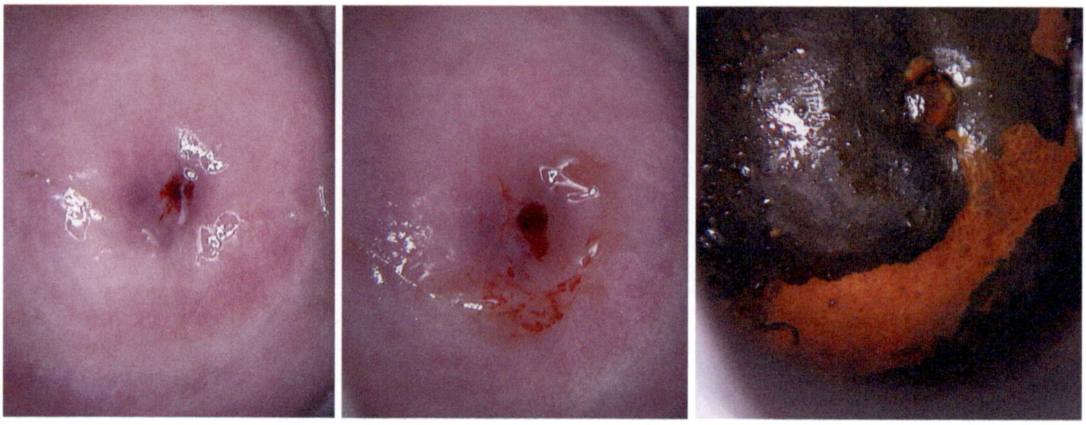

Fig. 3.34 A 41-year-old patient with HSIL of the vulva and a concomitant minor change of the cervix. Biopsy of the Lugol-negative area reveals LSIL

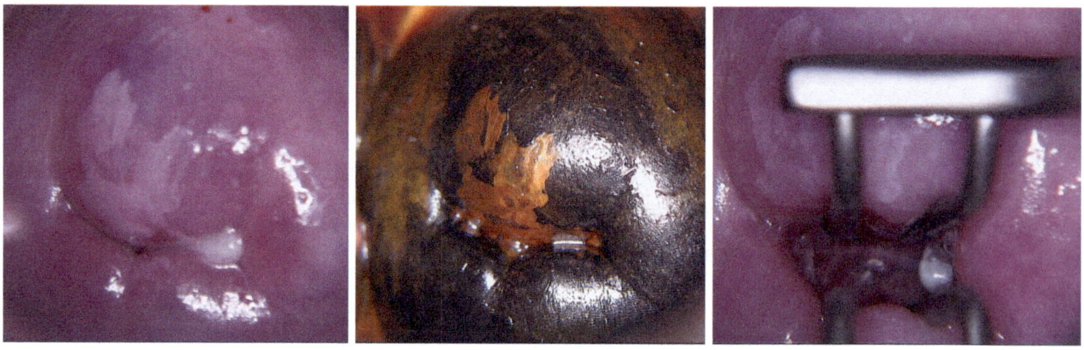

Fig. 3.35 A 32-year-old patient with biopsy-proven LSIL (minor change). The squamocolumnar junction can be visualized with the Kogan speculum

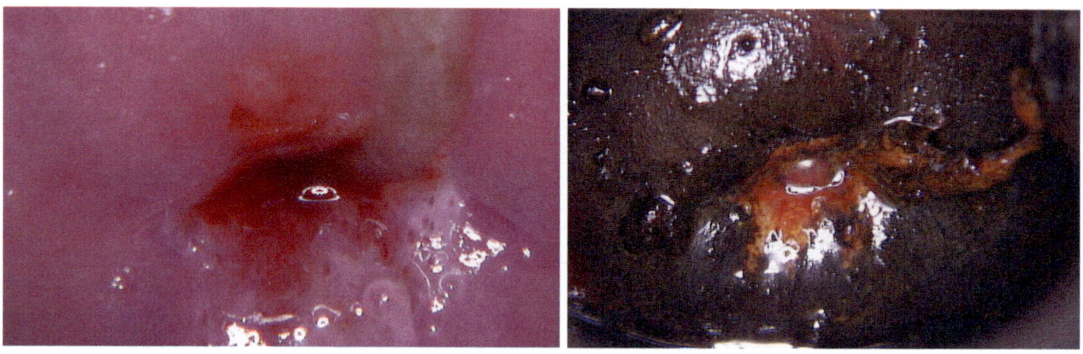

Fig. 3.36 Biopsy-proven LSIL in a 32-year-old nulligravid patient (minor change)

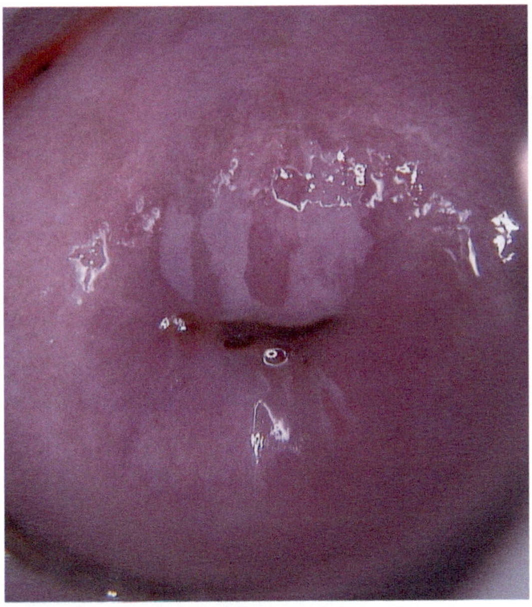

Fig. 3.37 Typical minor change in a 17-year-old patient without cervical dysplasia

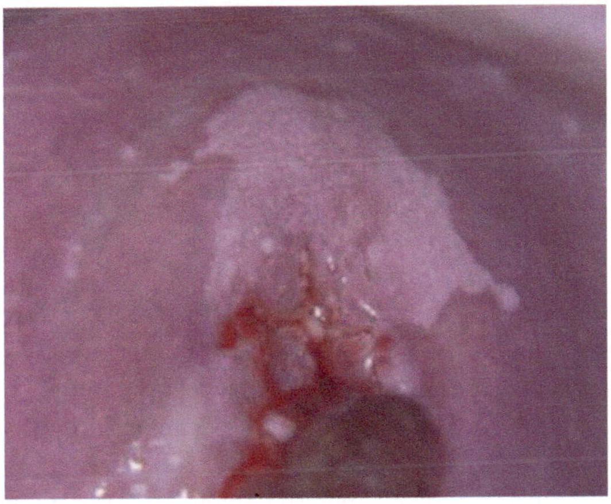

Fig. 3.38 A 27-year-old nulligravid patient with LSIL Pap smear. The biopsy obtained at 12 o'clock close to the squamocolumnar junction is negative

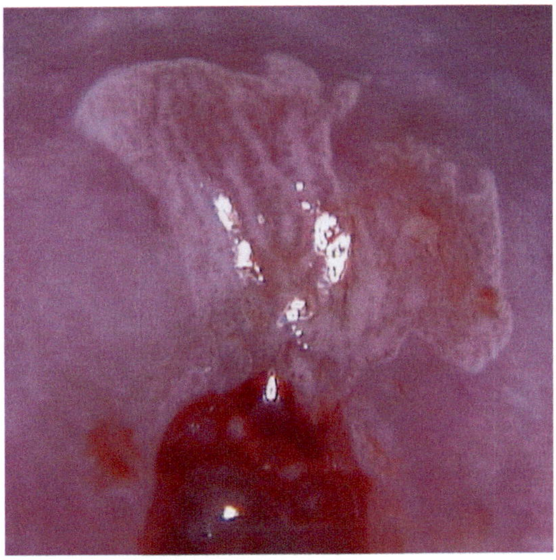

Fig. 3.39 Minor change with regular punctation. The 27-year-old patient, nulligravida, has no cervical dysplasia

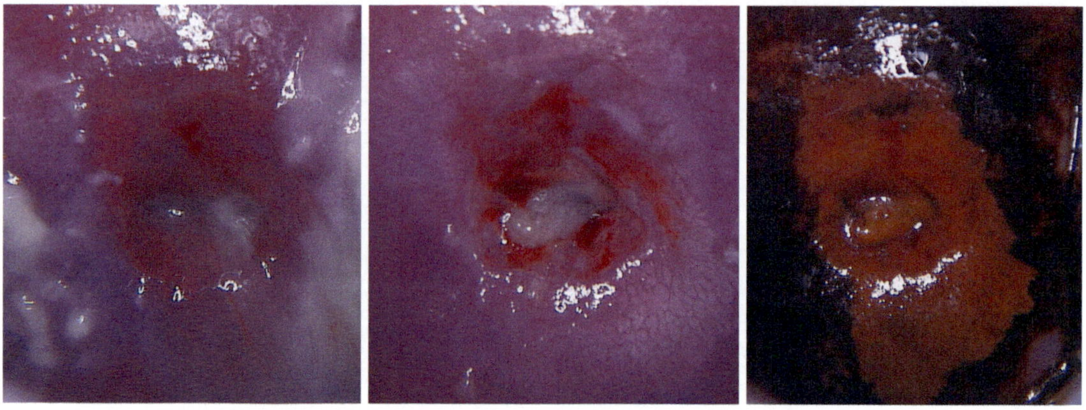

Fig. 3.40 Minor change with transparent regular mosaic

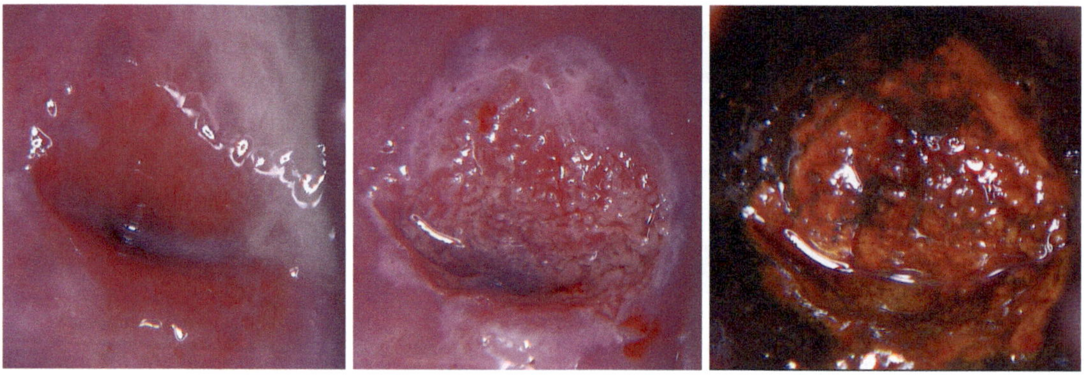

Fig. 3.41 Ectopy with transparent acetowhite epithelium close to the anterior (ventral) squamocolumnar junction

3.2.2 High-Grade Dysplasia

3.2.2.1 Pathogenesis

As pointed out earlier, the expression "high-grade squamous intraepithelial neoplasia" or HSIL is used for both CIN2 and CIN3 lesions.

The dramatic decline of the cervical cancer incidence is primarily due to the correct diagnosis and treatment of high-grade cervical dysplasia. The previous practice of surgical treatment of only cytopathologically diagnosed lesions led to significant overtreatment, which may be particularly harmful to younger women of childbearing age.

From a clinical point of view, it is important to clearly differentiate low-grade (LSIL) from high-grade changes (HSIL). Furthermore, the cytological and histological differences between CIN2 and CIN3 are less distinctive than the differences between LSIL and HSIL. Also, the cancer risk for CIN2 and CIN3, which are based on infection with the same HPV high-risk types, is similar.

HSIL assumingly has a significant risk of progression to invasive carcinoma. However, some evidence suggests that the diagnosis of CIN2/CIN3, based solely on morphological criteria, does not adequately reflect the biological progression potential of the cells. Due to genetic variations, the individual risk of developing cancer from a high-grade precancer may be quite low.

The same applies to the presence of high-risk HPV types in women without abnormal findings who overall have a low cancer risk. If precancer and cancer does occur, this may be due to a yet unidentified genetic variation. In the following discussion about the association of HPV infection and high-grade cervical dysplasia, it should be kept in mind that in a large percentage of sexually active women, DNA of human papillomaviruses can be detected without any evidence of disease. This has been known for a long time. Moscicki et al. (1990) demonstrated that more than 60% of sexually active adolescents are diagnosed with at least one of the following HPV high risk types: 16, 18, 31, 33, and/or 35.

Especially young women are able to eliminate the HP virus, whereas older women are more likely to develop persistent infection. This is of crucial importance as HPV persistence and not the transient HPV infection is responsible for the subsequent development of high-grade dysplasia and eventually invasive disease.

The most common HPV type 16 plays a special role as it may be harder to eliminate than other HPV high risk types (Moscicki et al. 1990).

It can be assumed that high-grade dysplasia originates from a small focus within an area of low-grade dysplasia within the cervix. This focus expands gradually and finally replaces the low-grade dysplastic epithelium. This so-called progression theory would explain the age distribution of patients with different degrees of dysplasia. Herrero et al. (2000) found that patients with CIN1 are younger than patients with CIN2 and CIN3, respectively.

Cervical lesions can be composed of both LSIL and HSIL (Fig. 3.42). This could be due to one of the two of these mechanisms (Park et al. 1998):

- Progression of CIN1 into CIN2/CIN3, in particular if two lesions found concomitantly on the cervix differ only by one grade of dysplasia (progression theory)
- Infection with more than one HPV type, especially if two concomitant lesions differ by more than one grade of dysplasia (CIN1 and CIN3 concomitantly)

The following cofactors can promote the development from low- to high-grade dysplasia (Brisson et al. 1994; Koutsky et al. 1992):

- Infection with HPV 16 (relative risk 8.7)
- Smoking (≥20 cigarettes per day)
- Hormonal contraception (relative risk 1.9)

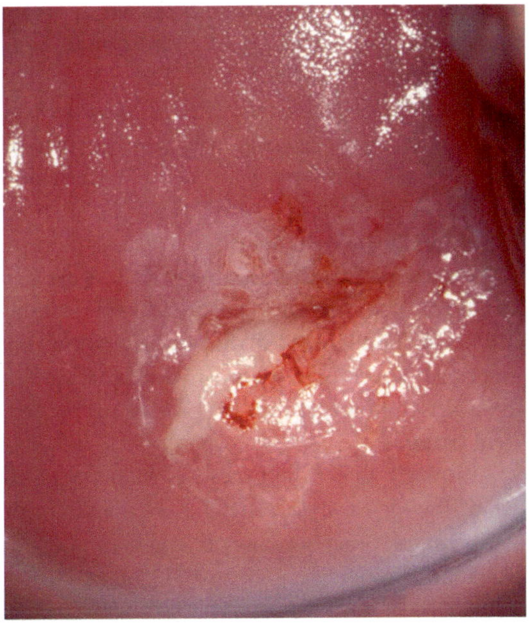

Fig. 3.42 A colposcopically guided biopsy from 12 o'clock showed high-grade dysplasia (CIN2 and CIN3). After loop resection of the abnormal transformation zone, all three grades of dysplasia (CIN1 to CIN3) were identified on histopathological exam

- Sexual intercourse with multiple partners (>4 sex partners: relative risk 1.4 for CIN2 and 2.3 for CIN3)
- Immunosuppression (due to medication, e.g. following transplant surgery, or disease related, e.g. HIV infection)

3.2.2.2 Colposcopic Appearance

The accuracy of colposcopic diagnosis of high-grade dysplasia is higher and more reliable compared to the abovementioned problematic discrimination between immature metaplastic changes and low-grade dysplasia. For the diagnosis of high-grade dysplasia, Hopman et al. (1995) found a reproducibility of 70% for the same investigator reevaluating previous colposcopic images and 76.9% agreement when different investigator evaluated the same cases. Similarly, the reliability and reproducibility of the histopathological diagnosis is also higher for the diagnosis of HSIL than for LSIL.

If colposcopic triage is used to further evaluate HSIL diagnosis on cytopathology, all

acetowhite lesions should be biopsied in order to increase the sensitivity of colposcopic diagnosis (Massad et al. 2009).

On the cervix, LSIL and HSIL can be present simultaneously. The aim of colposcopically guided tissue sampling is to identify the lesion with the highest degree of dysplasia in order to avoid inadequate treatment.

As a rule of thumb, high-grade lesions are frequently located close to the cervical canal and/or in the vicinity of the squamocolumnar junction. Therefore, when in doubt, biopsies should be taken from an area close to the cervical canal.

Assuming that a high-grade lesion develops out of low-grade dysplasia, the phenomenon of the so-called "inner border sign" can be explained. The inner border sign (Figs. 3.43 and 3.52) is defined as a dull, oyster white area, which is located within a less opaque acetowhite area (Scheungraber et al. 2009a, b; Vercellino et al. 2013). According to Scheungraber et al. (2009a, b), the inner border sign was identified in 7.6% of patients with an atypical transformation zone. In 70% of these patients, HSIL could be confirmed histopathologically. The sensitivity of the inner border sign for the presence of HSIL was 20% with a specificity of 97%. These observations were confirmed by Vercellino et al. (2013) who found a sensitivity and specificity of 20% and 99%, respectively.

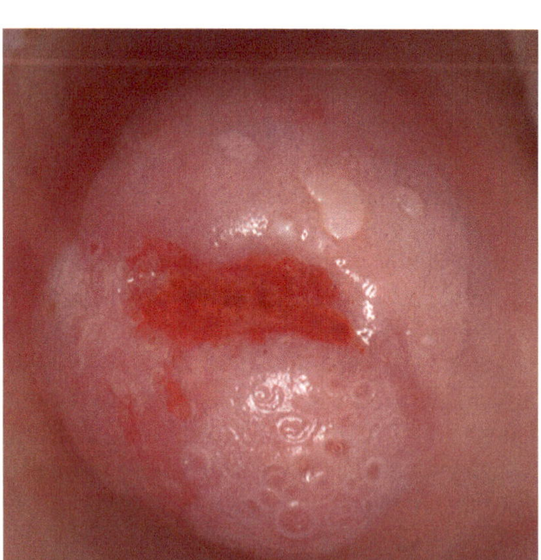

Fig. 3.43 Inner border sign. Biopsy reveals high-grade dysplasia (both CIN2 and CIN3)

Another colposcopic phenomenon that can be considered pathognomonic for high-grade dysplasia is the "ridge sign" (Fig. 3.48). The ridge sign is an opaque protuberance within the area of acetowhite epithelium located within the transformation zone. According to Scheungraber et al. (2009a, b), CIN2 or CIN3 were diagnosed in 63.8% of patients when the biopsy was taken from the area of the protuberant acetowhite epithelium. Sensitivity and specificity for HSIL diagnosis was 33.1% and 93.1%, respectively, compared to 52.5% and 96.4%, respectively (Vercellino et al. 2013).

Both the inner border sign and the ridge sign have been included in the 2011 colposcopic nomenclature of the International Federation for Cervical Pathology and Colposcopy (Bornstein et al. 2012).

A third pathognomonic colposcopic phenomenon of HSIL has been suggested by Vercellino et al. (2013), the "rag sign." The rag sign is defined as an iatrogenic erosion of the epithelium caused by mechanical trauma to the cervix, for example, when a Pap smear is obtained or acetic acid and iodine solution are applied using a cotton swab. Sensitivity and specificity for the prediction of high-grade dysplasia are 38.4% and 96.0%, respectively.

With colposcopic evaluation, a high degree of subjectivity is involved. However, inner border sign, ridge sign, and rag sign are three pathognomonic criteria strongly associated with the presence of high-grade dysplasia. In order to improve the sensitivity and specificity of colposcopically guided biopsy, pathognomic lesions should always be sampled.

The dynamics of acetic acid staining is different in high- compared to low-grade dysplasia: Acetowhite staining occurs more quickly and fades more slowly. The white color of high-grade dysplastic epithelium is very intense, and the abnormal epithelium becomes opaque, since the light rays are reflected completely due to the high density of dysplastic nuclei and the osmotic withdrawal of liquid caused by acetic acid (Fig. 3.44).

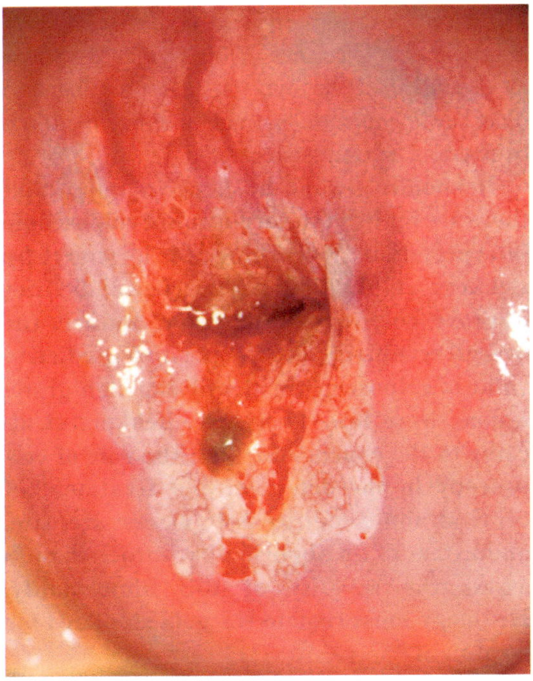

Fig. 3.44 A 32-year-old patient with biopsy-confirmed HSIL/CIN3. The characteristic features of a major change are seen with irregular mosaic, irregular punctation, and inner border lesion

Compared to the epithelium of low-grade dysplasia, the epithelium of CIN2/CIN3 lesions is thicker, and the acetowhite area will be slightly raised (Fig. 3.45). The margins of the abnormal epithelium are usually sharply demarcated.

Furthermore, atypical vascular phenomena may be seen after the application of acetic acid. As in low-grade dysplasia, the stroma capillaries will be more pronounced and may be visible as punctation and/or mosaic (Figs. 3.46, 3.47, 3.48, 3.49, 3.50, and 3.51). Both the pattern of punctation and of mosaic will be more irregular compared to low-grade lesions or immature metaplasia.

The atypical vascular phenomena described do not always occur. Elevated, coarse acetowhite areas without a recognizable vascular pattern such as punctation or mosaic are also indicative of high-grade dysplasia.

Sometimes, the raised and opaque epithelium surrounds the glandular openings within an atypical transformation zone (Figs. 3.52, 3.53 and 3.54). This is called "periglandular cuffing" and may also be an indication of high-grade dysplasia (Fig. 3.55).

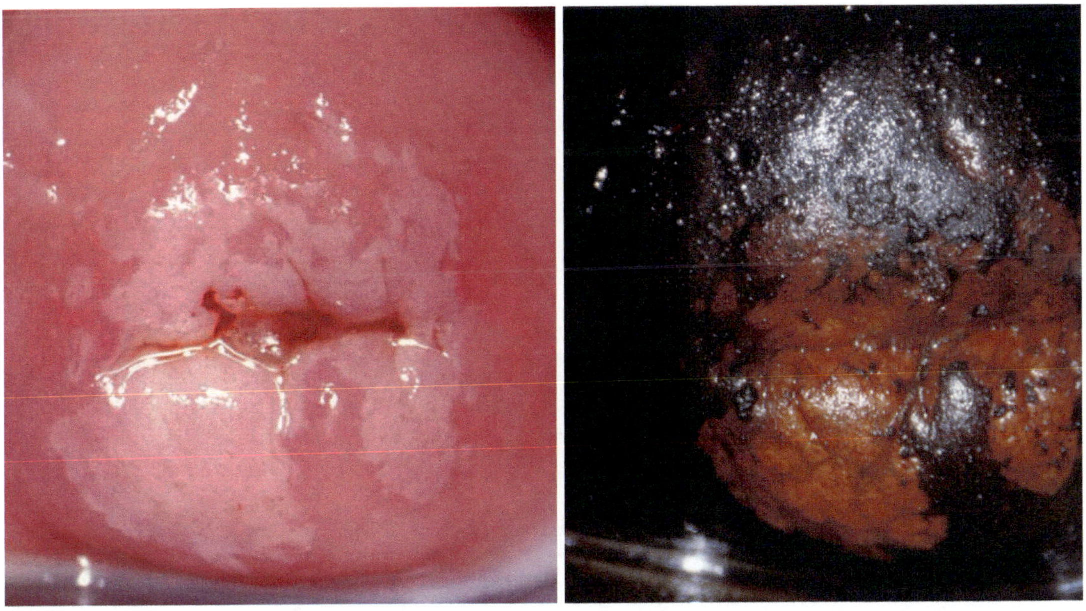

Fig. 3.45 CIN3 in a 40-year-old patient. There is opaque acetowhite staining with prominent blood vessels

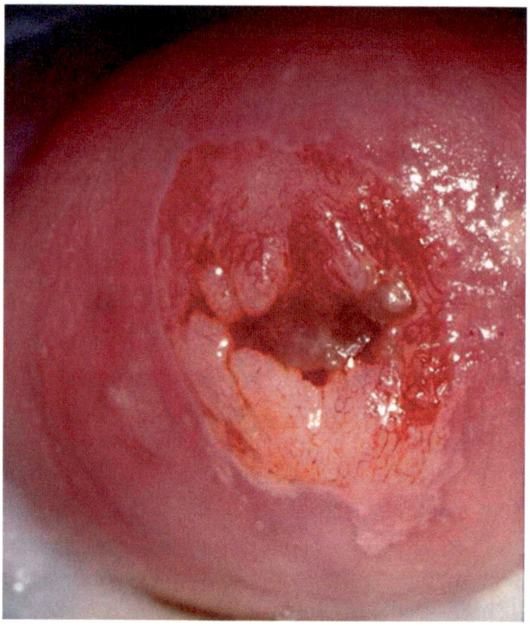

Fig. 3.46 CIN2 with intense acetowhite staining with sharp borders. The squamous epithelium is opaque and slightly raised

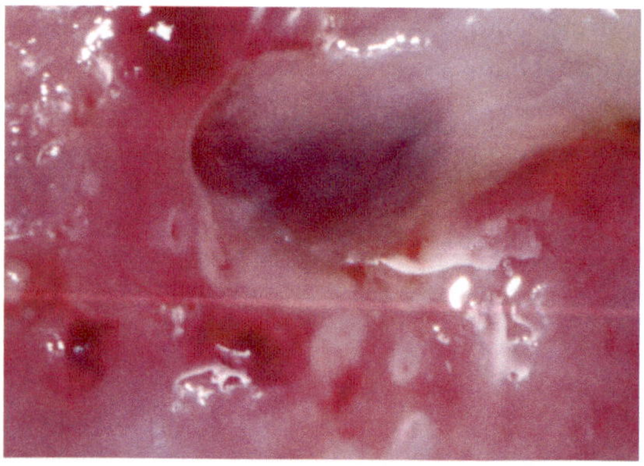

Fig. 3.47 CIN3 with coarse and irregular mosaic

Finally, it is important to note that the colposcopic characteristics of high-grade dysplasia as described above may be less prominent in older postmenopausal women and may therefore be overlooked or misinterpreted.

It should always be kept in mind that there are limits to the accuracy of colposcopic interpretation. According to a study by Bekkers et al. (2008), experience did not improve colposcopic accuracy. Rather, the overall sensitivity and the positive predictive value of colposcopy in identifying high-grade lesions were low. Therefore, Bekkers et al. came to the conclusion "that the role of colposcopy in the detection and treatment of cervical abnormalities is to assess size, site, and extent of an abnormality, rather than to assess the severity of this abnormality. Histology must remain the gold standard for treatment."

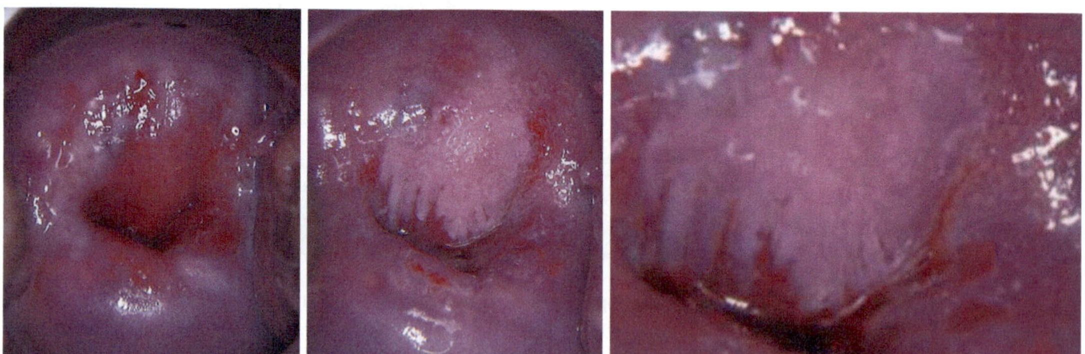

Fig. 3.48 Histologically confirmed HSIL/CIN3 of a 37-year-old patient: major change and ridge sign of the anterior (ventral) cervix

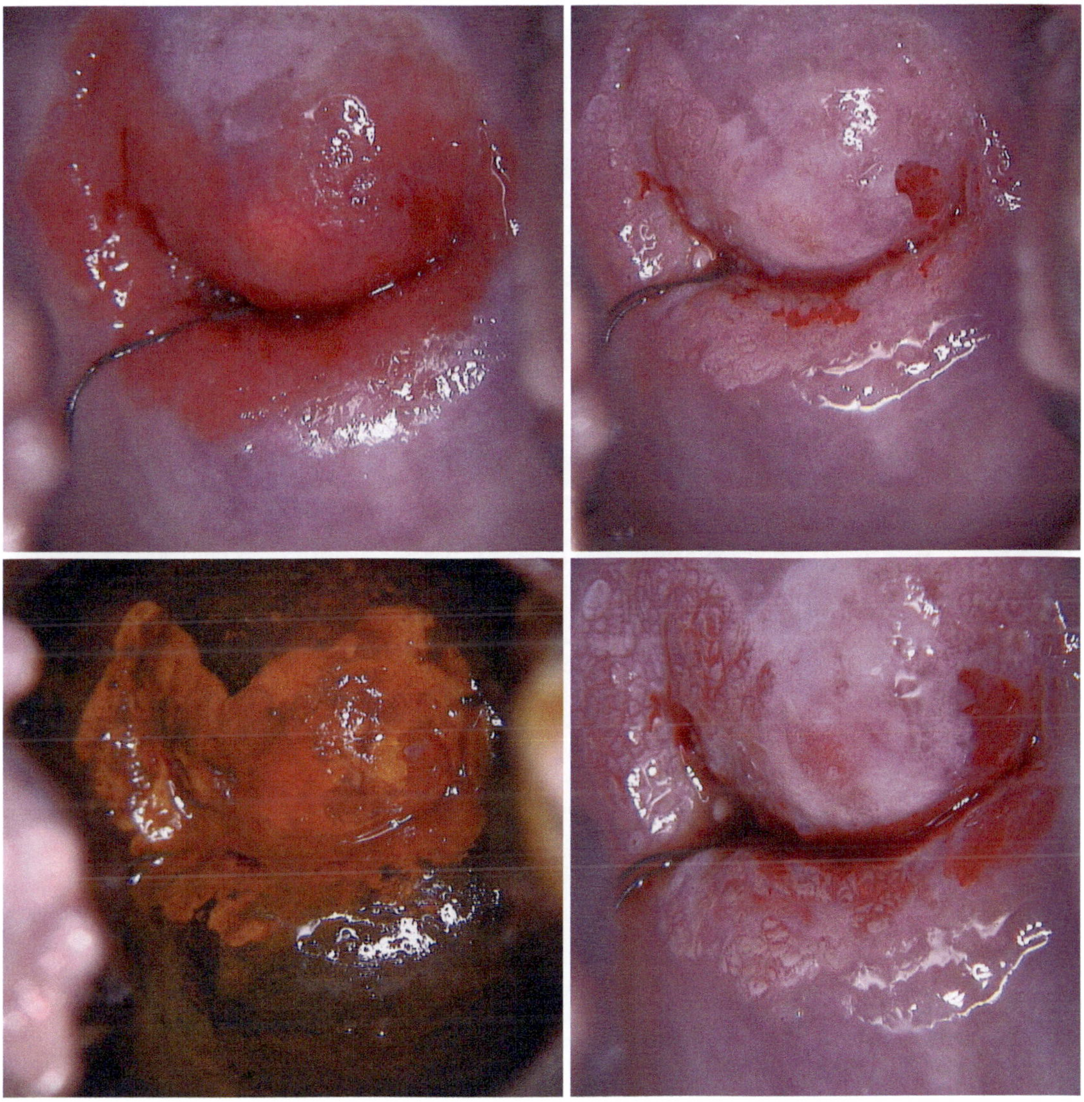

Fig. 3.49 A 28-year-old patient with biopsy-proven HSIL/CIN3. There is a major change of all four quadrants. When the acetic acid reaction slowly subsides, a characteristic irregular mosaic is visible

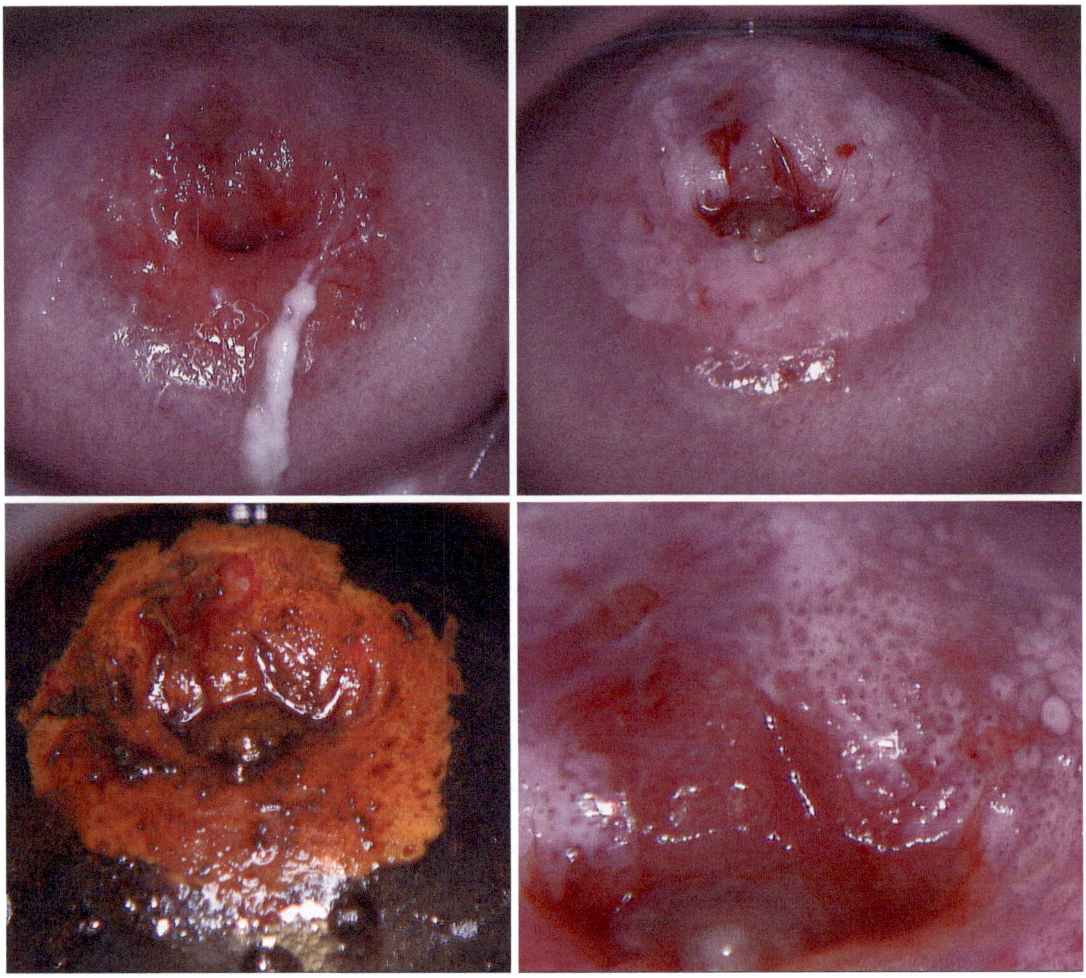

Fig. 3.50 Irregular mosaic and irregular punctation in a 29-year-old with HSIL/CIN3

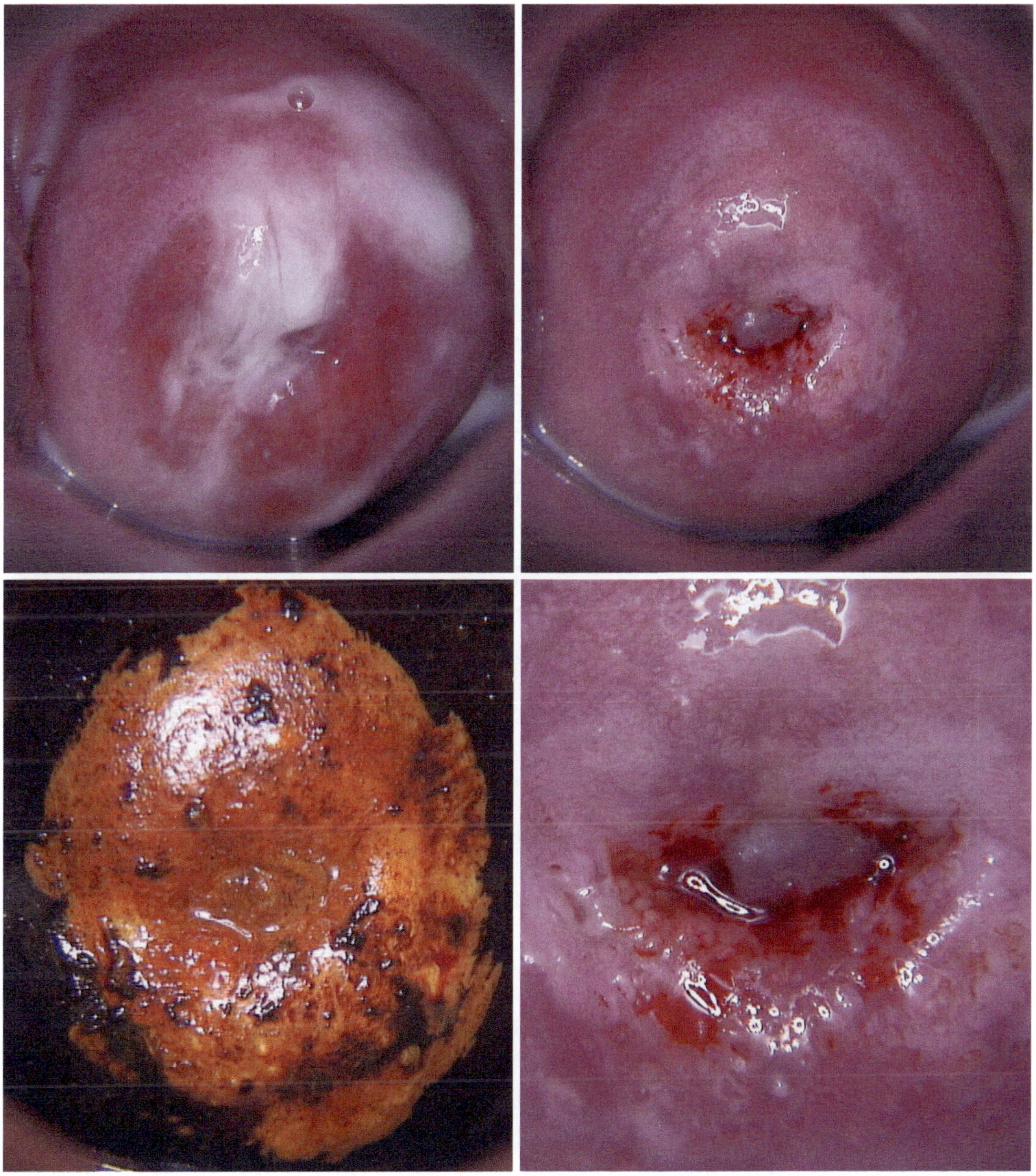

Fig. 3.51 Major change with discrete inner border lesion at 2 o'clock. Biopsy from the left ventral quadrant confirmed HSIL/CIN3 in this 26-year-old patient

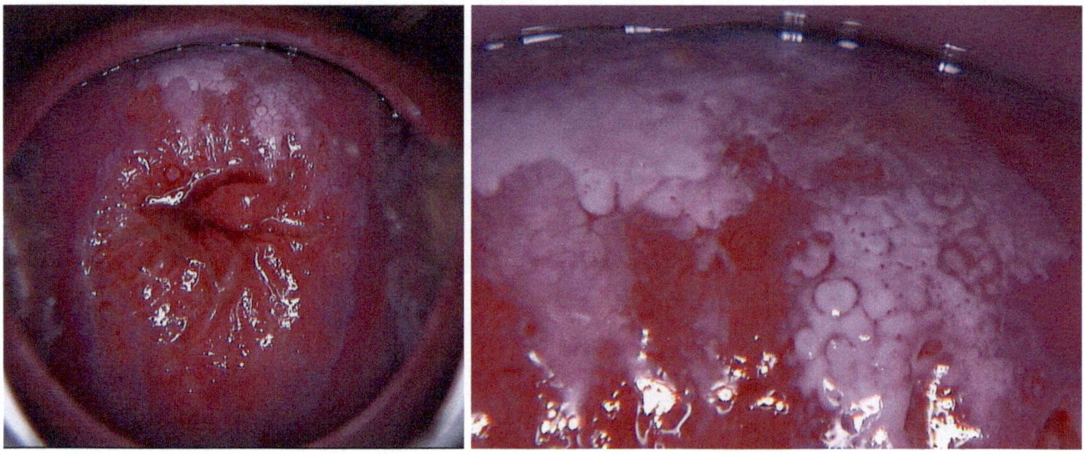

Fig. 3.52 CIN3 with raised opaque epithelium surrounding the glandular openings. This phenomenon is called "periglandular cuffing" and frequently associated with high-grade dysplasia

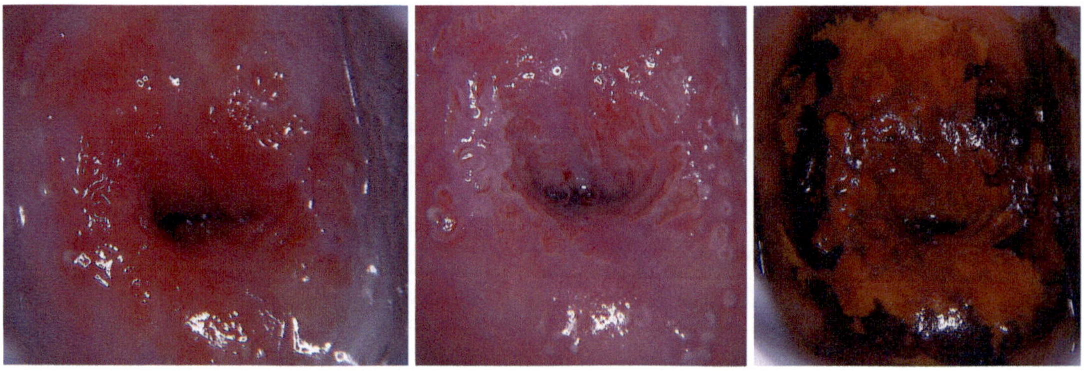

Fig. 3.53 Major change with periglandular cuffing

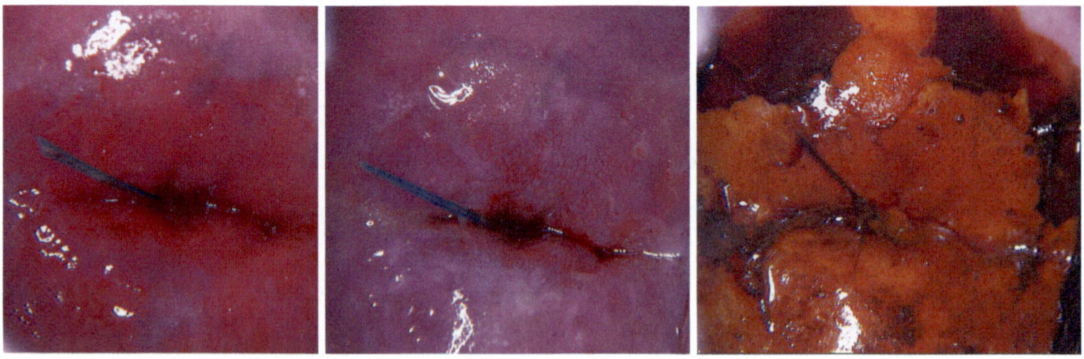

Fig. 3.54 Major change with irregular mosaic and inner border lesion. The mosaic pattern is more prominent after the acetic acid reaction has partially subsided

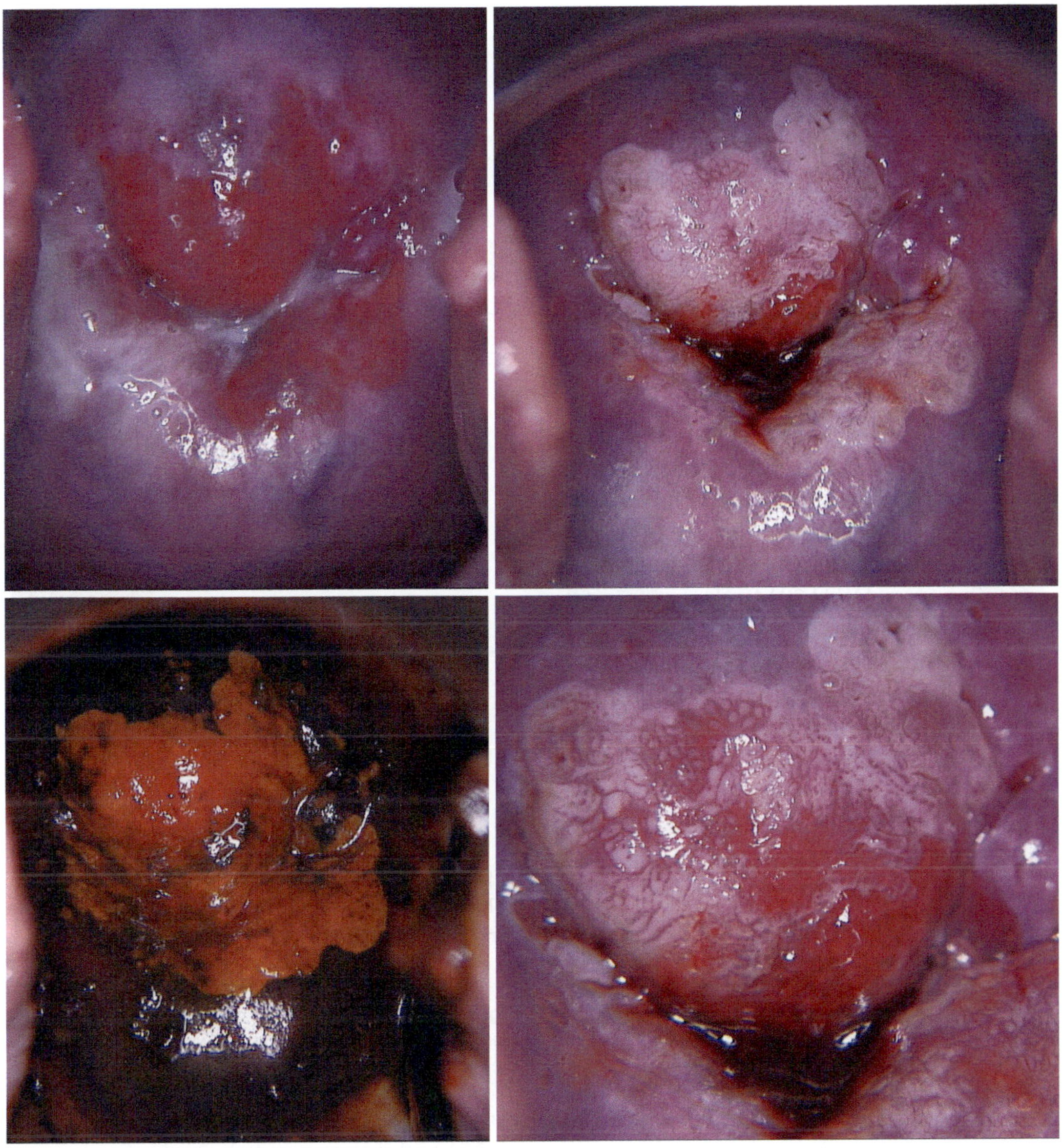

Fig. 3.55 Major change with prominent irregular mosaic

3.3 Carcinoma of the Cervix

3.3.1 Epidemiology and Clinical Presentation

The World Cancer Report published by the WHO in 2014 (Stewart and Wild 2014) shows a worldwide cervical carcinoma incidence of 7.9% of all women who develop cancer (Fig. 3.56). Thus, cancer of the cervix ranks fourth after cancers of the breast (25.2%), colorectum (9.2%), and lung (8.7%).

These four sites also represent the most common causes of cancer death in women: 14.7% (breast), 3.8% (lung), 9.0% (colorectum), and 7.5% (cervix).

Unlike other cancer types, incidence and mortality of cervical cancer is unevenly distributed

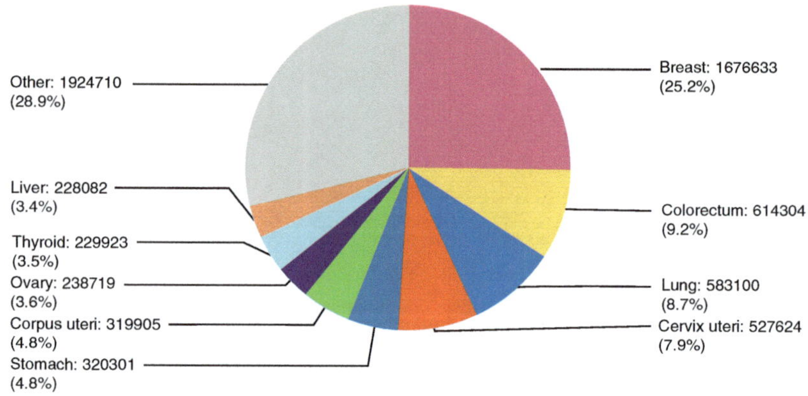

Fig. 3.56 Global cancer incidence proportions in women by cancer site. Cervical cancer ranks fourth (Stewart and Wild 2014)

between low- and high-resource countries due to the fact that cervical cancer and its precancerous lesions constitute a preventable disease as well as a type of cancer that benefits strongly from early detection. According to the WHO world cancer report (Stewart and Wild 2014), almost 70% of the global cervical cancer burden occurs in areas with low or medium levels of development. Although from a global perspective cancer of the breast, the colorectum, and the lung occurs more frequently, cervical cancer is the most common female cancer in 39 of 184 countries worldwide. In 45 countries, it is the leading cause of cancer deaths in women.

In recent decades, many countries in Europe and elsewhere have developed a sophisticated secondary prevention program based on cytological screening. A further decline of cervical cancer rates is to be expected when the positive effects of HPV vaccination will become more and more apparent.

Looking at the age-standardized rate of new cervical cancer cases in European countries and the United States, both incidence and mortality are low overall, although there are still differences between these countries (Fig. 3.57).

Data from Germany shall serve as an example for a typical industrialized nation that has introduced cytological screening as early as 1971, when health insurance providers began to cover screening expenses. The following data have been made available through regular reports published by the Robert Koch Institute (GEKID 2019).

With a population of roughly 83 million, 4380 patients have been diagnosed with cervical cancer in 2016. With regard to the percentage of female cancer (Fig. 3.58), cervical cancer ranks 13th (1.9%) with breast cancer being by far the most common malignant disease (29.5%). Other gynecological cancers such as endometrial and ovarian occupy rank 5 (4.7%) and 8 (3.1%), respectively.

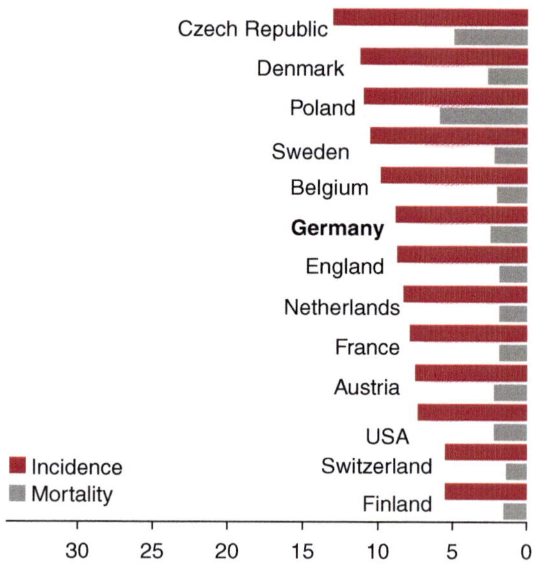

Fig. 3.57 Cervical cancer. Age-standardized rates of new diseases per 100,000 women in European countries and the United States (GEKID 2019)

While the incidence is already low, there has been a further decrease in recent years (Fig. 3.59). Mortality has also decreased. For 2020, 4400 new cases are projected. Thus, cervical cancer may even become less frequent than cancer of the vulva.

The mean age of cervical cancer patients in Germany is 55 years. The age-specific incidence is highest in the group of 40 to 44-year-olds (Fig. 3.60). Five- and 10-year survival rates are 67% and 63%, respectively.

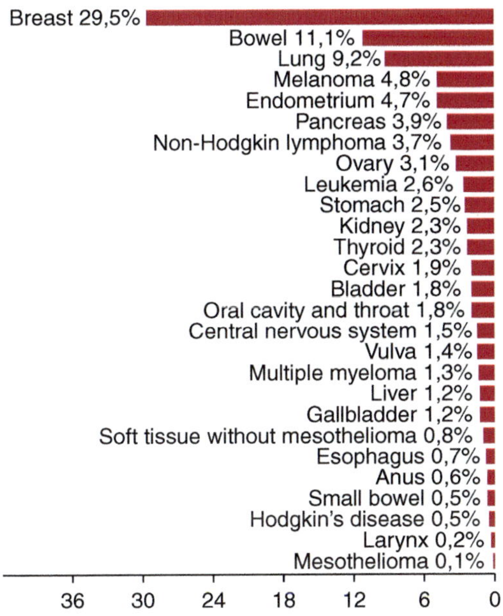

Fig. 3.58 Percentage of new cancer cases among women in Germany. Cancer of the cervix ranks 13th with 1.9% (GEKID 2019)

Forty-four percent of patients have FIGO stage I disease (Fig. 3.61), where surgical treatment is still feasible.

Colposcopy should be used for triage of cytological abnormalities and not for screening. However, historically, colposcopy has played a role for primary screening especially in the eastern states of the Federal Republic of Germany. A Health Technology Assessment Report of the German Institute for Medical Documentation and Information (DIMDI, Deutsches Institut für Medizinische Dokumentation und Information) has demonstrated unequivocally the superiority of cytological screening by a systematic literature review (Nocon et al. 2007). Four studies were identified that have compared sensitivity and specificity of colposcopic and cytological screening. In all of these studies, sensitivity of colposcopy screening was lower than that of cytopathology. The HTA report states:

The gold standard for the diagnosis of cervical carcinoma is colposcopy with biopsy.

- The most important goals of colposcopy are:
  - To rule out invasive disease (most importantly during pregnancy)
  - Histological confirmation by targeted biopsies
  - Gentle and targeted removal of microinvasive disease under colposcopic guidance
  - Early detection of recurrent disease during follow-up

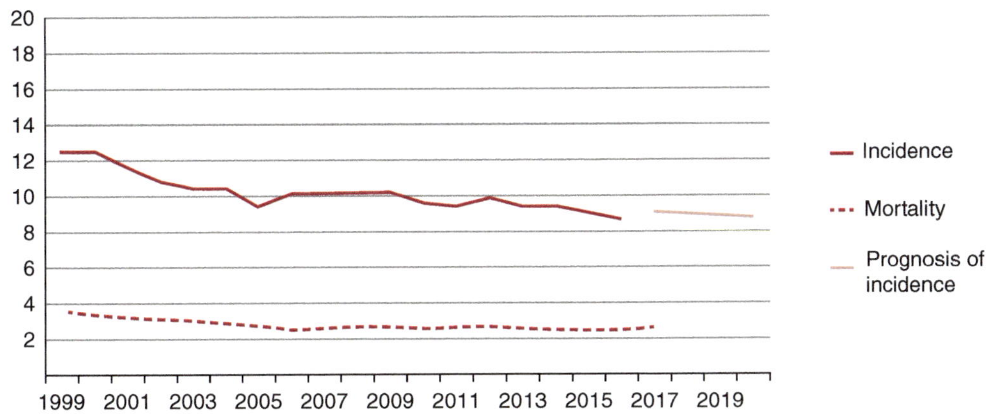

Fig. 3.59 Cervical cancer: age-standardized incidence and mortality per 100,000 women in Germany 1999 to 2017 including the incidence prognosis until 2020 (GEKID 2019)

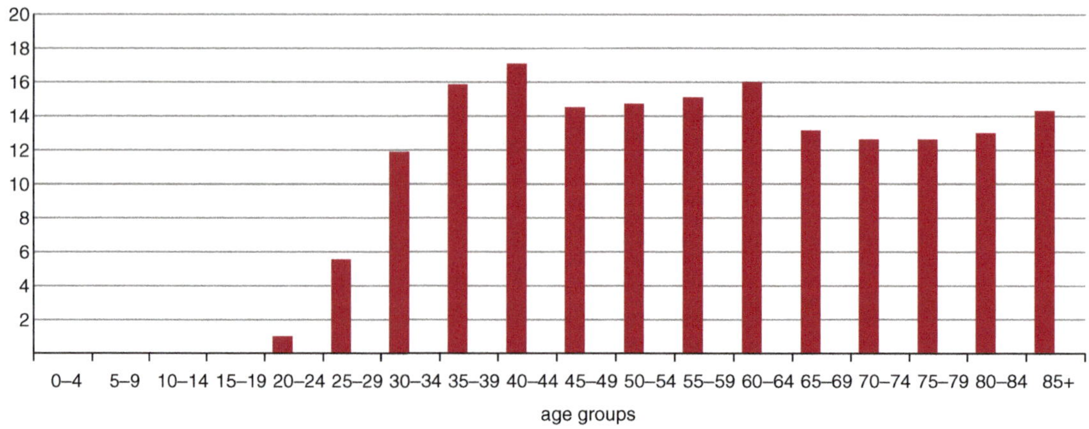

Fig. 3.60 Cervical cancer: age-specific incidence in Germany 2015 and 2016 (new cases per 100,000 women of the respective age group) (GEKID 2019)

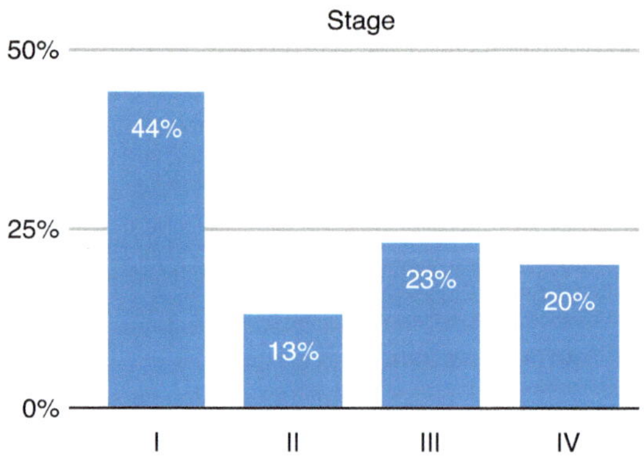

Fig. 3.61 Cervical cancer: distribution of UICC stages I to IV in Germany for 2015 and 2016 (UICC stages include local tumor spread as well as local and distant metastases at the time of initial diagnosis) (GEKID 2019)

The early diagnosis of invasive cervical carcinoma is of paramount importance. The sooner the cancer is detected, the higher the cure rate. The chances of preserving the uterus, especially in young patients, are also better. In FIGO stage IA1 disease, conization may be sufficient. In the case of more advanced carcinoma, radical cervical removal of the cervix (trachelectomy) can be carried out in selected cases (Halaska et al. 2015). In trachelectomy, the uterine corpus is preserved and thus fertility. Also, the parametrial and pelvic lymph nodes are removed to rule out metastatic involvement.

In 2006, Hertel et al. (2006) demonstrated a 90.8% recurrence-free survival with a median follow-up of 29 months in 108 patients who underwent trachelectomy for invasive tumors with a diameter of up to 2 cm and without lymph node involvement.

3.3.2 Colposcopic Appearance

Histologically, microinvasive carcinoma has a similar appearance as high-grade dysplasia. However, the cells already begin to penetrate the basal lamina and invade the underlying stroma (Fig. 3.62).

The expression "carcinoma in situ," which is sometimes used to describe an undifferentiated type of severe dysplasia, can be misleading to both patients as well as doctors. By definition, "carcinoma in situ" does not yet constitute cancer as the cells are still "in situ," i.e., "in their place" within the epithelium, and there is no stromal invasion.

The majority of malignant cervical tumors that present as FIGO stage IB or higher can be diagnosed with the naked eye. The macroscopic appearances can be quite variable (Figs. 3.63, 3.64, 3.65, 3.66, 3.67, 3.68, 3.69, 3.70, 3.71, 3.72, 3.73, 3.74, 3.75, 3.76, 3.77, 3.78, and 3.79). In any case, it is advisable to take a tissue sample at the initial gynecological examination when invasive disease is suspected macroscopically. The biopsy of tumor tissue is not painful. Occasionally, there is increased bleeding from

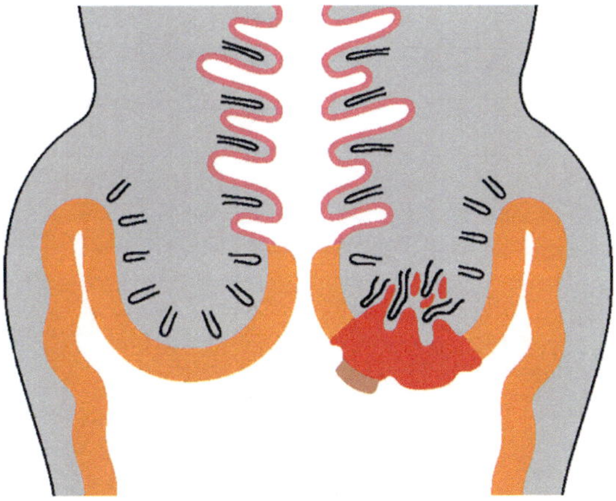

Fig. 3.62 Carcinoma of the cervix. There is invasion through the basal lamina into the stroma. Also, there may be hyperkeratosis indicative of keratinizing squamous cell carcinoma

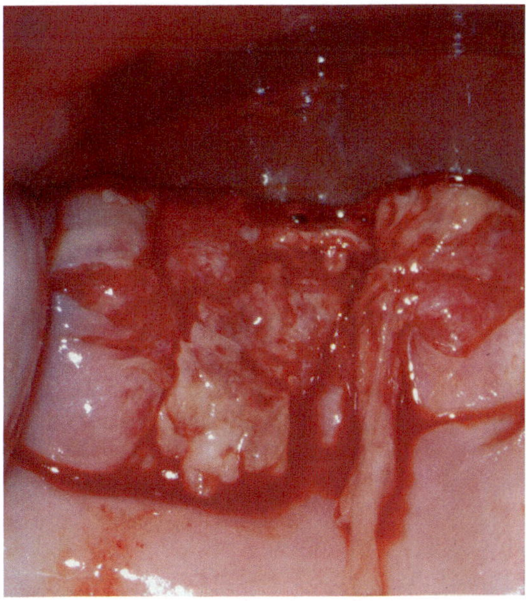

Fig. 3.64 Squamous cell carcinoma of the cervix. Instead of a cervix, only fragile tumor tissue is seen that disintegrates and bleeds on contact with the speculum

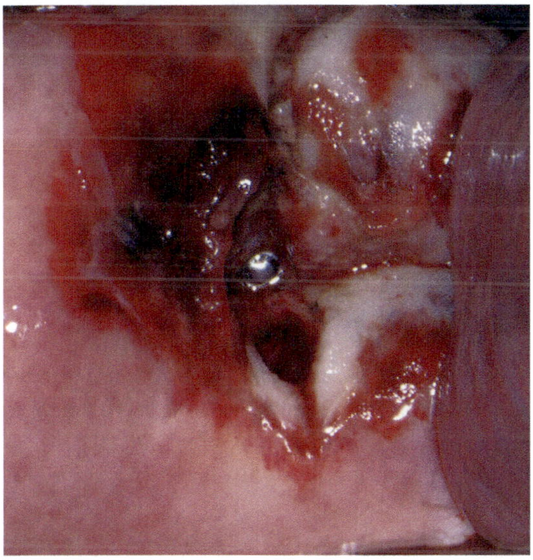

Fig. 3.63 A 60-year-old patient with moderately differentiated keratinizing squamous cell carcinoma FIGO stage IB1. A significant tissue defect is seen, which is due to ulceration

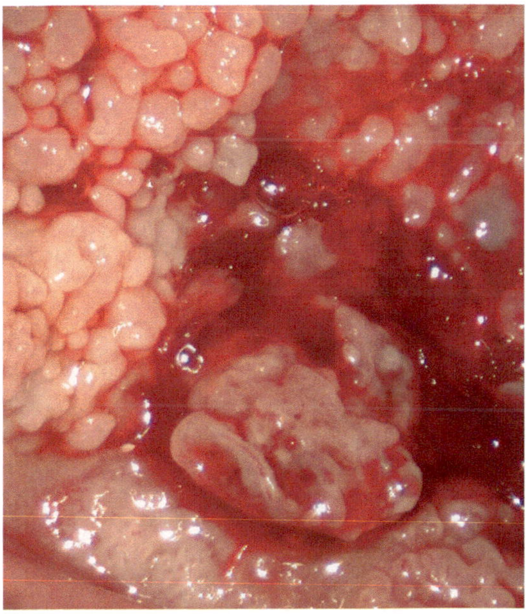

Fig. 3.65 Squamous cell carcinoma of the cervix with a papillary-like appearance

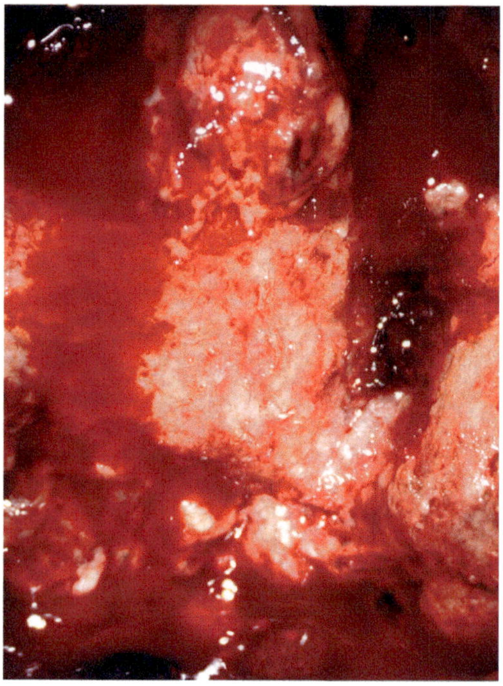

Fig. 3.66 Advanced adenocarcinoma of the cervix. The 24-year-old patient suffered from a heavy vaginal bleeding 10 weeks after cesarean section and had been diagnosed with a 5 cm cervical mass

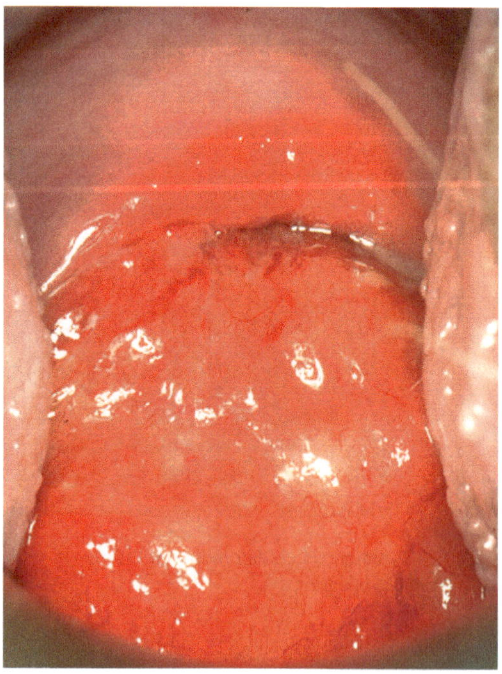

Fig. 3.67 Adenocarcinoma located on the posterior cervix in a 32-year-old patient who presented with heavy postcoital hemorrhage

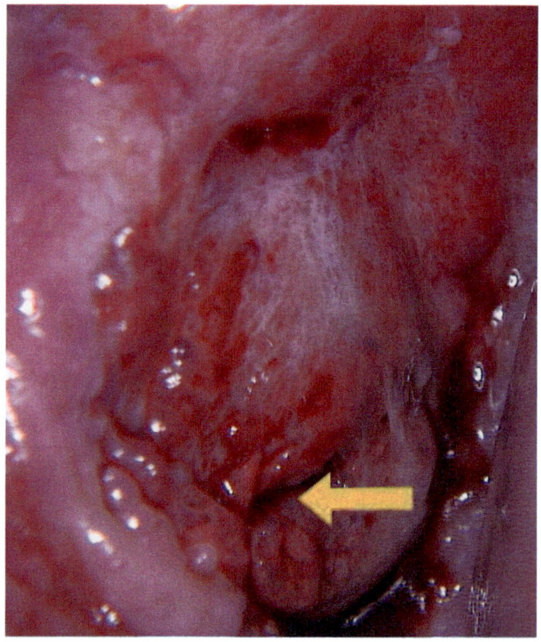

Fig. 3.68 A 26-year-old patient with a 6.1 cm adenocarcinoma of the cervix (FIGO stage IB3) with ulceration and atypical vessels. The appearance of the ectocervix is distorted. The arrow indicates the opening of the cervical os

the biopsy site as well as from the tumor itself. However, this can be easily controlled by vaginal tampon.

Histological confirmation of invasive disease should always be the first step before any further diagnostic and therapeutic measures are taken. In Chap. 17, clinical diagnosis of advanced cervical carcinoma within a low-resource environment is discussed in detail.

There are limits to the macroscopic and/or colposcopic diagnosis of invasive cervical carcinoma as one of the early manifestations and sometimes even more advanced tumors are not accessible to visual diagnosis when they are located within the cervical canal. This is particularly true for adenocarcinoma of the cervix.

Furthermore, microcarcinoma of the cervix is frequently impossible to diagnose based on colposcopic criteria alone. Usually, only high-grade dysplasia is suspected. According to a literature review by Hopman et al. (1998), approximately half of microinvasive carcinomas of the cervix are not recognized based on colposcopic criteria

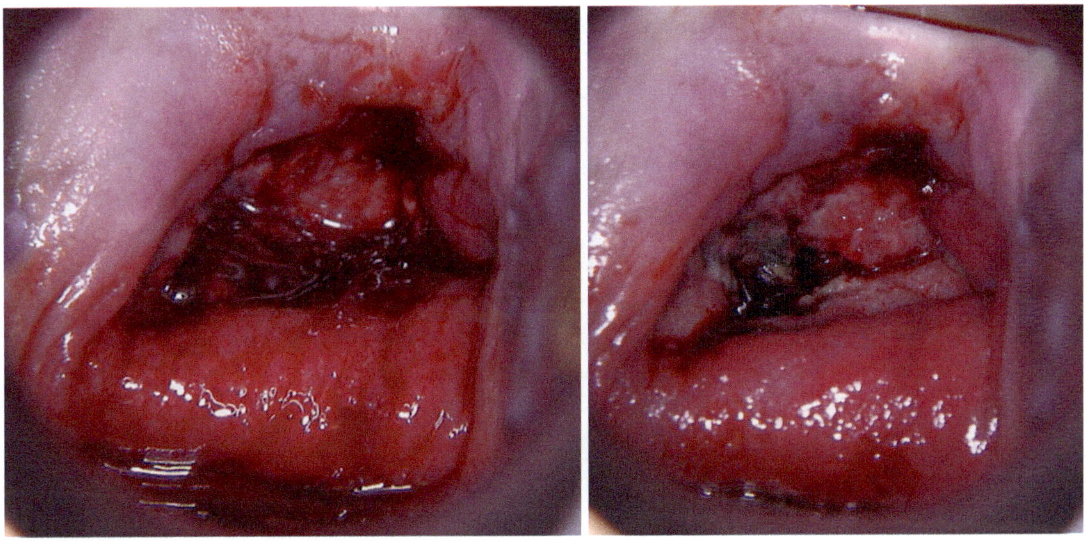

Fig. 3.69 Carcinoma of the cervix in a 49-year-old patient before and after acetic acid

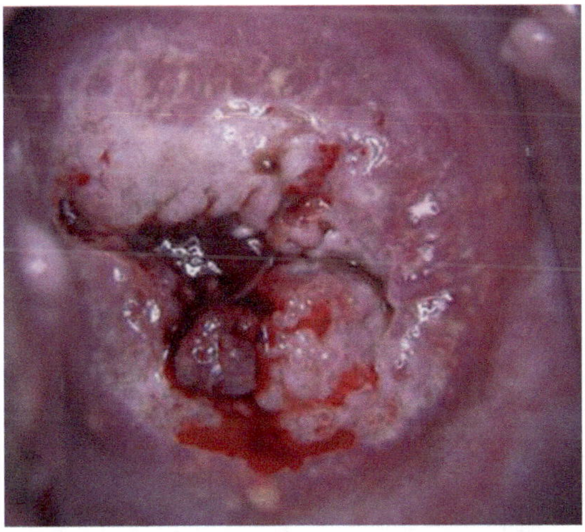

Fig. 3.70 Squamous cell carcinoma of the cervix in a 38-year-old patient arising from CIN3 (ventral quadrants)

alone. Even an experienced colposcopist will be faced with these problems because of the non-specificity of the colposcopic features of microcarcinoma.

Table 3.2 lists colposcopic features that may indicate invasive cervical disease. However, specificity is low, and no single criterion can be used to conclusively diagnose cervical carcinoma.

Microinvasive tumors with a depth of invasion of less than 3 mm do not necessarily induce neovascularization. Rather, the tumor cells are still supplied by diffusion from the surrounding tissue. Therefore, atypical vessels or ulceration/necrosis as a manifestation of insufficient blood supply due to rapid tumor growth are not seen. Instead, colposcopic findings are consistent with intraepithelial neoplasia: acetowhite and iodine-negative epithelium, as well as punctation and mosaic.

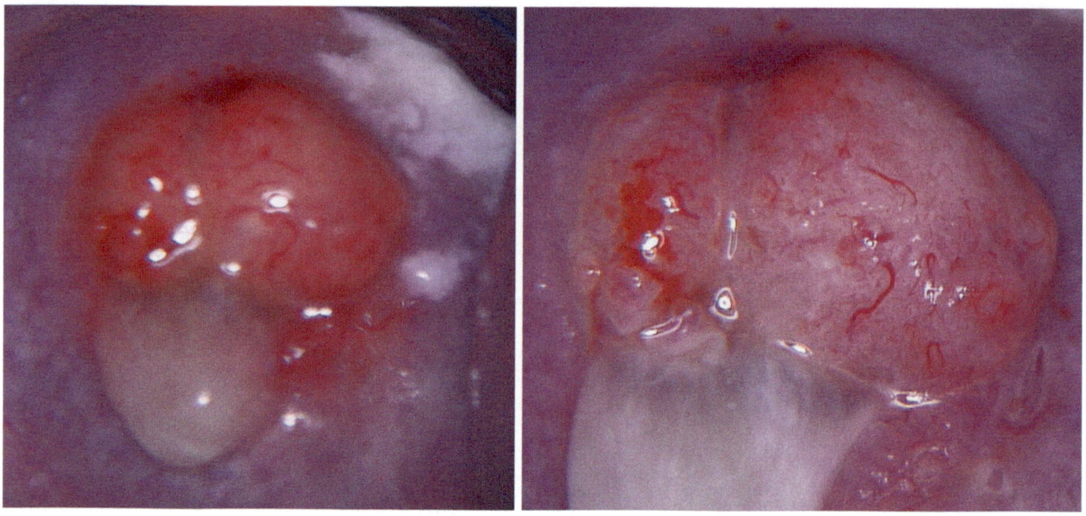

Fig. 3.71 Atypical vessels in a 32-year-old patient with adenocarcinoma of the cervix before and after acetic acid

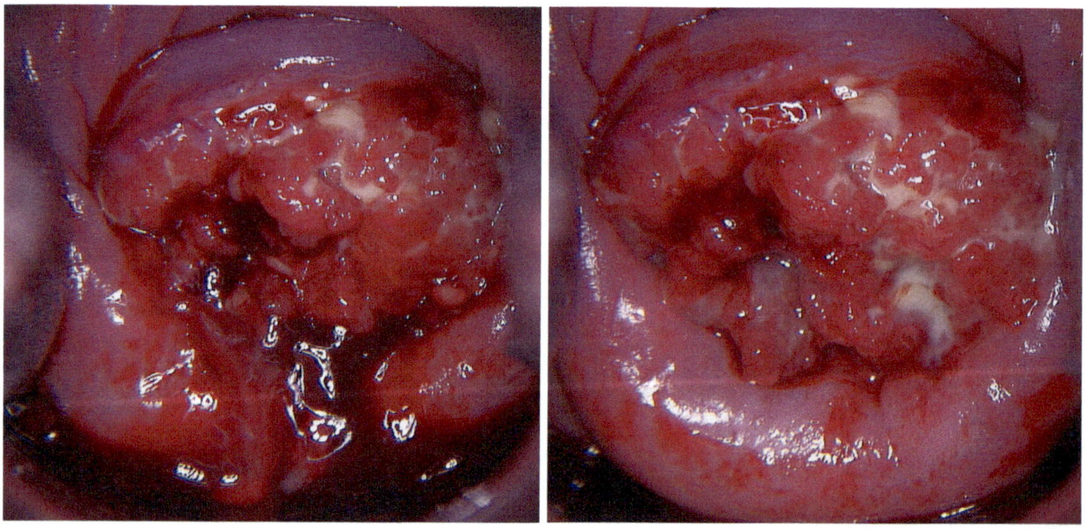

Fig. 3.72 A 29-year-old patient with adenocarcinoma of the cervix. Although in advanced cervical carcinoma there are no colposcopically distinguishable features between squamous and glandular carcinoma, the papillary appearance of the tumor suggests adenocarcinoma

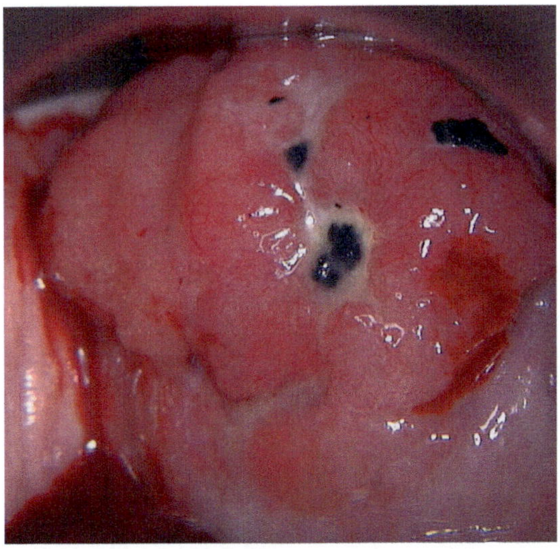

Fig. 3.73 A 30-year-old patient with advanced squamous cell carcinoma. The cervix is replaced by a large exophytic tumor

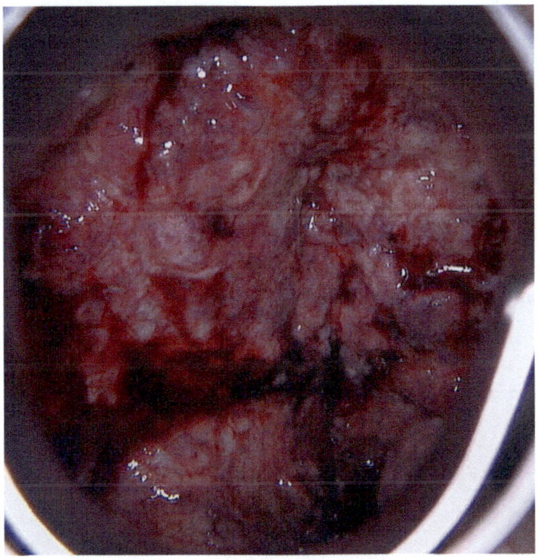

Fig. 3.74 A 52-year-old patient with a 7 × 7 cm squamous cell carcinoma of the cervix (FIGO stage IB3)

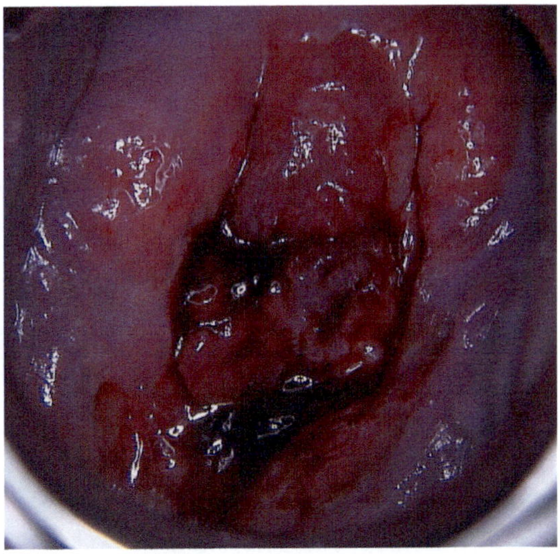

Fig. 3.75 A 32-year-old patient with a FIGO IB1 squamous cell carcinoma with clearly recognizable tissue defect

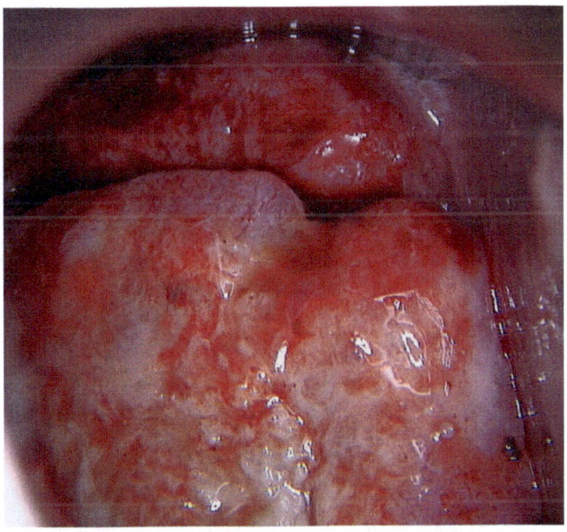

Fig. 3.76 A 52-year-old patient with locally advance squamous cell carcinoma of the cervix

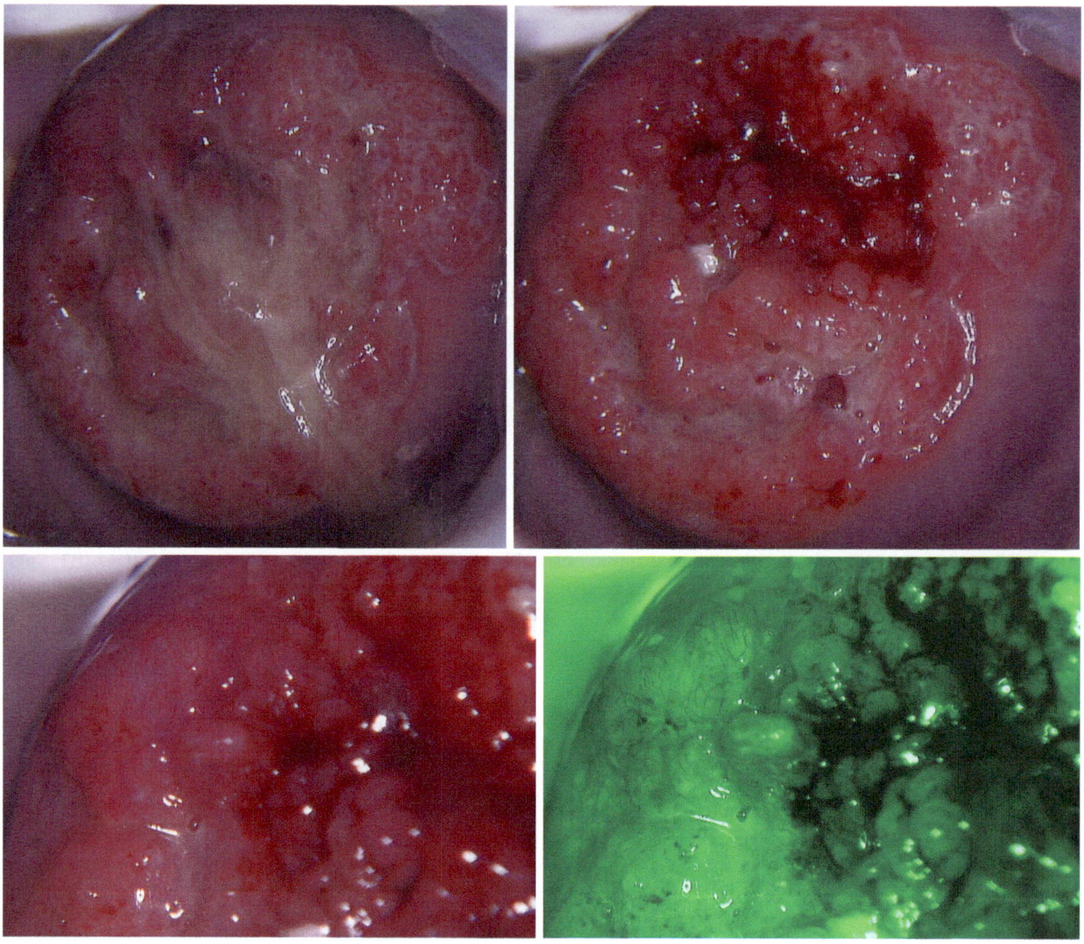

Fig. 3.77 A 31-year-old patient with FIGO stage IB1 squamous cell carcinoma. Atypical vessels are seen with the green filter

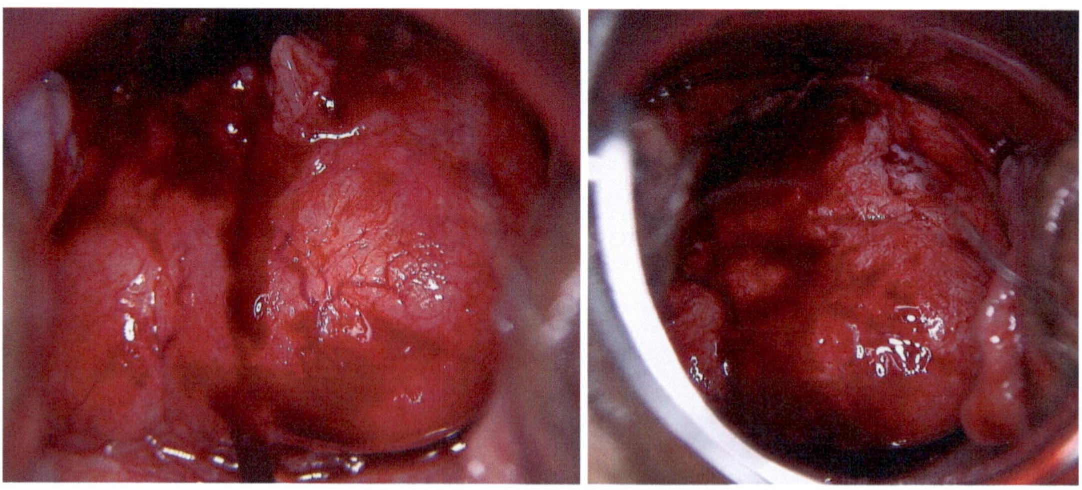

Fig. 3.78 Locally advanced adenosquamous carcinoma of the cervix in a 60-year-old patient

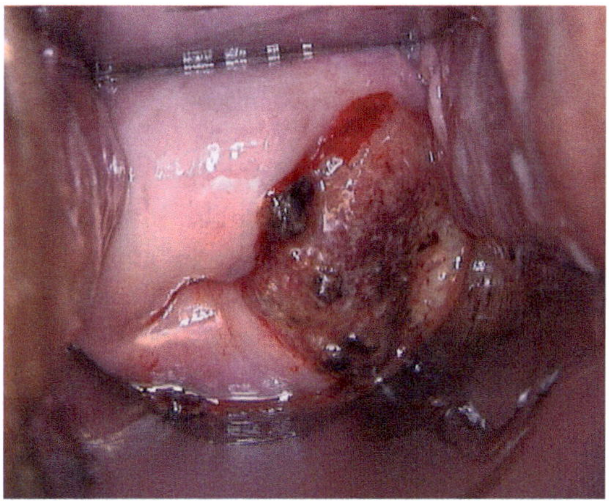

Fig. 3.79 A 49-year-old patient with a cervical metastasis from carcinoma of the sigmoid colon with widespread metastatic disease (ovaries, liver). The biopsy reveals adenocarcinoma. The colposcopic image would be highly unusual for primary carcinoma of the cervix and is explained by the fact that it is a metastatic lesion

Table 3.2 Differential diagnosis of colposcopic features that may be associated with invasive disease

Colposcopic observation	Differential diagnosis
Abnormal vessels	Prominent vessels overlying Nabothian cysts: gradual tapering toward the periphery, regular branching
Exophytic growth	Cervical condylomata acuminata
Hyperkeratosis	Hyperkeratosis due to condyloma or inflammation
Friable tissue	Inflammation, atrophy
Tissue defects (ulceration, necrosis)	True erosion: superficial sloughing of the squamous epithelial layer
	Obstetrical trauma: cervical defect without hemorrhage or other abnormal findings

The colposcopic evaluation of an atypical cervical lesion alone is not sufficient to rule out invasive disease. A targeted biopsy is always required. If invasive disease is suspected, multiple biopsies are appropriate. Surgical methods that do not allow comprehensive histopathologic evaluation, such as CO_2 laser vaporization or cryotherapy, are contraindicated.

Carcinoma of the cervix is staged clinically using the FIGO system (Bhatla et al. 2018) (Table 3.3). Treatment decisions

Table 3.3 FIGO classification of early stage cervical carcinoma (Bhatla et al. 2018) and therapeutic options

Stage	Definition	Therapy
I	The carcinoma is strictly confined to the cervix (extension to the corpus should be disregarded).	Surgery (or primary chemoradiation)
IA	Invasive carcinoma that can be diagnosed only by microscopy, with maximum depth of invasion <5 mm	(Nonradical) surgery
IA1	Measured stromal invasion of <3 mm in depth	Simple hysterectomy (no vascular or lymphatic system involvement)
		or
		trachelectomy (if fertility preservation is desired)
		or
		therapeutic conization
IA2	Measured stromal invasion of ≥3 mm and <5 mm in depth	Modified radical hysterectomy
IB	Invasive carcinoma with measured deepest invasion ≥5 mm (greater than stage IA), lesion limited to the cervix uteri	Radical hysterectomy (Wertheim-Meigs)
		or
		primary chemoradiation
IB1	Invasive carcinoma ≥5 mm depth of stroma invasion and <2 cm in greatest dimension	Radical hysterectomy (Wertheim-Meigs)
		or
		primary chemoradiation
		or
		trachelectomy (if fertility preservation is desired and tumor ≤2 cm, no lymph node involvement)
IB2	Invasive carcinoma ≥2 cm and <4 cm in greatest dimension	Radical hysterectomy (Wertheim-Meigs)
		or
IB3	Invasive carcinoma ≥4 cm in greatest dimension	primary chemoradiation

(surgery versus radiation therapy) are based on clinical examination as well as imaging techniques.

3.4 Special Considerations on Cervical Adenocarcinoma and Adenocarcinoma In Situ (AIS)

The majority of cervical carcinomas originates from squamous epithelium. However, an increasing number of adenocarcinomas are diagnosed. According to the FIGO report (Benedet et al. 2003), about 16% of cervical cancers are adenocarcinomas. Bray et al. (2005) reviewed epidemiological data from 13 European countries. The age-adjusted incidence rates of adenocarcinoma had increased within all European countries studied. The rate of increase was ranging from 0.5% per year in Denmark, Sweden, and Switzerland to more than or equal to 3% in Finland, Slovakia, and Slovenia.

The observed increase of adenocarcinoma may be due to shifting risk factors. On the other hand, cytology-based screening programs are less effective in detecting glandular precursors. According to Bray et al. (2005), cytological screening may have had at least some impact in reducing cervical adenocarcinoma incidence in some of the countries studied.

HPV-based screening is more effective preventing adenocarcinoma as shown by a review of four European randomized controlled trials comparing cytology-based screening and HPV-based screening (Ronco et al. 2014).

With HPV vaccines and especially the nonavalent type (Joura et al. 2015), prevention of premalignant and invasive glandular neoplasia should be as effective as the prevention of the squamous variety.

Analogous to squamous cell carcinoma, cervical adenocarcinoma develops from a precursor, adenocarcinoma in situ (AIS). Adenocarcinoma in situ is also related to HPV infection, mostly the HPV high risk types 18 and 45. It is assumed that gland cells are particularly susceptible to the transformational effect of these two HPV types (Iwasawa et al. 1996). Jakob et al. (2000) observed expression of two different HPV subtypes in a synchronous squamous cell and adenocarcinoma: the squamous component expressed HPV 33 while the adenocarcinoma was associated with HPV 18.

Both the cytological and the colposcopic diagnosis of adenocarcinoma in situ is a diagnostic challenge. Frequently, squamous dysplasia is diagnosed first, as CIN and AIS may occur concurrently, whereas the glandular component is much more difficult to detect.

Colposcopically, the acetic acid test has only a limited diagnostic significance, whereas Schiller's test is of no value at all as both normal and abnormal glandular epithelium are consistently Lugol-negative. In addition, adenocarcinoma in situ and early invasive adenocarcinoma without significant neoplastic growth and/or ulceration will not change the texture of the surface epithelium, as neoplastic changes may be embedded within the glandular crypts or may be located altogether within the cervical canal. Punctation or mosaic are no features of intraepithelial glandular neoplasia.

Costa et al. (2007) analyzed cytological and colposcopic findings from 42 patients with AIS. In less than half of patients (42.9%), atypical cells were identified. Results from the colposcopic evaluation were also disappointing: In 54.8% of patients, the squamocolumnar junction was not visible. In 16.7% of all colposcopic exams, no abnormality was seen.

Despite these difficulties, V. Cecil Wright (2008) has attempted to define the colposcopic features of glandular changes. Wright distinguishes three appearances (reproduced in descending order):

1. Resemblance to immature metaplasia
2. Patchy red and white areas, again resembling an immature transformation zone
3. A single isolated densely acetowhite and elevated lesion. This area may not be in contact with the squamocolumnar junction.

Thus, the first two phenomena of AIS resemble an immature transformation zone. As in cytological diagnosis, concomitant squamous dysplasia, which is present in about half of the cases, may distract from the more subtle features of glandular dysplasia.

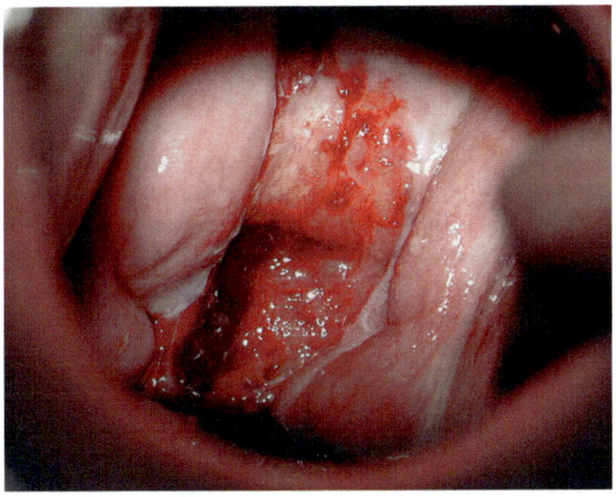

Fig. 3.80 Carcinoma of the endometrium with cervical involvement mimicking cervical cancer. There is a significant tissue defect due to tumor necrosis

For advanced adenocarcinomas of the cervix, no characteristic features exist that distinguishes them colposcopically from squamous carcinomas. Occasionally, endometrial carcinoma extending to the cervix may mimic cervical adenocarcinoma (Fig. 3.80).

References

Alam S, Conway MJ, Chen HS, Meyers C (2007) Cigarette smoke carcinogen benzo[a]pyrene enhances human papillomavirus synthesis. J Virol 82:1053. https://doi.org/10.1128/JVI.01813-07. JVI.01813-07 [pii]

ALTS (2000) Human papillomavirus testing for triage of women with cytologic evidence of low-grade squamous intraepithelial lesions: baseline data from a randomized trial. The Atypical Squamous Cells of Undetermined Significance/Low-Grade Squamous Intraepithelial Lesions Triage Study (ALTS) Group. J Natl Cancer Inst 92(5):397–402

Bekkers RL, van de Nieuwenhof HP, Neesham DE, Hendriks JH, Tan J, Quinn MA (2008) Does experience in colposcopy improve identification of high grade abnormalities? Eur J Obstet Gynecol Reprod Biol 141(1):75–78. https://doi.org/10.1016/j.ejogrb.2008.07.007. S0301-2115(08)00279-0 [pii]

Benedet JL, Odicino F, Maisonneuve P, Beller U, Creasman WT, Heintz AP et al (2003) Carcinoma of the cervix uteri. Int J Gynaecol Obstet 83(Suppl 1): 41–78

Bhatla N, Aoki D, Sharma DN, Sankaranarayanan R (2018) Cancer of the cervix uteri. Int J Gynaecol Obstet 143(Suppl 3):22–36. https://doi.org/10.1002/ijgo.12611

Bornstein J, Bentley J, Bosze P, Girardi F, Haefner H, Menton M et al (2012) 2011 Colposcopic terminology of the International Federation for Cervical Pathology and Colposcopy. Obstet Gynecol 120(1):166–172. https://doi.org/10.1097/AOG.0b013e318254f90c

Bray F, Loos AH, Mccarron P, Weiderpass E, Arbyn M, Møller H et al (2005) Trends in cervical squamous cell carcinoma incidence in 13 European countries: changing risk and the effects of screening. Cancer Epidemiol Biomark Prev 14(3):677–686. https://doi.org/10.1158/1055-9965.EPI-04-0569

Brisson J, Morin C, Fortier M, Roy M, Bouchard C, Leclerc J et al (1994) Risk factors for cervical intraepithelial neoplasia: differences between low- and high-grade lesions. Am J Epidemiol 140(8):700–710

Cantor SB, Atkinson EN, Cardenas-Turanzas M, Benedet JL, Follen M, MacAulay C (2005) Natural history of cervical intraepithelial neoplasia: a meta-analysis. Acta Cytol 49(4):405–415

Castle PE, Gage JC, Wheeler CM, Schiffman M (2011) The clinical meaning of a cervical intraepithelial neoplasia grade 1 biopsy. Obstet Gynecol 118(6):1222–1229. https://doi.org/10.1097/AOG.0b013e318237caf4

Costa S, Negri G, Sideri M, Santini D, Martinelli G, Venturoli S et al (2007) Human papillomavirus (HPV) test and PAP smear as predictors of outcome in conservatively treated adenocarcinoma in situ (AIS) of the uterine cervix. Gynecol Oncol 106:170

Doerfler D, Bernhaus A, Kottmel A, Sam C, Koelle D, Joura EA (2009) Human papilloma virus infection prior to coitarche. Am J Obstet Gynecol 200(5):487.e1–487.e5. https://doi.org/10.1016/j.ajog.2008.12.028

Duggan MA, McGregor SE, Stuart GC, Morris S, Chang-Poon V, Schepansky A, Honore L (1998) The natural history of CIN I lesions. Eur J Gynaecol Oncol 19(4):338–344

Fakokunde B, Selo-Ojeme D (2008) Impact of prolonged referral interval on colposcopic outcomes in women with moderate or severe dysplasia. Int J Gynaecol Obstet 101(3):245–247. https://doi.org/10.1016/j.ijgo.2007.11.014. S0020-7292(07)00734-5 [pii]

GEKID (2019) Krebs in Deutschland für 2015/2016. Robert Koch Institut, Berlin, p 12

Halaska MJ, Robova H, Pluta M, Rob L (2015) The role of trachelectomy in cervical cancer. Ecancermedicalscience 9:1–8. https://doi.org/10.3332/ecancer.2015.506

Hellberg D, Nilsson S (1990) 20-year experience of follow-up of the abnormal smear with colposcopy and histology and treatment by conization or cryosurgery. Gynecol Oncol 38(2):166–169

Herrero R, Hildesheim A, Bratti C, Sherman ME, Hutchinson M, Morales J et al (2000) Population-based study of human papillomavirus infection and cervical neoplasia in rural Costa Rica. J Natl Cancer Inst 92(6):464–474

Hertel H, Köhler C, Grund D, Hillemanns P, Possover M, Michels W, Schneider A (2006) Radical vaginal trachelectomy (RVT) combined with laparoscopic pelvic lymphadenectomy: prospective multicenter study of 100 patients with early cervical cancer. Gynecol Oncol 103(2):506–511

Ho GY, Bierman R, Beardsley L, Chang CJ, Burk RD (1998) Natural history of cervicovaginal papillomavirus infection in young women. N Engl J Med 338(7):423–428

Hopman EH, Voorhorst FJ, Kenemans P, Meyer CJ, Helmerhorst TJ (1995) Observer agreement on interpreting colposcopic images of CIN. Gynecol Oncol 58(2):206–209

Hopman EH, Kenemans P, Helmerhorst TJ (1998) Positive predictive rate of colposcopic examination of the cervix uteri: an overview of literature. Obstet Gynecol Surv 53(2):97–106

Iwasawa A, Nieminen P, Lehtinen M, Paavonen J (1996) Human papillomavirus DNA in uterine cervix squamous cell carcinoma and adenocarcinoma detected by polymerase chain reaction. Cancer 77(11): 2275–2279

Jakob C, Schlotter CM, Bosse U, Fuzesi L (2000) Human papillomavirus genotypes in cervical cancer with different histological features. Gynecol Obstet Investig 50(3):214–216

Joura EA, Giuliano AR, Iversen OE, Bouchard C, Mao C, Mehlsen J et al (2015) A 9-valent HPV vaccine against infection and intraepithelial neoplasia in women. N Engl J Med 372(8):711–723. https://doi.org/10.1056/NEJMoa1405044

Koliopoulos G, Arbyn M, Martin-Hirsch P, Kyrgiou M, Prendiville W, Paraskevaidis E (2007) Diagnostic accuracy of human papillomavirus testing in primary cervical screening: a systematic review and meta-analysis of non-randomized studies. Gynecol Oncol 104:232–46

Koss LG, Durfee GR (1956) Unusual patterns of squamous epithelium of the uterine cervix. Cytologic and pathologic study of koilocytotic atypia. Ann N Y Acad Sci 63:1245–1261

Koutsky LA, Holmes KK, Critchlow CW, Stevens CE, Paavonen J, Beckmann AM et al (1992) A cohort study of the risk of cervical intraepithelial neoplasia grade 2 or 3 in relation to papillomavirus infection. N Engl J Med 327(18):1272–1278

Massad LS, Jeronimo J, Katki HA, Schiffman M (2009) The accuracy of colposcopic grading for detection of high-grade cervical intraepithelial neoplasia. J Low Genit Tract Dis 13(3):137–144. https://doi.org/10.1097/LGT.0b013e31819308d4. 00128360-200907000-00004 [pii]

Moscicki AB, Palefsky J, Gonzales J, Schoolnik GK (1990) Human papillomavirus infection in sexually active adolescent females: prevalence and risk factors. Pediatr Res 28(5):507–513

Naylor B (2000) The century for cytopathology. Acta Cytol 44(5):709–725

Nocon M, Mittendorf T, Roll S, Greiner W, Willich SN, von der Schulenburg JM (2007) Welchen medizinischen und gesundheitsökonomischen Nutzen hat die Kolposkopie als primäres Screening auf das Zervixkarzinom? DIMDI, Cologne

Östör AG (1993) Natural history of cervical intraepithelial neoplasia: a critical review. Int J Gynecol Pathol 12(2):186–192

Park J, Sun D, Genest DR, Trivijitsilp P, Suh I, Crum CP (1998) Coexistence of low and high grade squamous intraepithelial lesions of the cervix: morphologic progression or multiple papillomaviruses? Gynecol Oncol 70(3):386–391

Petry KU, Menton S, Menton M, van Loenen-Frosch F, de Carvalho Gomes H, Holz B et al (2003) Inclusion of HPV testing in routine cervical cancer screening for women above 29 years in Germany: results for 8466 patients. Br J Cancer 88(10):1570–1577

Raffle AE, Alden B, Quinn M, Babb PJ, Brett MT (2003) Outcomes of screening to prevent cancer: analysis of cumulative incidence of cervical abnormality and modelling of cases and deaths prevented. BMJ 326(7395):901

Ronco G, Dillner J, Elfström KM, Tunesi S, Snijders PJF, Arbyn M et al (2014) Efficacy of HPV-based screening for prevention of invasive cervical cancer: follow-up of four European randomised controlled trials. Lancet 383(9916):524–532. https://doi.org/10.1016/S0140-6736(13)62218-7

Sankaranarayanan R, Wesley RS (2003) A practical manual on visual screening for cervical neoplasia. IARC Press, Lyon

Scheungraber C, Glutig K, Fechtel B, Kuehne-Heid R, Duerst M, Schneider A (2009a) Inner border-a specific and significant colposcopic sign for moderate or severe dysplasia (cervical intraepithelial neoplasia 2 or 3). J Low Genit Tract Dis 13(1):1–4. https://doi.org/10.1097/LGT.0b013e31817ff92a

Scheungraber C, Koenig U, Fechtel B, Kuehne-Heid R, Duerst M, Schneider A (2009b) The colposcopic feature ridge sign is associated with the presence of cervical intraepithelial neoplasia 2/3 and human papillomavirus 16 in young women. J Low Genit Tract Dis 13(1):13–16. https://doi.org/10.1097/LGT.0b013e318180438a

Shew ML, Weaver B, Tu W, Tong Y, Fortenberry JD, Brown DR (2013) High frequency of human papillomavirus detection in the vagina before first vaginal intercourse among females enrolled in a longitudinal cohort study. J Infect Dis 207(6):1012–1015. https://doi.org/10.1093/infdis/jis775

Stewart BW, Wild CP (2014) World cancer report 2014. International Agency for Research on Cancer, WHO, Geneva

Vercellino GF, Erdemoglu E, Chiantera V, Vasiljeva K, Drechsler I, Cichon G et al (2013) Validity of the colposcopic criteria inner border sign, ridge sign, and rag sign for detection of high-grade cervical intraepithelial neoplasia. Obstet Gynecol 121(3):624–631. https://doi.org/10.1097/AOG.0b013e3182835831

Wright VC (2008) Cervical glandular disease: adenocarcinoma in situ and adenocarcinoma. In: Apgar BS, Brotzman GL, Spitzer M (eds) Colposcopy - principles and practice. An integrated textbook and atlas, Saunders, Philadelphia, PA

zur Hausen H (2009) Papillomaviruses in the causation of human cancers - a brief historical account. Virology 384(2):260–265. https://doi.org/10.1016/j.virol.2008.11.046

4 International Nomenclature of Colposcopy

Contents

The colposcopic nomenclature was last updated in 2011/2012 by the International Federation of Cervical Pathology and Colposcopy (IFCPC). This system is used to describe and classify findings of the cervix as well as of the vagina and vulva.

4.1 Cervix

At the 14th IFCPC World Congress in Rio de Janeiro, the colposcopic terminology was updated by the nomenclature committee under the direction of Jacob Bornstein (Bornstein et al. 2012a; Quaas et al. 2013). The Rio classification system of the cervix is divided into five sections: general assessment, normal colposcopic findings, abnormal colposcopic findings, suspicious for invasion, and miscellaneous findings (Table 4.1).

The first step of colposcopic assessment should be a statement regarding the quality of this assessment. The terms "adequate" and "inadequate" are used. This should be the first statement of any written colposcopic evaluation. If colposcopy is considered inadequate, a reason is given. For example, due to extreme obesity, the cervix might not be visible at all. Also, when inflammation or atrophy are present, no adequate colposcopic evaluation is possible.

When colposcopy is considered inadequate, a follow-up examination should be carried out, for example, after local treatment of inflammation and atrophy or after suitable instruments have been procured (obesity).

Next, the visibility of the squamocolumnar junction is described. Formerly, the descriptors "satisfactory" and "unsatisfactory" have been used. A colposcopic exam was deemed unsatisfactory, if the transformation zone was not completely visible. However, the definitions of adequate/inadequate and satisfactory/unsatisfactory are not identical. According to the Rio 2011 nomenclature, adequacy and the type of transformation zone observed are separate statements. In fact, the IFCPC has abandoned the description of a colposcopic exam as "unsatisfactory"

R. J. Lellé, V. Küppers, *Colposcopy*, https://doi.org/10.1007/978-3-030-85388-4_4

Table 4.1 2011 International Federation of Cervical Pathology and Colposcopy terminology of the cervix (Bornstein et al. 2012a)

Section	
General assessment	• Adequate or inadequate for the reason (e.g., cervix obscured by inflammation, bleeding, or scar) • Squamocolumnar junction visibility: completely visible (type 1), partially visible (type 2), not visible (type 3)
Normal colposcopic findings	• Original squamous epithelium: mature, atrophic • Columnar epithelium: ectopy/ectropion • Metaplastic squamous epithelium: Nabothian cysts, crypt (gland) openings • Deciduosis in pregnancy
Abnormal colposcopic findings	• Location of the lesion: by clock position, inside or outside the transformation zone • Size of the lesion: number of cervical quadrants the lesion covers and/or as percentage of cervix • Grade 1 (minor change): fine mosaic, fine punctation, thin acetowhite epithelium, irregular, geographic border • Grade 2 (major change): sharp border, inner border sign, ridge sign, dense acetowhite epithelium, coarse mosaic, coarse punctation, rapid appearance of acetowhitening, cuffed crypt (gland) openings • Nonspecific: leukoplakia (keratosis, hyperkeratosis), erosion Lugol's staining (Schiller's test): stained or nonstained
Suspicious for invasion	• Atypical vessels • Additional signs: fragile vessels, irregular surface, exophytic lesion, necrosis, ulceration (necrotic), tumor or gross neoplasm
Miscellaneous findings	• Congenital transformation zone, condyloma, polyp (ectocervical or endocervical), inflammation, stenosis, congenital anomaly, posttreatment changes, endometriosis

altogether as it has the connotation of an insufficient exam that needs to be repeated.

In section two, normal colposcopic findings are described. This includes both original squamous and columnar/glandular epithelium as well as the phenomena of metaplasia such as gland openings or Nabothian cysts. Deciduosis, when it occurs in pregnancy, is also considered a normal finding.

In the third section, abnormal colposcopic findings are listed starting with the location and size of the abnormal lesion. By projecting a clock face onto the cervix, the approximate position and extent of a distinct area can be indicated. Although the dysplastic epithelium will usually be located within the transformation zone, any abnormality should be described in relation to its location regarding the transformation zone. "Inside the transformation zone" means that a lesion is located medial to the original squamocolumnar junction. However, in patients with a mature transformation zone, the original squamocolumnar junction may be difficult to identify.

The size of a lesion, which is relevant both for follow-up exams as well as treatment planning, can be given as the number of quadrants involved, the percentage of the cervix affected, or both. Quadrants are usually called right/left and anterior/posterior although the correct anatomical term would be "ventral" and "dorsal."

When abnormal colposcopic findings are described, the distinction between low-grade (CIN1) and high-grade (CIN2 and CIN3) precancer are most important as this will be decisive for further clinical management. In colposcopic nomenclature, the terms "minor" and "major" lesion are used, sometimes also called "grade 1" and "grade 2" lesions, respectively. Whenever appropriate, expressions such as "fine punctation/mosaic" versus "coarse punctation/mosaic" and "regular" versus "irregular pattern" should be used. In addition to the Rio nomenclature, the distinction between "transparent" and "opaque" acetowhite areas is helpful.

Inner border sign and ridge sign—possibly also rag sign—are considered to be pathognomonic for high-grade disease and will support the colposcopic diagnosis of a major/grade 2 lesion (Scheungraber et al. 2009; Vercellino et al. 2013).

For the colposcopic identification of a major lesion, not only the high intensity of acetowhite staining is important but also the rapid development of the acetic acid reaction.

However, even a slow reaction to the acetic acid, which in some cases may take up to 3 min, may be associated with major changes, especially if other criteria for a grade 2 lesion are met.

Periglandular cuffing, i.e., raised and opaque epithelium surrounding the glandular openings within an atypical transformation zone, may also be an indication of high-grade dysplasia.

The classification of Lugol's test (Schiller's test) as an unspecific reaction underlines the necessity of prior acetic acid application, especially preoperatively in order to determine the extent of the excision, as the Lugol reaction alone is not a suitable criterium. Leukoplakia (keratosis, hyperkeratosis) is also considered nonspecific.

The fourth section describes all phenomena that are suspicious for invasion, especially atypical and fragile vessels, an irregular surface, and ulceration and exophytic growth.

According to the Rio nomenclature, the presence of atypical vessels is considered to be pathognomonic for invasive disease, and histopathological clarification by colposcopically guided biopsy is mandatory.

Finally, in the fifth section, several colposcopic findings are summarized including condylomata and cervical polyps.

The IFCPC has added an addendum to its nomenclature regarding surgical treatment. The aim is to avoid poorly defined terms such as cone biopsy, conization, or small and large loop excision. Instead, three excision types are defined, which correspond to the three types of transformation zone T1, T2, and T3. Whereas a type 1 excision will resect a completely visible transformation zone, a type 2 excision includes a small area of endocervical tissue that can be visualized colposcopically. With a type 3 excision, a larger amount of endocervical tissue is resected. The type 3 excision is also used to effectively treat adenocarcinoma in situ or microinvasive disease.

The type of excision that depends on the length of the surgical specimen, its thickness, and its circumference should be reported by the pathologist.

4.2 Vagina

The IFCPC nomenclature also includes a classification system for the vagina, which is analogous to that of the cervix (Bornstein et al. 2012a). The aim of this nomenclature is to create an evidence-based terminology with relevance to management and especially to treatment of colposcopically diagnosed changes of the vagina.

The colposcopic nomenclature of the vagina is similar to that of the cervix (Table 4.2). Initially, the adequacy of the examination is evaluated. If it is considered to be "inadequate," an appropriate reason is given such as inflammation or hemorrhage.

Normal findings are classified either as "mature" or "atrophic." If an abnormality is identified, its location is given using descriptors such as "lower third of the vagina/upper two-thirds, anterior/posterior, and left/right vaginal wall." As with the uterine cervix, the abnormal findings are divided into "minor or grade 1 changes" and "major or grade 2 changes." As for the cervix, leukoplakia and the results of Lugol's test (Schiller's test) are classified as "nonspecific."

Nonspecific findings also include the presence of columnar epithelium in the vagina, so-called vaginal adenosis.

The diagnosis "suspicious for invasion" is part of the "abnormal colposcopic findings" section. Diagnosis is based on the same criteria as for suspected cervical cancer.

Table 4.2 2011 International Federation of Cervical Pathology and Colposcopy terminology of the vagina (Bornstein et al. 2012a)

Section	
General assessment	• Adequate or inadequate because of (e.g., inflammation, bleeding, or scar) • Transformation zone
Normal colposcopic findings	• Normal squamous epithelium: mature, atrophic
Abnormal colposcopic findings	• Location of the lesion: Upper third or lower two-thirds, anterior, posterior, or lateral (right or left) • Grade 1 (minor change): fine mosaic, fine punctation, thin acetowhite epithelium • Grade 2 (major change): coarse mosaic, coarse punctation, dense acetowhite epithelium • Suspicious for invasion: fragile vessels, irregular surface, exophytic lesion, necrosis, ulceration (necrotic), tumor or gross neoplasm • Nonspecific: columnar epithelium (adenosis) • Lugol's staining (Schiller's test): stained or nonstained, leukoplakia
Miscellaneous findings	• Erosion (traumatic), condyloma, polyp, cyst, endometriosis, inflammation, vaginal stenosis, congenital transformation zone

4.3 Vulva

The terminoloy system for the vulva as published by the International Federation of Cervical Pathology and Colposcopy (IFCPC) has been established in collaboration with the International Society for the Study of Vulvovaginal Diseases (ISSVD). However, since the IFCPC publication by Bornstein et al. in 2012, the ISSVD has published a modification of its terminology for vulvar intraepithelial neoplasia (VIN) (Bornstein et al. 2016). In the following section, the nomenclature of the IFCPC terminology is discussed in detail.

Compared to colposcopy of the cervix and vagina, colposcopic evaluation and nomenclature of the vulva differ significantly:

- **Evaluation of the vulva is more complex.**

There is a vast range of different dermatologic diseases that may affect the vulva. Due to the complexity of vulvar diagnosis, the reporting of vulvar lesions is frequently inconsistent.

- **The colposcope is not an indispensable tool for diagnosis of the vulva.**

Many experts on vulvar diseases will use only a magnifying glass or no magnification at all. The IFCPC has taken this into account calling its terminology "colposcopic" as well as "clinical".

- **The vulvar nomenclature is also applicable to the anus.**

- **The acetic acid test plays only a limited role compared to its value in the diagnosis of the cervix, and Lugol's test is not used at all.**

Acetowhitening of the vulva is not as specific as it is for the cervix, where the acetic acid test is mandatory for any colposcopic evaluation. In some circumstances, when intraepithelial neoplasia (VIN) is suspected, acetic acid may help to better delineate the abnormal area and choose an appropriate biopsy site. For all other vulvar diseases, acetic acid does not contribute to diagnosis. As Lugol's test is based on the presence or absence of glycogen with the intermediate cells of nonkeratinizing squamous epithelium, it is not applicable to the vulva.

As Bornstein et al. (2016) point out, the vulvar epithelium is more varied compared to the cervix and vagina as it encompasses both skin and mucosa. The skin is further divided into "hairy" such as the labia majora and "nonhairy" such as the clitoris. Some diseases may be limited to the skin or the mucosa alone, whereas others affect both types of epithelium. The description of the structures constitutes the first section of vulvar nomenclature.

Hirsuties papillaris (micropapillomatosis), which is sometimes confused with condylomata acuminata, sebaceous glands, and a mild

vestibular redness, are classified as normal findings and therefore should not be treated.

In order to appropriately describe abnormal findings, the dermatologic terminology is applied. Besides lesion size and location, the lesion type (macule, patch, papule, etc.) as well as the secondary morphology such as eczema or lichenification is given.

A weakness of present ISSVD nomenclature is the fact that no distinction is made between symptomatic and asymptomatic vulvar lesions. In the differential diagnosis of diseases of the vulva, the consideration of symptoms is decisive.

References

Bornstein J, Bentley J, Bosze P, Girardi F, Haefner H, Menton M et al (2012a) 2011 colposcopic terminology of the international federation for cervical pathology and colposcopy. Obstet Gynecol 120(1):166–172. https://doi.org/10.1097/AOG.0b013e318254f90c

Bornstein J, Bogliatto F, Haefner HK, Stockdale CK, Preti M, Bohl TG, Reutter J (2016) The 2015 International Society for the Study of Vulvovaginal Disease (ISSVD) terminology of vulvar squamous intraepithelial lesions. Obstet Gynecol 127(2):264–268. https://doi.org/10.1097/AOG.0000000000001285

Quaas J, Reich O, Frey Tirri B, Küppers V (2013) Erläuterung und Anwendung der kolposkopischen Nomenklatur der IFCPC (International Federation for Cervical Pathology and Colposcopy) Rio 2011 Zu den grundsätzlichen Hinweisen für die Kolposkopie der Cervix uteri – adäquat/inadäquat. Plattenepithel-Zy 73:1–4

Scheungraber C, Koenig U, Fechtel B, Kuehne-Heid R, Duerst M, Schneider A (2009) The colposcopic feature ridge sign is associated with the presence of cervical intraepithelial neoplasia 2/3 and human papillomavirus 16 in young women. J Low Genit Tract Dis 13(1):13–16. https://doi.org/10.1097/LGT.0b013e318180438a

Vercellino GF, Erdemoglu E, Chiantera V, Vasiljeva K, Drechsler I, Cichon G et al (2013) Validity of the colposcopic criteria inner border sign, ridge sign, and rag sign for detection of high-grade cervical intraepithelial neoplasia. Obstet Gynecol 121(3):624–631. https://doi.org/10.1097/AOG.0b013e3182835831

5 Indications for Colposcopy

Contents

Colposcopy is most frequently used for triage of patients with an abnormal cytological cervical smear and/or a positive HPV test result. In addition, there are special indications independent from cytological or HPV testing. Besides diagnostic colposcopy, all surgical procedures of the cervix and vagina are performed under colposcopic guidance.

5.1 General Objectives

The indication for colposcopy should be broad. The colposcope as a magnification device is a valuable tool for the inspection of the lower genital tract. In addition to the early detection of gynecological malignancies, the diagnosis of dermatologic and infectious diseases is improved.

Colposcopy has three basic objectives:

1. Assessment of the vulva, anus, vagina, and cervix uteri in the context of cancer screening as well as follow-up examination of patients who did or did not undergo surgical treatment of dysplasia
2. Performance of operations on lower genital tract diseases under colposcopic guidance
3. Differential diagnosis of dermatologic and infectious diseases of the lower genital tract including colposcopically guided biopsies

R. J. Lellé, V. Küppers, *Colposcopy*, https://doi.org/10.1007/978-3-030-85388-4_5

Colposcopy is mostly used to evaluate the cervix. If intraepithelial neoplasia is suspected, the most important task of colposcopy is grading of a lesion, i.e., the distinction between minor change/grade 1 and major change/grade2 according to the Rio 2011 colposcopic terminology (see Chap. 4). Usually, one or more colposcopically guided biopsies are obtained.

If no lesions are found despite cytological suspicion of HSIL and/or HPV16/18 infection, random biopsies of the transformation zone are helpful (Massad 2006; Massad et al. 2009) as well as endocervical curettage (Pretorius et al. 2012). Huh et al. (2014) found that a single random biopsy could increase the sensitivity of colposcopy to detect HSIL by about 20%, when colposcopy was considered to be adequate and no obvious lesion was identified. This was particularly true for patients positive for HPV16/18 on the cobas® HPV test.

By determining the type of transformation zone and by delineating the exact location and extent of the cervical lesion, appropriate treatment planning is possible.

The sensitivity of any single parameter of colposcopic evaluation is far from perfect. Sensitivity of colposcopic diagnosis is estimated to be 30–70% according to Huh et al. (2014).

Therefore, when all the test results from an individual patient have been gathered, a decision on further management is made based on the overall picture rather than any single parameter such as colposcopic grading or biopsy.

5.2 Triage of Abnormal Cytological Findings

The most common use of colposcopic triage is an abnormal cytologic screening result. Colposcopy is indicated if there is a 10% or higher probability of CIN3 and/or AIS. In addition, colposcopy may be useful in individual cases for reassurance of a patient with a lower likelihood of high-grade disease, e.g., when a low-grade squamous intraepithelial lesion (LSIL) is suspected for the first time. If the Pap smear result is repeatedly classified as unsatisfactory, colposcopy is also required.

Colposcopy indications based on abnormal Pap test results using the Bethesda classification (Nayar and Wilbur 2015) are as follows:

- Recurring atypical squamous cells of undetermined significance (ASC-US)
- Recurring low-grade squamous intraepithelial lesion (LSIL)
- Atypical squamous cells favor high grade (ASC-H)
- High-grade squamous intraepithelial lesion (HSIL)
- Atypical glandular cells (AGC)
- Adenocarcinoma in situ (AIS)
- Cytology suspicious for cancer

Decision-making for surgical procedures of the cervix such as a cone biopsy should not be based on the result of a cytological screening diagnosis alone but rather on thorough colposcopic evaluation including targeted biopsy.

5.3 Colposcopy as Triage of a Positive HPV Test Result

When a cytological ASC-US result is obtained for the first time, HPV testing can be used for triage. ASC-US/HPV positivity is considered an indication for colposcopy in women who are older than 30 years.

When primary HPV screening is performed (≥30 years), cytology can also be used as triage of a positive HPV test result. If the HPV test is able to identify HPV types 16 and 18 such as the cobas® test, the screening algorithm as suggested by Huh et al. (Huh et al. 2015) could be as follows (Fig. 5.1): If the test is HPV16/18 positive, the likelihood of a patient already having or developing a high-grade lesion or cancer is high. According to the trial data regarding the cobas® test (Wright et al. 2015), the 3-year cumulative incidence rate

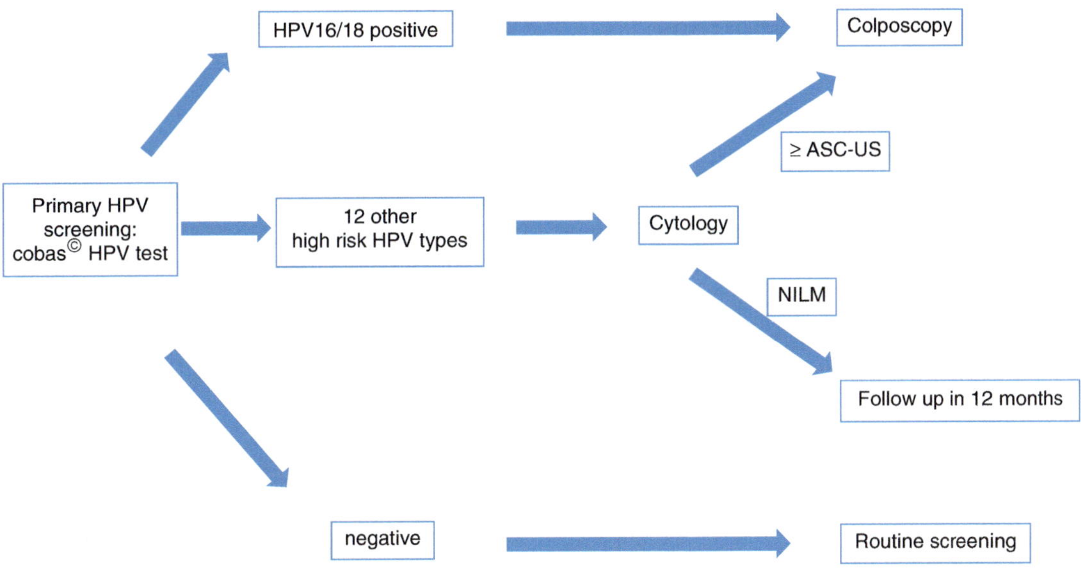

Fig. 5.1 Primary HPV screening algorithm based on the cobas® HPV test (Huh et al. 2015)

is as high as 21.16% (95% confidence interval 18.39–24.01%). Therefore, colposcopy without the need of preceding cytology is indicated. If the test is positive for other HPV high risk types (12 different HPV types are included in the cobas® test system), cytologic triage is required.

5.4 Other Indications

Besides triage of screening tests such as cytology, HPV test, or co-testing, colposcopy is indicated if any abnormality is identified without magnification with or without the use of acetic acid. Recurrent postcoital bleeding is also a frequent reason for colposcopic inspection of the cervix.

Patients with conditions involving immunosuppression due to HIV/AIDS or following transplant surgery are at higher risk for developing lower genital tract neoplasia. Therefore, colposcopy in combination with Pap smear and HPV testing at regular intervals is advisable.

Other indications for colposcopy include:

- Follow-up after surgical treatment of intraepithelial cervical disease
- Follow-up after HSIL cytology without identification of a lesion on initial colposcopic triage
- Young patients with HSIL that have not been treated initially and instead are followed at regular intervals for spontaneous regression

5.5 Contraindications

It should always be kept in mind that colposcopic triage, although not an invasive procedure such as surgery for actual or suspected cervical dysplasia, is still uncomfortable for most patients, both physically and psychologically (O'Connor et al. 2017). However, in many instances, colposcopy will be helpful to avoid unnecessary or even harmful surgical procedures. Therefore, no absolute contraindications for colposcopy exist.

Relative contraindications include atrophy and inflammation, as hormonal or anti-inflammatory pretreatment may be appropriate. Menstruation may also be a relative contraindication depending on the particular clinical circumstances. For example, bleeding might be due to malignant disease. Also, if there is only minor menstrual bleeding, colposcopic evaluation may still be possible.

5.6 Summary of Colposcopy Indications of the Cervix

- Colposcopy indications due to cytological findings
  - Recurring atypical squamous cells of undetermined significance (ASC-US)
  - Recurring low-grade squamous intraepithelial lesion (LSIL)
  - Atypical squamous cells favor high grade (ASC-H)
  - High-grade squamous intraepithelial lesion (HSIL)
  - Atypical glandular cells (AGC)
  - Adenocarcinoma in situ (AIS)
  - Cytology suspicious for cancer
- Colposcopy indications related to HPV test results
  - HPV high-risk positivity in combination with equivocal cytology (ASC-US)
  - HPV16/18 positivity in women ≥30 years of age
- Colposcopy due to other findings
  - Postcoital bleeding
  - Cervical abnormality when viewed without magnification
  - Immunocompromised patients (e.g., HIV/AIDS or following transplant surgery)
  - After surgical treatment of CIN
  - After HSIL cytology without a visible lesion
  - Follow-up for possible spontaneous regression of CIN
- Relative contraindications
- Atrophy
- Inflammation
- Menstrual bleeding

As an example for a practical approach to colposcopic triage, the algorithms for cervical screening in Germany are given (Figs. 5.2 and 5.3).

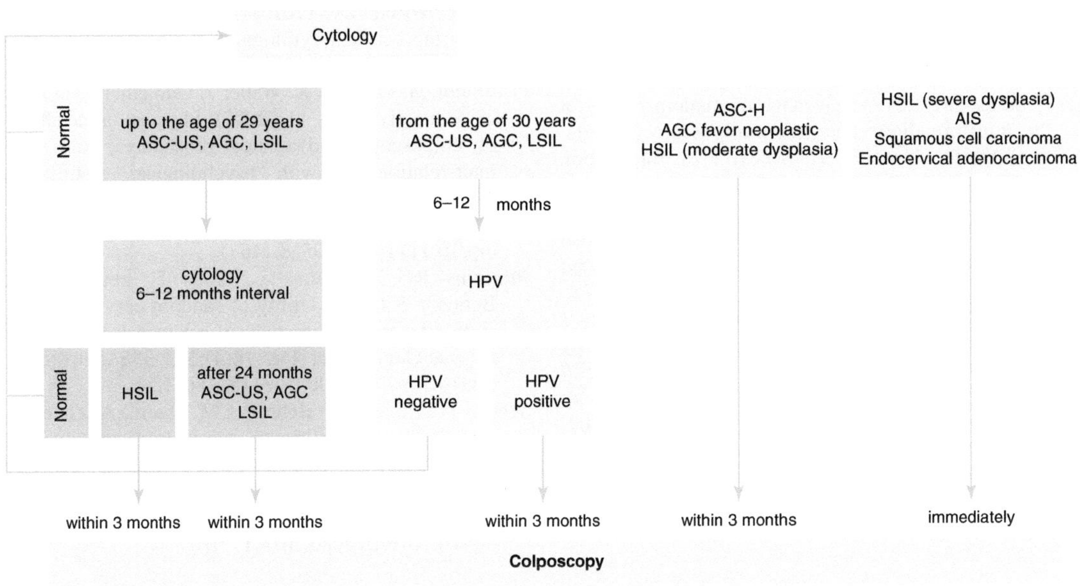

Fig. 5.2 Algorithm for cervical screening in German. Women 20–34 years are screened by annual Pap tests

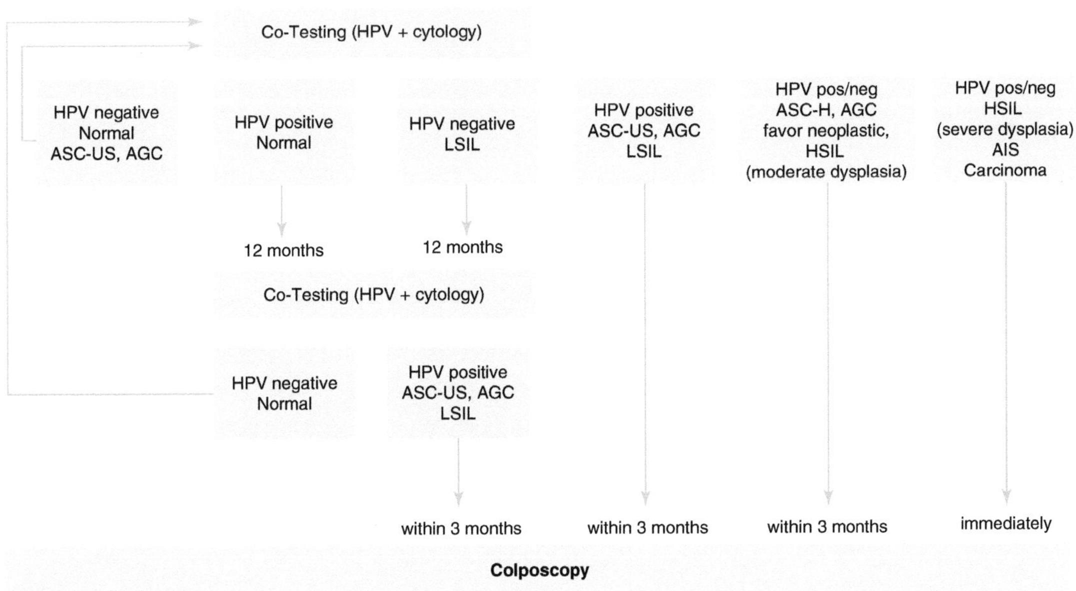

Fig. 5.3 Algorithm for cervical screening in German. Women from the age of 35 years are screened by co-testing

References

Huh WK, Sideri M, Stoler M, Zhang G, Feldman R, Behrens CM (2014) Relevance of random biopsy at the transformation zone when colposcopy is negative. Obstet Gynecol 124(4):670–678. https://doi.org/10.1097/AOG.0000000000000458

Huh WK, Ault KA, Chelmow D, Davey DD, Goulart RA, Garcia FA et al (2015) Use of primary high-risk human papillomavirus testing for cervical cancer screening: interim clinical guidance. Gynecol Oncol 136(2):178–182. https://doi.org/10.1016/j.ygyno.2014.12.022

Massad LS (2006) More is more: improving the sensitivity of colposcopy. Obstet Gynecol 108(2):246–247. https://doi.org/10.1097/01.AOG.0000229430.04828.83

Massad LS, Jeronimo J, Katki HA, Schiffman M (2009) The accuracy of colposcopic grading for detection of high-grade cervical intraepithelial neoplasia. J Low Genit Tract Dis 13(3):137–144. https://doi.org/10.1097/LGT.0b013e31819308d4

Nayar R, Wilbur DC (2015) The Bethesda system for reporting cervical cytology: definitions, criteria, and explanatory notes. Springer

O'Connor M, O'Brien K, Waller J, Gallagher P, D'Arcy T, Flannelly G et al (2017) Physical after-effects of colposcopy and related procedures, and their inter-relationship with psychological distress: a longitudinal survey. BJOG: an international. J Obstetr Gynaecol 124(9):1402–1410. https://doi.org/10.1111/1471-0528.14671

Pretorius RG, Belinson JL, Azizi F, Peterson PC, Belinson S (2012) Utility of random cervical biopsy and endocervical curettage in a low-risk population. J Low Genit Tract Dis 16(4):333–338. https://doi.org/10.1097/LGT.0b013e3182480c18

Wright TC, Stoler MH, Behrens CM, Sharma A, Zhang G, Wright TL (2015) Primary cervical cancer screening with human papillomavirus: end of study results from the ATHENA study using HPV as the first-line screening test. Gynecol Oncol 136(2):189–197. https://doi.org/10.1016/j.ygyno.2014.11.076

6 The Significance of Cytology, Biopsy, and HPV Testing

Contents

> Cytology is recognized as the gold standard of cervical screening that has led to a significant reduction of cervical cancer cases in numerous countries. However, Pap smear results alone do not provide a reliable diagnosis. Therefore, colposcopic triage is required, which includes target biopsy. HPV testing plays an important role as a screening tool either alone or in combination with cytology. For the colposcopist, knowledge of the strengths and limitations of these methods are indispensable.

6.1 Cytology

Cytology as a screening tool has been at the core of screening for cervical cancer and its precursors. It is responsible for a significant reduction in cervical cancer cases and thus has saved numerous lives. In the year 2000, Bernard Naylor, himself a former co-worker of George N. Papanicolaou, wrote about the impact of cytologic diagnosis (Naylor 2000) and concluded: "These and other events and achievements in cytopathology, from its meager beginnings in the early twentieth century to its worldwide use and acceptance today, mark this century as the 'century for cytopathology'." Although during the twenty-first century, the role of cytology, especially as the sole screening tool, will change significantly, cytology will continue to play an important role in cervical cancer prevention in the foreseeable future.

Colposcopy training courses require a basic knowledge in the field of morphology and additional methods based on molecular biology. Therefore, the following text will present the knowledge that is indispensable in the context of colposcopy.

The following explanations refer to the cervix. The statements made here only partially apply to other regions of the genital tract as well as the anus.

Currently, the Pap smear is the best documented screening procedure for early diag-

R. J. Lellé, V. Küppers, *Colposcopy*, https://doi.org/10.1007/978-3-030-85388-4_6

nosis of cervical carcinoma and especially its precursors. Colposcopy including targeted tissue removal, however, is used for triage, i.e. for further clarification of abnormal cytological findings and treatment planning.

In Germany, the country of origin of colposcopy, there has been a discussion whether cytology or rather colposcopy is the most effective screening tool. This dispute has long been settled, and cytology has become internationally accepted as the screening method of choice. As summarized in a Health Technology Assessment report (Nocon et al. 2007), colposcopy has a lower sensitivity compared to cytology for detecting cervical dysplasia.

In everyday clinical practice, Pap smears are frequently taken from the vagina and vulva. While the Pap test after hysterectomy for benign disease is not always required (Fox et al. 1999), vaginal intraepithelial neoplasia (VAIN) may occur after a previous diagnosis of cervical intraepithelial neoplasia. Therefore, Pap smear screening is indicated in the latter situation.

Conversely, the usefulness of vulvar cytology is less well documented, as the keratinizing squamous epithelium of the external genitalia is much more difficult to evaluate cytologically as are cells from the non-keratinizing epithelium including glandular tissue. In vulva smears, the cell yield is usually much lower, and the morphological assessment of keratocytes may be inconclusive.

If an abnormal or suspicious vulvar lesion is seen, a punch biopsy should be performed to rule out vulvar intraepithelial neoplasia (VIN) or invasive carcinoma, as vulvar cytology may yield a false negative result.

6.1.1 Cytological Morphology

The normal squamous epithelium of the cervix consists of basal cells, parabasal cells, small and large intermediate cells, and superficial cells. Keratinization does not usually occur on the cervical epithelium.

In the cytological smear, with the exception of basal cells, all the above-mentioned cell groups can be found. In non-atrophic epithelium consisting of multiple layers of squamous cells, the smear shows mainly superficial and intermediate cells, while in the case of atrophy only parabasal cells may be present.

In normal squamous epithelium, the cells become larger and the nuclei smaller the further they are from the basal layer. Therefore, superficial and large intermediate cells have a large amount of cytoplasm with a small round and pyknotic nucleus. In the Papanicolaou stain, the superficial cells are eosinophilic (red), while other cells are usually basophilic (blue) (Fig. 6.1).

In addition to the squamous epithelial cell component, endocervical glandular cells are found in the cervical smear (Fig. 6.2). The Pap smear report has to include a statement, whether endocervical or metaplastic cells are identified. The presence of these cell types signifies that the smear was taken from the transformation zone. Such a smear is more likely to be representative and therefore more sensitive/reliable as a smear containing squamous epithelial cells only.

Cervical intraepithelial neoplasia (CIN) leads to changes of both the cell nucleus as well as the cytoplasm. In higher grade CIN, the cell nucleus is larger and has a more abnormal chromatin structure (uneven distribution, coarseness, clumping), while at the same time the cytoplasmic volume decreases. This results in an increase in the nuclear-to-cytoplasmic ratio (N/C ratio).

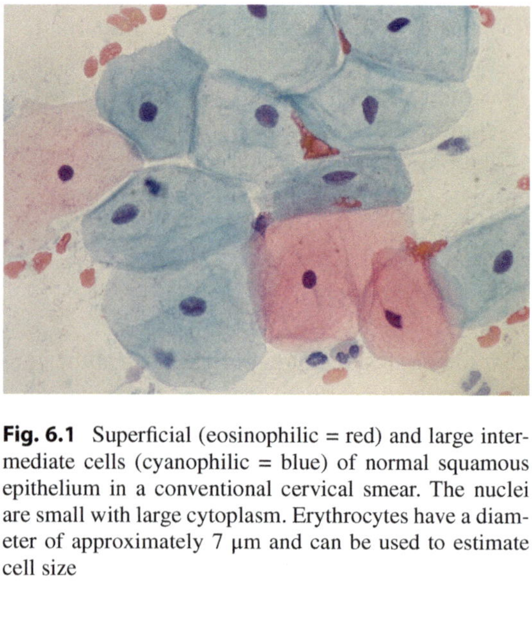

Fig. 6.1 Superficial (eosinophilic = red) and large intermediate cells (cyanophilic = blue) of normal squamous epithelium in a conventional cervical smear. The nuclei are small with large cytoplasm. Erythrocytes have a diameter of approximately 7 μm and can be used to estimate cell size

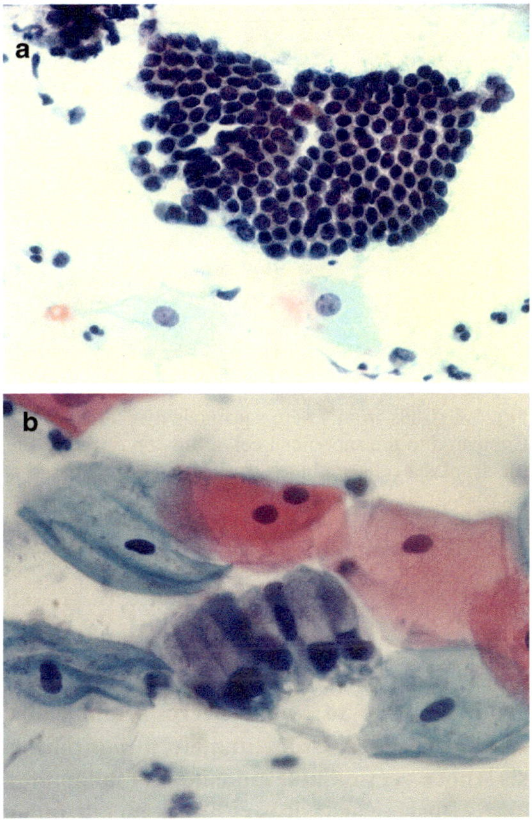

Fig. 6.2 Endocervical cells in a conventional Pap smear. When viewed from above, (**a**) endocervical cells form a honeycomb pattern. When viewed from the side, cells have a palisade-like appearance (**b**)

Table 6.1 summarizes the features of mild (CIN1), moderate (CIN2), and severe dysplasia (CIN3) (Flenker 2003; Lellé et al. 2007a, b).

Figures 6.3, 6.4, 6.5, and 6.6 show examples of the different degrees of dysplasia. It is important to note that grading of dysplastic changes always involves a certain amount of subjectivity on the part of the cytopathologist. Also, it is not uncommon for cells of different grades of dysplasia to coexist within the same smear. Of course, the final cytologic diagnosis is always based on the highest grade of dysplasia observed.

An unequivocal cytological diagnosis of malignant disease is not possible. The morphological proof of cancer is the presence of invasion, i.e. the presence of atypical cells within the stroma after these cells have broken through the basal membrane. Such a diagnosis is possible only on tissue sections and not on cytological smears. Therefore, cytological diagnosis, or rather suspicion of malignancy is primarily based on the presence of severely abnormal cells, particularly those with prominent nuclear changes. However, similar cells may be present in high grade squamous dysplasia (CIN3).

Therefore, cytological suspicion of malignancy always includes indirect signs of potential invasive disease such as fresh or hemolyzed blood cells and cellular debris (Figs. 6.7 and

Table 6.1 Cytological features of the three grades of dysplasia (CIN1–3) (Flenker 2003; Lellé et al. 2007a, b)

	CIN1 (LSIL)	CIN2 (HSIL)	CIN3 (HSIL)
Cytoplasm	Similar to superficial cells or large intermediate cell, koilocytosis	Similar to intermediate cells	Similar to parabasal cells
Nucleus	2–3 times larger than in large intermediate cells, irregular and hyperchromatic; chromatin evenly distributed	2–3 times larger than in large intermediate cells, marked increase of N/C ratio, irregular nuclei, indentations of the nuclear membrane, hyperchromasia with slightly coarsened and granular chromatin	Slightly smaller than in mild (CIN1) or moderate (CIN2) dysplasia, further increase of N/C ratio, severe deformation of the nucleus with indentations and invaginations of the nuclear membrane, severe invagination of the nuclear membrane, increased hyperchromasia with coarse and granular chromatin

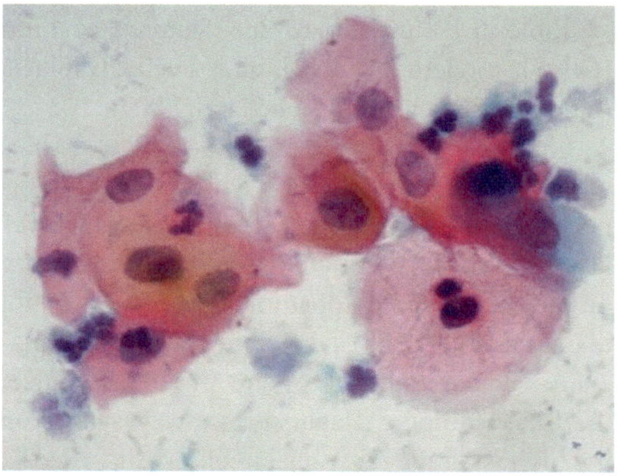

Fig. 6.3 Cells of low grade squamous dysplasia (CIN1). Superficial cells with enlarged nuclei with anisokaryosis and pleomorphism. The cytoplasm has turned orange in the Papanicolaou stain due to atypical keratinization

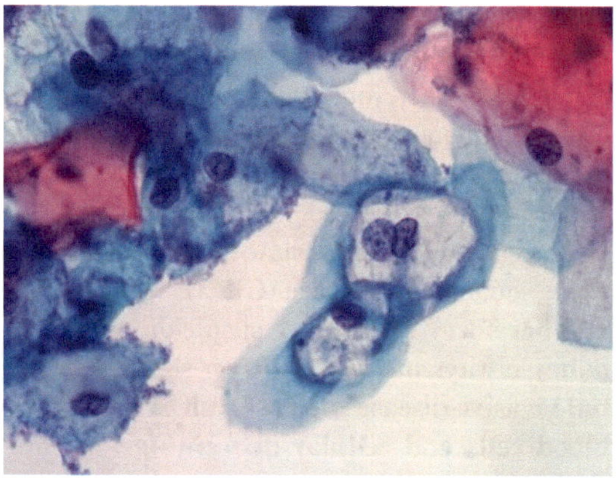

Fig. 6.4 Typical koilocytes. There is bright cytoplasm around the nuclei. One of the koilocytes has two nuclei. Koilocytes are the morphological sign of HPV infection and are frequently associated with low grade dysplasia (CIN1)

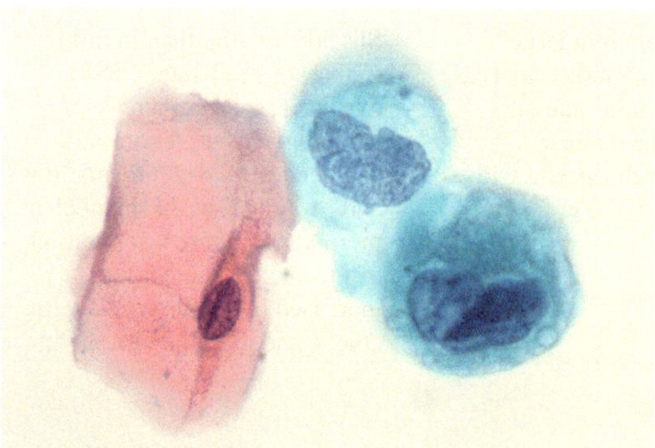

Fig. 6.5 Cells from moderate squamous dysplasia (CIN2). Next to a red superficial cell with a slightly enlarged nucleus are two smaller intermediate cells with enlarged nuclei and nuclear pleomorphism. The N/C ratio is increased

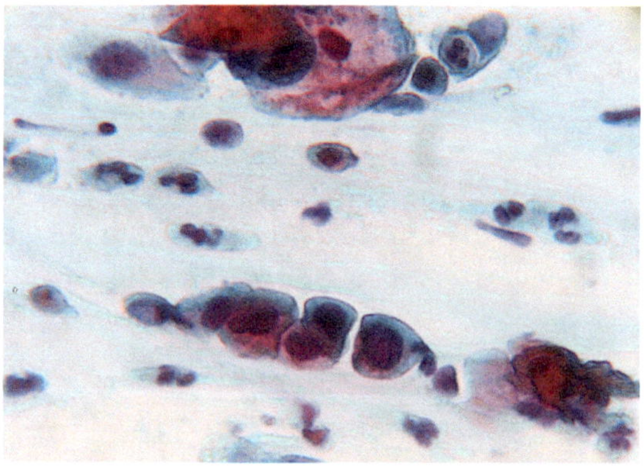

Fig. 6.6 Cells from severe squamous dysplasia (CIN3). Compared to the superficial cell at the top of the image, the dysplasia cells are much smaller and have a basal- or parabasal-cell like appearance. The nuclei almost fill out the cells with only a narrow cytoplasmic margin remaining. The dysplastic cells are arranged in a "cobblestone road manner"

6.8). This so-called malignant or dirty background is due to tumor necrosis and called tumor diathesis.[1] Unfortunately, tumor diathesis is not a very reliable indicator of malignancy.

As Rushing and Cibas (1997) point out, tumor diathesis is only present in about half of cytological smears obtained from squamous cell carcinomas. Also, there is a positive correlation between the presence of tumor diathesis and the depth of invasion, i.e. tumor diathesis is absent when the depth of invasion is less than 5 mm.

In summary, the accuracy of cytological diagnosis of malignancy is far from that of histological assessment. This should always be kept in mind when management decisions are made based on cytologic findings.

Examples of dysplasia and carcinoma depicted here all refer to squamous epithelium. The cytological diagnosis of precancerous lesions of the endocervical columnar epithelium (AIS, adenocarcinoma in situ) as well as invasive tumors (adenocarcinoma) is much more difficult and is less accurate than the cytological diagnosis of squamous lesions.

The morphology of abnormal cells from the keratinizing epithelium is far more difficult to interpret compared to the non-keratinizing cervi-

[1] "Diathesis" from Greek means "arrangement".

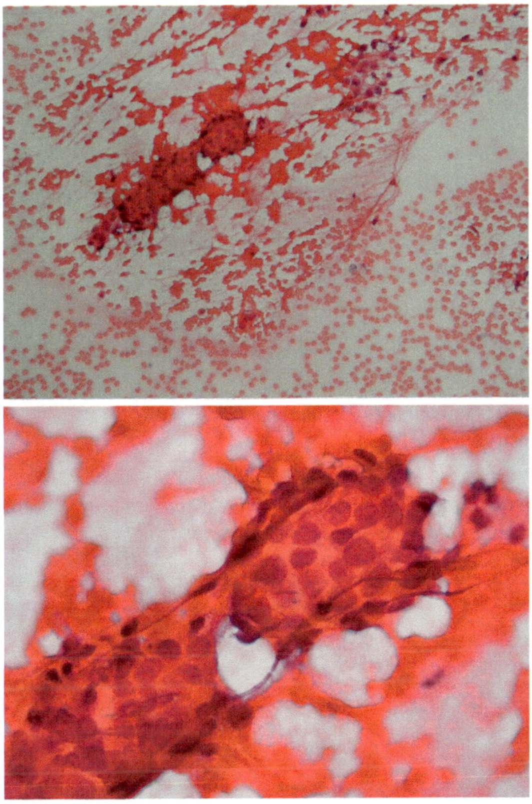

Fig. 6.7 Squamous cell carcinoma of the cervix. In this conventional smear, the background is bloody and inflammatory (tumor diathesis). A group of tumor cells clings to the erythrocytes. The N/C ratio of these cell is increased

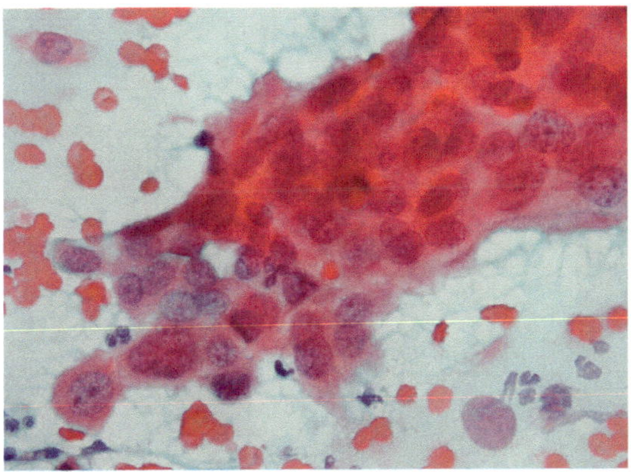

Fig. 6.8 Squamous cell carcinoma of the cervix. Tumor cell nuclei are enlarged with prominent macronucleoli. Characteristics of isolated cells may be identical to those of severe dysplasia (CIN3) (Table 6.1). The cytological suspicion of malignancy is based on a subjective impression of an experienced cytopathologist

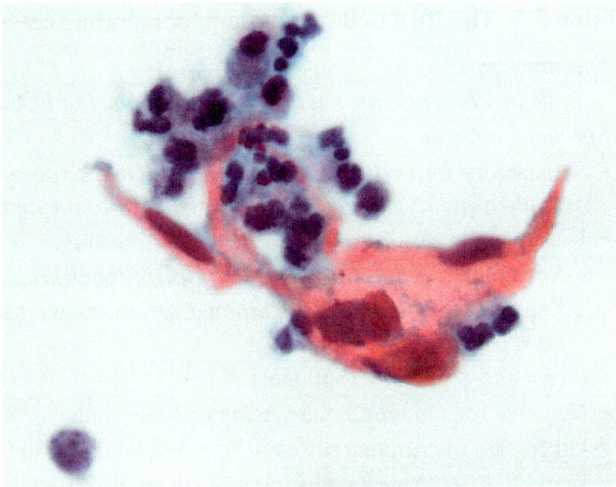

Fig. 6.9 Squamous cell of the vulva (ThinPrep® cytopathology). The tumor cells, which are called "dyskeratocytes," show prominent pleomorphism, both of the nucleus and the cytoplasm, the latter sometimes taking on bizarre cell forms. The N/C ratio shifted in favor of the cytoplasm, and not the other way around as with squamous epithelial dysplasia or carcinoma of non-keratinizing epithelium, where the nucleus pushes the cytoplasm towards the cell periphery

cal epithelium (Fig. 6.9). In Nauth's textbook and atlas "Gynecological Cytology" (Nauth 2007), vulvar cytology is discussed in detail. Otherwise, the literature is sparse, and the discussion about its relevance continues (Bae-Jump et al. 2007; Dennerstein 2009; Jimenez-Ayala and Jimenez-Ayala 2002; van den Einden et al. 2012).

In summary, there is no cytological screening of the vulva for the detection of vulvar intraepithelial neoplasia or early vulvar cancer. If a suspicious lesion of the vulva is seen, a punch biopsy should be obtained rather than a Pap smear.

6.1.2 Cytological Nomenclature

In the USA as well as in many other countries worldwide, the original cytological classification system using five Pap groups has been replaced by the Bethesda classification first established in 1988 (Table 6.2), last updated in 2014 (Nayar and Wilbur 2015). Instead of Pap groups, emphasis is placed on a descriptive morphological diagnosis. Instead of the designations CIN1 to CIN3, the term "squamous intraepithelial lesion" (SIL) is used, which applies not only to squamous precan-

Table 6.2 The 2014 Bethesda system for reporting cervical cytology (Nayar and Wilbur 2015)

Specimen type
Indicate conventional smear (Pap smear) vs. *liquid-bused preparation* vs. *other*
Specimen adequacy
• Satisfactory for evaluation (*describe presence or absence of endocervical/transformation zone component and any other quality indicators,* e.g., *partially obscuring blood, inflammation,* etc.)
• Unsatisfactory for evaluation … (*specify reason*)
– Specimen rejected/not processed (*specify reason*)
– Specimen processed and examined, but unsatisfactory for evaluation of epithelial abnormality because of (*specify reason*)
General categorization (optional)
• Negative for Intraepithelial Lesion or Malignancy
• Other: See Interpretation/Result (e.g., *endometrial cells in a woman ≥45 years of age*)
• Epithelial Cell Abnormality: See Interpretation/Result (*specify* 'squamous' *or* 'glandular' *as appropriate*)
Interpretation/result
Negative for intraepithelial lesion or malignancy
(*When there is no cellular evidence of neoplasia, state this in the General Categorization above and/or in the Interpretation/Result section of the report--whether or not there are organisms or other non-neoplastic findings*)
Non-neoplastic findings (*optional to report optional to report: List not inclusive*)
• Non-neoplastic cellular variations
– Squamous metaplasia
– Keratotic changes
– Tubal metaplasia
– Atrophy
– Pregnancy-associated changes
• Reactive cellular changes associated with:
– Inflammation (includes typical repair)
Lymphocytic (follicular) cervicitis
– Radiation
– Intrauterine contraceptive device (IUD)
• Glandular cells status post hysterectomy
Organisms
• *Trichomonas vaginalis*
• Fungal organisms morphologically consistent with *Candida* spp.
• Shift in flora suggestive of bacterial vaginosis
• Bacteria morphologically consistent with *Actinomyces* spp.
• Cellular changes consistent with herpes simplex virus
• Cellular changes consistent with cytomegalovirus
Other
• Endometrial cells (*in a woman ≥ 45 years of age*)
(*Specify if "negative for squamous intraepithelial lesion"*)
Epithelial cell abnormalities
Squamous cell
• Atypical squamous cells
– of undetermined significance (ASC-US)
– cannot exclude HSIL (ASC-H)
• Low-grade squamous intraepithelial lesion (LSIL)
(*encompassing: HPV/mild dysplasia/CIN 1*)

Table 6.2 (continued)

• High-grade squamous intraepithelial lesion (HSIL)
(*encompassing: moderate and severe dysplasia, CIS; CIN 2 and CIN 3*)
– with features suspicious for invasion (*if invasion is suspected*)
• Squamous cell carcinoma
Glandular cell
• Atypical
– endocervical cells (NOS *or specify in comments*)
– endometrial cells (NOS *or specify in comments*)
– glandular cells (NOS *or specify in comments*)
• Atypical
– endocervical cells, favor neoplastic
– glandular cells, favor neoplastic
• Reactive cellular changes associated with:
– Inflammation (includes typical repair)
• Lymphocytic (follicular) cervicitis
– Radiation
– Intrauterine contraceptive device (IUD)
• Glandular cells status post hysterectomy
Organisms
• *Trichomonas vaginalis*
• Fungal organisms morphologically consistent with *Candida* spp.
• Shift in flora suggestive of bacterial vaginosis
• Bacteria morphologically consistent with *Actinomyces* spp.
• Cellular changes consistent with herpes simplex virus
• Cellular changes consistent with cytomegalovirus
Other
• Endometrial cells (*in a woman ≥45 years of age*)
(*Specify if "negative for squamous intraepithelial lesion"*)
Epithelial cell abnormalities
Squamous cell
• Atypical squamous cells
– of undetermined significance (ASC-US)
– cannot exclude HSIL (ASC-H)
• Low-grade squamous intraepithelial lesion (LSIL)
(*encompassing: HPV/mild dysplasia/CIN 1*)
• High-grade squamous intraepithelial lesion (HSIL)
(*encompassing: moderate and severe dysplasia, CIS; CIN 2 and CIN 3*)
– with features suspicious for invasion (*if invasion is suspected*)
• Squamous cell carcinoma
Glandular cell
• Atypical
– endocervical cells (NOS *or specify in comments*)
– endometrial cells (NOS *or specify in comments*)
– glandular cells (NOS *or specify in comments*)
• Atypical
– endocervical cells, favor neoplastic
– glandular cells, favor neoplastic

(continued)

Table 6.2 (continued)

• Endocervical adenocarcinoma in situ
• Adenocarcinoma
– endocervical
– endometrial
– extrauterine
– not otherwise specified (NOS)
Other malignant neoplasms: (*specify*)
Adjunctive testing
Provide a brief description of the test method(s) and report the result so that it is easily understood by the clinician
Computer-assisted interpretation of cervical cytology
If case examined by an automated device, specify device and result
Educational notes and comments appended to cytology reports (*optional*)
Suggestions should be concise and consistent with clinical follow-up guidelines published by professional organizations (references to relevant publications may be included)

cer of the cervix but also to preinvasive lesions of the vagina, vulva, and anus.

Furthermore, squamous intraepithelial lesions are subdivided into LSIL (low grade squamous intraepithelial lesion) and HSIL (high grade squamous intraepithelial lesion). This dichotomy satisfies the clinical requirements better than the classification of CIN1 to CIN3, which has been in use since the 1970s. LSIL therefore stands for minor cell abnormalities that need to be followed rather than treated surgically, whereas HSIL may require treatment.

Another advantage of the Bethesda classification is the fact that the same nomenclature can be applied to both cytological and histological findings.

Occasionally, HSIL and CIN3 are called "carcinoma in situ," especially when the mitotic activity is high, and the basal-type dysplastic cells are not stratified anymore. In carcinoma in situ, the basal membrane is still intact. Consequently, it is not a "carcinoma." Moreover, due to its potential for spontaneous regression, albeit rarely, the term "carcinoma in situ" is not justified. Unfortunately, "squamous cell carcinoma in situ" is still mentioned as "acceptable terminology" for "HSIL (CIN3)" in the 2020 WHO classification update (WHO Classification of Tumours Editorial Board 2020). Also, TNM and FIGO staging systems recognize "in situ cancer" as Tis (TNM) and stage 0 (FIGO), respectively (Compton et al. 2012).

Some countries such as Germany have not adopted the Bethesda classification. Based on the traditional Papanicolaou Pap groups I to V, an update has been published in 2013 called the Munich III classification (Griesser et al. 2013) (Table 6.3).

Table 6.3 German system for reporting cervical cytology using the traditional Pap groups in relation to the Bethesda system

Pap group	Bethesda
0	Unsatisfactory for evaluation
I	NILM
II-a	NILM
II-p	ASC-US
II-g	AGC endocervical NOS
II-e	Endometrial cells
III-p	ASC-H
III-g	AGC endocervical favor neoplastic
III-e	AGC endometrial
III-x	AGC favor neoplastic
IIID1	LSIL
IIID2	HSIL
IVa-p	HSIL
IVa-g	AIS
IVb-p	HSIL with features suspicious for invasion
IVb-g	AIS with features suspicious for invasion
V-p	Squamous cell carcinoma
V-g	Endocervical adenocarcinoma
V-e	Endometrial adenocarcinoma
V-x	Other malignant neoplasms

p squamous, *g* glandular (endocervical), *e* endometrial, *x* unknown. *II-a* patient with a history of previous abnormal cytological/histological/colposcopic findings (Griesser et al. 2013)

Designations such as *p* ("plattenepithelial" = squamous), *g* (glandular/endocervical), *e* (endometrial), and *x* (unknown) are used for the presumed origin of cells. This may potentially overstretch the accuracy of cytological diagnosis. In contrast to the Bethesda classification, the Pap group system tries to make a clear distinction between CIN2 and CIN3 (Pap IIID2 and Pap IVa-p).

If a cytological sample is classified as Pap IVa-p, there is indeed a very high likelihood that CIN3 is present. According to Hilal et al. (2015), in 22 out of 25 patients CIN3 was confirmed histologically (85%). Marquardt and Ziemke (2018), who analyzed 4162 Pap smears classified as abnormal according to Munich III from 3396 women, found similar results: Pap IVa-p had a high specificity of 87.47% for CIN3+ and 98.07% für CIN2+. Compared to Pap IVa-p, the respective percentages for Pap IIID2 (suspecting CIN2) were 45.80% and 62.44% and for Pap IIID1 (suspecting CIN1/LSIL) 17.07% and 9.32%. The CIN2+ group of Pap IVa-p consisted of 10.60% histologically confirmed CIN2 lesions, 84.82% CIN3, 0.24% AIS, and 2.4% squamous cell carcinomas.

One should be aware that a clear distinction between CIN2 and CIN3 is difficult, both cytologically and histologically. As no evidence exists that CIN2 can be considered a distinct intermediate state between CIN1 and CIN3, it may as well be a mix of true CIN1 and CIN3 (Kurman et al. 2014**; WHO Classification of Tumours Editorial Board 2020**)**. Despite these limitations, an effort should be made to identify CIN2 as a subgroup with a certain potential for spontaneous regression, thus limiting overtreatment especially in younger patients with the intention to avoid pregnancy-related complications.**

6.1.3 Cytology as a Screening Tool

The effectiveness of cervical cytology, i.e. its sensitivity and specificity, is far from ideal. Screening error is estimated to be between 10% and 67%, and sampling error occurs at a rate of 20% to 39% (quoted from Bergeron et al. 1997). This is also demonstrated by Marquardt et al. (2007, 2011). The previous Pap smear history from 617 patients, who were eventually diagnosed with invasive cervical cancer, was documented. Most of these cancer patients (60%) had not had a Pap smear taken within the previous 5 years. In 31% of the patients, gynecological examinations had been done at irregular intervals. However, 9% of patients with a cervical cancer diagnosis participated regularly in the annual screening program.

Another retrospective analysis of cytology examinations prior to the histopathological diagnosis of "carcinoma in situ" (CIN3) was done by Bergeron et al. (1997). Whereas the smear immediately preceding the biopsy-proven diagnosis of CIS had been positive in 518 out of 585 women (88.5%), 20% of previous smears were false negative as they were found to be positive for HSIL on review.

Doctors, patients, and cytopathologists tend to overestimate the sensitivity of exfoliative cytology.

Despite its proven effectiveness in secondary cervical cancer prevention, cytological screening has a surprisingly low sensitivity. A meta-analysis by Cuzick et al. (2006) found a sensitivity of only 53%, whereas specificity was 96%. The authors conclude that purely cytology-based screening can only be effective if two or three consecutive annual examinations are performed before the screening interval may be extended. Statistically, sensitivity (based on the detection of CIN2+ lesions) will improve from 53% to 76%, when two consecutive Pap smears are obtained and improve up to 88% after three Pap tests.

Due to the low sensitivity of the cytological examination, every effort must be made to minimize potential sources of error.

- The following factors can be the cause of false negative cytological results:
  - Sampling from the wrong area.
  - No intracervical collection.
  - Insufficient transferral of cells to the slide.
  - Blood.
  - Inflammation.
  - Poor fixation.
  - Interpretation error.

The choice of the sampling device plays an important role in the quality and representativeness of the cell sample. In cervical screening, both the ectocervix and the endocervix need to be sampled, in order to cover the entire transformation zone. The European Guidelines for Quality Assurance in Cervical Cancer are giving recommendations on sampling methods (Arbyn et al. 2007). The use of a cotton tip applicator is considered inappropriate. Instead, three devices or combination of devices are recommended (Fig. 6.10):

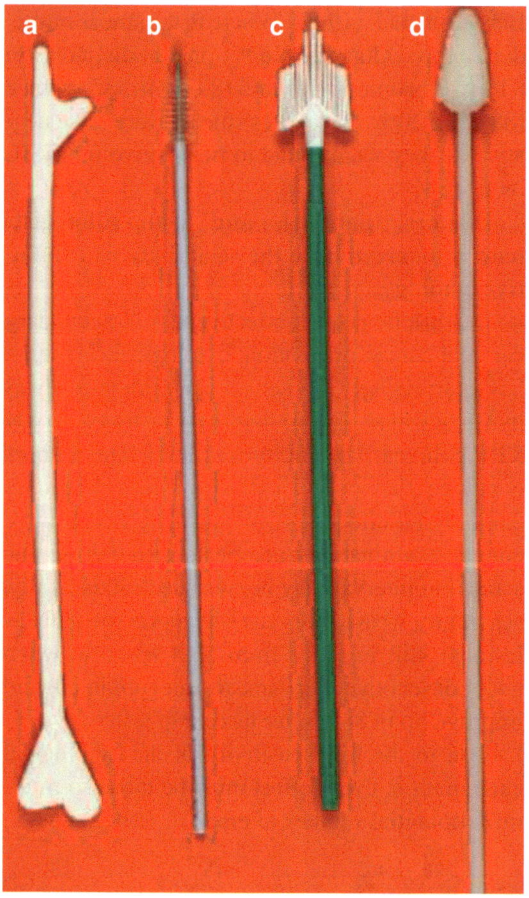

Fig. 6.10 Three of the cytological sampling devices that are recommended by the European Guidelines for Quality Assurance in Cervical Cancer Screening as well as the so-called PapCone®. (**a**) extended tip (Szalay) spatula (top) and Ayre spatula (bottom). (**b**) endocervical brush. (**c**) cervical broom (Cervex® brush). (**d**) PapCone® (Arbyn et al. 2007; Kaur and Kushtagi 2013; Petruzziello et al. 2011)

- The cervical broom.
- A spatula (wooden or plastic) in combination with an endocervical brush.
- The extended tip spatula.

There are certain national and certain individual preferences regarding the use of sampling devices. For example, the extended tip spatula is the preferred device in the UK.

Another device used is the PapCone®, a soft polyurethane foam swab which is compressible and can be used for both ectocervical and endocervical sampling (Petruzziello et al. 2011). When there is any doubt that a representative intracervical sample has been obtained, the additional use of the cervical brush is recommended. Conversely, the endocervical brush should not be used by itself.

The presence of a cellular component from the transformation zone (endocervical and/or metaplastic cells) is a valuable quality assurance measure. However, it is not required for the adequacy of each individual sample.

Several studies (Elias et al. 1983; Luzzatto and Boon 1996) showed that the presence or absence of cellular transformation zone components correlates with the reliability of the detection of dysplasia, since dysplastic cells from squamous epithelium always occur within the transformation zone, which may be located partially or completely within the cervical canal. However, women with Pap smears lacking the endocervical/metaplastic component do not develop cervical dysplasia more frequently (Bos et al. 2001; Kivlahan and Ingram 1986). The Bethesda cytological terminology takes this into account (Nayar and Wilbur 2015). The presence or absence of the transformation zone components should still be reported as a quality indicator. However, its absence should not lead to early repeat Pap smear testing as can be concluded from a Canadian meta-analysis (Elumir-Tanner and Doraty 2011).

If there already is a cytological suspicion of high grade dysplasia (HSIL) or even carcinoma, the presence or absence of a transformation zone component is irrelevant. Also, HPV testing in women 30 years and older is independent of transformation zone sampling.

6.1.4 Liquid-Based Cytology

Liquid-based cytology (LBC) has become increasingly popular over the last 20 years. Many cytology labs are using LBC as an alternative to conventional cytology. Most studies show that its performance is at least as good as the standard methodology. The major advantage of LBC is the fact that several cell samples can be obtained from one vial and then used for additional studies such as HPV testing or immunocytochemical analyses.

6.1.4.1 Principle of LBC

Several methods of cell preparations for LBC are available. They all use the same principle, i.e. transfer of the cell sample into a vial with a preservative medium by rinsing the collection device instead of spreading cells directly onto a glass slide. Thus, cell fixation is optimized and there are no drying artifacts.

For Pap testing, only an aliquot from the vial is needed. A representative cell sample is prepared and transferred onto a glass slide. There are several automated or semi-automated methods for cell preparation, some of which are described below. The two major principles of cell preparation are centrifugation and filtration.

LBC has the potential to significantly improve the quality of the Pap test. Almost the entire cell specimen is transferred into the vial by rinsing the collection device. Blood cells, inflammatory cells, or mucus, which may all interfere with cytological evaluation, are dissolved in the transport medium or removed by filtration. LBC also standardizes the distribution of cells onto the glass slide. Ideally, a cell sample resembling a monolayer is achieved.

6.1.4.2 LBC Procedures

Several LBC procedures have been developed. These are all based on one or more of the following principles:

- filtration
- density gradient centrifugation
- cell sedimentation

Not all LBC procedures that are available have been adequately tested in clinical trials. Although approval by the Food and Drug Administration (FDA) is not required outside of the USA, the use of FDA-approved methods only should be considered.

In Europe no institution comparable to the FDA exists, and there are no binding approval criteria for medical devices to assure that only scientifically tested methods are used. Bollmann et al. (2006) and Bollmann and Jordan (2005) have tried to establish criteria for the use of LBC methods in cytological screening. These criteria are fulfilled by both ThinPrep® and SurePath®. Both cell preparation systems have been studied extensively and are the only two procedures which obtained FDA approval (in 1996 and 1999, respectively). The FDA accepted that these techniques were significantly more effective compared with conventional Pap smear (ThinPrep®) or at least of similar efficiency (SurePath®) (Gibb and Martens 2011). Furthermore, both tests were recognized by the FDA to improve specimen adequacy and HSIL detection.

Several alternative LBC methods have been developed using similar slide preparation methods as ThinPrep® or SurePath®. However, none of these methods has been studied on large cohorts of patients and therefore are not FDA approved. Although these methods are legal in many countries, they should not be used.

Presently, LBC (ThinPrep® or SurePath®) is the preferred methodology for cytological testing in the USA. Also, the British National Health System has been officially using ThinPrep® and SurePath® testing since 2004.[2]

The two FDA-approved LBC methods, ThinPrep® and SurePath®, are described in more detail below.

6.1.4.2.1 ThinPrep® (Hologic)

ThinPrep® specimen preparation is based on filtration. The cells are collected as described

[2] https://assets.publishing.service.gov.uk/government/uploads/system/uploads/attachment_data/file/436647/lbc02.pdf.

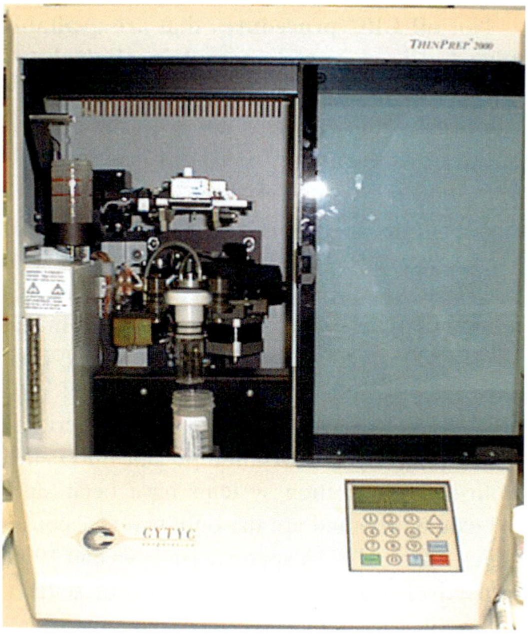

Fig. 6.11 ThinPrep® 2000 processor

above. The FDA certified collection device for ThinPrep® is the Cervex Brush®, which is rinsed in the so-called PreservCyt® medium, which contains methanol. However, its precise composition has not been published by Hologic.

In the cytologic laboratory, the cell sample is processed by the ThinPrep® processor (Fig. 6.11), a semi-automated slide preparation unit. A plastic cylinder, which is closed at the bottom with a filter membrane, is used for each sample. These filters are manufactured by shooting neutrons through a membrane, thus producing irregularly distributed pores, which all have the same diameter (Fig. 6.12).

The filter is immersed into the vial and rotated to produce a homogenized cell solution. Larger cell conglomerates are dissolved. A vacuum is then applied, and cells are aspirated onto the filter surface. Smaller particles such as erythrocytes, leukocytes, and part of the cell detritus are sucked through the filter pores and do not reach the slide. Some of the cells adhere to the filter membrane and close the pores. The ThinPrep® unit measures the relaxation time of the vacuum. These steps—aspiration and measurement of relaxation times—are repeated several times until

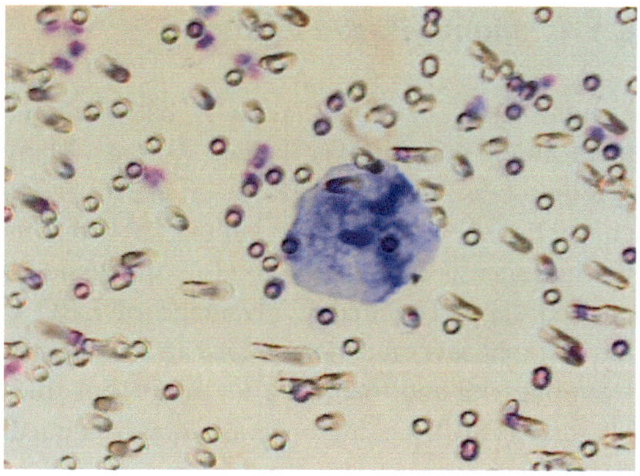

Fig. 6.12 ThinPrep® filter after cell preparation. After stamping the filter onto the slide, some of the cells still remain on the filter membrane. The filter pores are generated by shooting neutrons through a membrane. Thus they all have the same diameter

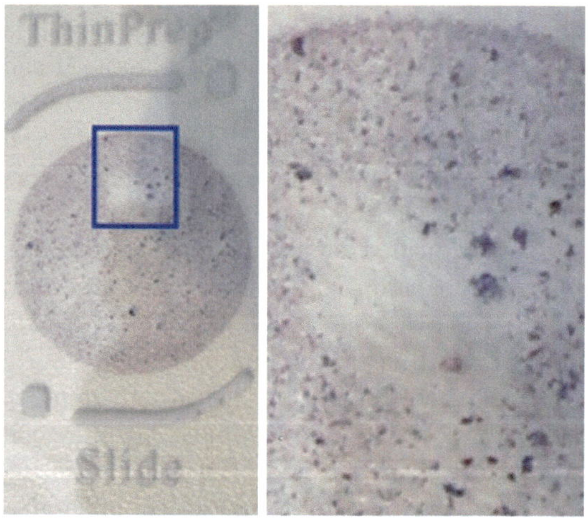

Fig. 6.13 ThinPrep® glass slide. The enlarged area shows a typical cell distribution after stamping the cylinder onto the glass slide with conglomerates of cells and cell-free areas. Therefore, the term "monolayer cytology" is not really appropriate

a sufficient amount of cells adheres to the filter. The filter is then pressed against the glass slide in order to transfer the cell sample into a 20 mm circle (Fig. 6.13). Finally, the slide is ejected into the fixative and stained in the usual manner.

6.1.4.2.2 SurePath® (Becton Dickinson)

In contrast to rinsing the collection devices in the transport medium as with the ThinPrep® technique, SurePath® requires to leave the tip of the collection devices in the vial in order to increase cell yield.

The storage medium contains ethanol. Its exact composition has not been published by Becton Dickinson. The cell preparation process is quite different from that of the ThinPrep® method. SurePath® uses repeated density gradient centrifugation with subsequent sedimentation instead of filtration (Figs. 6.14 and 6.15). During the first centrifuge step, mucus, erythrocytes, and leucocytes are removed. Slide preparation is automated and carried out by a slide processor.

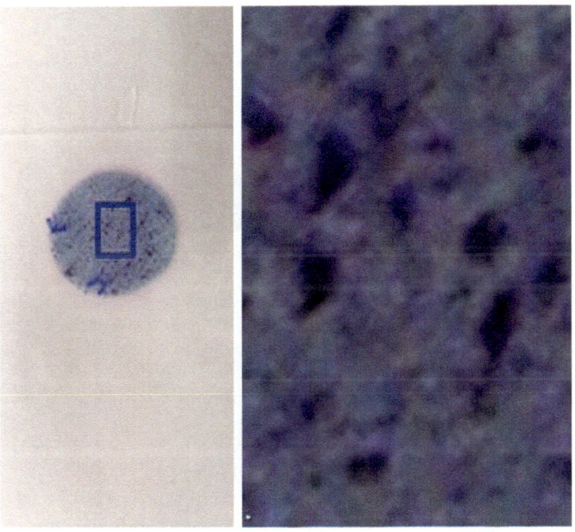

Fig. 6.14 SurePath® slide. The circular cell area is smaller than that of the ThinPrep® procedure. The cell sample is obtained by sedimentation. Cell aggregates are still present

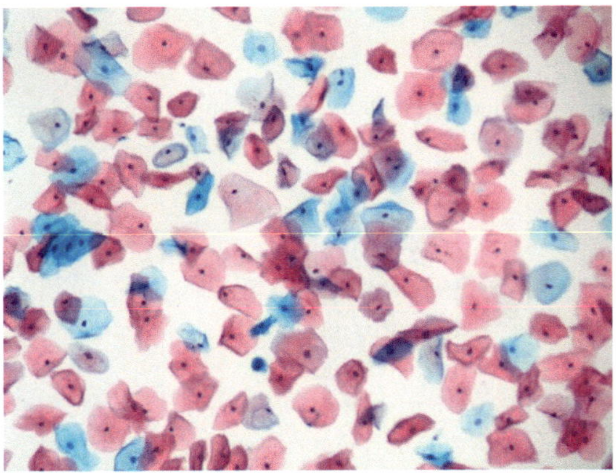

Fig. 6.15 Normal squamous epithelium using the SurePath® method. In this example, a cellular monolayer is almost achieved. However, the terms "liquid-based cytology" or "thin layer cytology" are more appropriate

Table 6.4 Comparison of the two validated and FDA-approved LBC methods

	ThinPrep®	SurePath®
Manufacturer	Hologic	BD (Becton, Dickinson and Company)
Website	www.hologic.com	www.surepath.com
Technical principle	Filtering via a computer-controlled vacuum	Density gradient centrifugation and sedimentation
Cell collection	Sampling device is rinsed in the vial and then removed	Sampling device is left in the vial
Computerized screening option	Location guided screening (ThinPrep® imager)	Ranking of slides (FocalPoint imaging)

Table 6.4 compares the properties of the two liquid-based cytological procedures ThinPrep® and SurePath®.

6.1.4.3 Morphological Features of Liquid-Based Cytology

The staff performing cytological assessment on conventional Pap smears must be trained when LBC is introduced in the cytology laboratory. Furthermore, when changing the LBC method, formal training is required again, as there are important differences in the morphology of cells and cell elements. A lack of appropriate knowledge may result in screening errors. Some of these morphological peculiarities are explained below for ThinPrep®.

A purified but still representative sample of the cell material is transferred to the slide. Although LBC is frequently called "monolayer cytology," a preparation of individual cells lying side by side without any overlap is rarely achieved. Instead, small and large cell conglomerates are seen, which are usually not as thick as in conventional smear. The expression "thin layer" is therefore more appropriate than "monolayer."

Compared to conventional smears, cell numbers and cell density are lower with ThinPrep®.

Therefore, the diagnosis of dysplasia may be based on a rather small number of diagnostic cells. ThinPrep® preparations have to be screened extra careful and more slowly than conventional slides (Fig. 6.16). The potential disadvantage of a longer screening time per slide is offset by the fact that a smaller area has to be assessed.

Although LBC procedures remove part of the background material, detection of specific inflammatory changes such as mycosis (Fig. 6.17) or trichomonas is as good as in conventional cytology. Sometimes these microbiological elements may even be more prominent against the "clean" background compared to conventional cytology (Renshaw et al. 2004).

The recognition of HPV-related as well as dysplastic cell changes is facilitated by optimal fixation of the cell sample. This is especially true for preservation of the chromatin structure (Figs. 6.18 and 6.19).

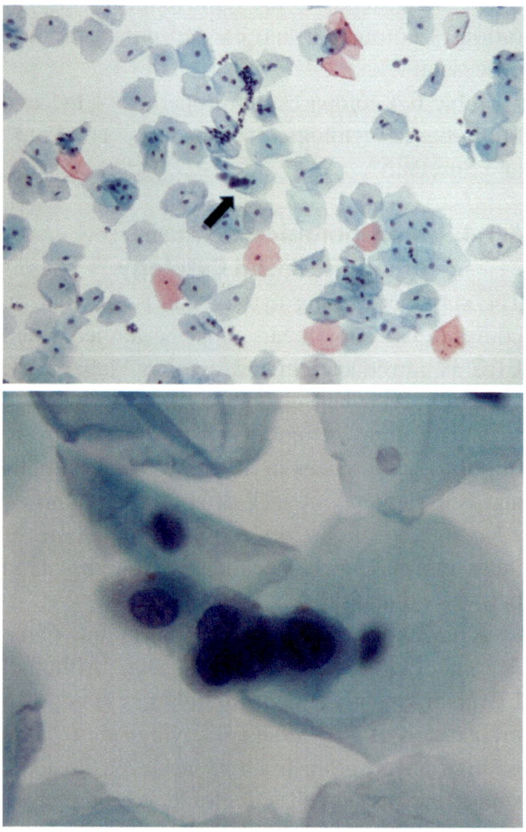

Fig. 6.16 HSIL/CIN3 ThinPrep®. The background is clean. Most of the cells are from the intermediate and some from the superficial layer of normal squamous epithelium. In between are a few small conglomerates of basal-type dysplastic cells, which might be overlooked

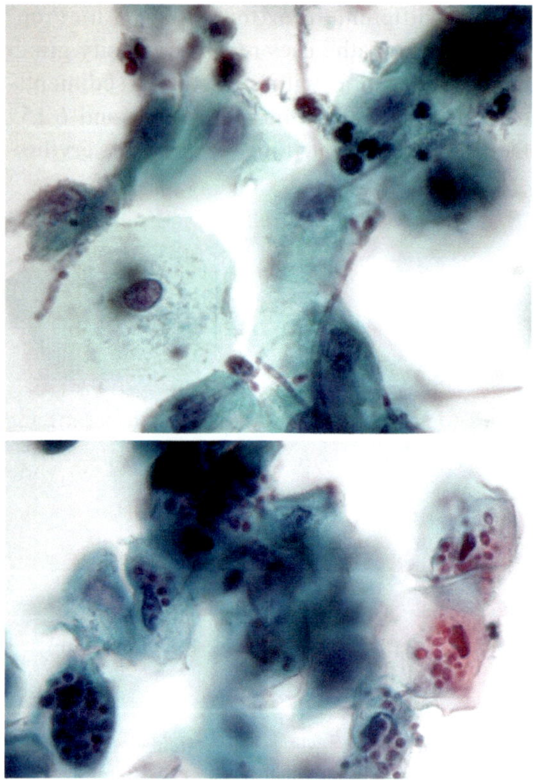

Fig. 6.17 Candida infection ThinPrep®. Hyphae and spores are easily recognized

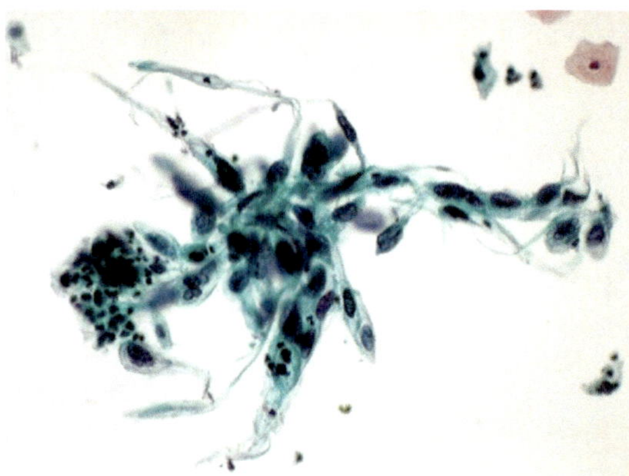

Fig. 6.18 HSIL/CIN3 ThinPrep®. The pleomorphic nuclei have a well-defined chromatin structure. Many nuclei are hyperchromatic

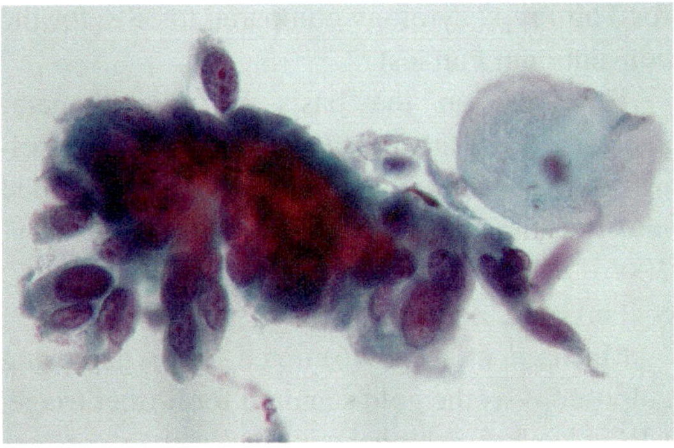

Fig. 6.19 Adenocarcinoma in situ (AIS) ThinPrep®. The chromatin structure of the abnormal endocervical cells is well preserved. Macronucleoli and chromocenters are easily visible

Cells tend to be slightly smaller and rounder than in conventional Pap smears, due to rounding of the cells when transferred into the liquid medium. Therefore, cells of squamous epithelial dysplasia may sometimes be misinterpreted as glandular (Renshaw et al. 2006). However, the N/C ratio remains unchanged.

Also, the cytoplasmic details are better visible in LBC, which is helpful for diagnosis of HPV-related changes such as koilocytosis. Some diagnostic patterns that result from manual spreading of cells onto the glass slide as, for example, the arrangement of CIN3 cells in a cobblestone road manner (Fig. 6.6) are not seen in LBC.

Most importantly, tumor diathesis is preserved in liquid-based slide preparations, although it has a slightly different morphological appearance compared to conventional cytology. Tumor diathesis, i.e. a "dirty" cell background due to hemolyzed blood and cellular debris, is helpful to establish the cytological diagnosis of cancer when highly abnormal and possibly malignant cells are present. Squamous cell carcinoma typically presents with "clinging tumor diathesis" as blood and cellular debris are attached to epithelial cells (Fig. 6.20).

A study by the College of American Pathologists comparing conventional and ThinPrep® educational slides (Renshaw et al. 2004) also suggested some difficulty of participants to identify squamous cell carcinoma on ThinPrep® slides.

Clark and Dawson (2002) observed a pattern of decreased cell coverage in ThinPrep® slides

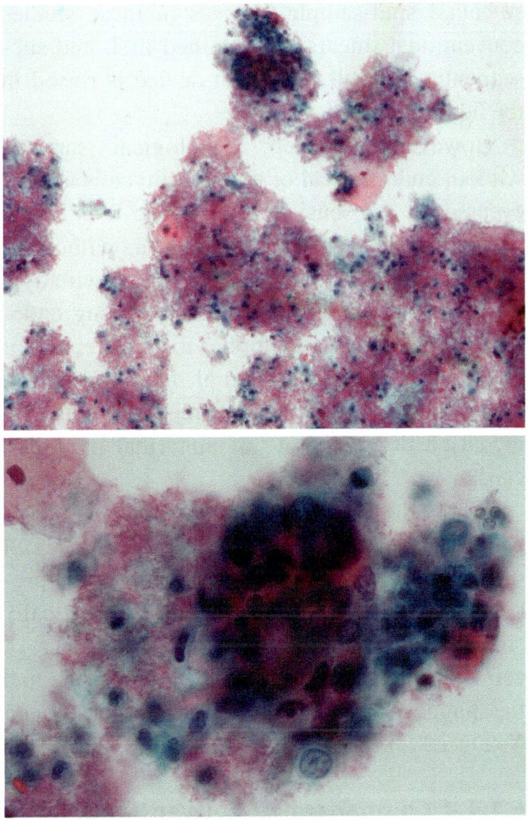

Fig. 6.20 Squamous cell carcinoma ThinPrep®. "Clinging tumor diathesis" is seen consisting of a "dirty" background of hemolyzed blood and cellular debris that are attached to the tumor cells

from squamous cell carcinomas and hypothesize that cellular particles of tumor diathesis and inflammation may decrease cellularity by blocking filter coverage by epithelial cells. They suggest that low cellularity in combination with tumor diathesis is a useful clue for the diagnosis of squamous cell carcinoma.

As stated above, the presence of endocervical cells is considered to be a marker for adequate cervical cell sampling and is correlated with the detection of dysplasia (Elias et al. 1983; Luzzatto and Boon 1996). Similarly, the presence of metaplastic cells also indicates adequate cell collection from the transformation zone. Compared to conventional slides, ThinPrep® slides more frequently do not contain endocervical or metaplastic cells (Lellé et al. 2007a, b): 11.6% versus 2.3%, respectively. This may partly be due to the so-called split-sample bias, as in these studies conventional smears are obtained first, and subsequently, the cell collection device is rinsed in the liquid medium.

However, ThinPrep® cytological samples without endocervical or metaplastic cells are not necessarily less sensitive. According to Selvaggi and Guidos (2002), ThinPrep® smears without an endocervical component are diagnosed with dysplasia as frequently as smears containing endocervical cells. This also applies to the detection of glandular lesions (Ashfaq et al. 1999). The FDA has even attributed the ThinPrep® procedure an increased detection rate of abnormal glandular cells.

While the discussion on the importance of endocervical cells in ThinPrep® slides is still ongoing, the routine use of the SurePath® procedure in the UK has revealed a statistically significant correlation between the presence of cell components of the transformation zone and the diagnosis of dysplastic changes (Narine and Young 2007).

6.1.4.4 Comparison of Conventional Cytology, ThinPrep®, and SurePath®

Numerous studies suggest that ThinPrep® and SurePath® identify high grade dysplasia significantly more often than conventional cytology and reduce the number of unsatisfactory samples.

The so-called Rhine-Saar study (Klug et al. 2012) is of particular relevance for Germany with non-organized opportunistic screening and evaluation of samples by a large number of different cytology laboratories operated by gynecologists or pathologists without centralized quality control. A total of 20 gynecologists in private practice participated in this study. Overall, 20,627 women were examined. At weekly intervals, conventional smear preparation and ThinPrep® procedure were alternated. For positive cytological findings, colposcopy was performed, and the detection rates of the two methods were compared with respect to CIN2+ lesions. The relative sensitivity of ThinPrep® cytology was significantly higher by a factor of 2.74. The positive predictive value for CIN2+ lesions was 48% for ThinPrep® cytology compared to 38% for the conventional Pap test.

However, on the basis of several meta-analyses, these advantages of liquid-based cytology over conventional cytology have been called into question (Arbyn et al. 2008; Davey et al. 2006; Sawaya 2008; Sawaya and Sox 2007; Siebert et al. 2003).

Macharia et al. (2016) noted, that when using colposcopy as the gold standard for further triage, LBC also has a higher specificity than conventional Pap tests. They therefore recommend that for repeat Pap tests liquid-based cytology is used.

Another study using the Dutch registry for histopathology and cytology analyzed data from 3,118,685 conventional Pap smears, 1,313,731 SurePath® samples, and 1,584,587 ThinPrep® samples (Rozemeijer et al. 2015). Compared to conventional cytology, SurePath® led to an increased probability to detect CIN2+. However, the number of CIN1 diagnoses also increased resulting in overdiagnosis.

6.1.4.5 Computer-Aided Cytological Evaluation

Computer-aided evaluation systems have been developed to increase the accuracy of cytological examinations as well as overall efficiency. Such systems exist for conventional cytology as well as for ThinPrep® and SurePath® (Ikenberg 2011). The BD FocalPoint GS Imaging System is able to analyze both SurePath® and conventional Pap smears.

A computer algorithm assigns the cytology samples to specific groups according to the statistical probability that abnormal cells are present. 25% of slides that are assigned to the category with the lowest risk do not need to be reviewed. Thus, the laboratory staff can focus on the highest risk groups and review those slides more thoroughly.

Hologic has developed the ThinPrep® Imaging System. It uses an automated microscope attached to a computer (Fig. 6.21) that uses algorithms, which results in location guided screening. After the imager has screened the entire slide, 22 areas of special interest are marked. These areas are reviewed manually. Only when abnormal cells are detected, the entire slide is reviewed.

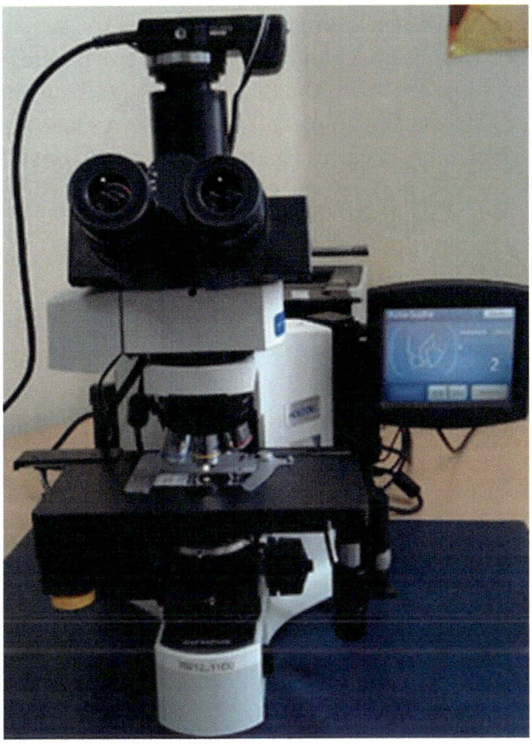

Fig. 6.21 ThinPrep® Imaging System. A computer algorithm marks 22 visual fields, which may contain abnormal cells and need to be reviewed manually

Both the FocalPoint GS Imaging System® and the ThinPrep® Imager are at least as sensitive as manual screening and make the workflow more efficient. Studies with both systems provide evidence of a higher sensitivity for detection of high grade cervical dysplasia without increasing the number of ASC-US or LSIL (Wilbur et al. 2009; Davey et al. 2007), whereas other authors found equal HSIL detection rates for the ThinPrep® Imaging System without increasing ASC-US or AGUS rates (Quddus et al. 2009; Thrall et al. 2008).

The Rhine-Saar study cited above (Klug et al. 2012), which showed a higher detection rate of CIN2+ lesions by ThinPrep®, also included an imager study arm. No additional improvement in the detection rate of HSIL lesions (CIN2+) could be demonstrated under the conditions of the German screening system.

Computerized optimization of cytology-based screening will become increasingly important, as the HPV vaccine effect will decrease the prevalence of cervical dysplasia. Statistically, this will reduce the predictive value of the screening test. In other words, dysplastic cell changes may be overlooked more easily.

Summary: Liquid-Based Cytology

The aim of liquid-based cytology is to improve the quality of cell preparations by

- increasing the number of cells transferred from the collection device to the transport medium
- optimizing cell distribution on the slide (thin layer)
- removal of mucus, blood, and cell debris
- optimal fixation without drying artifacts

Two LBC methods are available: ThinPrep® based on cell filtration and SurePath® based on centrifugation and sedimentation. Both methods have been extensively studied and approved by the American Food and Drug Administration (FDA).

With liquid-based cytology, several cell samples can be obtained so that additional tests can be carried out, such as testing for human papillomavirus ("reflex testing").

The superiority of LBC over conventional cytology by diagnosing more high grade lesions is controversial in the literature. For the German screening system, the Rhine-Saar study demonstrated a significantly higher detection rate for CIN2+ lesions using the ThinPrep® method. However, a computer-assisted evaluation using the ThinPrep® imager did not result in further improvement of sensitivity.

Computer-assisted evaluation methods, which are available for both LBC methods and conventional cytology, will become increasingly important in the future as the prevalence of high grade dysplasia decreases due to the anticipated effects of HPV vaccination.

6.1.5 Adjunctive Cytological Tests

According to Pinto et al. (2012), it is likely that a better understanding of HPV effects on cell cycle control will one day lead to the "ideal biomolecular Papanicolaou test." Numerous adjunctive tests are already available which complement morphological evaluation of a cytological sample with Papanicolaou staining. However, none of these tests is yet incorporated in screening algorithms.

From the many adjunctive cytological markers that are available, three tests will be discussed in more detail: DNA ploidy analysis, HPV L1 capsid protein detection, and p16/Ki67 dual stain (CINtecPLUS®). The most important of all biomarkers, HPV testing, will be discussed separately.

All three methods can be carried out on conventional cytological preparations after destaining of the slide. With liquid-based cytology additional slides can be obtained from the cell suspension, so that the original slides remain available for morphological evaluation.

The biomarkers available should not yet be incorporated into routine clinical practice. Presently, there is no sufficient evidence to justify the use of these tests for primary screening or triage.

As Pinto et al. (2012) point out, those biomarkers need "to be evaluated in large prospective clinical trials with appropriate colposcopic, histological, and clinical endpoints as well as adequate follow-up."

6.1.5.1 DNA Ploidy Analysis

One of the first steps of carcinogenesis is genetic instability. Genetic instability results in cells with an aneuploid set of chromosomes. Several methods are available for measuring ploidy of a cell sample, such as Feulgen staining of the nucleic acids (Feulgen and Rossenbach 1924). Measurements are semi-automated using electronic image analysis. The area of the cell nucleus is directly proportional to DNA content and ploidy. Leukocyte nuclei, which have a diploid set of chromosomes, are used for standardization.

The degree of aneuploidy serves as an objective measure of dysplasia. This may be helpful to establish the correct morphological diagnosis. Conversely, aneuploidy may be used as a progression marker. According to Bocking and Nguyen (2004) and Bocking et al. (2004), DNA euploidy has a high negative predictive value of around 95% regarding progression of LSIL. Conversely, DNA aneuploidy has a positive predictive value of up to 100% with respect to the development of CIN3 within a follow-up period of 3 years.

Nghiem et al. (2015) calculated that DNA ploidy analysis may be more cost-effective for cervical screening than liquid-based cytology. As measurements of ploidy can be automated and do not need the highly skilled staff required for cytological screening, the authors suggest that it may be a promising alternative, feasible also in a low resource setting.

6.1.5.2 HPV L1 Capsid Protein Detection

The L1 protein is a major part of the HPV virus shell or capsid. The presence of the L1 capsid protein can be determined immunocytochemically on cytological samples (Cytoactiv test®, Cytoimmun Diagnostics GmbH, Pirmasens, Germany). If L1 is found to be positive in the case of HPV infection, the immune system is still capable to produce antibodies against the virus. If the L1 capsid is absent, cellular dysregulation may already be too advanced, and an adequate immune response is no longer possible. Thus, L1 protein detection may discriminate between true cervical precancer and transient HPV infection.

Mehlhorn et al. (2013) studied women with a positive HPV test and the cytological diagnosis of LSIL. The patients were subsequently followed by colposcopic examinations and biopsies for up to 54 months. If L1 was positive, only 20% of low grade lesions progressed to CIN3 compared to 84%, if L1 was negative. With a cytological HSIL/CIN2 diagnosis and L1 negativity, only 5% of patients had a spontaneous remission compared to 68% in the LSIL/L1 positive group.

L1 capsid protein detection on cytological samples may be combined with a rapid human papillomavirus type 16 L1 specific antibody test to improve risk assessment and clinical management of low risk dysplastic lesions, in order to avoid overtreatment, especially in women of reproductive age (Mehlhorn et al. 2014).

6.1.5.3 p16/Ki67 Dual Stain (CINtecPlus®)

The CINtecPlus® test (Roche) or p16/Ki67 dual stain may be the most interesting Pap test based assays which has been developed to date. CINtecPlus® is an immunocytochemical double stain (p16 and Ki67), which is preferably done on thin layer cytological specimens.

P16 (p16INK4a protein) is overexpressed in transforming HPV infections and cervical precancer, whereas Ki67 is a marker of cell proliferation. Under physiological conditions, the p16 protein serves as a cell cycle regulator that triggers a cascade of biochemical events which eventually lead to cell cycle arrest. In precancerous lesions of the cervix, p16 is overexpressed. Ki67 is expressed in several phases of the cell cycle and indicates active proliferation. When cells are found to express both p16 and Ki67 simultaneously, this is a clear indication of cell cycle dysregulation, as under normal circumstances, p16 positive cells are not able to proliferate. In normal cells, the expression of p16 and Ki67 is mutually exclusive. Simultaneous p16/Ki67 positivity is associated with HPV-induced oncogenic transformation. Therefore, a strong correlation exists between the presence of cells that are simultaneously positive for both biomarkers and the diagnosis of high grade cervical disease.

For CINtecPlus® testing, Ki67 is visualized by APAAP (alkaline phosphatase anti-alkaline phosphatase) staining, resulting in a red nucleus. For p16, which is located in the cytoplasm, DAB (diaminobenzidine) immunostaining is used. Positive cells have a brown colored cytoplasm.

One single dual-stained cell in the cytological sample already indicates cell cycle dysregulation and oncogenic transformation (Figs. 6.22 and 6.23), and the CINtecPLUS® test is considered to be positive.

Nevertheless, the number of dual-stained cells is also significant as it correlates with the grade of dysplastic changes of the cervix (Yoshida et al. 2011): The more p16/Ki67 positive cells are present, the more likely is the diagnosis of high grade dysplasia.

For the p16/Ki67 dual stain, intra- and interobserver agreement is very good for both pathologists and cytotechnologists (Goh et al. 2017; McMenamin et al. 2017).

Wentzensen et al. (2012) performed the CINtecPlus® test on patients referred for colposcopy and found a statistically significant correlation between different grades of CIN and CINtecPlus® positivity: When histopathology was found to be negative, 26.8% of cytological preparations were positive compared to 46.5% for CIN1, 82.8% for CIN2, and 92.8% for CIN3.

In addition, the CINtecPlus® test could improve the detectability of glandular lesions. According to Ravarino et al. (2012), 92.5% of the

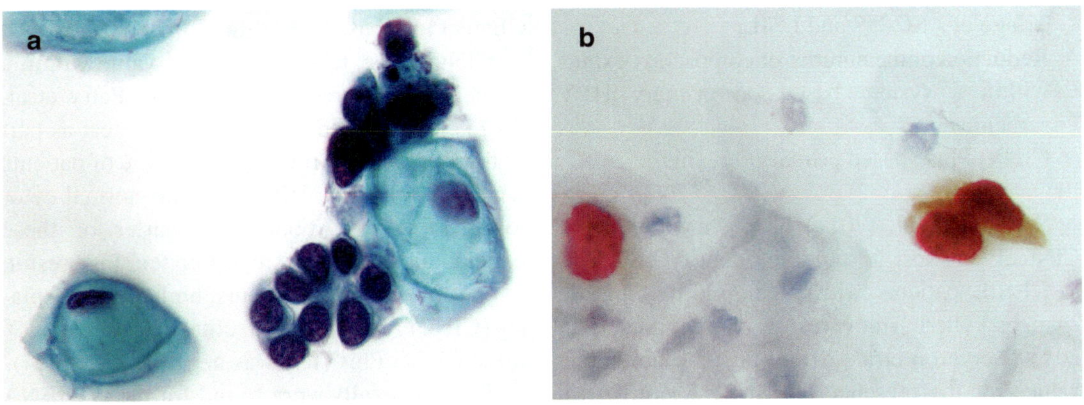

Fig. 6.22 CINtecPlus® and HSIL/CIN3. Basal-type cells with increased N/C ratio indicate HSIL/CIN3 (**a**), and the immunohistochemical double stain (**b**) is positive for both p16 (brown) and Ki67 (red)

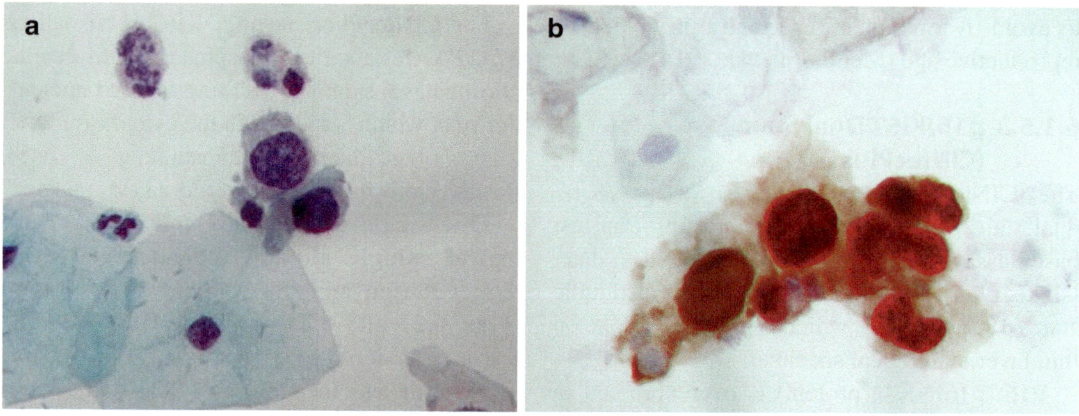

Fig. 6.23 CINtecPlus® and HSIL/CIN3. The atypical cells (**a**) are simultaneously positive for p16 and Ki67 (**b**)

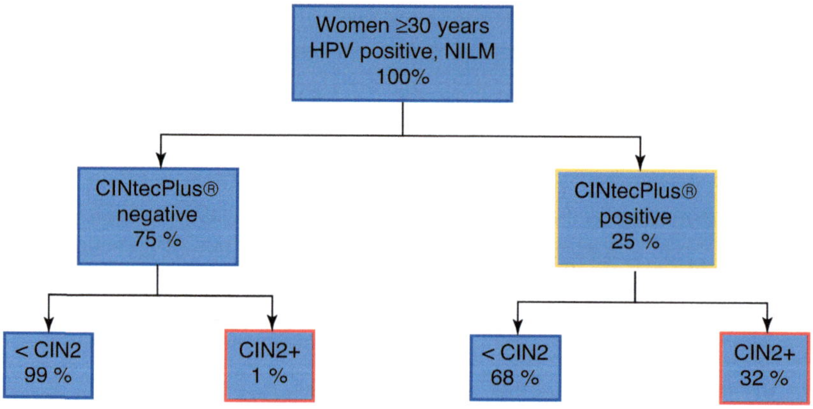

Fig. 6.24 CINtecPlus® Triage of patients screened HPV positive (HC2) and normal Pap smear result (NILM) in the Wolfsburg trial. Almost all CIN2+ diagnoses fall within the CINtecPlus® positive group (Petry et al. 2011)

cytologic preparations with glandular lesions are p16/Ki67 positive.

Presently, three indications for the CINtecPlus® test are discussed:

- Triage of ASC-US and LSIL.
- Reduction of the number of colposcopy exams within a system based on primary HPV screening.
- CINtecPlus® based primary screening.

Schmidt et al. (2011) have shown that the CINtecPlus® test is able to identify ASC-US and LSIL patients with high grade dysplastic changes. These study results were updated in 2015 (Bergeron et al. 2015). Positive predictive values for the presence of CIN2+ lesions were significantly higher for CINtecPlus® positivity than for the HPV positive test (HC2): 78.7% versus 60.4% for ASC-US and 53.3% versus 15.6% for LSIL, respectively. Thus, the number of colposcopy referrals for ASC-US and LSIL triage could be greatly reduced by introducing a CINtecPlus® based algorithm.

CINtecPlus® testing is also of value within a primary HPV screening algorithm. Petry et al. (2011) investigated the CINtecPlus® test as part of the Wolfsburg project for the triage of patients who had a positive HPV test with normal cytological finding. About one quarter of these patients also had a positive CINtecPlus® result. In one-third of these patients, high grade dysplasia (CIN2+) was detected, compared to only 1% if the CINtecPlus® test was negative (Fig. 6.24).

Similar results were found for the ATHENA trial using the cobas® HPV test (Wright et al.

2017). Referral for colposcopy of all HPV 16/18 positive women combined with p16/Ki67 dual stain triage of women positive for 12 other HPV genotypes detected by the cobas® test provides the highest sensitivity for the detection of CIN3+ lesions (86.8%; 95% CI: 81.9–90.8).

Wentzensen et al. (2017) also used HPV16 and 18 genotyping. Within a group of 7124 HPV positive women, 315 CIN3 lesions were detected. 88.9% of these patients were CINtecPlus® positive, whereas only 55.9% were positive for HPV16 or 18.

Sun et al. (2018), who performed a meta-analysis on p16/Ki67 dual immunostaining, found a pooled sensitivity for the detection of HSIL of 0.88 (95% CI 0.86–0.90) and a pooled specificity of 0.58 (95% CI 0.56–0.60). The sensitivity of the HPV test (0.94; 95% CI 0.93–0.96) is comparable, whereas its specificity is lower (0.32; 95% CI 0.29–0.34). Sun et al. therefore suggest that CINtecPlus® should be evaluated as an initial screening assay.

6.2 Biopsy

Colposcopy requires a basic understanding of histopathological methods, particularly the interpretation, validity, and reliability of cervical biopsy, which plays a central role in colposcopic triage.

Early on, Rudolf Virchow (1821–1902), the father of anatomical histopathology, and his contemporaries recognized the problem of representativeness of tissue samples that are only a few millimeters in size. It has been said that early pathologists flatly refused to evaluate tissue fragments such as from uterine curettage. At the time it was argued that histopathological diagnosis should only be made on the organ that has been removed completely. Eventually, this so-called "Stückchendiagnstostik" (fragment diagnostics) was taken up by Carl Ruge (1846–1926), a nephew of Virchow. Ruge took care of numerous gynecological patients as part of his general medicine practice in Berlin, Germany (Becker 1979). In 1881, Ruge published the world's first comprehensive textbook on cervical cancer (Ruge and Veit 1881) (Fig. 6.25), which includes detailed histopathological drawings (Fig. 6.26).

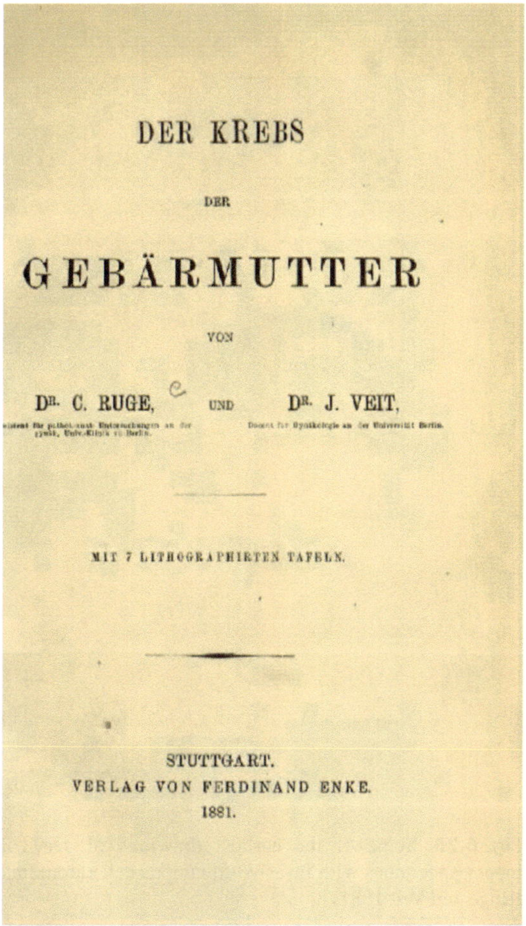
DER KREBS

DER

GEBÄRMUTTER

VON

DR. C. RUGE, UND DR. J. VEIT,

MIT 7 LITHOGRAPHIRTEN TAFELN.

STUTTGART.
VERLAG VON FERDINAND ENKE.
1881.

Fig. 6.25 "Der Krebs der Gebärmutter" (Cancer of the Uterus) by Ruge and Veit in 1881 was the world's first comprehensive monograph on cervical cancer (Ruge and Veit 1881)

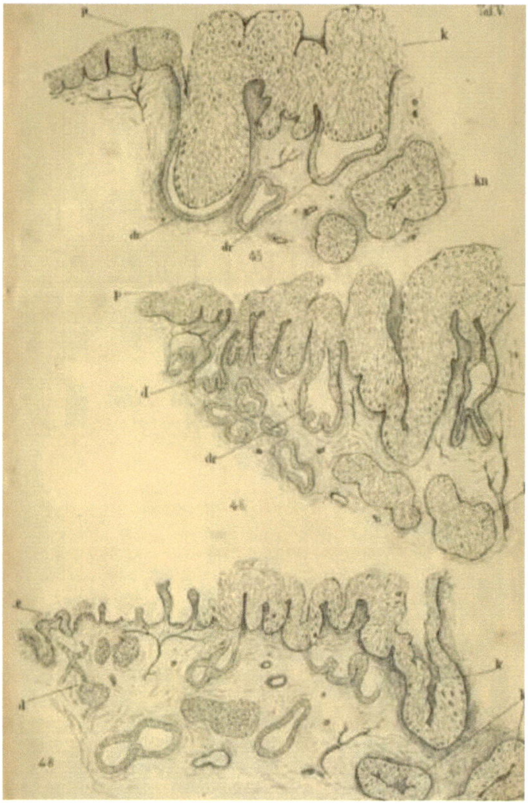

Fig. 6.26 Some of the earliest drawings of cervical biopsy specimens with invasive squamous cell carcinoma (Ruge and Veit 1881)

6.2.1 Histological Morphology

Histopathological assessment of cervical lesions is standardized and based on the WHO publication "Female Genital Tumors" last published in 2020 (WHO Classification of Tumours Editorial Board 2020). Cervical dysplasia is subdivided into three grades of severity, CIN1, CIN2, and CIN3, based on evaluation of hematoxylin-eosin stained slides. As with all such grading systems, a high degree of subjectivity is involved, especially since CIN constitutes a continuum of abnormal changes. According to the WHO classification, a system of LSIL and HSIL is both more biologically relevant and more reproducible than the three-tier CIN1 to 3 terminology.

Cervical dysplasia is characterized as follows:

LSIL (CIN1)
- proliferation of the basal/parabasal cell layer to no more than one-third of the epithelium
- mitotic figures confined to the lower one-third of the epithelium, usually not abnormal
- differentiation/maturation towards the surface of the epithelium with an increasing amount of cytoplasm
- enlargement of nuclei with an increased N/C ratio
- koilocytic atypia

HSIL (CIN2 and CIN3)
- less cytoplasmatic differentiation with extension of the proliferating cells up into the middle (CIN2) or the upper third (CIN3).
- mitotic figures more abundant, more frequently abnormal, extending into the middle or upper third of the epithelium (Fig. 6.27).
- increased nuclear size, irregular nuclear membranes, and a further increase of the N/C ratio.

Unfortunately, the designation "carcinoma in situ" ("Tis") as a distinct form of high grade cervical dysplasia is still used according to the official histopathological WHO classification (Kurman et al. 2014; WHO Classification of Tumours Editorial Board 2020), not however by FIGO (Pecorelli 2009).

If cervical carcinoma is not yet visible macroscopically, it is called microcarcinoma. Depth of invasion should not exceed 5 mm, whereas the lateral extent of the tumor is no longer considered (Bhatla et al. 2018). FIGO stage IA is subdivided into stage IA1 and IA2, depending on whether the depth of invasion is <3 mm or ≥3 mm.

For glandular preinvasive disease, only one grade of severity is defined: high grade cervical glandular intraepithelial neoplasia (HGCGIN) or as it is more frequently called: adenocarcinoma in situ (ACIS or AIS).

Diagnosis of AIS on cytological slides can be challenging and is associated with a significant

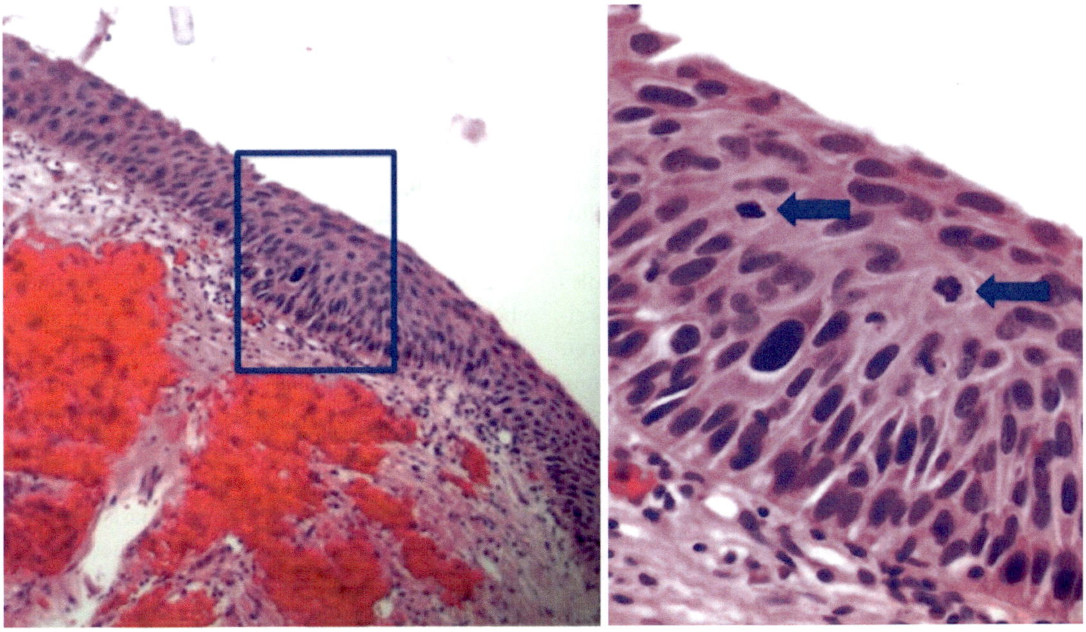

Fig. 6.27 Severe squamous dysplasia (CIN3). The abnormal cells extend to the upper one-third with several mitotic figures within the middle and upper third of the squamous epithelium (arrow)

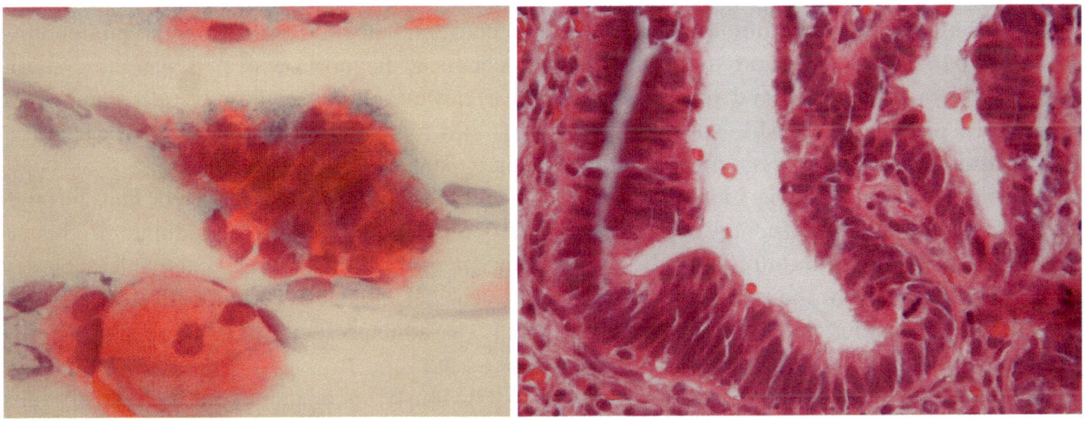

Fig. 6.28 Adenocarcinoma in situ (AIS) of the cervix. The Pap smear shows a dense group of abnormal endocervical cells with washed-out chromatin und fuzzy margins, which is adjacent to a normal superficial squamous cell. Histopathology shows densely packed partially superimposed nuclei. Characteristically, areas of AIS are juxtaposed to normal endocervical epithelium

degree of uncertainty. In comparison, AIS diagnosis on histopathological slides (Kurman et al. 2014; WHO Classification of Tumours Editorial Board 2020) is less difficult (Fig. 6.28).

Manifestations of AIS are confined to areas of pre-existing normal endocervical epithelium. AIS may be located on the endocervical surface or within endocervical glands. Nuclei are enlarged with hyperchromatic and coarse chromatin structure. Prominent nucleoli may be present. Usually, mitotic figures are found. AIS may be of the usual/endocervical type, or it may show intestinal or endometrioid differentiation.

In contrast to carcinoma, in adenocarcinoma in situ there is no desmoplastic stromal reaction, and no neoplastic glands are found beyond the deepest normal gland.

In invasive adenocarcinoma, a variety of subtypes are distinguished, including mucinous, endometrial, clear cell, mesonephric, and villoglandular adenocarcinoma.

According to the current FIGO staging rules (Bhatla et al. 2018), the definition of microcarcinoma as quoted above also applies to adenocarcinomas, even though the depth of invasion is more difficult to determine in glandular neoplasms as there is no basal membrane for reference.

6.2.1.1 p16 (p16INK4a Protein) Immunohistochemistry

As has already been explained in connection with the p16/Ki67 dual stain, p16 is a cell-regulating protein which is overexpressed in HPV transformed cells under the influence of high risk HPV-associated oncoproteins. The abnormal p16 protein can no longer trigger cell cycle arrest.

Of the multitude of immunohistochemical markers, p16 has been found to be particularly useful in diagnosing and grading squamous intraepithelial dysplasia, especially when only a limited amount of tissue is available as is the case with colposcopic biopsy material. Therefore, a number of pathology departments are routinely using p16 immunohistochemistry for tissue samples from the cervix.

As in the CINtecPlus® test, immunoperoxidase p16 staining is used, which results in a brown color of the cytoplasm, if p16 is overexpressed.

Under normal conditions, only isolated squamous epithelial cells are p16 positive. In LSIL, only cells in the basal epithelium are stained. In HSIL, also the middle (CIN2) and upper third (CIN3) are involved (Fig. 6.29). Figures 6.30, 6.31, and 6.32 show p16 staining examples in moderate and severe intraepithelial neoplasia and Fig. 6.33 in invasive squamous cell carcinoma. Moderate dysplasia (CIN2) may be diagnosed, when the middle third is also p16 positive. In severe dysplasia (CIN3), the entire depth of the epithelium may be p16 positive (Fig. 6.31).

Diagnosis and grading of cervical dysplasia should by not be based exclusively on p16 staining. According to a meta-analysis by Tsoumpou et al. (2009), biopsies with normal squamous epithelium may be diffusely p16-positive in 2% of cases (82% in CIN3 lesions). P16 positivity in LSIL does not have any predictive value, i.e. p16 is not a potential progression marker for low grade disease (Sagasta et al. 2016). Therefore, in LSIL/CIN1 lesions, p16 immunostaining should be used in equivocal cases only.

Galgano et al. (2010) studied 1455 cervical biopsies and used the conventional slide diagnosis as the gold standard for a consensus diagnosis of three experienced pathologists. In comparison to conventional slide evaluation, the immunohistochemical diagnosis with p16 was more sensitive, however less specific. Overall, staining for p16 was found to be a useful adjunct for identifying patients with CIN2+ lesions.

Stoler et al. (2018) reported that through p16 immunostaining as an adjunct to hematoxylin and eosin staining, diagnostic accuracy of cervical biopsies is higher. Both sensitivity (11.5%) and specificity (3.0%) are significantly increased.

Obviously, p16 immunohistochemistry can also be helpful in cervical screening of HIV infected women. As an adjunctive test, p16 immunostaining increases specificity and the positive predictive value of HPV and VIA for CIN2/CIN3 (McGrath et al. 2017).

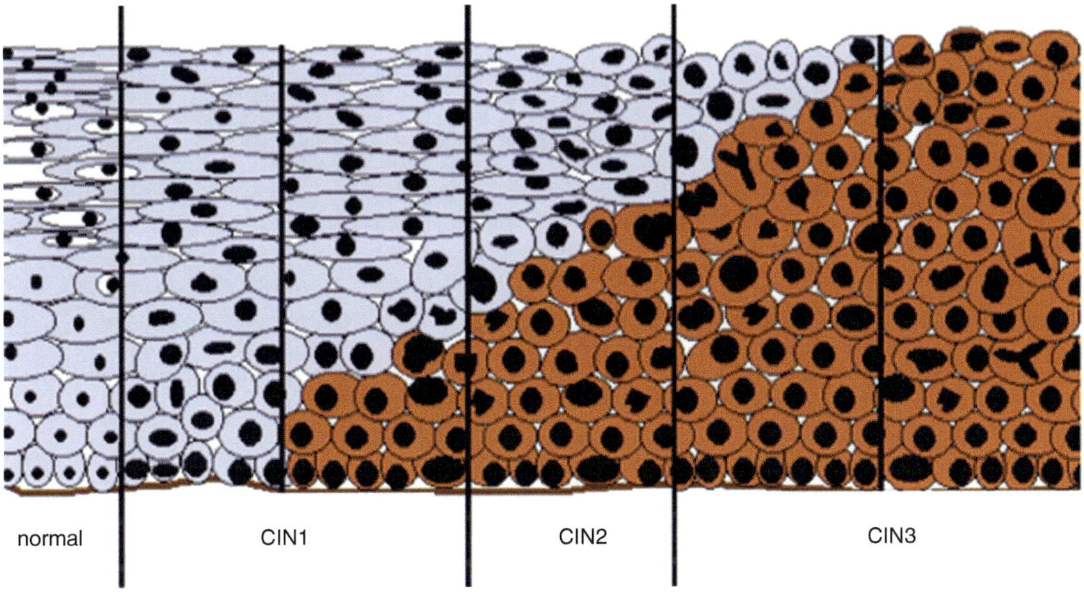

Fig. 6.29 p16 immunostaining of different grades of squamous dysplasia. In accordance with the WHO definition of CIN1–3, in CIN1 the lower one-third of the squamous epithelium is p16 positive. In CIN2, positive cells are also present in the middle one-third, and in CIN3, all cell layers stain positive

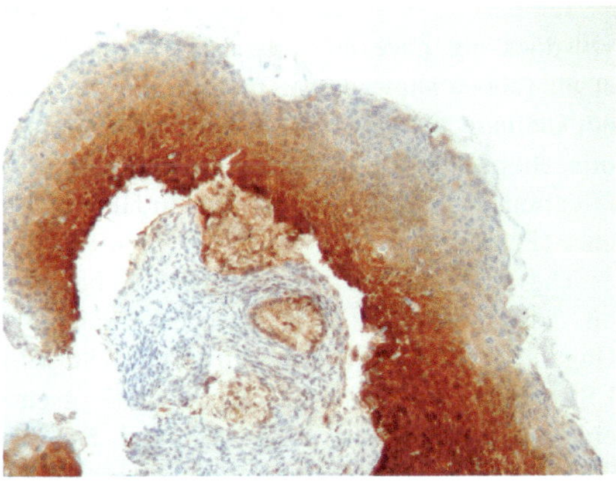

Fig. 6.30 p16 immunohistochemistry in CIN2. The lower and the middle one-third of the squamous epithelium are p16 positive

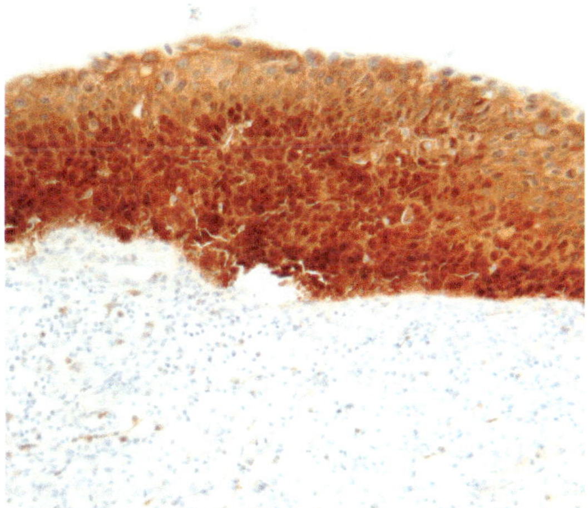

Fig. 6.31 p16 immunohistochemistry in CIN3. The epithelium is homogeneously p16 positive

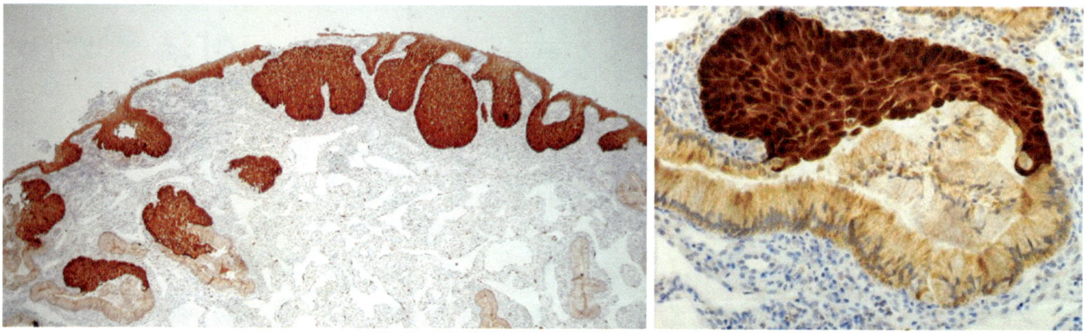

Fig. 6.32 p16 immunohistochemistry of CIN3. The dysplastic epithelium, which is homogeneously p16 positive, extends into the endocervical glands. This may not be confused with true invasion

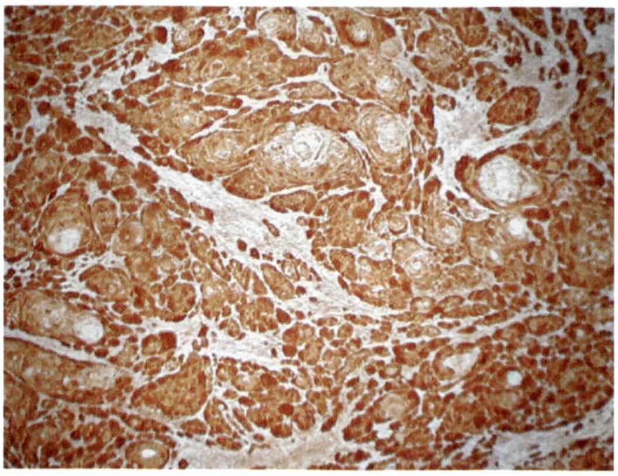

Fig. 6.33 p16 immunohistochemistry of invasive squamous cell carcinoma. Numerous nests of p16 positive tumor cells infiltrate the stroma

6.2.1.2 Reliability of Colposcopically Guided Biopsy Sampling

Histological diagnosis of dysplasia is subject to considerable intra- and interobserver variability (Ceballos et al. 2008). These inaccuracies can be improved to some extent by p16 immunohistochemistry.

However, both cervical biopsies (Fig. 6.34) and endocervical curettage (ECC) (Fig. 6.35) are small volume samples and will not always be representative. Nevertheless, colposcopically guided cervical biopsy is considered to be the gold standard of cervical diagnosis, a fact that has been called into question by cytopathologists such as Mangold and Nauth (2008) and Nauth and Mangold (2009). However, in practice not all cytological abnormalities can be clarified by diagnostic conization, as this procedure usually requires general anesthesia, has a significant risk of bleeding, and may lead to complications of future pregnancies. Therefore, in the context of dysplasia diagnosis, colposcopy and targeted biopsy is the best available triage at present (Versi 1992), although its sensitivity and specificity are well below 100%.

Taking one or several biopsies from the cervix does not have any adverse effects. Castle et al. (2009) showed that multiple biopsies do not increase the risk of subsequent HPV infection. Biopsies may even induce clearance of HPV infections and/or shorten the time to HPV clearance (Petry et al. 2018).

The influence of the number of biopsies on diagnostic sensitivity has been studied by Gage et al. (2006). Patients from the ASC-US/LSIL triage study who developed CIN3 or carcinoma within 2 years were identified. By taking two instead of one biopsy, sensitivity can be increased significantly: 68% and 82%, respectively. However, three or more biopsies do not lead to any further increase of sensitivity.

Interestingly, the overall accuracy of colposcopic diagnosis was similar across people with different types of medical training, such as nurse practitioners, general gynecologists, and gynecologic oncologists.

According to these data, about one-third of diagnoses based on a single targeted biopsy do not accurately reflect the findings on subsequent LEEP resection or cone biopsy. Several other studies have led to similar results. Stoler et al.

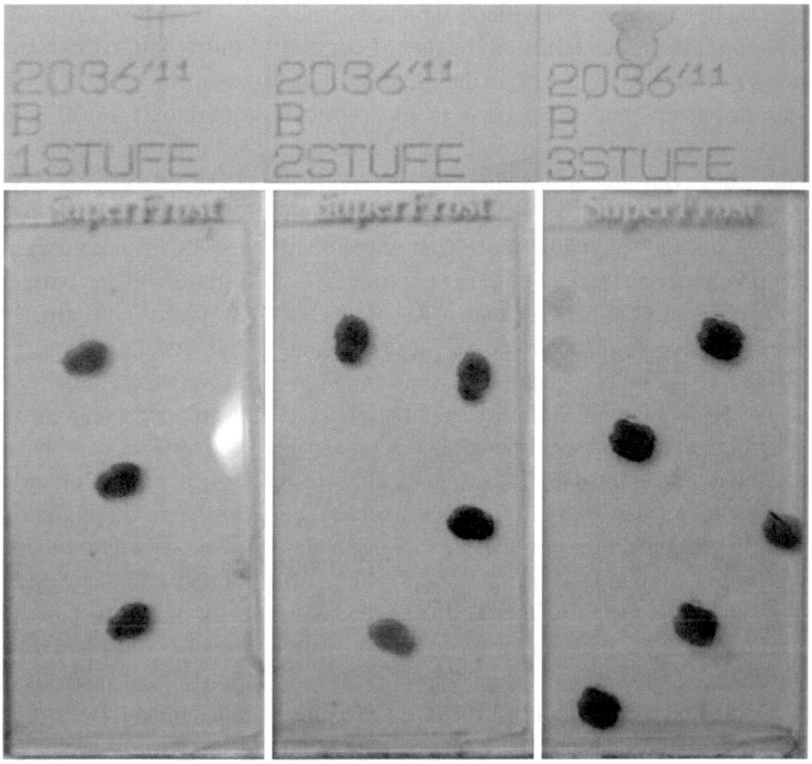

Fig. 6.34 Cervical biopsy specimen. The tissue sample is only a few millimeters in size and has been cut into 12 sections

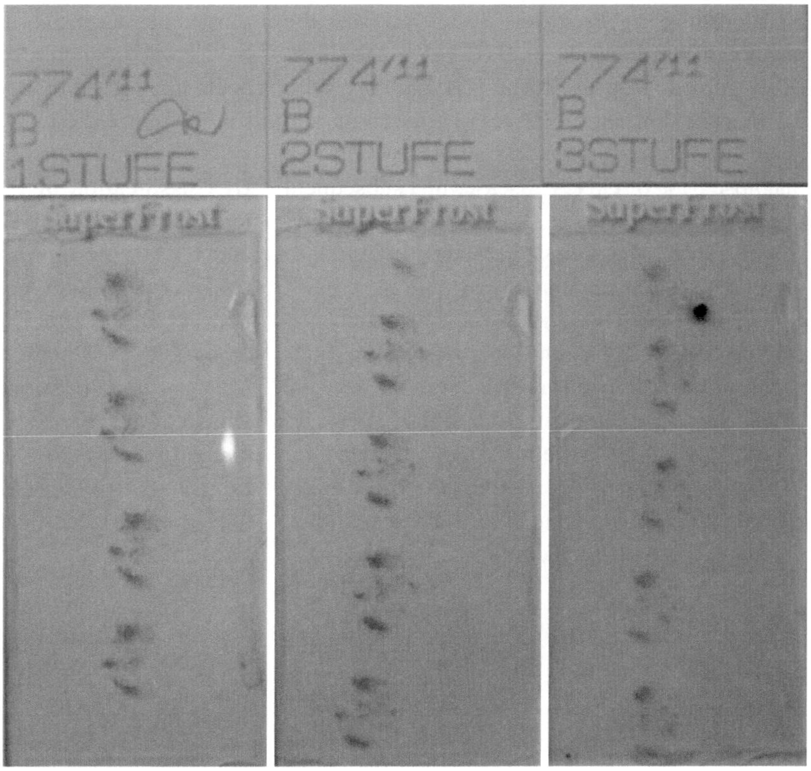

Fig. 6.35 Endocervical curettage specimen. Endocervical curettage has been performed with the Stiefel® curette. Nevertheless, the amount of tissue is small, which is a contributing factor of the low sensitivity of ECC

(2011a, b) examined 594 patients who had one or more target biopsies taken on the day of conization. Dysplasia (CIN or AIS) in the cone specimen was frequently underdiagnosed in the cervical biopsy or biopsies. The overall agreement was only 56% with underestimation of CIN2/CIN3/AIS being 57%. In accordance with the data from Gage et al. (2006), taking more than one biopsy improved the accuracy of colposcopic triage.

Zuchna et al. (2010) found a sensitivity of 52.0% for the detection of CIN2+ lesions when taking a single biopsy, and 65.2% when two biopsies were obtained. A third biopsy did not lead to a significant improvement in sensitivity, again in accordance with the data from Gage et al.

Byrom et al. (2006) found a sensitivity of 74% for the detection of CIN2+ by taking a single biopsy immediately prior to conization. All patients had a type T1 or T2 transformation zone. Two out of three microinvasive carcinomas were not detected by biopsy.

Data from Stubbe et al. (2011) are very similar: In 240 correlations between biopsies and confirmational result, only 67% of the patients had an exact match.

According to Pretorius et al. (2004), the diagnosis was correct in 57% of colposcopically guided biopsies from 364 patients with a CIN2+ lesion and a T2 or T3 transformation zone. Interestingly, a random biopsy would still diagnose 37% of CIN2+ disease. In a subsequent publication, Pretorius et al. (2012) found that 61 out of 295 CIN3+ cases (21%) were diagnosed with CIN2+ after random biopsy and/or ECC.

Endocervical tissue removal, i.e. endocervical curettage, is by definition a blind biopsy. Its accuracy is much lower than targeted cervical biopsy/biopsies (Driggers and Zahn 2008). In Chap. 7, a Stiefel® curette is recommended for ECC. However, whether significantly more material can be obtained compared to a conventional curette has not yet been confirmed by a study.

According to data derived from the ALTS study (ASC-US/LSIL triage), CIN2+ was diagnosed in only 3.7% of patients by ECC compared to 21.7% of patients who were diagnosed by biopsy (Solomon et al. 2007). Thus, sensitivity of ECC was only 12.2% compared to 72.5% for the biopsy. The relative contribution of ECC to the diagnosis of CIN2+ lesions was higher in older patients: 13.0% among women 40 years and older versus 2.2% in women younger than 40.

Fan et al. (2017) tried to correlate accuracy of colposcopically directed cervical biopsy with clinical factors. The agreement between histological results of biopsy and cone was 74.1% (78.2% for high grade lesions). Univariate analysis showed that underdiagnosis was significantly more frequent in older patients (≥50 years of age), postmenopause and transformation zone type T3, and when fewer biopsies were taken. On multivariate analysis, cone width was the only independent factor correlated with the accuracy of cervical biopsy.

Based on the limited sensitivity of cervical biopsies, Massad (2006) suggests to consider immediate loop excision in older women who have completed childbearing when cytology suspects high grade disease without prior confirmation by targeted biopsy.

As pointed out above, the German Munich III classification of Pap groups places particular emphasis on the distinction between CIN2 and CIN3 cytology (Pap IIID2 and Pap IVa-p, respectively). Specificity of a Pap IVa-p diagnosis is high with 85% to 87% for a CIN3 diagnosis and 98% for CIN2+ (Hilal et al. 2015; Marquardt and Ziemke 2018). In contrast, as shown above, biopsies are only concordant with conization diagnosis in 52% to 74%. Therefore, biopsy—but not colposcopy—may be omitted prior to therapeutic resection in selected patients.

Summary: Target Biopsy

- Colposcopically guided biopsy as the sole diagnostic criterion would be unreliable and deviates from the definitive diagnosis in about one-quarter to one-third of patients.
- Taking two biopsies instead of one significantly improves accuracy.
- Technically, endocervical curettage constitutes a "blind biopsy" and has a low negative predictive value.
- Cervical biopsy and ECC are only two of the several decision criteria, and their interpretation in the context of clinical decision-making must take into account the inherent error rate.
- Prior to the colposcopic triage decision, an overall assessment is required including.
  - age
  - reproductive desire
  - previous and present cytological results
  - colposcopic evaluation (T1-T3, minor versus major change)
  - individual risk factors (immunosuppression)
  - individual patients preferences

6.3 HPV Test

The HPV test plays an important role, both in screening as a primary test option or as a co-test in combination with cytology. Also, the HPV test can be used as triage of ASC-US and as a test of cure following treatment of preinvasive cervical disease. The following chapter focuses on basic requirements for HPV tests that are used in clinical decision-making.

6.3.1 HPV Assays Suitable for Clinical Use

Test sensitivity is one of the most important issues.

***Analytical sensitivity*, i.e. the detection of a very low number of viruses, is less important than *clinical sensitivity*, i.e. the capability to detect CIN2+ lesions. Therefore, an HPV assay is only useful for screening, if it has a certain accuracy to predict the presence of HSIL.**

The Hybrid Capture 2 test (HC2), which is discussed in more detail below, can be considered the benchmark assay, as most clinical studies on CIN2+ detection are based on HC2. Newer and more advanced tests have to prove their efficacy through comparison with HC2 data. Therefore, these newer assays need to be calibrated, so that their thresholds of high risk HPV detection corresponds with CIN2+ detection. The oversensitive detection of an HPV infection per se is not clinically useful (de Thurah et al. 2018). Rather, this could lead to an unnecessary increase in the number of colposcopic triage examinations, as Kinney et al. (2010) pointed out when the FDA-approved Cervista test (Hologic) was found to be two to four times more often positive than the other FDA-approved tests.

> *"Misguided attempts to achieve the lofty goal of perfect clinical sensitivity (via increasing analytic sensitivity) have the potential to result in significant patient harm from unnecessary clinical follow-up, unnecessary diagnostic procedures, and unnecessary treatment of healthy women."*
>
> (Kinney et al. 2010)

Results from different HPV assays do not necessarily have to be concordant. However, in the presence of CIN2+ disease, the concordance between different HPV test procedures is as high as 84%, compared to only 29% of the entire screening population. This has been shown by Rebolj et al. (2016) who compared four different assays (HC2, CLART®, cobas®, APTIMA®).

- The following basic guidelines have been established for the requirements of HPV tests that are applied clinically, especially when used for primary cervical screening:
- (Stoler et al. 2007; Meijer et al. 2009)
  - The test should be capable of detecting the following 13 HPV high risk types: 16, 18, 31, 33, 35, 39, 45, 51, 52, 56, 58, 59, and 68.
  - Sensitivity to detect CIN2+ should be at least 90% compared to an established and clinically validated HPV test.
  - Specificity to diagnose CIN2+ should be at least 98% compared to an established and clinically validated HPV test.

6.3.1.1 Hybrid Capture II Test (HC2)

The hybrid capture assay is a signal-amplifying hybridization assay for the qualitative detection of DNA of human papillomaviruses. The assay can distinguish two HPV groups: the A probe identifies the low risk HPV types 6, 11, 42, 43, and 44 and the B probe the high risk HPV types 16, 18, 31, 33, 35, 39, 45, 51, 52, 56, 58, 59, and 68.

Overall, 13 high risk HPV types are qualitatively analyzed with the Hybrid Capture II test. Identification of individual virus types (genotyping) is not possible. Nor can the viral load be quantified. The test is positive, when at least 5000 viral copies/ml (1 pg DNA) are present.

During gynecological examination, the specimen is obtained from the cervix or from the posterior vaginal vault using a brush-like sampling device. The brush is placed into the transport medium and sent to the laboratory without the need for refrigeration. The sample can be stored for up to 2 weeks at room temperature.

In the laboratory, the DNA is released from the cells using sodium bicarbonate and then hybridized with the specific HPV RNA probes A and B. In this step, DNA–RNA hybridization occurs if the sample contains the HPV DNA target sequences.

The next phase involves the so-called capture step, as the DNA–RNA hybrids are bound to the surface of a microtiter plate. Each well of the microtiter plate contains on its surface anti-RNA–DNA antibodies which capture the hybrids. Subsequently, antibodies are added, which are conjugated with alkaline phosphatase and bind specifically to DNA–RNA hybrids.

Finally, hybridization is detected by chemiluminescence. A special reagent serves as a substrate of alkaline phosphatase. As a result of this enzymatic reaction, light is emitted, which is measured in the luminometer and reported as "relative light units" (RLU). By comparison with a positive and a negative sample serving as a standard, it is determined whether the sample is positive for either the A or B probe or both.

Although the A probe, which identifies four different HPV low risk viruses is still available, no clinical indication for its use does exist. Rather, the diagnosis of HPV low risk types, which are of no diagnostic or therapeutic consequence, may only be disconcerting to the patient and should therefore be avoided.

6.3.1.2 Other HPV Assays

Although FDA approval is not required outside the USA, FDA certification can still be considered a quality criterion. FDA approval of laboratory tests, that are used for clinical decision making, requires extensive documentation.

Presently, the following four HPV tests are FDA approved:

- Digene Hybrid Capture 2 High Risk HPV DNA Test (Qiagen, Gaithersburg, MD, USA). HPV types 16, 18, 31, 33, 35, 39, 45, 51, 52, 56, 58, 59, and 68 (antigen: DNA, whole genome).

- Cobas® HPV Test (Roche Diagnostics). HPV 16/18 (genotyping), 31, 33, 35, 39, 45, 51, 52, 56, 58, 59, 66, and 68 (antigen: DNA, L1).
- Cervista® HPV HR and GenFind DNA Extraction (Kit) (Hologic). HPV 16, 18, 31, 33, 35, 39, 45, 51, 52, 56, 58, 59, 66, and 68 (antigen: DNA, E6/E7/L1).
- APTIMA® HPV Assay (Hologic). HPV 16, 18, 31, 33, 35, 39, 45, 51, 52, 56, 58, 59, 66, and 68 (antigen: RNA, E6/E7).

A more comprehensive list of commercially available HPV tests is given in Table 6.5.

Table 6.5 List of commercial HPV tests (Poljak et al. 2012, updated 2018)

hrHPV DNA tests Hybrid Capture® 2 (HC2) HPV DNA Test (QIAGEN Inc., Gaithersburg, MD; USA (previously Digene Corp.)) EIA kit HPV GP HR (Diassay, Rijswijk, The Netherlands) Cervista® HPV HR Test (Hologic, Madison, WI) CareHPV™ Test (QIAGEN Inc., Gaithersburg, MD; USA)	Current status US FDA-approved (2003) clinically validated US FDA-approved (2009) clinically validated
hrHPV DNA tests with concurrent or reflex partial genotyping for the main hrHPV types Tests with concurrent partial genotyping for the main hrHPV types cobas® 4800 HPV Test (Roche Molecular Systems Inc., Alameda, CA, USA) RealTime High Risk HPV test (Abbott Molecular, Des Plaines, IL) Tests with reflex partial genotyping for the main hrHPV types Cervista HPV 16/18 Test (Hologic, Madison, WI) digene® HPV Genotyping PS Test, RUO (Qiagen, Hilden, Germany)	US FDA-approved (2011) clinically validated US FDA-approved (2009)
HPV DNA full genotyping tests Strip, filter or microtiter-well hybridization based full genotyping tests Linear Array® HPV Genotyping Test (Roche Molecular Systems Inc., Alameda, CA, USA) INNO-LiPA HPV Genotyping Extra (Innogenetics NV, Gent, Belgium) HPV SPF10 LiPA25$_{\text{version 1}}$ (Labo Bio-Medical Products, Ev Rijswijk, The Netherlands) digene HPV Genotyping RH Test (Qiagen, Hilden, Germany) Medium or low density microarray-based full genotyping tests PapilloCheck® HPV Screening Test/High risk Test (Greiner Bio-One, Frickenhausen, Germany) Clart® HPV 2 - Papillomavirus Clinical Arrays (Genomica, Coslada, Spain) Microsphere beads based full genotyping tests Gel electrophoresis based full genotyping tests Capillary electrophoresis based full genotyping tests Real-time PCR based full genotyping tests PCR combined with matrix-assisted laser desorption/ionization time-of-flight mass spectrometry	Widely used test widely used test widely used test widely used test Clinically validated widely used test
HPV DNA type- or group-specific genotyping tests Real-time PCR based tests Gel electrophoresis based test	
hrHPVE6/E7 mRNAtests APTIMA® HPV Test (Gen-Probe Inc., San Diego, CA) PreTect HPV-Proofer (NorChip, Klokkarstua, Norway)/NucliSENS EasyQ® HPV (Biomerieux, Marcy l'Etoile, France)	US FDA-approved (2011) widely used test
In situ based hybridization HPV tests	

HPV human papillomavirus, *hrHPV* high risk human papillomavirus, *PCR* polymerase chain reaction

6.3.2 Clinical Application of HPV Testing

HPV tests play an important role in the present concepts of secondary cervical cancer prevention (Arbyn et al. 2012). In the USA and elsewhere, HPV testing as a primary screening strategy has been approved for women of ≥30 years. In other countries, such as Germany, co-testing with cytology has been introduced for women of ≥35 years.

Besides primary screening, HPV testing is useful for the triage of equivocal (ASC-US) or LSIL Pap smear result. Also, in post-LEEP or conization follow-up, the HPV test can is considered as a "test of cure."

As a general rule, women under the age of 30 years should not be tested for HPV, regardless of the indication for the HPV test, as there are too many incident HPV infections which are not clinically significant.

6.3.2.1 HPV Triage of ASC-US and LSIL

The HPV test can successfully triage women with equivocal or low grade cytological abnormalities at screening. Thus, the number of referrals to colposcopy can be reduced (Solomon et al. 2001). This is particularly true for ASC-US cytology, whereas in women with LSIL its value is less obvious (Arbyn et al. 2012). Figure 6.36 shows the recommendations of the Italian Group for Cervical Cancer Screening for management of women with HPV positive ASC-US (Carozzi et al. 2015). For LSIL, the same triage algorithm is proposed with the HPV test result playing a limited role only.

However, Kyrgiou et al. (2016) state that immediate colposcopy for LSIL does not increase the detection of CIN2+ lesions, compared to repeat cytology over 2 years. Unfortunately, compliance decreases with the length of follow-up, so that immediate colposcopy might be considered for women with LSIL/HPV+ findings.

For triage of glandular cytological abnormalities, HPV testing plays only a very limited role. According to a systematic review by Verdoodt et al. (2016), the risk for high grade squamous and/or glandular dysplasia or invasive disease (CIN2+/AIS+) in women with atypical glandular cells (AGC) was 19.8%, and as high as 55.7% in women with concurrent squamous lesions (AGC/ASC-US+). Therefore, a cytological AGC diagnosis warrants referral to colposcopy regardless of HPV status. However, a negative HPV test in

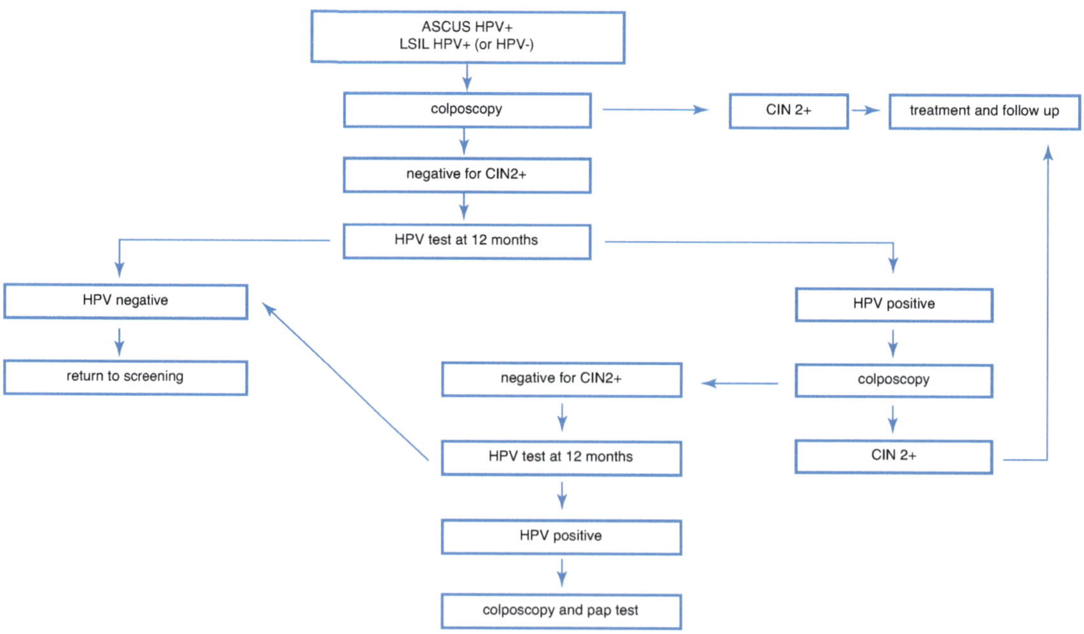

Fig. 6.36 Recommendations of the Italian Group for Cervical Cancer Screening for management of women with ASC-US using HPV triage and LSIL with or without HPV testing (Carozzi et al. 2015)

patients with atypical glandular cells is linked with an 18% chance of extra-cervical neoplasia such as endometrial, fallopian tube, or ovarian malignancy.

6.3.2.2 HPV Test for Post-Treatment Follow-Up ("Test of Cure")

HPV tests are useful in post-treatment follow-up (Alonso et al. 2006; Bae et al. 2007; Prato et al. 2007) since numerous studies have shown that after successful surgical dysplasia treatment the HPV test frequently becomes negative. When the HPV test is negative, most likely the precancerous lesion has been removed completely.

In fact, a negative HPV test result is more reliable than a negative margin on histopathological examination, or a normal Pap smear obtained during follow-up (Verguts et al. 2006). Alonso et al. (2006) found that 11.8% of patients with a negative resection margin still developed a relapse, whereas 63.6% with a positive margin had no recurrence.

According to a meta-analysis by Arbyn et al. (2012), the summary accuracy estimates for the HPV test 6 months after treatment were higher than for cytology (Fig. 6.37).

However, it has to be kept in mind that a positive HPV test on follow-up is not necessarily associated with persistent CIN. According to the study by Verguts et al. (2006), 23% of women who did not relapse within a two-year follow-up continued to be positive for high risk HPV.

In patients treated conservatively for cervical adenocarcinoma in situ, post-treatment monitoring by colposcopy and cytology is even less effective than for squamous lesions, and an additional parameter such as the HPV test is advantageous. Costa et al. (2007) found a diagnostic sensitivity of 90% for a combination of cytology and HPV testing (HC2) with a specificity of 50% for follow-up of adenocarcinoma in situ.

Globally, an increasing number of algorithms incorporate HPV testing as a "test of cure" during post-treatment follow-up.

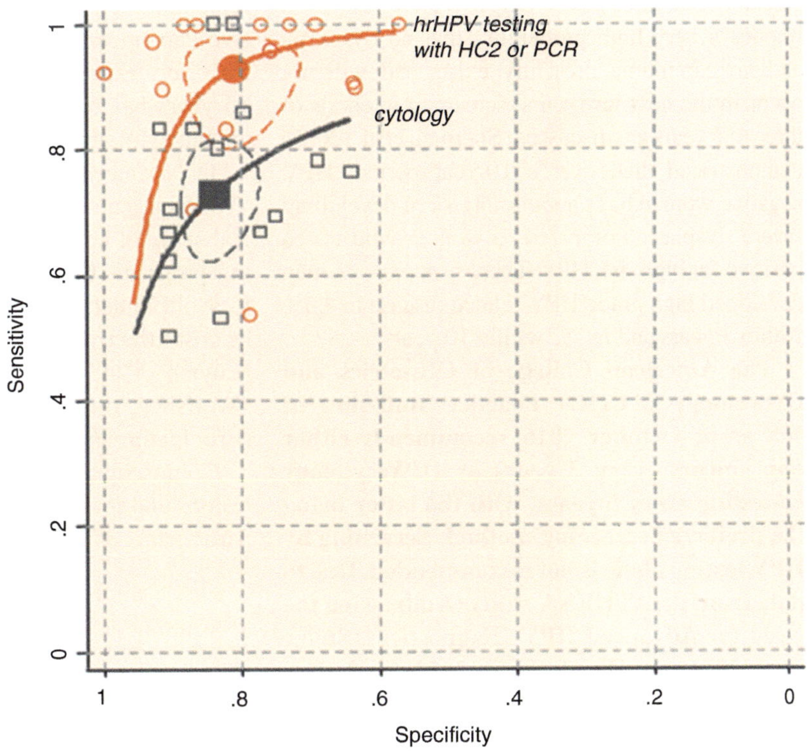

Fig. 6.37 Sensitivity and specificity of HPV testing versus cytological surveillance following treatment of HSIL to predict treatment failure. The summary accuracy estimates for the HPV test (filled orange circle) and cytology (filled gray square) 6 months after treatment are given together with the 95% confidence interval as an ellipse around the summary estimates. According to this review, HPV testing is superior to cytology in the post-treatment follow-up (Arbyn et al. 2012)

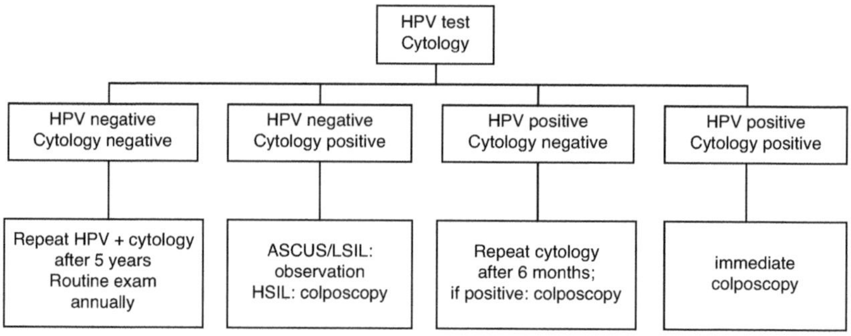

Fig. 6.38 Primary HPV screening project in Wolfsburg, Germany, with cytology co-testing for women ≥30 years (Luyten et al. 2009)

6.3.2.3 Primary HPV Screening

Although Pap smear based screening has been proven to be very effective in secondary prevention of cervical cancer, additional or alternative testing is needed in order to increase test sensitivity, especially in a population that has a low prevalence of HPV-related cervical disease due to previous screening effort as well as the effects of HPV vaccination. Primary HPV screening, either alone or in combination with cytology, has been shown to decrease false negative screening results and improve test sensitivity (Mayrand et al. 2007; Naucler et al. 2007). As a negative HPV test result implies a very high probability that no dysplasia and no carcinoma presently exists and will not occur in the next few years, screening intervals of three to 5 years are discussed. Sherman et al. (2003) demonstrated that, over a 10-year period, HPV negative women have a minimal risk of developing severe dysplasia compared to women who tested positive for high risk HPV. These groups of women developed high grade HPV-related disease in 4.3% within 3 years and in 7% within 10 years.

The American College of Obstetrics and Gynecology (ACOG) Practice Bulletin Nr. 168 as of October 2016 recommends either Pap smears every 3 years or HPV/cytology co-testing every 5 years, with the latter being the preferred screening method. Screening by HPV testing alone is not recommended. Due to data from the ATHENA study (Addressing the Need for Advanced HPV Diagnostics) (Stoler et al. 2011a, b; Wright et al. 2012), and after interim suggestions for using the cobas® HPV test, the U.S. Preventive Services Task Force (USPSTF) in 2017 published new cervical cancer screening recommendations for public review.[3] According to this proposal, co-testing is no longer recommended. Instead, women aged 30 to 65 years should receive primary HPV testing every 5 years as an alternative to cervical cytology every 3 years.

Similar to the USA, there is an increasing number of national cervical screening programs and guidelines that incorporate HPV testing into primary screening. However, in some countries such as Germany that has a tendency to overdiagnose cytological abnormalities by performing Pap tests every year, health care officials are reluctant to change the current practice of exclusive Pap smear screening. Eventually, starting in 2020, co-testing every 3 years from the age of 35 years has been approved as an alternative to annual cytological screening.[4]

In Germany, Petry et al. (2003) initiated the "Wolfsburg model," a long-term prospective clinical study of an HPV and cytology-based screening program (Fig. 6.38), which has been shown to avoid unnecessary surgical procedures and to be cost-effective due to longer screening intervals (Luyten et al. 2009). Also, acceptance for the "Wolfsburg model" is high for both patients and participating gynecologists.

Colposcopic triage for the detection of CIN3 lesions and invasive disease appears to be safe in participants of primary HPV screening programs

[3] https://www.acog.org/Clinical-Guidance-and-Publications/Practice-Advisories/Practice-Advisory-Cervical-Cancer-Screening.

[4] https://www.g-ba.de/downloads/39-261-2713/2016-09-15_Aenderung_Beauftragung-IQWiG_Einladung_Zervixkarzinom-Screening_vom-2015-03-19.pdf.

with an acceptable failure rate of 4.7% (Petry et al. 2013).

Although genotyping of all 13 HPV types included in primary screening assays is not required as it does not increase clinical sensitivity, some assays (Table 6.5) will report HPV 16 and/or HPV 18 infection separately. Patients who are positive for either HPV 16 or 18 have a significantly increased risk of developing CIN3 disease or cancer over the next several years and should undergo colposcopic triage regardless of a concomitant Pap test result.

References

Alonso I, Torne A, Puig-Tintore LM, Esteve R, Quinto L, Campo E et al (2006) Pre- and post-conization high-risk HPV testing predicts residual/recurrent disease in patients treated for CIN 2-3. Gynecol Oncol 103(2):631–636

Arbyn M, Herbert A, Schenck U, Nieminen P, Jordan J, McGoogan E et al (2007) European guidelines for quality assurance in cervical cancer screening: recommendations for collecting samples for conventional and liquid-based cytology. Cytopathology 18(3):133–139. https://doi.org/10.1111/j.1365-2303.2007.00464.x

Arbyn M, Bergeron C, Klinkhamer P, Martin-Hirsch P, Siebers AG, Bulten J (2008) Liquid compared with conventional cervical cytology: a systematic review and meta-analysis. Obstet Gynecol 111(1):167–177. https://doi.org/10.1097/01.AOG.0000296488.85807.b3

Arbyn M, Ronco G, Anttila A, Meijer CJLM, Poljak M, Ogilvie G et al (2012) Evidence regarding human papillomavirus testing in secondary prevention of cervical cancer. Vaccine 30:F88–F99. https://doi.org/10.1016/j.vaccine.2012.06.095

Ashfaq R, Gibbons D, Vela C, Saboorian MH, Iliya F (1999) ThinPrep Pap Test. Accuracy for glandular disease. Acta Cytol 43(1):81–85

Bae JH, Kim CJ, Park TC, Namkoong SE, Park JS (2007) Persistence of human papillomavirus as a predictor for treatment failure after loop electrosurgical excision procedure. Int J Gynecol Cancer 17(6): 1271–1277

Bae-Jump VL, Bauer M, Van Le L (2007) Cytological evaluation correlates poorly with histological diagnosis of vulvar neoplasias. J Low Genit Tract Dis 11(1):8–11. https://doi.org/10.1097/01.lgt.0000229566.57482.f3

Becker V (1979) Carl Ruge: 100 Jahre Stückchen-Diagnose. Arch Gynecol 227(3):193–204

Bergeron C, Debaque H, Ayivi J, Amaizo S, Fagnani F (1997) Cervical smear histories of 585 women with biopsy-proven carcinoma in situ. Acta Cytol 41(6):1676–1680. https://doi.org/10.1159/000333167

Bergeron C, Ikenberg H, Sideri M, Denton K, Bogers J, Schmidt D et al (2015) Prospective evaluation of p16/Ki-67 dual-stained cytology for managing women with abnormal Papanicolaou cytology: PALMS study results. Cancer Cytopathol 123(6):373–381. https://doi.org/10.1002/cncy.21542

Bhatla N, Aoki D, Sharma DN, Sankaranarayanan R (2018) Cancer of the cervix uteri. Int J Gynaecol Obstet 143(Suppl.3):22–36. https://doi.org/10.1002/ijgo.12611

Bocking A, Nguyen VQ (2004) Diagnostic and prognostic use of DNA image cytometry in cervical squamous intraepithelial lesions and invasive carcinoma. Cancer 102(1):41–54. https://doi.org/10.1002/cncr.11889

Bocking A, Nguyen VQH, Reich O, Pickel H (2004) Abnormer Pap-Abstrich: DNA-Bildzytometrie ermittelt Progressionsrisiko. Frauenarzt 45:194–196

Bollmann R, Jordan B (2005) Technische Voraussetzungen einer validierten Flüssigkeitszytologie. Frauenarzt 46:405–420

Bollmann R, Bocking A, Ikenberg H, Jordan B (2006) Stellungnahme zu Methoden der Flüssigkeitszytologie. Frauenarzt 47:136–139

Bos AB, Ballegooijen M van, Marle ME van den A, Hanselaar AG, Oortmarssen GJ van, Habbema JD (2001) Endocervical status is not predictive of the incidence of cervical cancer in the years after negative smears. Am J Clin Pathol 115:851–5.

Byrom J, Douce G, Jones PW, Tucker H, Millinship J, Dhar K, Redman CW (2006) Should punch biopsies be used when high-grade disease is suspected at initial colposcopic assessment? A prospective study. Int J Gynecol Cancer 16(1):253–256. https://doi.org/10.1111/j.1525-1438.2006.00344.x

Carozzi FM, Iossa A, Scalisi A, Sideri M, Prev KAE (2015) Hr-HPV testing in the management of women with ASC-US+ and in the follow-up of women with cytological abnormalities and negative colposcopy. Recommendations of the Italian group for cervical cancer screening (GISCi). Epidemiol Prev 39(3 Suppl 1): 84–90

Castle PE, Wentzensen N, Wheeler CM, Rydzak G, Schiffman M (2009) Effect of the number of biopsies on the subsequent acquisition of new human papillomavirus infections. Obstet Gynecol 114(5):1057–1062. https://doi.org/10.1097/AOG.0b013e3181bb5632

Ceballos KM, Chapman W, Daya D, Julian JA, Lytwyn A, McLachlin CM, Elit L (2008) Reproducibility of the histological diagnosis of cervical dysplasia among pathologists from 4 continents. Int J Gynecol Pathol 27(1):101–107. https://doi.org/10.1097/pgp.0b013e31814fb1da

Clark SB, Dawson AE (2002) Invasive squamous-cell carcinoma in ThinPrep® specimens: diagnostic clues in the cellular pattern. Diagn Cytopathol 26(1):1–4. https://doi.org/10.1002/dc.10033

Compton CC, Byrd DR, Garcia-Aguilar J, Kurtzman SH, Olawaiye A, Washington MK (eds) (2012) AJCC cancer staging atlas, 2nd edn. Springer, New York, NY, pp 1–621. https://doi.org/10.1007/978-1-4614-2080-4

Costa S, Negri G, Sideri M, Santini D, Martinelli G, Venturoli S et al (2007) Human papillomavirus (HPV) test and PAP smear as predictors of outcome in conservatively treated adenocarcinoma in situ (AIS) of the uterine cervix. Gynecol Oncol 106(1):170–176

Cuzick J, Clavel C, Petry KU, Meijer CJ, Hoyer H, Ratnam S et al (2006) Overview of the European and north American studies on HPV testing in primary cervical cancer screening. Int J Cancer 119(5):1095–1101. https://doi.org/10.1002/ijc.21955

Davey E, Barratt A, Irwig L, Chan SF, Macaskill P, Mannes P, Saville AM (2006) Effect of study design and quality on unsatisfactory rates, cytology classifications, and accuracy in liquid-based versus conventional cervical cytology: a systematic review. Lancet 367(9505):122–132

Davey E, D'Assuncao J, Irwig L, Macaskill P, Chan SF, Richards A, Farnsworth A (2007) Accuracy of reading liquid based cytology slides using the ThinPrep imager compared with conventional cytology: prospective study. BMJ 335(7609):31

de Thurah L, Bonde J, Lam JUH, Rebolj M (2018) Not all HPV nucleic acid tests are equal: only those calibrated to detect high grade lesions matter for cervical screening: response to "concordant testing results between various human papillomavirus assays in primary cervical cancer screening: systematic review" by de Thurah, Bonde, Uyen, Lam and Rebolj. Published 27 May, 2017. Clin Microbiol Infect 24(4):438–439. https://doi.org/10.1016/j.cmi.2017.12.001

Dennerstein G (2009) Vulvar cytology: useful or not? J Low Genit Tract Dis 13(3):192. https://doi.org/10.1097/LGT.0b013e31818e159a

Driggers RW, Zahn CM (2008) To ECC or not to ECC: the question remains. Obstet Gynecol Clin N Am 35(4):583–597.; viii. https://doi.org/10.1016/j.ogc.2008.09.007

Elias A, Linthorst G, Bekker B, Vooijs PG (1983) The significance of endocervical cells in the diagnosis of cervical epithelial changes. Acta Cytol 27(3): 225–229

Elumir-Tanner L, Doraty M (2011) Management of Papanicolaou test results that lack endocervical cells. Can Med Assoc J 183(5):563–568. https://doi.org/10.1503/cmaj.101156

Fan A, Zhang L, Wang C, Wang Y, Han C, Xue F (2017) Analysis of clinical factors correlated with the accuracy of colposcopically directed biopsy. Arch Gynecol Obstet 296(5):965–972. https://doi.org/10.1007/s00404-017-4500-z

Feulgen R, Rossenbach H (1924) Mikroscopisch-chemischer Nachweis einer Nucleinsäure vom Typus der Thymonucleinsäure. Hoppe Seylers Z Physiol Chem 135:203

Flenker H (2003) Taschenatlas der gynäkologischen Zytologie. IDwerk, Bremen

Fox J, Remington P, Layde P, Klein G (1999) The effect of hysterectomy on the risk of an abnormal screening Papanicolaou test result. Am J Obstet Gynecol 180(5):1104–1109

Gage JC, Hanson VW, Abbey K, Dippery S, Gardner S, Kubota J et al (2006) Number of cervical biopsies and sensitivity of colposcopy. Obstet Gynecol 108(2):264–272. https://doi.org/10.1097/01.AOG.0000220505.18525.85

Galgano MT, Castle PE, Atkins KA, Brix WK, Nassau SR, Stoler MH (2010) Using biomarkers as objective standards in the diagnosis of cervical biopsies. Am J Surg Pathol 34:1077–87

Gibb RK, Martens MG (2011) The impact of liquid-based cytology in decreasing the incidence of cervical cancer. Rev Obstet Gynecol 4(Suppl 1):S2–S11

Goh ST, Tay T, Lim KL, Song LH, Thika AA, Mantoo S (2017) Inter-observer variabilty of CINtec PLUS dual staining for p16/ki67. J Am Soc Cytopathol 6(5):S30. https://doi.org/10.1016/j.jasc.2017.06.074

Griesser H, Marquardt K, Jordan B, Kuhn W, Neis K, Neumann H et al (2013) Gynäkologische Zytodiagnostik der Zervix. Münchner Nomenklatur III. Frauenarzt 54(11):1042–1048

Hilal Z, Tempfer C, Schiermeier S, Reinecke J, Ruppenkamp C, Hilal Z (2015) Progression or regression? – strengths and weaknesses of the New Munich nomenclature III for cervix cytology. Geburtshilfe Frauenheilkd 75(10):1051–1057. https://doi.org/10.1055/s-0035-1557904

Ikenberg H (2011) Computer-assisted diagnostics in cervical cytology. Pathologe 32(6):476–483. https://doi.org/10.1007/s00292-011-1477-4

Jimenez-Ayala M, Jimenez-Ayala B (2002) Terminology for vulvar cytology based on the Bethesda system. Acta Cytol 46(4):645–650

Kaur P, Kushtagi P (2013) Plastic spatula with narrow long tip provides higher satisfactory smears for pap test. J Cytol Ind Acad Cytologist 30(3):159–161. https://doi.org/10.4103/0970-9371.117654

Kinney W, Stoler MH, Castle PE (2010) Special commentary: patient safety and the next generation of HPV DNA tests. Am J Clin Pathol 134(2):193–199. https://doi.org/10.1309/AJCPRI8XPQUEAA3K

Kivlahan C, Ingram E (1986) Papanicolaou smears without endocervical cells. Are they inadequate? Acta Cytol 30(3):258–260

Klug SJ, Neis KJ, Harlfinger W, Malter A, Konig J, Spieth S et al (2012) A randomized trial comparing conventional cytology to liquid-based cytology and computer assistance. Int J Cancer J Inter Du Cancer. https://doi.org/10.1002/ijc.27955

Kurman RJ, Carcangiu ML, Harrington CS, Young RH (2014) WHO classification of tumours of female reproductive organs. IARC Press, Lyon

Kyrgiou M, Kalliala I, Mitra A, Ng B, Raglan O, Fotopoulou C et al (2016) Immediate referral to colposcopy vs. cytological surveillance for low-grade cervical cytological abnormalities in the absence of HPV test: a systematic review and a meta-analysis of the literature. Int J Cancer 140(1):216–223. https://doi.org/10.1002/ijc.30419

Lellé RJ, Bettendorf O, Eltze E (2007a) Forum Zytologie: Die zervikale intraepitheliale Neoplsie (CIN) - 5. Teil. Praktische Gyn 12:30–32

Lellé RJ, Cordes A, Regidor M, Maier E, Flenker H (2007b) Comparison of the ThinPrep monolayer technique and conventional cervical Pap smears in a high-risk population using the Munich II nomenclature. Gynakol Geburtshilfliche Rundsch 47(2):81–87. https://doi.org/10.1159/000100337

Luyten A, Scherbring S, Reinecke-Luthge A, Braun BE, Pietralla M, Theiler K, Petry KU (2009) Risk-adapted primary HPV cervical cancer screening project in Wolfsburg, Germany - experience over 3 years. J Clin Virol 46(S3):S5–S10

Luzzatto R, Boon ME (1996) Contribution of the endocervical Cytobrush sample to the diagnosis of cervical lesions. Acta Cytol 40(6):1143–1147

Macharia C, Cheserem J, Bukusi E, Muchiri L (2016) A comparative analysis of conventional Pap smear cytology, liquid based cytology and colposcopy clinical impression with colposcopy biopsy histology as gold standard in women undergoing colposcopy in Kenyatta National Hospital. Int J Reprod Contracept Obstet Gynecol 3(1):58–63. https://doi.org/10.4236/ojog.2013.33058

Mangold BR, Nauth HF (2008) Konisation oder kolposkopisch gesteuerte Portiobiopsie? Vergleich der Wertigkeit der beiden Verfahren bei zytologischem Verdacht auf CIN III. Frauenarzt 49:522–527

Marquardt K, Ziemke P (2018) Munich nomenclature III: classification according to risk : follow-up for conspicuous squamous findings. Pathologe 39(1):57–64. https://doi.org/10.1007/s00292-017-0382-x

Marquardt K, Broschewitz U, Büttner HH, Barten M (2007) Zervixkarzinom trotz Früherkennungsprogramm - Analyse von Teilnahmeraten und Tumorstadium. Der Frauenarzt 48(11):1086–1088

Marquardt K, Büttner HH, Broschewitz U, Barten M, Schneider V (2011) Persistent carcinoma in cervical cancer screening: non-participation is the most significant cause. Acta Cytol 55(5):433–437. https://doi.org/10.1159/000331811

Massad LS (2006) More is more: improving the sensitivity of colposcopy. Obstet Gynecol 108(2):246–247. https://doi.org/10.1097/01.AOG.0000229430.04828.83

Mayrand MH, Duarte-Franco E, Rodrigues I, Walter SD, Hanley J, Ferenczy A et al (2007) Human papillomavirus DNA versus Papanicolaou screening tests for cervical cancer. N Engl J Med 357(16):1579–1588. https://doi.org/10.1056/NEJMoa071430

McGrath CJ, Garcia R, Trinh TT, Richardson BA, John-Stewart GC, Nyongesa-Malava E et al (2017) Role of p16 testing in cervical cancer screening among HIV-infected women. PLoS One 12(10):e0185597. https://doi.org/10.1371/journal.pone.0185597

McMenamin M, McKenna M, McDowell A, Dawson C, McKenna R (2017) Intra- and inter-observer reproducibility of CINtec® PLUS in ThinPrep® cytology preparations. Cytopathology 28(4):284–290. https://doi.org/10.1111/cyt.12426

Mehlhorn G, Obermann E, Negri G, Bubendorf L, Mian C, Koch M et al (2013) HPV L1 detection discriminates cervical precancer from transient HPV infection: a prospective international multicenter study. Mod Pathol Off J U S Canad Acad Pathol. https://doi.org/10.1038/modpathol.2012.233

Mehlhorn G, Hautmann SK, Koch MC, Strehl JD, Hartmann A, Hilfrich R et al (2014) HPV16-L1-specific antibody response is associated with clinical remission of high-risk HPV-positive early dysplastic lesions. Anticancer Res 34(9):5127–5132

Meijer CJ, Berkhof J, Castle PE, Hesselink AT, Franco EL, Ronco G et al (2009) Guidelines for human papillomavirus DNA test requirements for primary cervical cancer screening in women 30 years and older. Int J Cancer 124(3):516–520. https://doi.org/10.1002/ijc.24010

Narine N, Young W (2007) Transformation zone sampling rate is a useful performance indicator for practitioners collecting cervical samples using SurePath(TM) liquid-based cytology system. Cytopathology 18(4):220–224

Naucler P, Ryd W, Tornberg S, Strand A, Wadell G, Elfgren K et al (2007) Human papillomavirus and Papanicolaou tests to screen for cervical cancer. N Engl J Med 357(16):1589–1597. https://doi.org/10.1056/NEJMoa073204

Nauth HF (2007) Gynecological cytology. Thieme Stuttgart

Nauth HF, Mangold BR (2009) Klinische Konsequenzen bei positiven gynäkologischen Abstrichbefunden. Gynäkol Prax 33:265–276

Nayar R, Wilbur DC (2015) The Bethesda system for reporting cervical cytology: definitions, criteria, and explanatory notes. Springer

Naylor B (2000) The century for cytopathology. Acta Cytol 44(5):709–725

Nghiem VT, Davies KR, Beck JR, Follen M, MacAulay C, Guillaud M, Cantor SB (2015) Economic evaluation of DNA ploidy analysis vs liquid-based cytology for cervical screening. Br J Cancer 112(12):1951–1957. https://doi.org/10.1038/bjc.2015.95

Nocon M, Mittendorf T, Roll S, Greiner W, S N, W., & Schulenburg, von der, J. M. (2007) Welchen medizinischen und gesundheitsökonomischen Nutzen hat die Kolposkopie als primäres Screening auf das Zervixkarzinom? Dimdi

Pecorelli S (2009) Revised FIGO staging for carcinoma of the vulva, cervix, and endometrium. Int J Gynaecol Obstet 105:103–4.

Petruzziello L, Relucenti M, D'Aluisio D, Iannaccio S, Giovagnoli MR, Lukic A et al (2011) The PapCone® as a valid cervical sampling device: a comparative ultrastructural and semiquantitative study. Italian Journal of Anatomy and Embryology 116(2):142. https://doi.org/10.13128/IJAE-10166

Petry KU, Menton S, Menton M, van Loenen-Frosch F, de Carvalho Gomes H, Holz B et al (2003) Inclusion of HPV testing in routine cervical cancer screening for women above 29 years in Germany: results for 8466 patients. Br J Cancer 88(10):1570–1577

Petry KU, Schmidt D, Scherbring S, Luyten A, Reinecke-Luthge A, Bergeron C et al (2011) Triaging Pap cytology negative, HPV positive cervical cancer screening results with p16/Ki-67 dual-stained cytology. Gynecol Oncol 121(3):505–509. https://doi.org/10.1016/j.ygyno.2011.02.033

Petry KU, Luyten A, Scherbring S (2013) Accuracy of colposcopy management to detect CIN3 and invasive cancer in women with abnormal screening tests: results from a primary HPV screening project from 2006 to 2011 in Wolfsburg, Germany. Gynecol Oncol 128(2):282–287. https://doi.org/10.1016/j.ygyno.2012.10.017

Petry KU, Horn J, Luyten A, Mikolajczyk RT (2018) Punch biopsies shorten time to clearance of high-risk human papillomavirus infections of the uterine cervix. BMC Cancer 18(1):318. https://doi.org/10.1186/s12885-018-4225-9

Pinto AP, Degen M, Villa LL, Cibas ES (2012) Immunomarkers in gynecologic cytology: the search for the ideal biomolecular Papanicolaou test. Acta Cytol 56(2):109–121. https://doi.org/10.1159/000335065

Poljak M, Cuzick J, Kocjan BJ, Iftner T, Dillner J, Arbyn M (2012) Nucleic acid tests for the detection of alpha human papillomaviruses. Vaccine 30(Suppl 5):F100–F106. https://doi.org/10.1016/j.vaccine.2012.04.105

Prato B, Ghelardi A, Gadducci A, Marchetti I, Di Cristofano C, Di Coscio G et al (2007) Correlation of recurrence rates and times with posttreatment human papillomavirus status in patients treated with loop electrosurgical excision procedure conization for cervical squamous intraepithelial lesions. Int J Gynecol Cancer. https://doi.org/10.1136/ijgc-00009577-200801000-00014

Pretorius RG, Zhang WH, Belinson JL, Huang MN, Wu LY, Zhang X, Qiao YL (2004) Colposcopically directed biopsy, random cervical biopsy, and endocervical curettage in the diagnosis of cervical intraepithelial neoplasia II or worse. Am J Obstet Gynecol 191(2):430–434. https://doi.org/10.1016/j.ajog.2004.02.065

Pretorius RG, Belinson JL, Azizi F, Peterson PC, Belinson S (2012) Utility of random cervical biopsy and endocervical curettage in a low-risk population. J Low Genit Tract Dis. https://doi.org/10.1097/LGT.0b013e3182480c18

Quddus MR, Neves T, Reilly ME, Steinhoff MM, Sung CJ (2009) Does the ThinPrep Imaging System increase the detection of high-risk HPV-positive ASC-US and AGUS? The Women and Infants Hospital experience with over 200,000 cervical cytology cases. Cytojournal 6(1):15. https://doi.org/10.4103/1742-6413.54917

Ravarino A, Nemolato S, Macciocu E, Fraschini M, Senes G, Faa G, Negri G (2012) CINtec PLUS immunocytochemistry as a tool for the cytologic diagnosis of glandular lesions of the cervix uteri. Am J Clin Pathol 138(5):652–656. https://doi.org/10.1309/AJCP00INMGIFYFNQ

Rebolj M, Bonde J, Preisler S, Ejegod D, Rygaard C, Lynge E (2016) Differential detection of human papillomavirus genotypes and cervical intraepithelial neoplasia by four commercial assays. J Clin Microbiol 54(11):2669–2675. https://doi.org/10.1128/JCM.01321-16

Renshaw AA, Young NA, Birdsong GG, Styer PE, Davey DD, Mody DR, Colgan TJ (2004) Comparison of performance of conventional and ThinPrep gynecologic preparations in the College of American Pathologists Gynecologic Cytology Program. Arch Pathol Lab Med 128(1):17–22

Renshaw AA, Mody DR, Wang E, Haja J, Colgan TJ (2006) Hyperchromatic crowded groups in cervical cytology--differing appearances and interpretations in conventional and ThinPrep preparations: a study from the College of American Pathologists Interlaboratory Comparison Program in Cervicovaginal Cytology. Arch Pathol Lab Med 130(3):332–336

Rozemeijer K, Penning C, Siebers AG, Naber SK, Matthijsse SM, van Ballegooijen M et al (2015) Comparing SurePath, ThinPrep, and conventional cytology as primary test method: SurePath is associated with increased CIN II<Superscript>+</Superscript> detection rates. Cancer Causes Control 27(1):15–25. https://doi.org/10.1007/s10552-015-0678-1

Ruge C, Veit J (1881) Der Krebs der Gebärmutter. Enke, Stuttgart

Rushing L, Cibas ES (1997) Frequency of tumor diathesis in smears from women with squamous cell carcinoma of the cervix. Acta Cytol 41(3):781–785. https://doi.org/10.1159/000332704

Sagasta A, Castillo P, Saco A, Torné A, Esteve R, Marimon L et al (2016) p16 staining has limited value in predicting the outcome of histological low-grade squamous intraepithelial lesions of the cervix. Mod Pathol 29(1):51–59. https://doi.org/10.1038/modpathol.2015.126

Sawaya GF (2008) Evidence-based medicine versus liquid-based cytology. Obstet Gynecol 111(1):2–3. https://doi.org/10.1097/01.AOG.0000298948.65284.d5

Sawaya GF, Sox HC (2007) Trials that matter: liquid-based cervical cytology: disadvantages seem to outweigh advantages. Ann Intern Med 147(9):668–669

Schmidt D, Bergeron C, Denton KJ, Ridder R, European CCSG (2011) p16/ki-67 dual-stain cytology in the triage of ASCUS and LSIL papanicolaou cytology: results from the European equivocal or mildly abnormal Papanicolaou cytology study. Cancer Cytopathol 119(3):158–166. https://doi.org/10.1002/cncy.20140

Selvaggi SM, Guidos BJ (2002) Endocervical component: is it a determinant of specimen adequacy? Diagn Cytopathol 26(1):53–55

Sherman ME, Lorincz AT, Scott DR, Wacholder S, Castle PE, Glass AG et al (2003) Baseline cytology, human papillomavirus testing, and risk for cervical neoplasia: a 10-year cohort analysis. J Natl Cancer Inst 95(1):46–52

Siebert U, Muth C, Sroczynski C, Velasco-Garrido M, Gerhardus A, Gibis BH (2003) Dünnschichtpräparationen und computergestützte Untersuchungen von Zervixabstrichen - Medizinische Effektivität, gesundheitsökonomische Evaluation und systematische Entscheidungsanalyse

Solomon D, Schiffman M, Tarone R (2001) Comparison of three management strategies for patients with atypical squamous cells of undetermined significance: baseline results from a randomized trial. J Natl Cancer Inst 93(4):293–299

Solomon D, Stoler M, Jeronimo J, Khan M, Castle P, Schiffman M (2007) Diagnostic utility of endocervical curettage in women undergoing colposcopy for equivocal or low-grade cytologic abnormalities. Obstet Gynecol 110(2 Pt 1):288–295. https://doi.org/10.1097/01.AOG.0000270154.69879.09

Stoler MH, Castle PE, Solomon D, Schiffman M, American Society for Colposcopy and Cervical Pathology (2007) The expanded use of HPV testing in gynecologic practice per ASCCP-guided management requires the use of well-validated assays. Am J Clin Pathol. https://doi.org/10.1309/RNF3C01JKADQCLKP

Stoler MH, Vichnin MD, Ferenczy A, Ferris DG, Perez G, Paavonen J et al (2011a) The accuracy of colposcopic biopsy: analyses from the placebo arm of the Gardasil clinical trials. Int J Cancer 128(6):1354–1362. https://doi.org/10.1002/ijc.25470

Stoler MH, Wright TC, Sharma A, Apple R, Gutekunst K, Wright TL, ATHENA (Addressing THE Need for Advanced HPV Diagnostics) HPV Study Group (2011b) High-risk human papillomavirus testing in women with ASC-US cytology: results from the ATHENA HPV study. Am J Clin Pathol 135(3):468–475. https://doi.org/10.1309/AJCPZ5JY6FCVNMOT

Stoler MH, Wright TC, Ferenczy A, Ranger-Moore J, Fang Q, Kapadia M, Ridder R (2018) Routine use of adjunctive p16 immunohistochemistry improves diagnostic agreement of cervical biopsy interpretation: results from the CERTAIN study. Am J Surg Pathol 1. https://doi.org/10.1097/PAS.0000000000001072

Stubbe M, Broschewitz U, Kramm G, Schmidt W, Radtke A (2011) Analyse der Konisationen im Zeitraum von 2005 - 2009 in Rostock. Geburtsh Frauenheilk 71:187–193

Sun M, Shen Y, Ren M-L, Dong Y-M (2018) Meta-analysis on the performance of p16/Ki-67 dual immunostaining in detecting high-grade cervical intraepithelial neoplasm. J Cancer Res Ther 14:S587–S593

Thrall MJ, Russell DK, Bonfiglio TA, Hoda RS (2008) Use of the ThinPrep® imaging system does not alter the frequency of interpreting Papanicolaou tests as atypical squamous cells of undetermined significance. Cytojournal 5(1):10. https://doi.org/10.1186/1742-6413-5-10

Tsoumpou I, Arbyn M, Kyrgiou M, Wentzensen N, Koliopoulos G, Martin-Hirsch P et al (2009) p16(INK4a) immunostaining in cytological and histological specimens from the uterine cervix: a systematic review and meta-analysis. Cancer Treat Rev 35(3):210–220. https://doi.org/10.1016/j.ctrv.2008.10.005

van den Einden LC, Grefte JM, van der Avoort IA, Vedder JE, van Kempen LC, Massuger LF, De Hullu JA (2012) Cytology of the vulva: feasibility and preliminary results of a new brush. Br J Cancer 106(2):269–273. https://doi.org/10.1038/bjc.2011.533

Verdoodt F, Jiang X, Williams M, Schnatz PF, Arbyn M (2016) High-risk HPV testing in the management of atypical glandular cells: a systematic review and meta-analysis. Int J Cancer 138(2):303–310. https://doi.org/10.1002/ijc.29424

Verguts J, Bronselaer B, Donders G, Arbyn M, Van Eldere J, Drijkoningen M, Poppe W (2006) Prediction of recurrence after treatment for high-grade cervical intraepithelial neoplasia: the role of human papillomavirus testing and age at conisation. BJOG 113(11):1303–1307

Versi E (1992) "Gold standard" is an appropriate term. BMJ 305(6846):187

Wentzensen N, Schwartz L, Zuna RE, Smith K, Mathews C, Gold MA et al (2012) Performance of p16/Ki-67 immunostaining to detect cervical cancer precursors in a colposcopy referral population. Clin Cancer Res Off J Am Assoc Cancer Res 18(15):4154–4162. https://doi.org/10.1158/1078-0432.CCR-12-0270

Wentzensen NA, Fetterman B, Bremer R, Castle P, Tokugawa D, Poitras N et al (2017) Abstract 5296: evaluation of p16/Ki-67 dual stain, cytology, and HPV16/18 genotyping for triage of HPV-positive women in a large screening population. Cancer Res 77(13 Suppl):5296–5296. https://doi.org/10.1158/1538-7445.AM2017-5296

WHO Classification of Tumours Editorial Board (2020) Female genital tumours. IARC Press, Lyon

Wilbur DC, Black-Schaffer WS, Luff RD, Abraham KP, Kemper C, Molina JT, Tench WD (2009) The Becton Dickinson FocalPoint GS Imaging System: clinical trials demonstrate significantly improved sensitivity for the detection of important cervical lesions. Am J Clin Pathol 132(5):767–775. https://doi.org/10.1309/AJCP8VE7AWBZCVQT

Wright TC Jr, Stoler MH, Behrens CM, Apple R, Derion T, Wright TL (2012) The ATHENA human papillomavirus study: design, methods, and baseline results. Am J Obstet Gynecol 206(1):46.e1–46.e11. https://doi.org/10.1016/j.ajog.2011.07.024

Wright TC, Behrens CM, Ranger-Moore J, Rehm S, Sharma A, Stoler MH, Ridder R (2017) Triaging HPV-positive women with p16/Ki-67 dual-stained cytology: results from a sub-study nested into the ATHENA trial. Gynecol Oncol 144(1):51–56. https://doi.org/10.1016/j.ygyno.2016.10.031

Yoshida T, Sano T, Kanuma T, Inoue H, Itoh T, Yazaki C et al (2011) Usefulness of CINtec(R) PLUS p16/Ki-67 double-staining in cytological screening of cervical cancer. Acta Cytol 55(5):413–420. https://doi.org/10.1159/000331047

Zuchna C, Hager M, Tringler B, Georgoulopoulos A, Ciresa-Koenig A, Volgger B et al (2010) Diagnostic accuracy of guided cervical biopsies: a prospective multicenter study comparing the histopathology of simultaneous biopsy and cone specimen. Am J Obstet Gynecol 203(4):321.e1–321.e6. https://doi.org/10.1016/j.ajog.2010.05.033

Colposcopic Examination

7

Contents

The colposcopic examination starts with the collection of relevant patient data followed by colposcopic inspection including cytological smear collection and then colposcopically guided biopsy or biopsies. In the following section, practical aspects of colposcopy are explained including the use of colposcopic instruments.

The main objective of colposcopic examination is the diagnosis of high-grade dysplastic disease, i.e., the identification of major changes. Most importantly, invasive disease must not be overlooked. Furthermore, the site or sites with the most abnormal changes are identified, and targeted biopsies are obtained.

7.1 History Taking

Prior to colposcopic examination, a detailed history is taken. Table 7.1 lists key points that are relevant to colposcopy. Usually, the patient herself will provide this information. However, it is advisable to obtain copies of prior medical reports, especially on previous Pap smears and HPV test results (type of HPV test).

Cervical dysplasia does not cause any symptoms. However, many patients are worried and anxious and may associate unspecific symptoms with serious disease and cancer. Vaginal bleeding during and after sexual intercourse does not necessarily indicate carcinoma and may occur because of a benign condition such as a large ectopy or inflammation. In the case

R. J. Lellé, V. Küppers, *Colposcopy*, https://doi.org/10.1007/978-3-030-85388-4_7

Table 7.1 Key points for history taking in colposcopy

Reason for referral to the colposcopy clinic/ presenting complaint	• Abnormal Pap smear, presently and in the past • HPV test results • Other relevant test results • Abnormal findings of cervix, vagina, vulva, and anus
Complaints	• Vaginal discharge (inflammatory, bloody) • Vaginal bleeding/spotting (intermenstrual bleeding) • Pain (dyspareunia) • Itching • Genital warts • Abnormal skin areas (including oral mucosa, scalp)
Past medical history (including medication)/previous surgery	• Particularly any diseases, conditions, or medications that may impair the immune system – Inflammatory bowel diseases (medication) – Transplant surgery (medication) – Rheumatic arthritis (medication) – HIV infection, etc. • Previous surgery • Gynecologic operations (see below) • Other operations (bowel, anus)
Previous (gynecologic) surgery	• Conization, LEEP, laser surgery • Sterilization of patient or partner • Hysterectomy (indication)
Pregnancies	• Gravidity and parity • Previous deliveries (cesarian section, obstetrical trauma to the lower genital tract) • Infertility treatment • Future family planning
Sexual history	• Age at first intercourse • Regular sexual partner, number of partners (male/female) • Types of sex (vaginal, oral, anal) • Condom use • Previous STDs • Sexually transmitted diseases (including partner, including drug or surgical condyloma removal)
Contraception/ hormones	• IUD with or without hormones • NuvaRing® • Oral contraceptive • Hormone replacement therapy • Topical estrogen treatment • Barrier contraception (condom)
Smoking	• For how many years • How many cigarettes a day
Allergies	• Iodine

of intermenstrual bleeding (metrorrhagia), however, invasive disease of the uterus needs to be considered.

In contrast to cervical precancer, HSIL of the vulva may cause local discomfort such as itching or pain. In cases of lichen planus of the vulva or vagina, the oral mucosa and/or scalp may also be affected, and the patient should be specifically asked if she has any symptoms in areas outside the lower genital tract.

The presence of an intrauterine device should be noted before the colposcopic examination, as well as vaginal contraceptive devices such as a NuvaRing®. The NuvaRing® should be removed before the examination and reinserted within 3 hours so as not to impair contraception.

The sexual history should be documented also. Considering anxiety and the negative association between dysplasia, HPV infection, and sexual activity, anything should be avoided that may cause or intensify feelings of guilt.

Smoking habits should be documented too, and the association between tobacco use and the risk of intraepithelial neoplasia, especially of the vulva, should be explained. Enrollment in a smoking cessation program should be offered.

Furthermore, it is important to find out if the patient wants to become pregnant in the near future. If the patient does not use hormonal contraception, condoms should be recommended until colposcopic diagnosis and possible surgical treatment have been completed.

Further important aspects of the patient's history are previous surgery, especially procedures directly related to the colposcopic examination, such as conization or hysterectomy. Also, comprehensive information should be gathered about the patient's past medical history. Any diseases or medications that may compromise the immune system are of particular interest.

7.2 Colposcopes

Since Hinselmann's invention in 1925, the basic design of the colposcope has not changed. With an optical colposcope, a magnification of up to 15 or 30 times is possible. For example, the Leisegang colposcope (Leisegang Feinmechanik Optik GmbH, Berlin, Germany) has three steps of magnification: 3.75, 7.5, and 15 times (Fig. 7.1). Usually, the focal length of colposcopes is such that the working distance is about 30 cm.

A more recent concept is the video colposcope. This device does not need complex optical lenses like the classical colposcope. As with laparoscopy, the person doing the colposcopy looks at the monitor while performing the examination, including tissue removal. Although in the year 2000 the majority of physicians still gave preference to the classical optical colposcope (Ferris et al. 2000), the present generation of gynecologists is well versed in laparoscopic techniques and is already used to working via a video screen.

Patients also react positively to video colposcopy, as it helps to explain the colposcopic findings and to improve communication between patient and doctor. Greimel et al. (1997) did a prospective randomized study on the effect of video colposcopy. Patient satisfaction was significantly higher when using video colposcopy. However, video colposcopy does not significantly reduce the anxiety levels of patients when tested in a controlled trial setting (Hilal et al. 2017; Ketelaars et al. 2017).

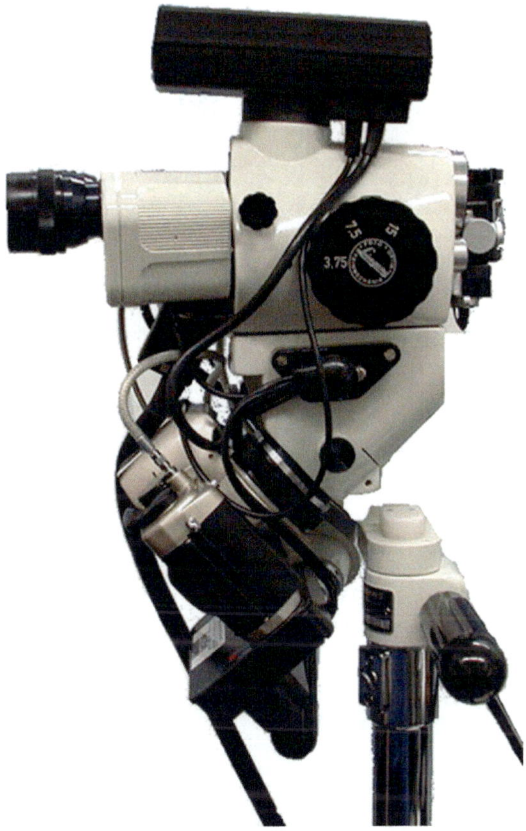

Fig. 7.1 A classic Leisegang colposcope (Leisegang Feinmechanik Optik GmbH, Berlin, Germany) with magnifications of 3.75, 7.5, and 15 times. The attached camera records three-dimensional images

In addition to his well-known colposcope, Hinselmann described the "von Eicken'sche Stirnlampe," a magnification device with a light source mounted on a headset (Fig. 7.2). A modern version of this device using a 4× magnification ("Muenster Colposcopic Magnification Device") can be used as a simple and economical alternative to the conventional colposcope (Lellé 2007), especially when performing surgery (Fig. 7.3).

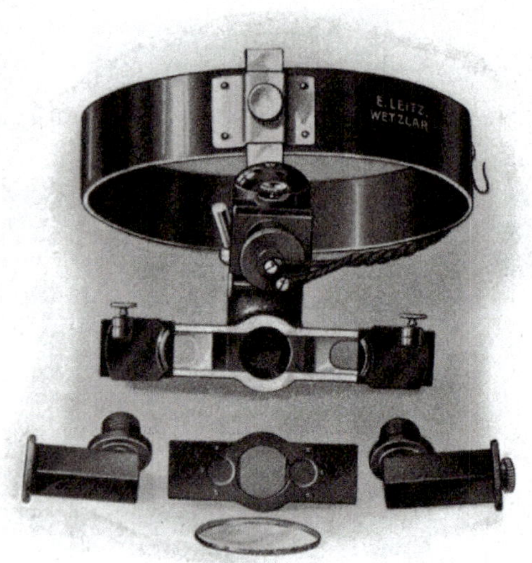

Fig. 7.2 "von Eicken'sche Stirnlampe" as described by Hinselmann in 1925 as an alternative to the classical colposcope (Hinselmann 1925)

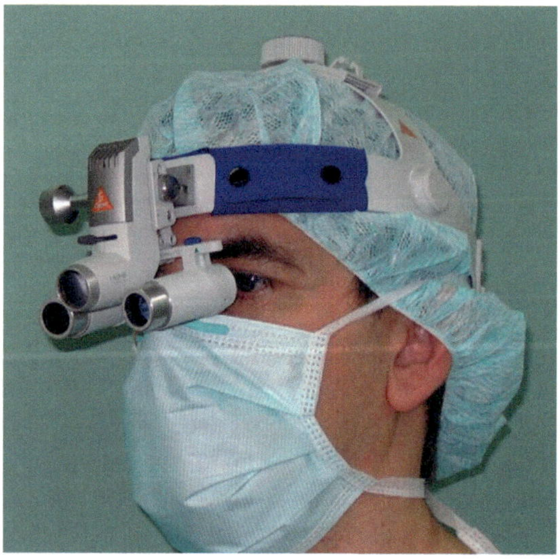

Fig. 7.3 "Muenster Colposcopic Magnification Device" as a modern version of Hinselmann's device (Fig. 7.2) with a 4× magnification. The headset design is particularly useful when performing surgery under colposcopic guidance (Lellé 2007)

With the improvement of digital imaging, a whole range of portable imaging devices has been developed based on smartphone technology (Chap. 17).

7.3 Handling of the Colposcope and Speculum

First, the colposcope needs to be adjusted to the person doing the exam. For the binocular colposcope, first the interpupillary distance is set. As with a microscope, the distance between the oculars is indicated on a scale located between the eyepieces. The diopter settings are initially set to "0," if the colposcopist has 20/20 vision or uses corrective glasses or contact lenses. Alternatively, the diopter settings are adjusted accordingly. Now, the colposcope is focused by moving the head of the colposcope back and forth. Focus is only accomplished when the distance to the target is within the range of the focal distance, which is usually about 30 cm. Some colposcopes are equipped with a mechanism to achieve final focus by moving the colposcope in small increments only.

When an optical colposcope is equipped with a video camera, both the optical and the digital image are brought into focus simultaneously by first adjusting to the image on the monitor. Subsequently, each eyepiece is focused separately using the diopter settings without moving the colposcope.

The colposcopic examination begins with the inspection of the vulva and anus. Occasionally, HSIL of the vulva is identified in an asymptomatic patient, who presents with cervical dysplasia.

Furthermore, the vagina should be carefully inspected. The upper (proximal) portion of the vagina can be evaluated together with the portio. The middle and lower (distal) portion is best examined by slowly retracting the speculum. The partially closed speculum is rotated in order to assess the anterior (ventral) and posterior (dorsal) aspects of the vagina. If there is suspicion of vaginal intraepithelial neoplasia (VAIN), Lugol's solution is applied.

Some colposcopists are using two separate specula for spreading the vagina (e.g., combining the *Seidl* speculum with the *Kristeller* speculum). However, "duckbill" specula such as the Cusco[1] type are better suited for colposcopy, as

[1] Edward Gabriel Cusco, French physician 1819–1894.

both hands remain free. The Grave speculum is also commonly used. In addition to a two-bladed mechanism similar to the Cusco speculum, the valves can be moved further apart.

The speculum chosen for colposcopy must be sufficiently large and adequately shaped. Usually, it is not the size of the speculum that causes discomfort to the patient but an insertion technique that does not take into account the anatomy of the lower genital tract. If the speculum is too small and/or too narrow, the lateral vaginal walls are not sufficiently unfolded and exposed and obstruct the view of the ectocervix (Fig. 7.4).

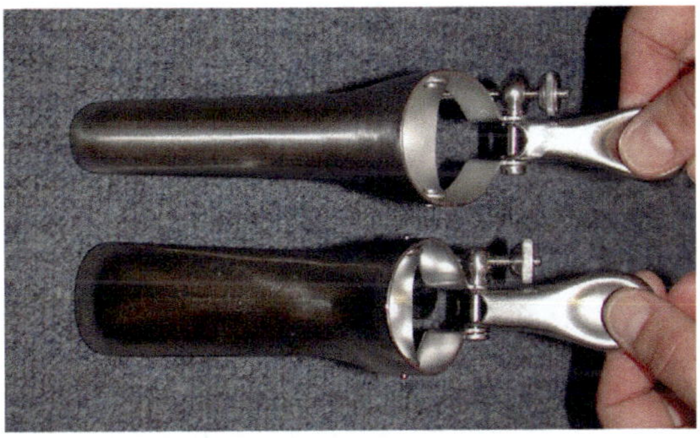

Fig. 7.4 Two Cusco type specula. The speculum in the upper part of the image may be too narrow so that the view of the ectocervix is partially obstructed as the lateral vaginal walls are not sufficiently unfolded

Sometimes, the vaginal walls may still not be sufficiently unfolded, for example, in very obese patients or during a second or third trimester pregnancy. In these situations, the use of a condom, which is pulled over the speculum and cut distally, can be helpful (Fig. 7.5).

Before inserting the speculum, the inside of the thigh is lightly touched with the back of the hand as the immediate contact of the vulva with the speculum may startle the patient. The small labia are spread using the left hand. Then the closed speculum is inserted under pressure in the direction of the posterior fourchette. As the vulvar opening has a vertical axis, the speculum is inserted accordingly. The closed speculum is then rotated clockwise by 90° and fixed by turning the screw (also see Chap. 17).

After inserting the speculum, the position of the examination chair is adjusted so that the colposcopist sits in a comfortable upright position. The patient is typically in a slight head-down position (Fig. 7.6).

First, the colposcope is set to its lowest magnification, as this facilitates focusing. All subsequent steps are now performed under colposcopic guidance.

The cervix and upper vagina are inspected before any manipulation of the cervix. However, excessive mucus may be initially removed using

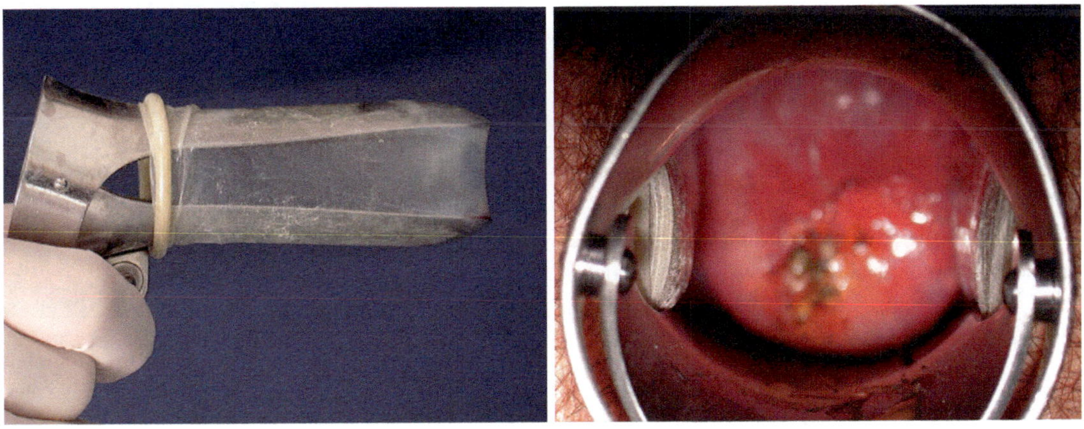

Fig. 7.5 A condom is pulled over the speculum to help to unfold the vaginal wall and improve visualization of the ectocervix

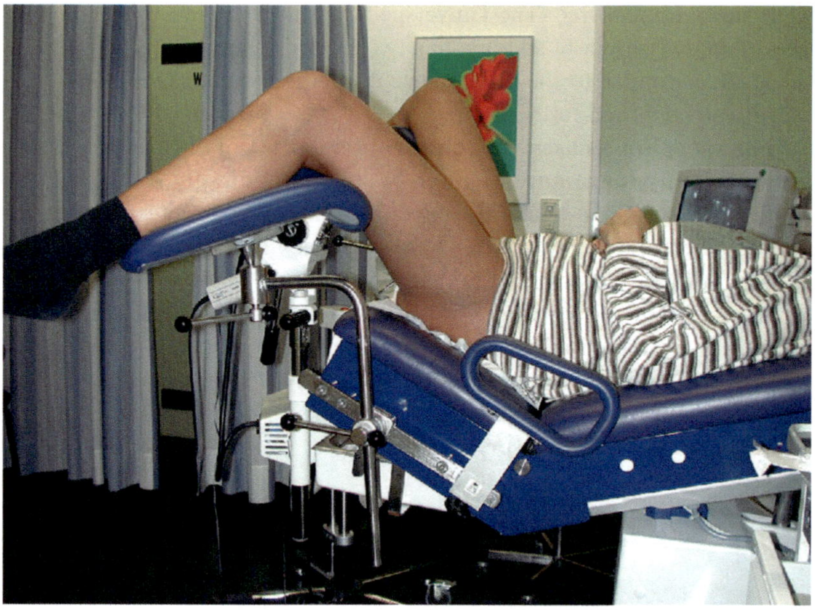

Fig. 7.6 The patient is positioned for colposcopy with the pelvis elevated

a cotton swab. If leukoplakia is identified, a biopsy is obtained after colposcopic inspection using acetic acid and then Lugol's solution has been completed.

Small abnormal vessels are best visualized prior to the application of acetic acid. Acetic acid has a mild vasoconstrictive effect on small blood vessels through tissue edema, thus making these vessels less visible. Some colposcopists use normal saline to remove mucus and improve visualization.

A cytological smear is now obtained. A 3–5% acetic acid solution is now abundantly applied using a cotton swab (Fig. 7.7). Alternatively, a spray bottle may be used.

Usually, application of acetic acid of up to 5% does not cause discomfort. Occasionally, patients will feel a temporary burning sensation.

Using a prospective study design with video documentation, Hilal et al. (2020) were able to determine optimal timing of colposcopic assessment following the application of acetic acid. A 5% acetic acid solution was used. From this well-designed study, the following conclusions can be drawn:

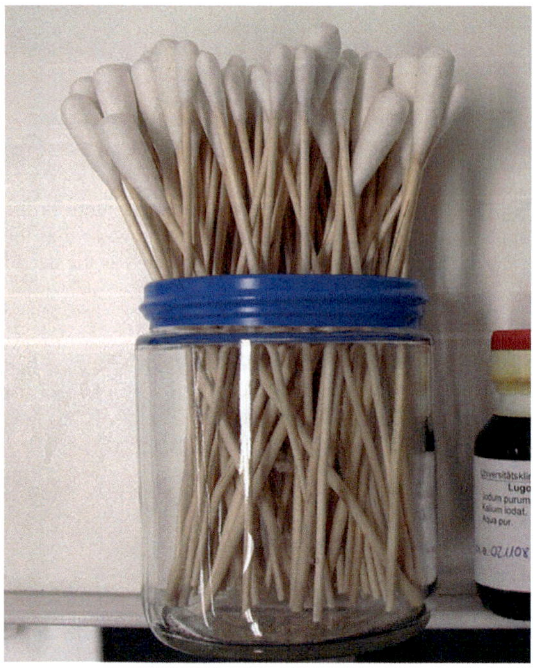

Fig. 7.7 Large and small cotton swabs for the removal of mucus and blood and for application of acetic acid and Lugol's solution

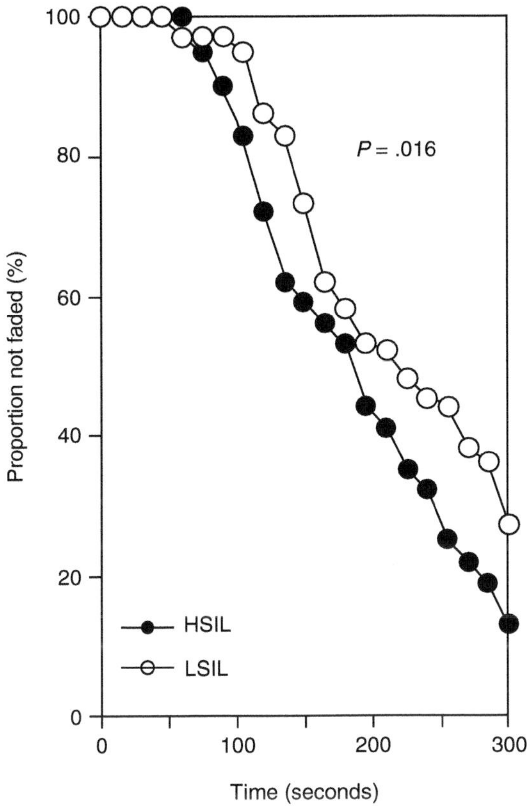

Fig. 7.8 Time dynamics of acetowhite staining and fading. HSIL lesions (filled circles) fade significantly more quickly than LSIL lesions (open circles). The optimal time for diagnosis is about 1 min after the application of acetic acid (Hilal et al. 2020)

- Acetowhite staining develops very quickly. HSIL lesions become visible after a median of 7 seconds, whereas LSIL is first recognized after a median of 19 s.
- Subsequently, staining of both LSIL and HSIL lesions intensifies and reaches its maximum after 50 s.
- A plateau is reached between 1 and 3 min. After that, fading of the acetic acid effect is observed that occurs significantly more quickly in HSIL as in LSIL (Fig. 7.8).

Thus, the optimal time to identify both HSIL and LSIL lesions is 1 min after the application of acetic acid, and colposcopic observation should not be longer than approximately 3 min because of fading of the acetowhite staining.

At this point of the examination, one should determine whether the area where the squamous and glandular epithelium meet (squamocolumnar junction) is completely visible (T1/T2). It may also be helpful to try to define the original squamocolumnar junction, before the physiological changes of metaplasia had occurred. This is only possible if there is still immature metaplasia or if gland openings and/or Nabothian cysts are visible, because, in older women with mature squamous metaplasia, identification of the original squamocolumnar junction is not possible anymore. The transformation zone, i.e., the area between the current and the original squamocolumnar junction, is the major area of interest, where squamous intraepithelial neoplasia is most likely to occur.

According to a survey from eight colposcopy centers (Luyten et al. 2015), the squamocolumnar junction can be visualized in the majority of patients (81%). A T3 transformation zone was found to be the most commonly reported type in women older than 50 years (70%).

Visualization of the entire squamocolumnar junction is usually accomplished by spreading the outer cervical canal with the Kogan endocervical speculum (Fig. 7.9) or by using two dry cotton swabs.

Visualization of vascular structures can be enhanced by using the green filter. The filter should be used both before and after the application of the acetic acid. Under the green filter, vessels appear black and have a better contrast to the surrounding tissue. Also, punctation and mosaic are seen more clearly, as these two phenomena are due to the peculiar morphology of subepithelial capillaries.

Now, Lugol's solution is applied to the cervix and upper vagina, if the patient is not allergic to iodine, as an anaphylactic-like reaction with vaginal and generalized pruritus, vaginal edema, hypotension, tachycardia, and breathing difficulties has been documented by Indraccolo et al. (2009).

Finally, any abnormal findings of the ectocervix or upper vagina are biopsied including endocervical curettage.

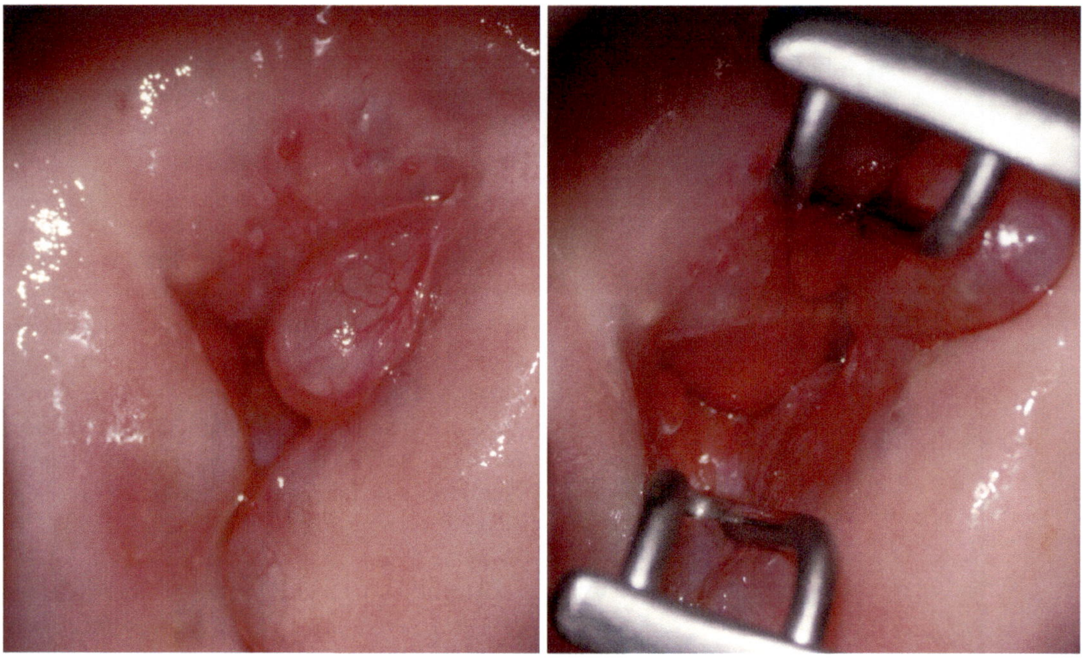

Fig. 7.9 Kogan speculum. A pedunculated Nabothian cyst is pushed aside to visualize the squamocolumnar junction (T2)

7.4 Cytological Smear

When colposcopic triage for an abnormal Pap smear is performed, repeat cytology is not required in the majority of cases.

The Pap test is intended for screening and not for definitive diagnosis, as it does not come close the specificity of histopathologic evaluation. Also, if the interval between two cytological smears is short, false-negative results seem to be more common. This problem has been known for a long time (Meisels 1990). Drescher et al. (1983) obtained a cytological smear immediately prior to colposcopic biopsy in 540 patients. Pap smears were false negative in 26.4% of patients. In a more recent study, Kolben et al. (2017) showed that the risk of a false-negative result of a second smear taken immediately after the first is not statistically significant, although a tendency toward a more benign outcome in the second smear was observed.

However, only 1.2–2.0% of repeat cytological examinations obtained during colposcopy have an influence on management decisions (Young et al. 1993; Panos et al. 2001). Panos et al. found a high false-negative rate of 19%. However, Zardawi and Rode (2002) saw some benefit of the repeat Pap test, if the previous smear had shown only mild dysplasia.

Hall et al. (2011) concluded that repeat cytology provides useful clinical information in only 3.6% of patients. However, when the patient is referred for evaluation of HSIL, the repeat Pap test provided potentially useful information in 41% of cases.

If the Pap test is repeated at the time of colposcopic triage, it should be obtained prior to the application of acetic acid.

After the acetic acid test, the cell yield is significantly lower and the rate of unsatisfactory false-negative results is higher (Griffiths et al. 1989; Cronje et al. 1997).

7.5 Tissue Sampling

Obtaining one or more colposcopically directed biopsies from the cervix or vagina and performing endocervical curettage are integral parts of colposcopy, as colposcopic assessment alone has a low specificity, even when done by an experienced colposcopist.

The procedure of tissue sampling should be explained to the patient in advance, and her consent should be obtained as for any surgical procedure. If the patient is relaxed and confidently goes into the examination, she will find colposcopy and tissue sampling less uncomfortable. It is also crucial that the medical assistant is well acquainted with the procedure and contributes to a anxiety-free atmosphere.

As biopsy results will only be available at a later date, these results have to be related to the patient in a timely fashion together with possible treatment or follow-up suggestions.

7.5.1 Biopsy

Colposcopic biopsy is usually done without local anesthesia as most patient will experience only minor discomfort. However, a recent prospective randomized trial suggests that injection of a local anesthetic makes the procedure less painful (Kiviharju et al. 2017). Another controlled prospective study has shown that forced coughing can also provide significant pain relief (Akavia et al. 2018).

Tissue samples are always "targeted," i.e., taken under direct colposcopic guidance. Biopsies are obtained from areas with the most severe changes. As a rule, higher-grade lesions are more likely located close to the squamocolumnar junction. Also, colposcopic phenomena that are considered to be pathognomonic for high-grade disease such as inner border sign, ridge sign, or rag sign should be biopsied.

Several biopsy forceps types are available such as Tischler (Figs. 7.10 and 7.11), Eppendorfer, Kevorkian, or Burke. The tips of these instruments are of different sizes and shapes. However, size is not decisive, as it is not necessary to make use of the entire cutting surface. For histological evaluation, a few millimeters of tissue are sufficient.

To prevent the biopsy forceps from slipping off a smooth and firm tissue surface, a hook-like instrument can be used to immobilize the cervix. Similar problems may be encountered in the vagina, especially on the lateral vaginal walls. By slightly closing and retracting the speculum, tension is released and the biopsy forceps can be applied to the slightly folded vaginal wall.

If the tissue sample is taken too superficially, only dysplastic epithelium that is detached from the stroma may be seen on histopathological examination so that possible invasion cannot be assessed. If ulceration is present, biopsies should not be limited to the ulcerating area. The lesion's margin also needs to be biopsied so that the pathologist is better able

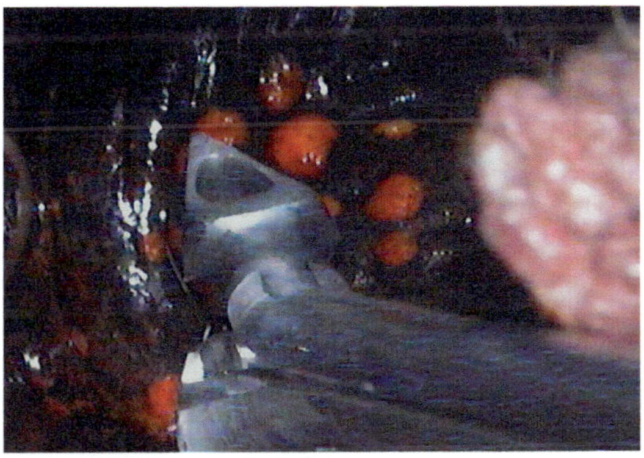

Fig. 7.11 Targeted biopsy under colposcopic guidance with a Tischler forceps

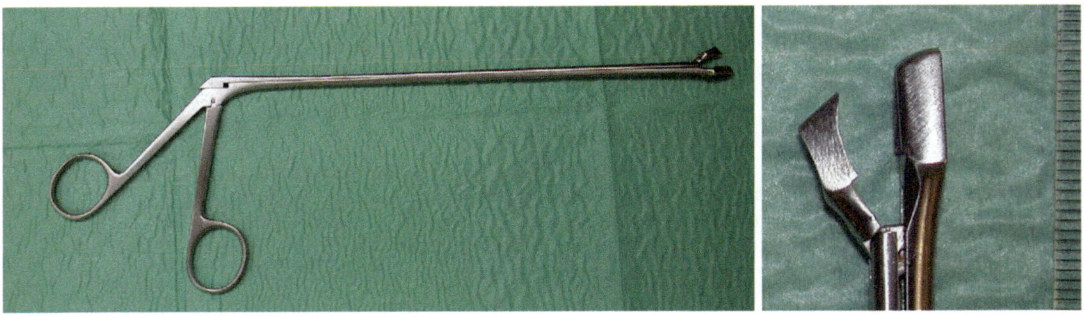

Fig. 7.10 Tischler biopsy forceps

to ascertain invasion of tumor cells through the basal membrane.

The cervix is well supplied with blood, and the amount of bleeding resulting from even a small biopsy can be upsetting to a less experienced colposcopist. However, satisfactory hemostasis can always be achieved if there are no coagulation disorders.

If one is uncomfortable with the amount of bleeding, especially during pregnancy, a loose tampon can be applied, which the patient can remove herself after a couple of hours.

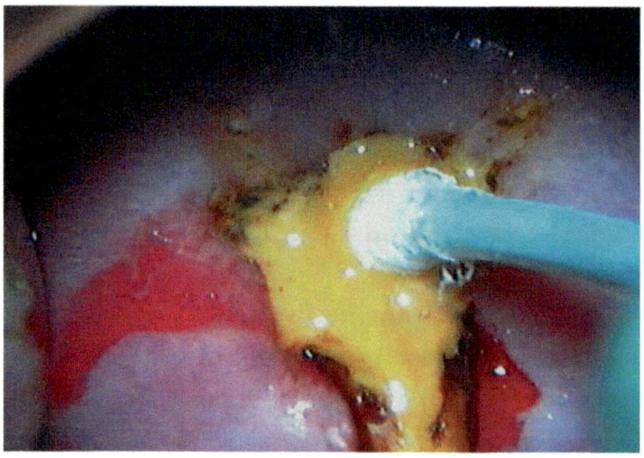

Fig. 7.12 Monsel's solution for hemostasis after cervical biopsy

For better control of bleeding during the procedure, the biopsy forceps is held in one hand and a cotton swab in the other to immediately apply pressure onto the biopsy site. A hemostatic agent such as Monsel's solution can then be used (Fig. 7.12). Monsel's solution is ferric subsulfate solution named after Léon Monsel, a military apothecary of Bordeaux, France, who in 1856 reported on its hemostatic effect (Monsel 1856).

There are different ways for preparing Monsel's solution or Monsel's paste. The procedure that is recommended by the World Health Organization (2014) is given in Table 7.2.

If necessary, a large tampon is inserted, the tip of which has been immersed in Monsel's solution. The patient must be made aware that she will have a greenish black discharge for some time after the biopsy.

Hilal et al. (2016) have tested the efficacy of Monsel's solution in a randomized trial setting. The control group did not receive any hemostatic agent. Overall, the clinical benefit of Monsel's

Table 7.2 Preparation of Monsel's solution (World Health Organization 2014)

Ingredients	Quantity
1. Ferric sulfate base	15 g
2. Ferrous sulfate powder	a few grains
3. Sterlle water for mixing	10 ml
4. Glycerol starch (see preparation on next page)	12 g

Preparation:

Take care, as the reaction is exothermic (emits heat).

1. Add a few grains of ferrous sulfate powder to10 ml of sterile water in a glass beaker. Shake.
2. Dissolve the ferric sulfate base in the solution by stirring with a glass stick. The solution should become crystal clear.
3. Weigh the glycerol starch (see preparation instructions below) in a glass mortar. Mix well.
4. Slowly add the ferric sulfate solution to the glycerol starch constantly mixing to get a homogeneous mixture.
5. Place in a 25-ml brown glass bottle.

Note: Most clinics prefer to leave the stopper of the bottle loose, to allow the mixture to evaporate until it has a sticky paste-like consistency and looks like mustard. This may take 2-3 weeks, depending on the environment. The top of the bottle can then be secured for storage. If necessary, sterile water can be added to the paste to thin it.

Label: Monsel's paste
Store in a cool place
For external use only
Use by: [day/month/year] (one year from date of preparation)

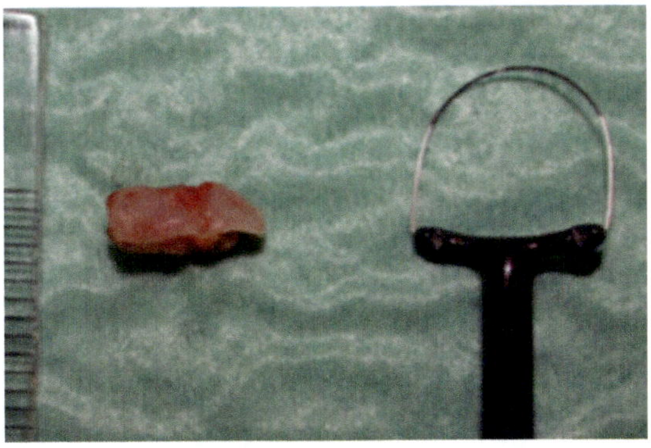

Fig. 7.13 Small electrosurgical loop for targeted biopsy, performed as in-office procedure (LEEP)

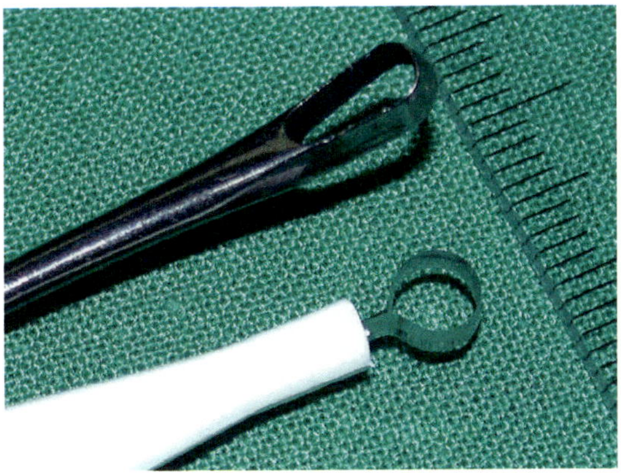

Fig. 7.14 Ring curette (Stiefel®) for endocervical curettage in comparison to a conventional instrument

solution was low. Although bleeding was reduced significantly for 6 h after biopsy, it did not reduce pain or increase overall satisfaction.

Targeted colposcopic biopsies may also be obtained by using a small electrosurgical loop (Fig. 7.13). In some cases, a small lesion can be removed completely as an in-office gynecological procedure.

7.5.2 Endocervical Curettage

If the squamocolumnar junction is not visible, or if there is cytologic evidence of abnormal endocervical gland cells, endocervical curettage (ECC) is performed. Usually, endocervical curettage is done without anesthesia, because the internal cervical os does not need to be dilated as with regular D&C. A narrow curette is used, which can be inserted into the cervical canal without resistance.

When pulling back the curette, pressure is applied. The curette is then washed out in normal saline, and the procedure is repeated three more times in order to sample all four quadrants before the tissue is transferred into the fixative. Endocervical curettage is always done while looking through the colposcope.

The use of a ring curette (Stiefel® curette) is recommended (Fig. 7.14). Originally, this type of curette has been designed for superficial skin biopsies in dermatology. Its sharp scalpel-like edge ensures that a sufficient amount of tissue is obtained. If the cervical canal is narrow, the ring of the curette can be compressed using a sterile clamp (Fig. 7.15).

Drescher et al. (1983) found a positive endocervical curettage result in 17.9% of patients with a visible squamocolumnar junction (T1/T2), including several patients with a normal-appearing ectocervix. While some colposcopists regularly perform endocervical curettage, others rely on the cytological smear, which is obtained by inserting a brush into the endocervical canal. According to Weitzman et al. (1988), the diagnostic information of both methods is comparable.

Liu et al. (2017) recommend routine ECC in women aged 45 years or older with HPV 16 infection. All women aged 30 years or older should receive endocervical curettage, if any of the following criteria are met:

- HSIL (or higher) or ASC-H
- Colposcopy: major change
- ASC-US or LSIL, when the entire transformation zone is not visible (T3)

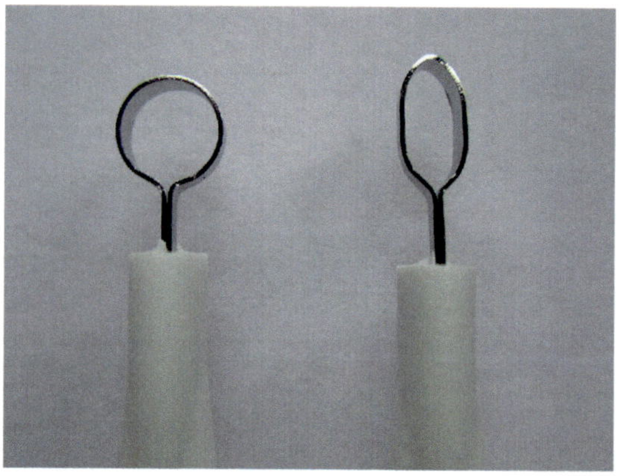

Fig. 7.15 If the cervical canal is narrow, the ring of the Stiefel® curette can be compressed using a sterile clamp

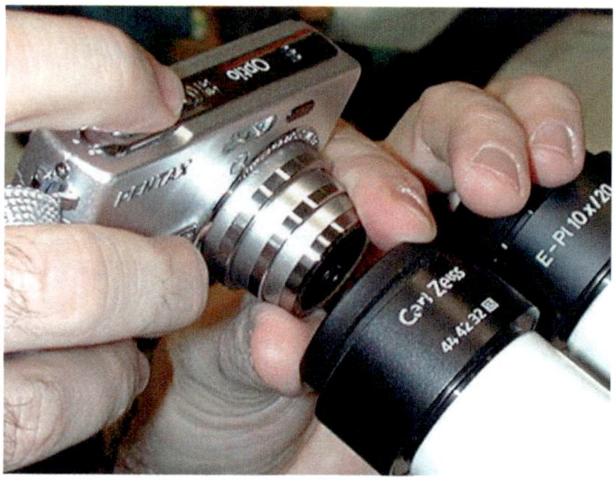

Fig. 7.16 Photographic documentation through the eyepiece of the colposcope

7.6 Documentation

To document colposcopic findings, a drawing can be made outlining the localization and shape of abnormal areas and illustrating the biopsy site. An essential component of all documentation is the localization of the squamocolumnar junction or a statement as to whether the junction is completely visible (T1) or can be visualized (T2).

Photographic documentation has many advantages. For continuous learning, the colposcopist should always compare colposcopic findings and histological results.

For image or video capture, several technical solutions are available, including the three-dimensional recording of slides. With most compact digital cameras, images can be taken directly through the eyepiece of the optical colposcope (Figs. 7.16 and 7.17). This works just as well with a microscope as with any colposcope.

Figure 7.18 depicts a custom-made smartphone adapter, which can be adjusted to both microscopes and colposcopes.

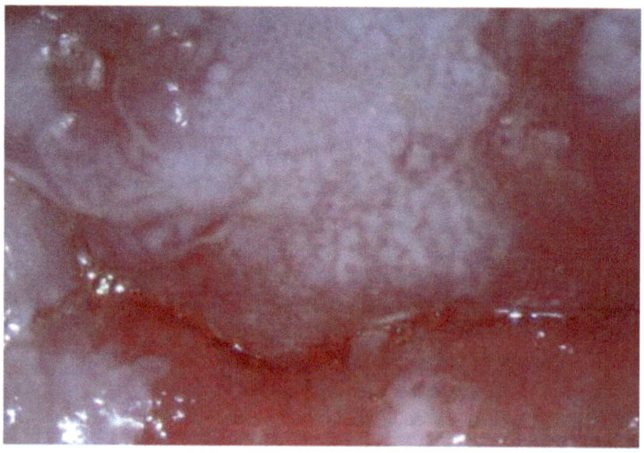

Fig. 7.17 Photographic documentation through the eyepiece of the colposcope. Major change with irregular punctation and coarse mosaic

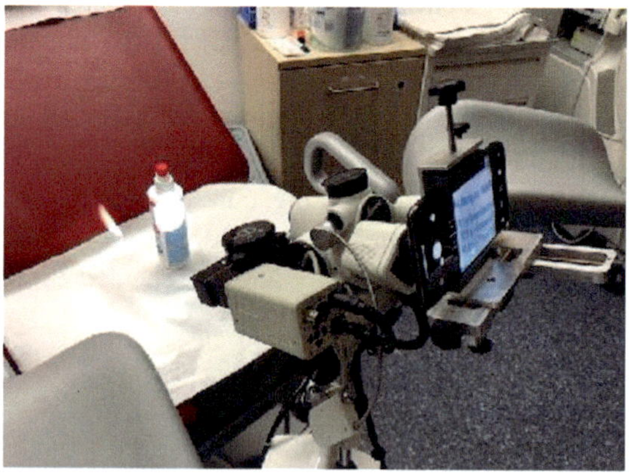

Fig. 7.18 Smartphone adapter attached to the eyepiece of a standard colposcope

7.7 Practical Colposcopic Examination Step by Step

Step #1	**Take patient's history**	See Table 7.1
Step #2	**Inform the patient about the exam and obtain informed consent**	Providing information and addressing the patient's concern (fertility, hysterectomy, cancer) prior to colposcopy will greatly reduce anxiety
Step #3	**Label the specimen containers and slides**	Always label containers prior to obtaining the specimens to avoid any mix-up
Step #4	**Inspect vulva and anus**	CIN, HSIL of the vulva, AIN, and condylomata acuminata are all HPV-associated and can occur simultaneously
Step #5	**Insert the speculum**	Use a Cusco or Grave speculum that is wide enough to allow adequate colposcopic assessment. Use a proper technique for handling the speculum to avoid unnecessary discomfort Change gloves. From now on, touch colposcope and instruments only
Step #6	**Adjust the position of the gynecologic exam chair and focus the colposcope**	Place the colposcope in a comfortable working position and adjust the patient's position on the examination chair accordingly (not vice versa)
Step #7	**Inspect cervix and upper vagina**	Use different magnifications. Use green filter. Start with photo or video documentation
Step #8	**Obtain Pap smear**	Remove cervical mucus and take Pap smear under colposcopic guidance See Sect. 7.4 about indications for Pap test during colposcopic triage
Step #9	**Apply 5% acetic acid solution**	The optimal time to identify HSIL and LSIL lesions is 1 min after the application of acetic acid. Colposcopic observation should not be longer than about 3 min because of fading of the acetic acid effect (Hilal et al. 2020)
Step #10	**Inspect cervix and upper vagina again**	Step #10 is the most important part of colposcopic assessment, as minor and major changes, and sometimes cancer, may be identified Spread the cervical canal with Kogan speculum or other suitable device if required
Step #11	**Photo/video documentation**	Alternatively, a drawing by hand is also acceptable
Step #12	**Apply Lugol's solution**	After Lugol's solution, repeat or continue photo/video documentation
Step #13	**Obtain biopsy and/or endocervical curettage under colposcopic guidance**	If in doubt, obtain tissue samples. Always consider biopsy of grade 1/minor change lesions
Step #14	**Ensure hemostasis**	Use Monsel's solution. In case of heavier bleeding, insert tampon
Step #15	**Inspect the vagina**	The middle and lower one-third of the vagina is inspected when slowly retracting and rotating the speculum. If VAIN is suspected, Lugol's solution is applied

Step #16	**Bimanual transvaginal and transrectal examination**	This is not a routine part of colposcopic triage when there is no evidence of malignant disease
Step #17	**Check for vasovagal reaction before the patient gets out of the examination chair**	Ask the patient if she has had a vasovagal reaction before. Watch for symptoms and be prepared
Step #18	**Document the colposcopic findings and explain them to the patient**	This is another important element to decrease patient's anxiety levels
Step #19	**Write final report with further management recommendations**	This should be done in a timely fashion. The patient should also receive a copy of the report

References

Akavia TG, Segev Y, Balan E, Siegler E (2018) The analgesic efficacy of forced coughing during cervical punch biopsy: a prospective randomised controlled study. Aust N Z J Obstet Gynaecol 52(2):342. https://doi.org/10.1111/ajo.12784

Cronje HS, Divall P, Bam RH, Cooreman BF, Niemand I (1997) Effects of dilute acetic acid on the cervical smear. Acta Cytol 41(4):1091–1094

Drescher CW, Peters WA III, Roberts JA (1983) Contribution of endocervical curettage in evaluating abnormal cervical cytology. Obstet Gynecol 62(3):343–347

Ferris DG, Ho TH, Guijon F (2000) A comparison of colposcopy using optical and video colposcopes. J Low Genit Tract Dis 4:65

Greimel ER, Gappmayer-Locker E, Girardi FL, Huber HP (1997) Increasing women's knowledge and satisfaction with cervical cancer screening. J Psychosom Obstet Gynaecol 18(4):273–279

Griffiths M, Turner MJ, Partington CK, Soutter WP (1989) Should smears in a colposcopy clinic be taken after the application of acetic acid? Acta Cytol 33(3): 324–326

Hall JM, Han JJ, Fadare O (2011) The value of repeated cytology at the time of first colposcopya retrospective analysis of 1,087 cases. Am J Clin Pathol 135(4):628–636. https://doi.org/10.1309/AJCP25UEVETXTNBF

Hilal Z, Rezniczek GA, Tettenborn Z, Hefler LA, Tempfer CB (2016) Efficacy of monsel solution after cervical biopsy: a randomized trial. J Low Genit Tract Dis 20(4):312–316. https://doi.org/10.1097/LGT.0000000000000234

Hilal Z, Alici F, Tempfer CB, Seebacher V, Rezniczek GA (2017) Video colposcopy for reducing patient anxiety during colposcopy: a randomized controlled trial. Obstet Gynecol 130(2):411–419. https://doi.org/10.1097/AOG.0000000000002127

Hilal Z, Tempfer CB, Burgard L, Rehman S, Rezniczek GA (2020) How long is too long? Application of acetic acid during colposcopy: a prospective study. Am J Obstet Gynecol. https://doi.org/10.1016/j.ajog.2020.01.038

Hinselmann H (1925) Verbesserung der Inspektionsmöglichkeiten von Vulva, Vagina und Portio. MMWR 72:1733

Indraccolo U, Palombino K, Greco P (2009) Anaphylactic-like reaction to lugol solution during colposcopy. South Med J 102(1):96–97. https://doi.org/10.1097/SMJ.0b013e31818894f4

Ketelaars PJW, Buskes MHM, Bosgraaf RP, van Hamont D, Prins JB, Massuger LFAG et al (2017) The effect of video information on anxiety levels in women attending colposcopy: a randomized controlled trial. Acta Oncol 56(12):1728–1733. https://doi.org/10.1080/0284186X.2017.1355108

Kiviharju M, Kalliala I, Nieminen P, Dyba T, Riska A, Jakobsson M (2017) Pain sensation during colposcopy and cervical biopsy, with or without local anesthesia: a randomized trial. J Low Genit Tract Dis 21(2):102–107. https://doi.org/10.1097/LGT.0000000000000292

Kolben TM, Bergauer F, Moeckel J, Boettcher B, Thaler CJ, Kolben T et al (2017) Short interval between two Pap smears: effect on the result of the second smear? A prospective randomized trial. Arch Gynecol Obstet 295(6):1427–1433. https://doi.org/10.1007/s00404-017-4369-x

Lellé RJ (2007) Die Münster-Kolposkopielupe - eine Alternative zum konventionellen Kolposkop. Geburtshilfe Frauenheilkd 67:154–155

Liu AH-C, Walker J, Gage JC, Gold MA, Zuna R, Dunn ST et al (2017) Diagnosis of cervical precancers by endocervical curettage at colposcopy of women with abnormal cervical cytology. Obstet Gynecol 130(6):1218–1225. https://doi.org/10.1097/AOG.0000000000002330

Luyten A, Buttmann-Schweiger N, Hagemann I, Scherbring S, Boehmer G, Gieseking F et al (2015) Utility and reproducibility of the international federation for cervical pathology and colposcopy classification of transformation zones in daily practice: a multicenter study of the German Colposcopy Network. J Low Genit Tract Dis 19(3):185–188. https://doi.org/10.1097/LGT.0000000000000069

Meisels A (1990) Are two smears better than one? Letter 34(3):459–460

Monsel ML (1856) Propriété hémostatique du sulfate de peroxyde de fer. Recueil Mémoirs Méd 17: 424–434

Panos JC, Jones BA, Mazzara PF (2001) Usefulness of concurrent Papanicolaou smear at time of cervical biopsy. Diagn Cytopathol 25(4):270–273

Weitzman GA, Korhonen MO, Reeves KO, Irwin JF, Carter TS, Kaufman RH (1988) Endocervical brush cytology. An alternative to endocervical curettage? J Reprod Med 33(8):677–683

World Health Organization (2014) Comprehensive cervical cancer control. A guide to essential practice, 2nd edn. Springer, New York

Young NA, Naryshkin S, Bowman RL (1993) Value of repeat cervical smears at the time of colposcopic biopsy. Diagn Cytopathol 9(6):646–649

Zardawi IM, Rode JW (2002) Clinical value of repeat Pap smear at the time of colposcopy. Acta Cytol 46(3):495–498

8 Operative Colposcopy

Contents

The term "operative colposcopy" refers to the use of the colposcope during ablative and/or destructive treatment of cervical, vaginal, and vulvar precancerous lesions. In the following chapter, various procedures such as cold-knife conization, LEEP, cryosurgery, and CO_2 laser vaporization are described. Also, follow-up assessment of successful removal of squamous and glandular precancerous lesions is discussed.

The term "operative colposcopy" refers to the use of the colposcope during all procedures for treatment of precancerous lesions of the lower genital tract including perianal or anal lesions. Under colposcopic magnification, the affected tissue can be completely and gently removed avoiding unnecessary tissue loss. Ideally, all gynecologists performing these procedures, which are often regarded as "minor surgery," should be trained in colposcopy.

The use of the colposcope during surgery for cervical intraepithelial lesions has a direct impact on the size of resection.

According to Heineman et al. (2016), colposcopic guidance led to significant reduction of the height and diameter of the excised specimen. However, in this retrospective study, no significant reduction of the rate of treatment failure could be demonstrated. A prospective randomized trial (Hilal et al. 2018) confirmed that intraoperative colposcopy significantly reduces the amount of tissue removed. At the same time, margin status is not compromised, i.e., in the groups with and without intraoperative colposcopy, R0 resection was achieved in more than 80% of patients.

To date, the treatment of precancerous lesions of the cervix is always done surgically, as there are no effective drugs for conservative treatment. A therapeutic HPV vaccine is not yet available.

Imiquimod, which is used for topical treatment of condylomata acuminata, is a potential candidate for medical treatment of HPV-induced precancer. A study on topical application of

R. J. Lellé, V. Küppers, *Colposcopy*, https://doi.org/10.1007/978-3-030-85388-4_8

imiquimod (Aldara®) showed that 73% of high-grade lesions of the cervix responded to treatment compared to 39% in the placebo group (Grimm et al. 2012). However, patients require imiquimod treatment for at least 16 weeks. In comparison, a colposcopically guided tissue-sparing cervical resection will take only a few minutes to perform and is much more effective with a success rate of over 90%.

Van de Sande et al. (2018) initiated a non-inferiority trial on imiquimod treatment of patients with recurrent cervical intraepithelial neoplasia in order to avoid potential adverse outcomes of future pregnancies caused by multiple cervical resections. A 5% imiquimod cream was used intravaginally three times a week for 16 weeks. Patients in the standard arm were treated by LLETZ. Ultimately, this prospective randomized trial concept had to be changed as not enough patients agreed to randomization (Koeneman et al. 2017). Obviously, a strong patient preference existed for either modality. Therefore, the study had to be continued in a nonrandomized open-label design. Treatment was successful in 95% of patients who opted for loop resection, whereas topical imiquimod treatment was successful in 59% only. Furthermore, all patients treated with imiquimod reported side effects, most frequently headaches and fatigue.

In summary, ablation or destruction of the dysplastic epithelium remains the treatment of choice for persistent high-grade squamous intraepithelial neoplasia of the cervix.

It is unclear how much cervical tissue should be removed as there are no reliable data available. However, Kolben et al. (2019) tried to evaluate limited excision of the dysplastic lesion (CIN3) in order to limit the amount of resected tissue. Limited resection was compared to the standard approach, i.e., removal of the entire transformation zone. Unfortunately, the prospective randomized trial was terminated early after inclusion of 50 patients in each group due to slow accrual. However, preliminary results seem to favor limited resection. As was to be expected, cone size was significantly lower in the limited resection group (1.02 ccm versus 1.97 ccm, respectively). After 6 months of follow-up, this patient group did not have a lower rate of HPV-negative test results compared to the standard resection group (80% versus 78%), although margins were more frequently involved (20% versus 8%).

8.1 Risks for Future Pregnancies

Kyrgiou et al. (2006) came to the conclusion that all ablative surgical procedures—with the exception of CO_2 laser vaporization alone—lead to a significantly increased rate of premature births with a relative risk of delivery before the 37th week of gestation of 2.59 after conization and 1.70 after loop resection (LEEP). Many clinicians and several national guidelines, including Germany, consider the classic cold-knife conization obsolete. Arbyn et al. (2008) also came to the conclusion that perinatal mortality is increased after cold-knife conization and presumably also following laser surgery or extensive electrosurgical resections.

Especially for treatment of reproductive age patients, the scalpel should not be used anymore.

Ortoft et al. (2010) found that conization increases perinatal mortality by a factor of 2.8. This is due to the fact that the likelihood of extreme prematurity (delivery before the 28th week) is increased by a factor of 4.9. Thirty-seven patients underwent two consecutive cervical resections. For those, the risk of premature delivery was tenfold higher than in women without previous conization.

Cone length appears to play an important role. If the specimen is longer than 1 cm, Simoens et al. (2012) found a statistically significant increase of premature births. According to Poon et al. (2012), the risk of premature birth can be estimated by measuring cervical length between the 20th and 24th week of gestation. However, obstetrical management of patients with a history of surgery for CIN is not clear (Quenby 2010).

In contrast to the studies mentioned above, Castanon et al. (2012), who analyzed data from the UK health system, did not find a significant increase in preterm deliveries following loop excision of cervical dysplasia and suggested that this might be related to British quality management and the fact that resection volume was kept to a minimum.

A systematic review and meta-analysis involving 36,954 patients treated during pregnancy and 1,794,174 controls still leaves several questions unanswered (Jin et al. 2013). LEEP was in fact associated with a risk of preterm delivery both before week 32 and week 28. However, although a cervical length of less than 3 cm occurred significantly more frequently in treated patients, a larger resection volume or depth was not found to be associated with an increased risk of preterm delivery. Also, perinatal mortality was not increased by prior LEEP.

Preoperative colposcopic diagnosis and colposcopically guided surgery are potentially able to reduce the rate of pregnancy complications. Despite the findings quoted above, it might still be useful to document the resection volume. The tissue volume can easily be measured by determining its fluid displacement according to Archimedes' principle immediately following the procedure (Fig. 8.1).

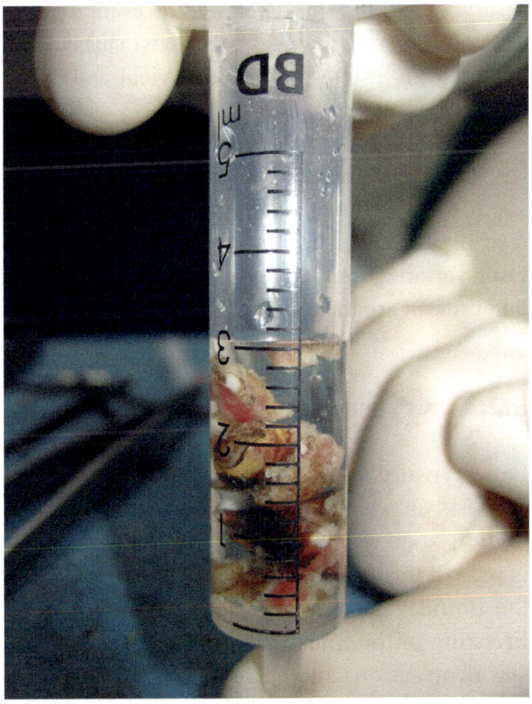

Fig. 8.1 Measurement of the resection volume of LEEP using the Archimedes' principle. From a sealed 5 or 10 ml syringe, the plunger is removed and half filled with saline. The removed tissue is placed into the saline. The increase of the fluid level is equal to the resection volume

The goal of all surgical procedures for premalignant disease of the lower genital tract is the complete removal of all dysplastic epithelium without excessive damage to healthy tissue. This can be achieved either by resection or tissue destruction or a combination of the two.

According to the recommendations of the IFCPC (Bornstein et al. 2012), nonstandardized terms such as "conization" or "loop excision" should be avoided. Instead, excision types 1, 2, and 3 are defined in analogy to the three types of transformation zones: T1, T2, and T3.

The goal of surgical treatment of premalignant disease of the cervix is to cause as little damage as possible to healthy tissue. This is especially important in reproductive age patients, as any type of cervical resection has the potential to significantly increase the risk of premature delivery and thus the risk of perinatal morbidity and mortality. In young patients, the resection volume should be as low as possible without compromising complete removal of disease. Wide resection margins, which are essential in oncologic surgery, must be considered overtreatment in precancerous lesions and should be avoided.

8.2 Surgical Procedures

8.2.1 Cold-Knife Conization

Through cold-knife conization, a more or less cone-shaped piece of cervical tissue is obtained by using either a regular scalpel or an angled conization scalpel. Usually, the goal of cold-knife conization is the complete removal of the transformation zone and not just a limited area of the cervix. This fairly bloody procedure cannot be performed under colposcopic guidance, and it is usually done under general or spinal anesthesia.

Staining with Lugol's iodine serves as a guide to the position of the transformation zone. Most surgeons place lateral cervical sutures at 3 and 9 o'clock to reduce bleeding by ligating the lower branches of the uterine artery. Instead of monopolar coagulation, the so-called Sturmdorf suture used to be performed for hemostasis. By placing sutures anteriorly and posteriorly, the edges of the remaining cervix are folded inward in order to compress the cervical surface for hemostasis. However, the Sturmdorf procedure will make it more difficult to evaluate the cervix during follow-up colposcopic exams so that it is preferably to use monopolar coagulation instead of sutures.

Kalliala et al. (2007) conducted a retrospective study over a 30-year period and determined that cold-knife conization is the least effective method compared to all other surgical treatment options with regard to prevention of recurrences (severe dysplasia or carcinoma). Santesso et al. (2016) compared data on cold-knife conization, LEEP, and cryotherapy for the treatment of CIN. The systematic review and meta-analysis were disappointing as mostly low-quality evidence was identified with a lack of prospective randomized studies, most importantly regarding pregnancy outcomes. Recurrence rate was 5.3% 12 months after LEEP or cryotherapy compared to only 1.4% following cold-knife conization. However, complications including long-term pregnancy-related problems appeared to occur more frequently after cold-knife conization.

8.2.2 Monopolar Loop Resection (LEEP)

With LEEP (*L*oop *E*lectrosurgical *E*xcision *P*rocedure) or LLETZ (*L*arge *L*oop *E*xcision of the *T*ransformation *Z*one), resection of either the entire transformation zone or of a specific lesion is possible using loops of different sizes (Fig. 8.2).

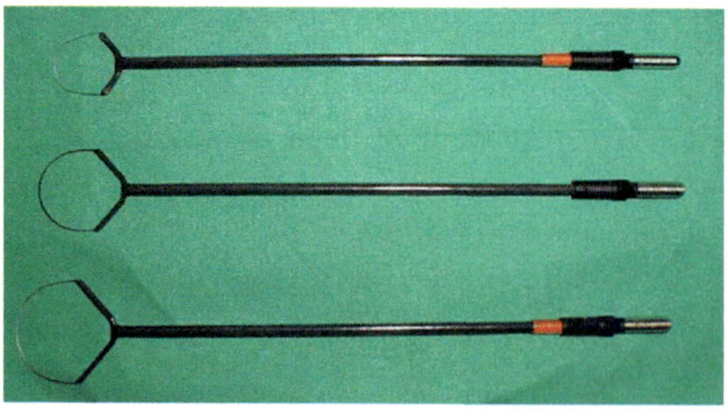

Fig. 8.2 Electrosurgical loops of different sizes for the "loop electrosurgical excision procedure" (LEEP)

LEEP can and should be performed under colposcopic guidance. Hemostasis is achieved by monopolar coagulation. For loop resection, the electrical generator should be set on a low coagulation current so that the coagulation zone of the tissue margins comprises only a small number of cell layers. Thus, histopathological assessment of resection margins will not be impaired.

There is no doubt anymore that loop resection is as effective as cold-knife conization for treatment of cervical intraepithelial neoplasia as shown by a meta-analysis (Jiang et al. 2016). This applies to all parameters studied: recurrence, positive margins, postoperative bleeding, and the occurrence of cervical stenosis.

Following tissue removal by LEEP/LLETZ, an endocervical curettage is performed. A narrow curette is used so that no cervical dilatation is required. Neither inspection of the uterine corpus (hysteroscopy) nor endometrial curettage is necessary and would only increase the complication rate. However, if the cytopathologist suspects an endometrial lesion, both endocervical and endometrial curettage are done.

In addition to cold-knife conization and LEEP/LLETZ, which preserve the resected tissue for further histopathologic evaluation, localized tissue destruction with cryosurgery or CO_2 laser vaporization is also acceptable, when certain criteria are met.

8.2.3 Cryosurgery

For cryosurgery of cervical lesions, a cryoprobe is chosen that covers the entire transformation zone. Nitrous oxide or liquid nitrogen is passed through this probe. Decompression of the liquid gas leads to very low temperatures. Freezing of the transformation zone causes tissue destruction, and the patient will notice a strong vaginal discharge in the days following the treatment.

Cryosurgery is an inexpensive method that is performed without general anesthesia. However, it is not suitable for treatment of large cervical lesions, although the exact extent of tissue destruction is difficult to control.

8.2.4 CO_2 Laser Vaporization

The CO_2 laser beam has similar physical properties as light beams from the visible spectrum. A system of mirrors is used to direct the laser beam from the generator tube to the manipulator device that is attached to the colposcope. With a joystick-controlled mirror, the laser beam can be directed onto the target tissue with a high degree of precision. Since the CO_2 laser beam itself is invisible, a red laser pointer is projected into the beam path (Fig. 8.3).

If the entire transformation zone is to be vaporized, it is treated from dorsal to ventral. The laser beam is set to 15–25 W and defocused as appropriate. The depth of vaporization should be 7 mm in order to treat all dysplastic tissue within the glandular crypts (Fig. 8.4).

Treatment modalities such as cryosurgery or CO_2 laser vaporization that destroy tissue rather than make it available for histopathologic evaluation are only acceptable, if the following prerequisites are met:

- The entire squamocolumnar junction must be visible (preferably T1).
- There should be no suspicion of invasive disease, neither on colposcopy, cytopathology, nor tissue biopsy.

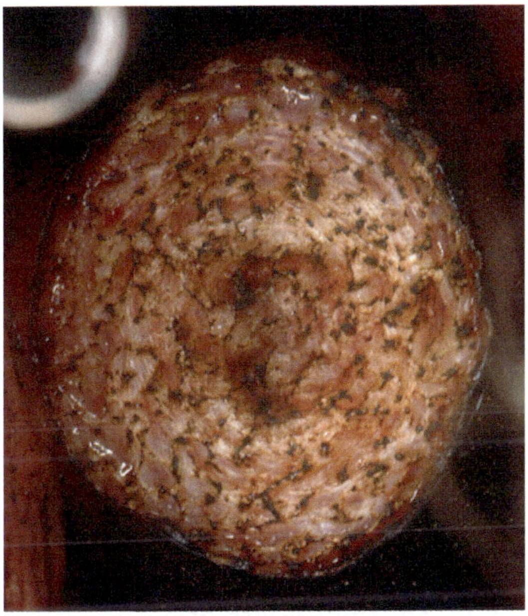

Fig. 8.4 Cervix immediately after CO_2 laser vaporization. Destruction of the tissue should be about 7 mm in depth

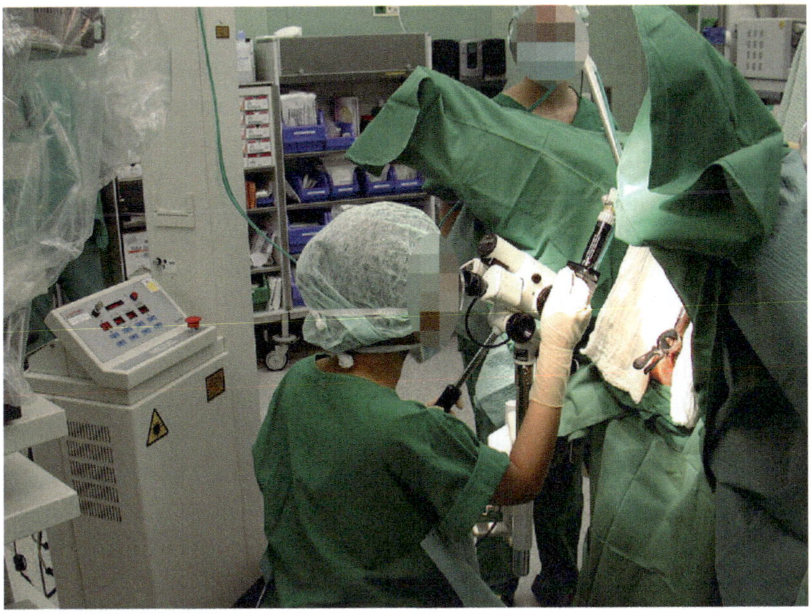

Fig. 8.3 CO_2 laser vaporization of the cervix. The laser is attached to the colposcope and can be controlled very precisely

- The area to be treated must be clearly identifiable und fully visible.
- HSIL/CIN2/CIN3 must have been unequivocally confirmed by targeted biopsy.
- There must be no significant disagreement between the different diagnostic modalities (cytopathology, colposcopy, histopathology).

LEEP resection may be combined with CO_2 laser vaporization. The peripheral part of the transformation zone can be vaporized, whereas the center is removed with the loop, as the area close to the cervical canal is more likely to be affected by high-grade dysplasia.

If the CO_2 laser beam is focused, it can also be used to excise the tissue instead of vaporizing it. Thus, "laser conization" is another alternative to cold-knife conization.

8.3 Assessment of Complete Removal of Cervical Dysplasia

8.3.1 Squamous Dysplasia

The primary goal of all surgical procedures described above is complete removal of all dysplastic epithelium. In invasive cancer treatment, histologically free margins are a benchmark for complete removal (R0). However, cervical dysplasia should not be treated like invasive cancer. Whereas CIN1 usually does not require treatment, HSIL (CIN2 and CIN3) should be surgically treated without removing too much of the surrounding healthy tissue, especially in reproductive age patients.

This can be best achieved by performing the resection using a colposcope. Under colposcopic guidance, the abnormal tissue is removed in its entirety, but without a wide safety margin. It is not uncommon that the dysplastic lesion reaches the resection margins of the histopathological specimen. However, this does not mean that the lesion has not been removed completely, as the cervix needs to be coagulated for hemostasis, so that additional tissue will be eliminated.

Depending on the location of a precancerous squamous epithelial lesion, resection by LEEP may be combined with localized tissue destruction using CO_2 laser vaporization. When using this approach, histological evaluation of the margin status is pointless.

If a positive resection margin is identified on histopathologic evaluation of squamous dysplasia, immediate repeat surgery is not indicated and should be avoided, especially in reproductive age patients.

Repeat resections are associated with a 1:36 risk of preterm birth before the 28th week of gestation in subsequent pregnancies (Ortoft et al. 2010). On the other hand, 78% of patients will no longer have high-grade dysplasia on follow-up, although specimen margins had been positive for CIN3 (Reich et al. 2002).

If the transformation zone is not fully visible postoperatively and/or low-grade dysplastic changes are present at the resection margins, this is not an indication for repeat surgery as it is unlikely that these patients still have CIN2+ disease, and a wait-and-see strategy is recommended (Day et al. 2008).

A meta-analysis of 97 eligible studies (Arbyn et al. 2008) found a recurrence rate of 6.6% for CIN2+ lesions. The recurrence rate was significantly higher if resection margins had been positive.

However, postoperative HPV positivity more accurately predicts recurrence risk than positive margins at the time of surgery.

In women beyond reproductive years, hysterectomy is sometimes recommended as a definitive treatment of cervical dysplasia. However, there is a significant risk of subsequent vaginal intraepithelial dysplasia.

Schockaert et al. (2008) conducted a retrospective analysis of women with a diagnosis of CIN2+ and no previous history of VAIN who underwent hysterectomy within 6 months of CIN diagnosis. The incidence rate of subsequent VAIN2+ was 7.4% including two patients with carcinoma of the vagina. Thus, Schockaert et al. came to the conclusion that hysterectomy in patients with CIN2+ cannot be considered as a definitive treatment.

Follow-up of patients treated for high-grade cervical lesions is crucial as there is an increased risk of death from cervical or vaginal carcinoma for patients treated for CIN3. Using the data of the Swedish Cancer Registry from 1958 to 2008, Strander et al. (2014) estimated a mortality risk of 2.35 (95% CI 2.11–2.61) compared to the general population.

Rather than using margin status as a predictor of persistent disease, the cervix should be reassessed colposcopically after it has healed completely, for example, after about 3 months. If the endocervical curettage had been positive for squamous dysplasia at the time of surgery, endocervical curettage should be performed. Alternatively, an intracervical brush cytology specimen may be obtained.

Integrating the HPV test into follow-up care is also helpful (Kocken et al. 2012), as demonstrated for the UK health-care system (Legood et al. 2012). The authors of the German guidelines for cervical cancer prevention presented a meta-analysis on the use of the HPV test for follow-up (https://www.awmf.org/uploads/tx_szleitlinien/015-027OLl_Praevention_Zervixkarzinom_2020-03-verlaengert.pdf; viewed April 2021). Seventeen relevant studies were identified, 15 of which were prospective studies. The sensitivity and specificity of Pap smear, HPV test, or combined testing for the prediction of persistent/recurrent disease were as follows:

Pap smear alone	
Sensitivity: 72.0%	95% CI: 65.6–77.5%
Specificity: 84.6%	95% CI: 80.7–87.9%
HPV test alone	
Sensitivity: 94.3%	95% CI: 88.4–97.3%
Specificity: 80.0%	95% CI: 74.2–84.8%
Pap smear plus HPV test	
Sensitivity: 95.3%	95% CI: 88.1–98.2%
Specificity: 69.6%	95% CI: 61.7–78.5%

The German guidelines recommend the combination of both tests as it traditionally relies heavily on cytological testing. However, there is no doubt that the much more sensitive of the two test modalities is the HPV test.

Follow-up recommendations will vary widely between different countries, and no definitive recommendation can be given on follow-up intervals. The German guideline quoted above recommends co-testing (Pap smear and HPV) after 6, 12, and 24 months, respectively. If either test is abnormal/positive, colposcopy is done.

8.3.2 Adenocarcinoma In Situ (AIS)

All the above considerations relate to squamous cell precancers. However, follow-up for adenocarcinoma in situ treated by loop resection is much more challenging. Several considerations, especially regarding surgical margin status and the role of hysterectomy, are different.

The safest treatment option for patients with adenocarcinoma in situ after childbearing age is still hysterectomy, especially for extensive and/or multifocal AIS.

Of course, for younger women who desire to preserve their fertility, this is not an acceptable treatment option.

In Australia, cold-knife conization is considered the standard of care for adenocarcinoma in situ in patients who wish to preserve fertility. However, according to a retrospective study by Munro et al. (2015), loop excision (LEEP) was equally effective. The only determinant of persistence or recurrence of AIS was the presence or absence of a positive margin.

With loop excision, the cervical lesion should be removed in its entirety. Ideally, surgical margins should be free of disease on histopathology (Hopkins 2000). Excision using an adequately sized loop is the treatment of choice, preferably applying a one-pass technique to avoid fragmentation of the specimen (van Hanegem et al. 2012).

In a meta-analysis of 1278 patients with cervical adenocarcinoma in situ (Salani et al. 2009), 19.4% of patients with positive margins developed recurrence compared to 2.6% of women with negative margins. In addition, the authors found a higher likelihood of invasive adenocarcinoma when margins were positive (5.2% versus

0.1%). Costa et al. (2007) report on 42 patients after conservative AIS treatment and a median follow-up of 40 months, of whom 17 (40.4%) relapsed. Even if the margins were negative on conization, the rate of recurrence was still 19%. On the other hand, Andersen and Nielsen (2002) argue against overvaluation of retrospective surgical margin assessment.

In any case, the recognizability of recurrence in AIS and possibly adenocarcinoma is significantly worse than in squamous epithelial lesions. The combination of cytological smear and HPV test is the most effective strategy for these patients, with the HPV test clearly having the strongest predictive value. According to Costa et al. (2012), sensitivity and specificity for the combined approach were 90.0% and 50.0%, respectively, for the first follow-up visit after 6 months. For the second follow-up visit another 6 months later, both sensitivity and specificity were 100%.

The Society of Gynecologic Oncology (SGO), in cooperation with the American Society of Colposcopy and Cervical Pathology (ASCCP), has published guidelines for the diagnosis and management of adenocarcinoma in situ (Teoh et al. 2020). According to these recommendations, margin status is decisive for the management of patients who wish to preserve the uterus. Fertility-sparing treatment is not acceptable if negative margins cannot be achieved, even with repeat excisions. Also, hysterectomy is recommended after childbearing age, unless HPV tests on follow-up exams are consistently negative.

Figure 8.5 summarizes the SGO recommendations.

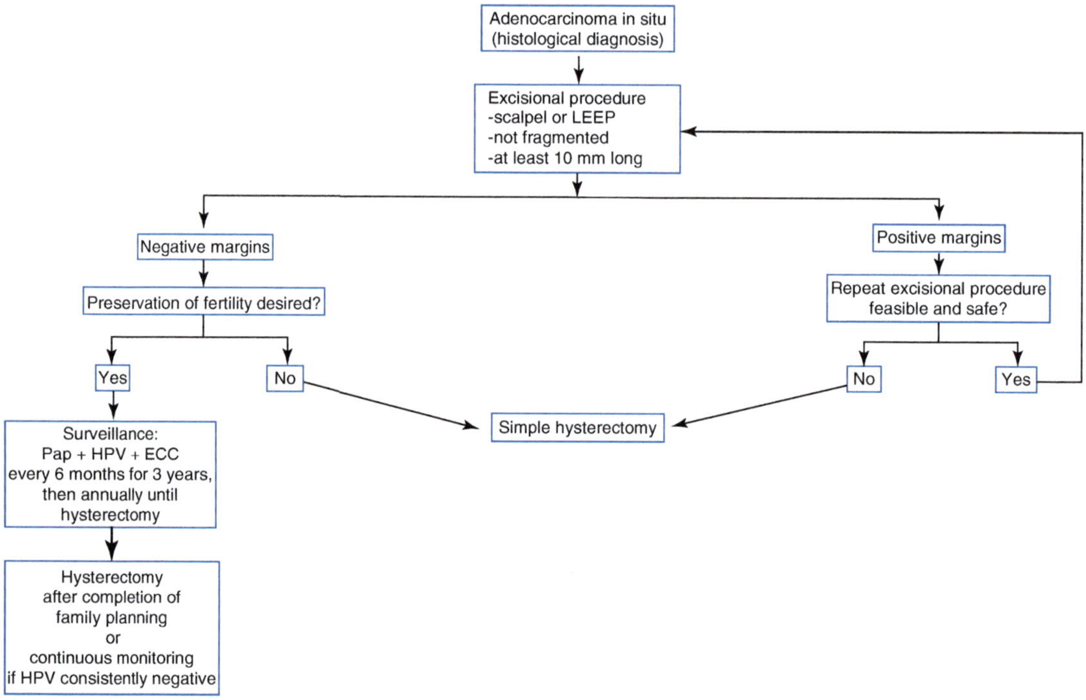

Fig. 8.5 Management of adenocarcinoma in situ of the cervix with or without negative margins after excision. According to these recommendations, a negative margin status is decisive for uterus-conserving treatment

References

Andersen ES, Nielsen K (2002) Adenocarcinoma in situ of the cervix: a prospective study of conization as definitive treatment. Gynecol Oncol 86(3):365–369

Arbyn M, Kyrgiou M, Simoens C, Raifu AO, Koliopoulos G, Martin-Hirsch P et al (2008) Perinatal mortality and other severe adverse pregnancy outcomes associated with treatment of cervical intraepithelial neoplasia: meta-analysis. BMJ 337:1284

Bornstein J, Bentley J, Bosze P, Girardi F, Haefner H, Menton M et al (2012) 2011 colposcopic terminology of the international federation for cervical pathology and colposcopy. Obstet Gynecol 120(1):166–172. https://doi.org/10.1097/AOG.0b013e318254f90c

Castanon A, Brocklehurst P, Evans H, Peebles D, Singh N, Walker P et al (2012) Risk of preterm birth after treatment for cervical intraepithelial neoplasia among women attending colposcopy in England: retrospective-prospective cohort study. BMJ 345:e5174. https://doi.org/10.1136/bmj.e5174

Costa S, Negri G, Sideri M, Santini D, Martinelli G, Venturoli S et al (2007) Human papillomavirus (HPV) test and PAP smear as predictors of outcome in conservatively treated adenocarcinoma in situ (AIS) of the uterine cervix. Gynecol Oncol 106(1):170–176

Costa S, Venturoli S, Negri G, Sideri M, Preti M, Pesaresi M et al (2012) Factors predicting the outcome of conservatively treated adenocarcinoma in situ of the uterine cervix: an analysis of 166 cases. Gynecol Oncol 124(3):490–495. https://doi.org/10.1016/j.ygyno.2011.11.039

Day T, Weitzen S, Cooper AS, Boardman LA (2008) Should unsatisfactory colposcopy necessitate treatment of cervical intraepithelial neoplasia 1? J Low Genit Tract Dis 12(1):11–15. https://doi.org/10.1097/lgt.0b013e318057f330

Grimm C, Polterauer S, Natter C, Rahhal J, Hefler L, Tempfer CB et al (2012) Treatment of cervical intraepithelial neoplasia with topical imiquimod: a randomized controlled trial. Obstet Gynecol 120(1):152–159. https://doi.org/10.1097/AOG.0b013e31825bc6e8

Heineman M, Mancini J, Villeret J, Agostini A, Houvenaeghel G, Boubli L, Carcopino X (2016) Treatment failure following excision therapy of CIN: the impact of direct colposcopic vision during procedure. Arch Gynecol Obstet 293(4):825–831. https://doi.org/10.1007/s00404-015-3887-7

Hilal Z, Rezniczek GA, Alici F, Kumpernatz A, Dogan A, Alieva L, Tempfer CB (2018) Loop electrosurgical excision procedure (LEEP) with or without intraoperative colposcopy: a randomized trial. Am J Obstet Gynecol. https://doi.org/10.1016/j.ajog.2018.07.023

Hopkins MP (2000) Adenocarcinoma in situ of the cervix–the margins must be clear. Gynecol Oncol 79(1):4–5.https://doi.org/10.1006/gyno.2000.5991S0090-8258(00)95991-2

Jiang Y-M, Chen C-X, Li L (2016) Meta-analysis of cold-knife conization versus loop electrosurgical excision procedure for cervical intraepithelial neoplasia. Onco Targets Ther 9:3907–3915. https://doi.org/10.2147/OTT.S108832

Jin G, LanLan Z, Li C, Dan Z (2013) Pregnancy outcome following loop electrosurgical excision procedure (LEEP) a systematic review and meta-analysis. Arch Gynecol Obstet 289(1):85–99. https://doi.org/10.1007/s00404-013-2955-0

Kalliala I, Nieminen P, Dyba T, Pukkala E, Anttila A (2007) Cancer free survival after CIN treatment: comparisons of treatment methods and histology. Gynecol Oncol 105(1):228–233

Kocken M, Uijterwaal MH, de Vries AL, Berkhof J, Ket JC, Helmerhorst TJ, Meijer CJ (2012) High-risk human papillomavirus testing versus cytology in predicting post-treatment disease in women treated for high-grade cervical disease: a systematic review and meta-analysis. Gynecol Oncol 125(2):500–507. https://doi.org/10.1016/j.ygyno.2012.01.015

Koeneman MM, Kruse AJ, Kooreman LFS, Hausen Z, Hopman AHN, Sep SJS et al (2017) Preliminary stop of the TOPical Imiquimod treatment of high-grade Cervical intraepithelial neoplasia (TOPIC) trial. BMC Cancer 17(1):110. https://doi.org/10.1186/s12885-017-3108-9

Kolben TM, Etzel LT, Bergauer F, Hagemann I (2019) A randomized trial comparing limited-excision conisation to large loop excision of the transformation zone (LLETZ) in cervical dysplasia patients. J Gynecol Oncol 30(3):e42

Kyrgiou M, Koliopoulos G, Martin-Hirsch P, Arbyn M, Prendiville W, Paraskevaidis E (2006) Obstetric outcomes after conservative treatment for intraepithelial or early invasive cervical lesions: systematic review and meta-analysis. Lancet 367:489–98.

Legood R, Smith M, Lew JB, Walker R, Moss S, Kitchener H et al (2012) Cost effectiveness of human papillomavirus test of cure after treatment for cervical intraepithelial neoplasia in England: economic analysis from NHS Sentinel Sites Study. BMJ 345:e7086. https://doi.org/10.1136/bmj.e7086

Munro A, Leung Y, Spilsbury K, Stewart CJR, Semmens J, Codde J et al (2015) Comparison of cold knife cone biopsy and loop electrosurgical excision procedure in the management of cervical adenocarcinoma in situ: what is the gold standard? Gynecol Oncol 137(2):258–263. https://doi.org/10.1016/j.ygyno.2015.02.024

Ortoft G, Henriksen T, Hansen E, Petersen L (2010) After conisation of the cervix, the perinatal mortality as a result of preterm delivery increases in subsequent pregnancy. BJOG 117(3):258–267. https://doi.org/10.1111/j.1471-0528.2009.02438.x

Poon L, Savvas M, Zamblera D, Skyfta E, Nicolaides K (2012) Large loop excision of transformation zone and cervical length in the prediction of spontaneous

preterm delivery. BJOG 119(6):692–698. https://doi.org/10.1111/j.1471-0528.2011.03203.x
Quenby S (2010) Obstetric management of women after treatment for CIN. BJOG 117(3):243–244. https://doi.org/10.1111/j.1471-0528.2009.02460.x
Reich O, Lahousen M, Pickel H, Tamussino K, Winter R (2002) Cervical intraepithelial neoplasia III: long-term follow-up after cold-knife conization with involved margins. Obstet Gynecol 99(2):193–196
Salani R, Puri I, Bristow RE (2009) Adenocarcinoma in situ of the uterine cervix: a metaanalysis of 1278 patients evaluating the predictive value of conization margin status. Am J Obstet Gynecol 200(2):182. https://doi.org/10.1016/j.ajog.2008.09.012
Santesso N, Mustafa RA, Wiercioch W, Kehar R, Gandhi S, Chen Y et al (2016) Systematic reviews and meta-analyses of benefits and harms of cryotherapy, LEEP, and cold knife conization to treat cervical intraepithelial neoplasia. Int J Gynaecol Obstet 132(3):266–271. https://doi.org/10.1016/j.ijgo.2015.07.026
Schockaert S, Poppe W, Arbyn M, Verguts T, Verguts J (2008) Incidence of vaginal intraepithelial neoplasia after hysterectomy for cervical intraepithelial neoplasia: a retrospective study. Am J Obstet Gynecol 199(2):113. https://doi.org/10.1016/j.ajog.2008.02.026
Simoens C, Goffin F, Simon P, Barlow P, Antoine J, Foidart JM, Arbyn M (2012) Adverse obstetrical outcomes after treatment of precancerous cervical lesions: a Belgian multicentre study. BJOG 119(10):1247–1255. https://doi.org/10.1111/j.1471-0528.2012.03429.x
Strander B, Hällgren J, Sparén P (2014) Effect of ageing on cervical or vaginal cancer in Swedish women previously treated for cervical intraepithelial neoplasia grade 3: population based cohort study of long term incidence and mortality. BMJ 348(1):7361. https://doi.org/10.1136/bmj.f7361
Teoh D, Musa F, Salani R, Huh W, Jimenez E (2020) Diagnosis and management of adenocarcinoma in situ: a society of gynecologic oncology evidence-based review and recommendations. Obstet Gynecol 135(4):869–878. https://doi.org/10.1097/AOG.0000000000003761
van de Sande AJM, Koeneman MM, Gerestein CG, Kruse AJ, van Kemenade FJ, van Beekhuizen HJ (2018) TOPical Imiquimod treatment of residual or recurrent cervical intraepithelial neoplasia (TOPIC-2 trial): a study protocol for a randomized controlled trial. BMC Cancer 18(1):655. https://doi.org/10.1186/s12885-018-4510-7
van Hanegem N, Barroilhet LM, Nucci MR, Bernstein M, Feldman S (2012) Fertility-sparing treatment in younger women with adenocarcinoma in situ of the cervix. Gynecol Oncol 124(1):72–77. https://doi.org/10.1016/j.ygyno.2011.09.006

9 Colposcopy of the Surgically Treated Cervix

Contents

Colposcopy plays a crucial role in the diagnosis of persistence or recurrence of intraepithelial neoplasia. As the appearance of the cervix changes significantly after surgical treatment of dysplasia, this presents an additional challenge for colposcopy.

The surgeon who performs the dysplasia treatment should see the patient at least once for follow-up colposcopy.

Thus, the surgeon can continuously check on his own technique, regarding the functional preservation of the cervix as well as the success rate of dysplasia treatment. The primary objective is complete removal of the dysplastic lesion. However, for all women of childbearing age, it is equally important to limit the amount of tissue resection. Naturally, the more tissue is removed, the less likely dysplasia will persist or recur. On the other hand, a large resection volume will be more likely to cause complications for future pregnancies. Therefore, a certain percentage of patients with recurrent disease is acceptable.

Soutter et al. (Soutter et al. 2006) found a recurrence rate of 3%. Recurrence was defined as CIN2+ disease. The authors recommend postoperative colposcopy as an adjunct to cytological examination to increase the sensitivity for the detection of high-grade disease. In this retrospective study, sensitivity was 91% for patients undergoing both colposcopy and Pap smear compared to only 64% for cytological follow-up only. With the combined approach, specificity dropped from 95% to 88%. Soutter et al. conclude that the benefit of colposcopy would be greater in women with a higher risk of treatment failure, for example, patients with involved tissue margins.

Colposcopic examination following treatment for dysplasia is best done after 10 to 12 weeks. At this time, it can be safely assumed that the cervix has healed completely (Fig. 9.1) and can be optimally assessed colposcopically.

R. J. Lellé, V. Küppers, *Colposcopy*, https://doi.org/10.1007/978-3-030-85388-4_9

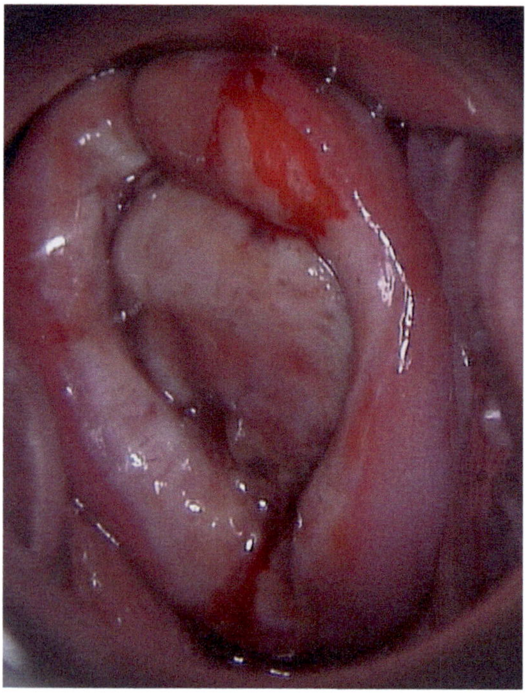

Fig. 9.1 Cervix 7 days after LEEP. The 25-year-old patient underwent surgery for microcarcinoma of the cervix (FIGO stage Ia1). As suturing of the cervix is avoided, there is an open wound. Any attempts of colposcopic or cytological assessment would be misleading

Colposcopic examination after surgical dysplasia treatment of the cervix should address the following questions:

- How well is the cervix preserved?
- Can the transformation zone visualized completely?
- Is there stenosis of the cervical canal?
- Is there any colposcopic evidence of persistent cervical dysplasia?
- Is there evidence for vaginal intraepithelial neoplasia?

If the colposcopic exam is normal, a Pap smear including an intracervical brush specimen is obtained. If the endocervical curettage during surgery had been positive, ECC should be repeated. All visible abnormalities that are identified colposcopically, including both major and minor changes, need to be biopsied.

9.1 State of Preservation of the Cervix

Postoperatively, the cervix of reproductive age women should still protrude above the level of the vagina and be shaped normally. Figure 9.2 shows an example of an acceptable postoperative result following cold-knife conization. In contrast, in Figs. 9.3 and 9.4, hardly any cervical tissue is visible, and the opening of the cervical canal is within the plane of the vaginal wall.

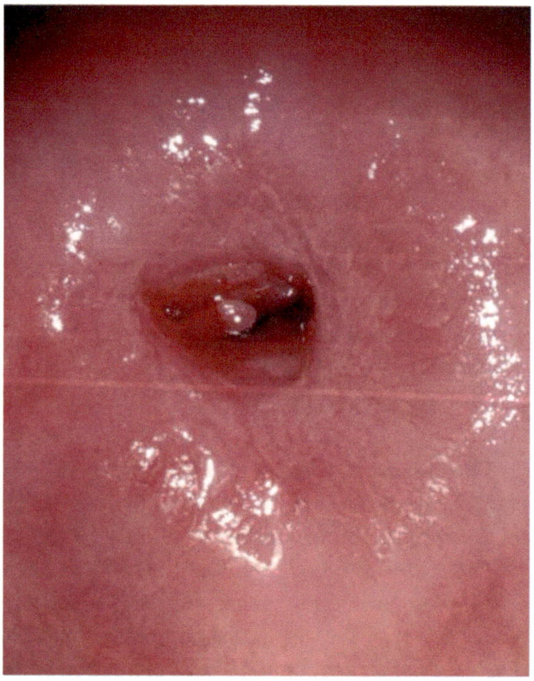

Fig. 9.2 Acceptable result after cold-knife conization of the cervix. The 39-year-old female had a CIN3 lesion removed 8 weeks ago

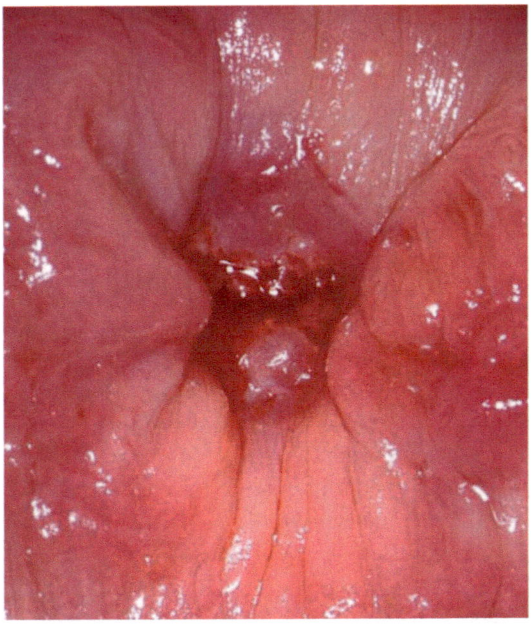

Fig. 9.3 Cervix after previous LEEP. The patient is only 26 years old and underwent surgery 3 years ago. Most of the ectocervix had been removed

9.2 Visibility of the Transformation Zone

Ideally, the entire transformation zone should be visible postoperatively with or without manipulation of the cervical os (T2 and T1, respectively). Unfortunately, this is not always possible regardless of the surgical technique used. In a Cochrane meta-analysis, Martin-Hirsch et al. (2000) were unable to identify a superior surgical technique. Also, the frequency of cervical stenosis did not differ. Only with CO_2 laser vaporization there was a tendency of less frequent stenosis and the more frequent visualization of the entire transformation zone.

In Figs. 9.5, 9.6, and 9.7, there has been optimal postoperative regeneration of the cervix so that the squamocolumnar junction is completely visible.

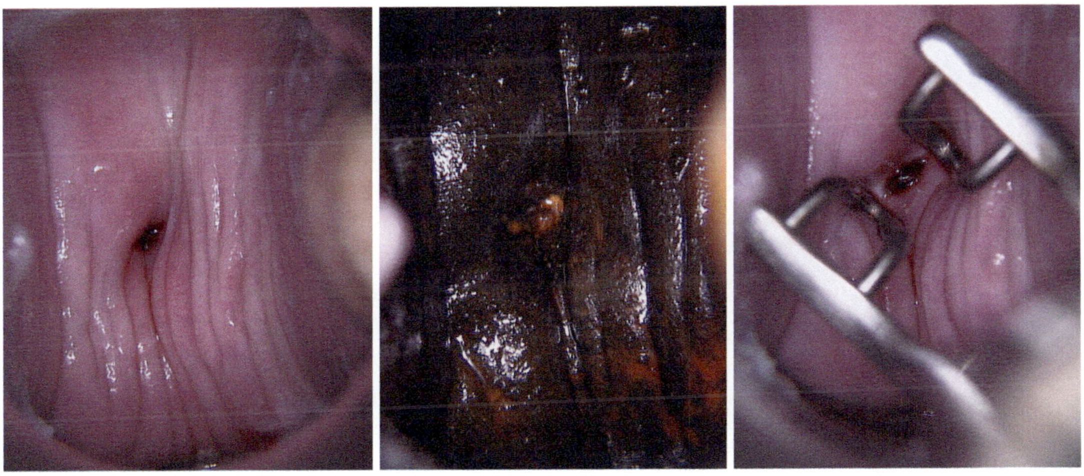

Fig. 9.4 Cervical stenosis after three previous LEEP in a 36-year-old patient

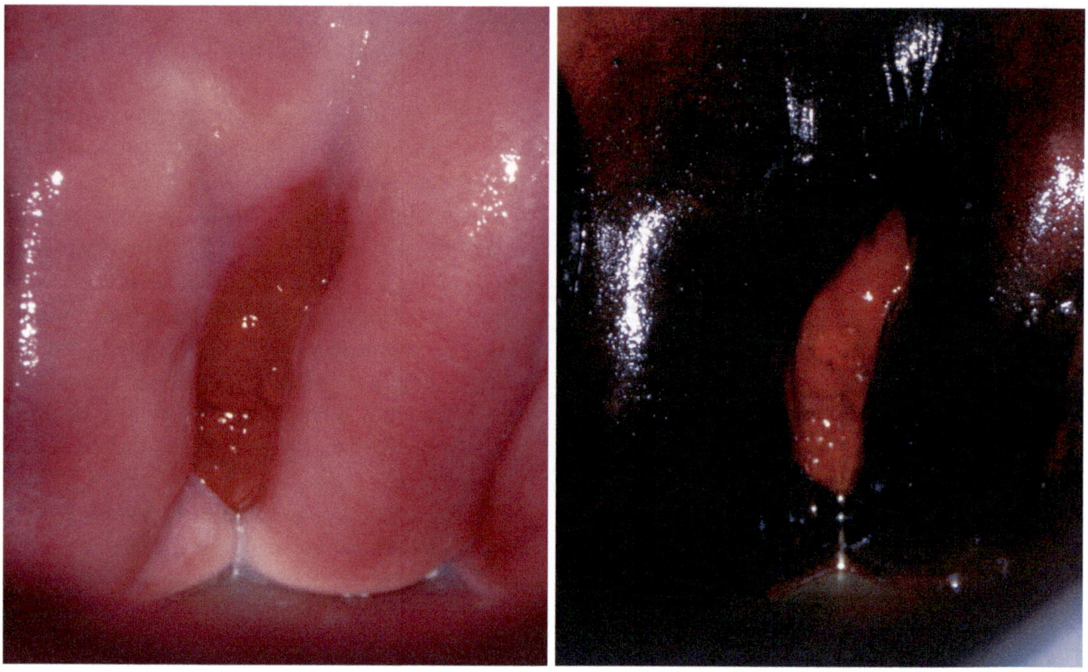

Fig. 9.5 Visible squamocolumnar junction (T1) 6 months after LEEP

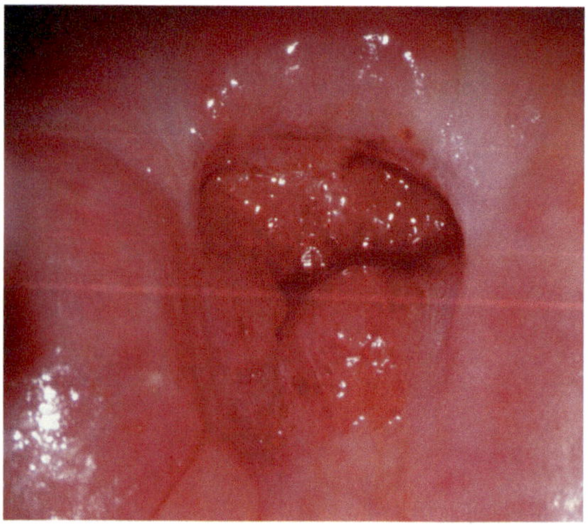

Fig. 9.6 New transformation zone 3 months after conization. The 34-year-old woman has been treated for CIN3. There is a significant tissue defect. The squamocolumnar junction is visible

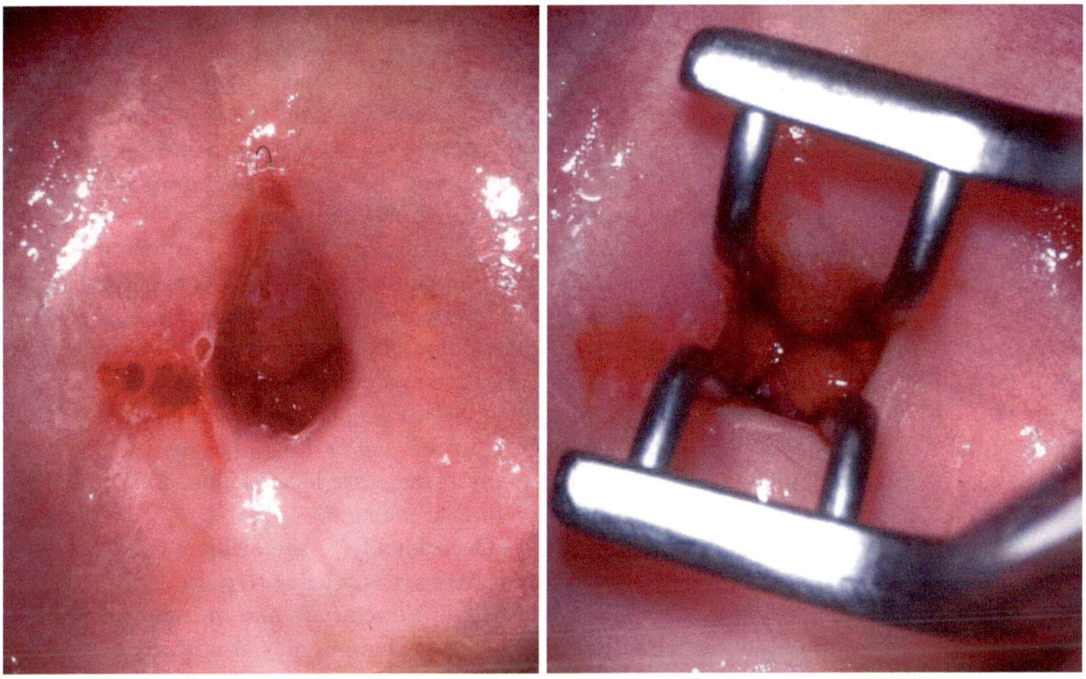

Fig. 9.7 Acceptable result 11 months after LEEP for HSIL/CIN3 in a 29-year-old patient. The squamocolumnar junction can be visualized with the Kogan speculum

9.3 Stenosis of the Cervical Canal

Narrowing of the cervical canal can be an unwelcome consequence of cervical tissue resections (Fig. 9.8).

Per definition, cervical stenosis is present when a 2.5 mm Hegar dilator cannot be inserted (Christianson et al. 2008). Thus, the cytological brush usually cannot pass the cervical os.

If follow-up Pap smears can only be obtained from the ectocervix, this information should be relayed to the cytopathologist, and the Pap smear result may be less accurate.

Retrospective data obtained by Hasegawa et al. (Hasegawa et al. 2016) show a high rate of cervical stenosis following conization. Stenosis occurred significantly more frequently in postmenopausal than in premenopausal patients (59.1% versus 8.3%). This may in part be related to cone size, as cone length was significantly greater in postmenopausal patients.

Christianson et al. (Christianson et al. 2008) summarized several articles on the frequency of

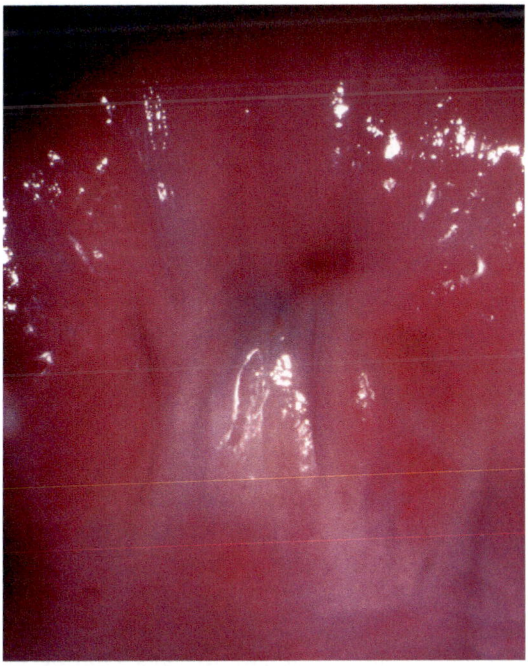

Fig. 9.8 Persistent cervical stenosis after conization. The 39-year-old patient underwent conization 6 years previously, and intracervical cytology could not be obtained anymore. A small loop resection (LEEP) was performed to reopen the cervical canal. But 7 months later, the cervix is stenotic again

cervical stenosis: 17% of patients following laser conization, 4–19% for loop resections, and 10% or more for cold-knife conizations. However, cervical stenosis that is severe enough that menstrual blood is blocked inside the uterus leading to severe dysmenorrhea is quite rare.

With cervical stenosis, it is difficult or impossible to obtain an intracervical cytological sample. However, if the screening Pap smear lacks an endocervical component, accelerated repeat examination is not recommended (Polanco Jacome et al. 2018), as the subsequent risk of high-grade dysplasia or cancer is not significantly higher compared to patients with Pap smears containing endocervical and/or metaplastic cells (Sultana et al. 2014).

Misoprostol, a prostaglandin E1 analog, is sometimes used intravaginally or orally for cervical ripening. In a meta-analysis (Pergialiotis et al. 2015), misoprostol was able to increase the rate of colposcopic exams that could visualize the transformation zone. This conversion rate ranged between 55.5% and 78.9%. However, numbers were too small to draw any definite conclusions.

Some patients, who are at high risk for developing intracervical CIN2+ disease, may have to undergo diagnostic/therapeutic LEEP. Also, hysterectomy might be an option in individual cases, as long as the patient knows about the significant risk of subsequent development of vaginal intraepithelial neoplasia.

In summary, cervical stenosis, especially following surgical procedures of the cervix, is still a challenging problem, and treatment recommendations are unsatisfactory, as no evidence-based algorithms can be established (Maier et al. 2017).

9.4 Colposcopic Diagnosis of Persistent or Recurrent Cervical Dysplasia

Immediate or premature repeat surgery for suspected persistent disease should be avoided, especially in women of childbearing age. As a rule, HSIL should be confirmed histologically by colposcopically guided biopsy prior to any surgical intervention. Low-grade dysplasia (LSIL/CIN1) is not an acceptable reason for repeat surgery and will unnecessarily increase the complication rate of subsequent pregnancies.

The recurrence rate after treatment for cervical intraepithelial neoplasia is between 5% and 7% (Arbyn et al. 2017; Santesso et al. 2016). The colposcopic assessment criteria after dysplasia treatment are basically the same as prior to surgery. Attention should be paid to acetowhite and/or Lugol-negative areas, especially if these are located close to the squamocolumnar junction.

Occasionally, acetowhite and Lugol-negative areas are due to postoperative regeneration. Punctation and mosaic resembling dysplastic changes may also be seen.

These findings (Figs. 9.9, 9.10, 9.11, and 9.12) may be colposcopically indistinguishable from actual recurrence (Figs. 9.13 and 9.14). Targeted biopsy will confirm or rule out recurrent or persistent disease.

If endocervical curettage performed as part of the initial surgical treatment had been positive for dysplasia, curettage should be repeated during the first colposcopic follow-up exam, especially if the squamocolumnar junction is not visible (T3). In addition, an intracervical Pap smear should be obtained with a brush.

In select cases, LEEP may be performed without prior histological confirmation of HSIL, when the Pap smear indicates CIN3 disease and colposcopy confirms a major change or the squamocolumnar junction is not visible. If no dysplasia is detected histologically, the possibility of vaginal intraepithelial dysplasia should be considered and the vagina carefully reexamined with particular attention to the vaginal wall adjacent to the cervix. All Lugol-negative areas should be biopsied.

The high value of HPV testing in the follow-up of dysplasia treatment has already been discussed

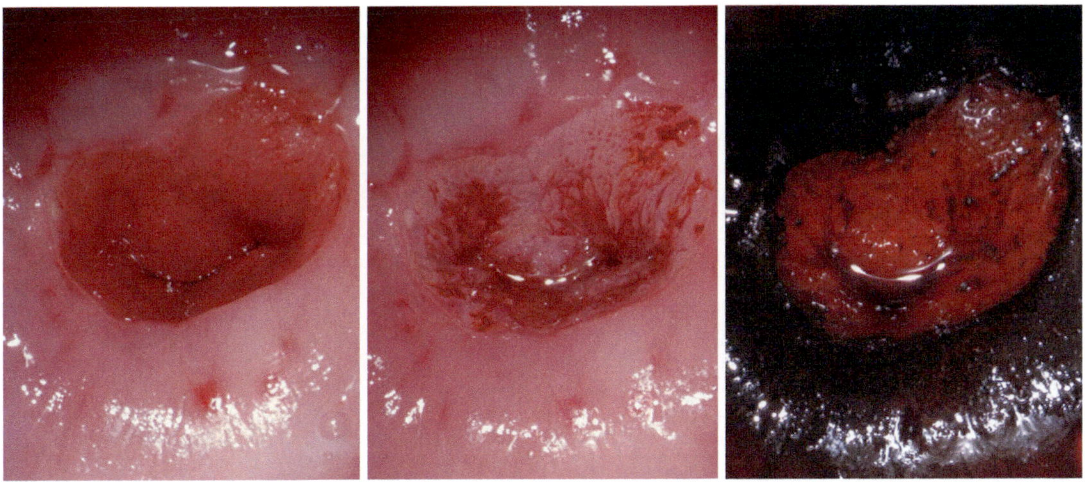

Fig. 9.9 Metaplastic changes 7 months after LEEP. After application of acetic acid (center), there is intense acetowhite staining with mosaic (major change). Biopsy from this area did not reveal dysplasia

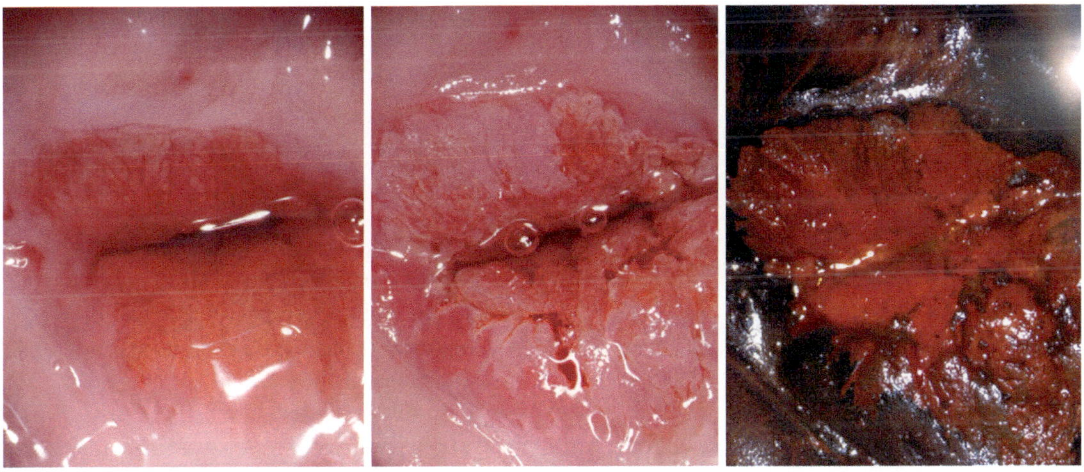

Fig. 9.10 New transformation zone/ectopy following CIN3 treatment (LEEP). The opaque acetowhite area at 12 o'clock with coarse mosaic (major change) suggests persistent or recurrent disease. However, biopsy is negative

previously (Chap. 6). Therefore, histopathologic evaluation as to whether a dysplastic lesion has been removed completely (free margins) has only a limited predictive value regarding persistence or recurrence of dysplasia. Rather, the result of the HPV test should be used to select patients who should undergo colposcopic follow-up after dysplasia treatment.

The benefit of routine colposcopic examination of all patients 12 months after LEEP has been questioned by Thompson and Marin (Thompson and Marin 2013). In a retrospective analysis, they came to the conclusion that the sensitivity of colposcopy is low whereas the likelihood of false-negative findings is high causing unnecessary follow-up exams.

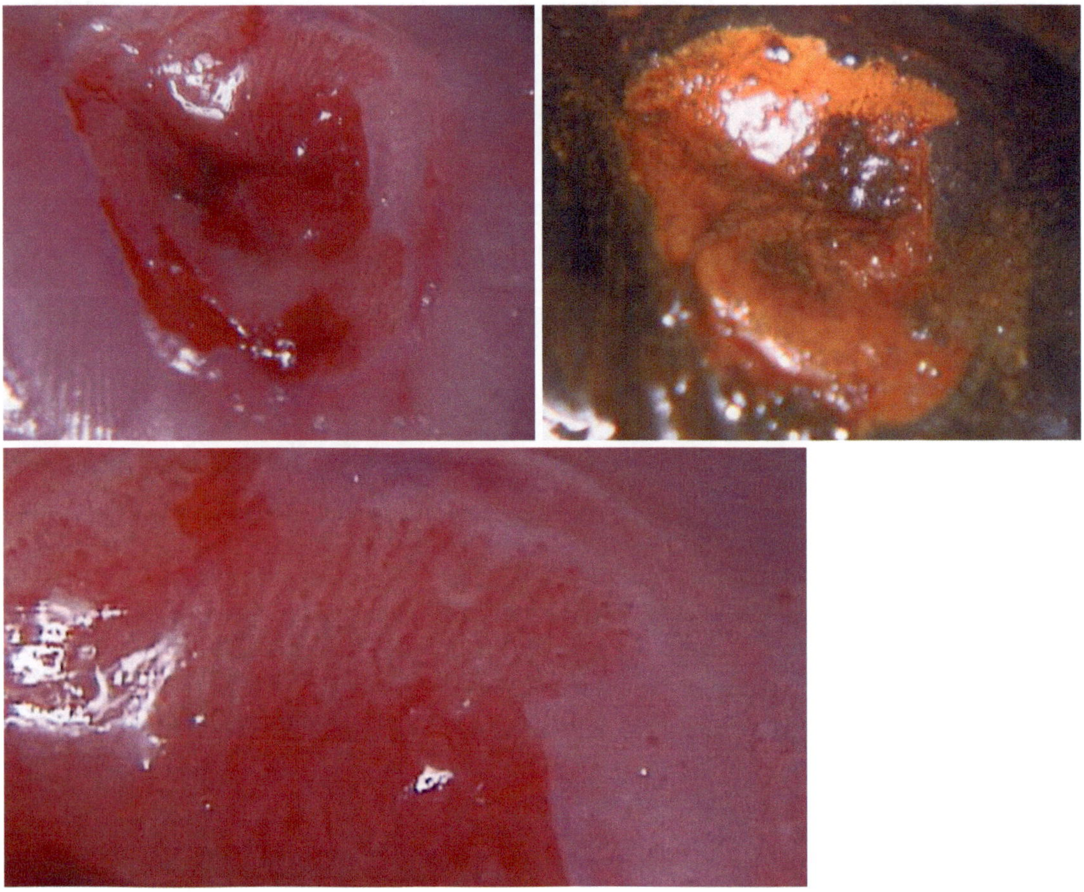

Fig. 9.11 Postoperative cervical mosaic resembling persistent CIN. The 31-year-old patient underwent LEEP twice. The last surgery for CIN3 was 3 months ago. There is irregular punctation at 12 o'clock. However, the acetowhite area is still transparent (minor change)

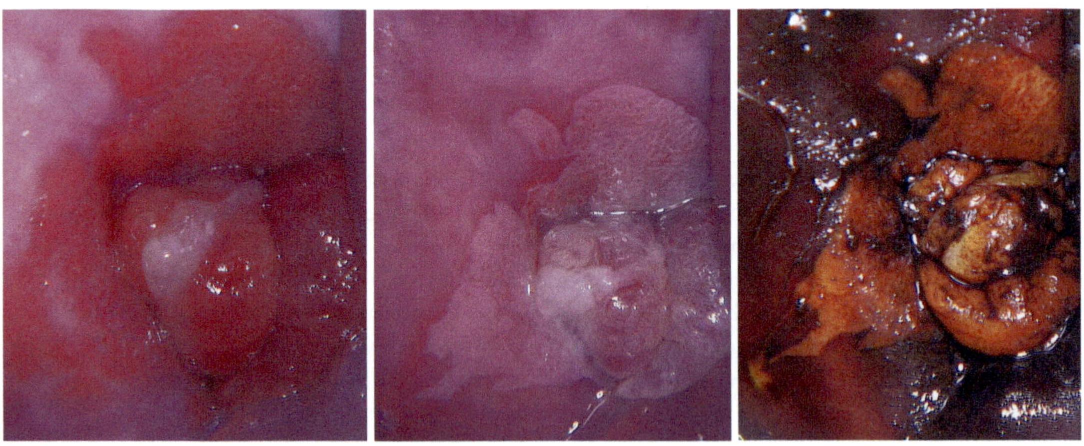

Fig. 9.12 Cervix with postoperative major change in pregnancy resembling HSIL. The 33-year-old patient is 22 weeks pregnant and has had LEEP resection for ACIS at 14 weeks of gestation. Biopsy of the major change does not confirm the suspicion of dysplasia, and the HPV test (HC2) is negative

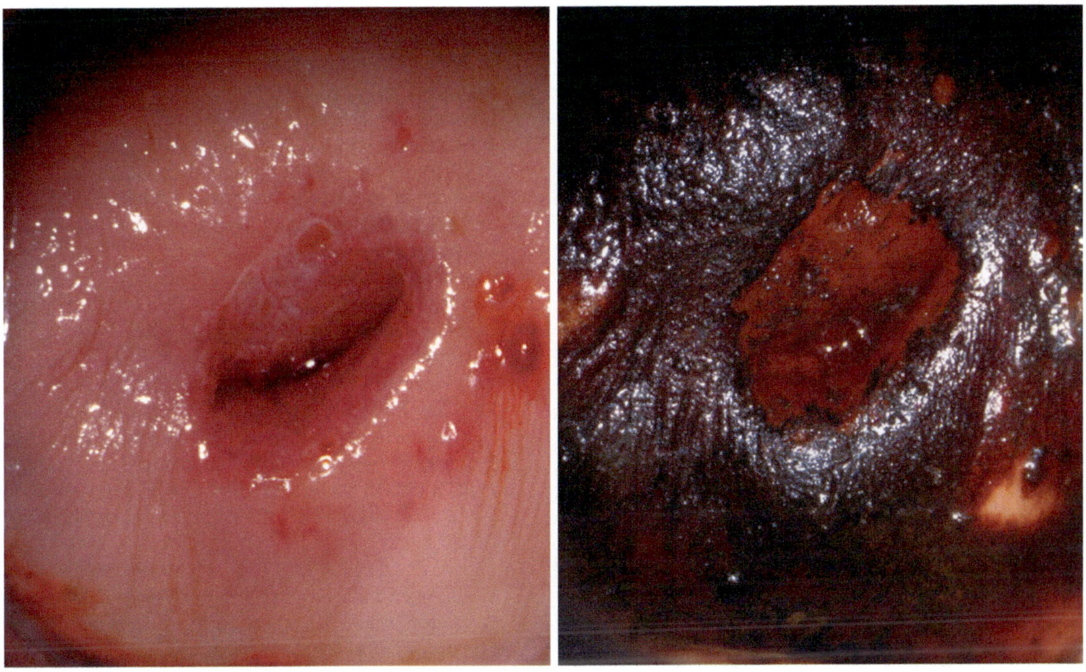

Fig. 9.13 HSIL/CIN3 recurrence 6 months after conization in a 31-year-old patient. At 12 o'clock, there is a small area of regular mosaic (minor change). A biopsy using the Stiefel® curette shows HSIL/CIN2 disease

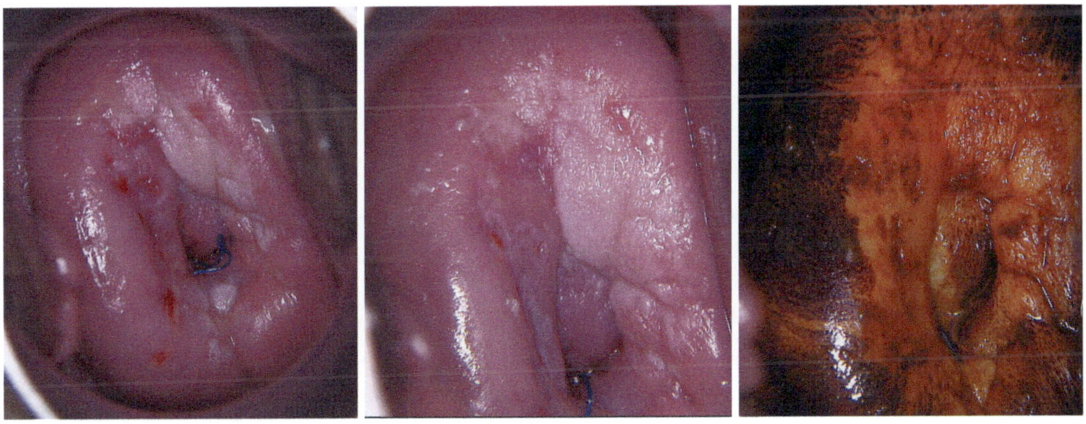

Fig. 9.14 A 38-year-old patient with recurrent HSIL/CIN3 7 months after LEEP. There is a significant tissue defect. At 12 o'clock, there is prominent leukoplakia, visible both before (left) and after (center) acetic acid application. Otherwise, the colposcopic features are uncharacteristic

References

Arbyn M, Redman CWE, Verdoodt F, Kyrgiou M, Tzafetas M, Ghaem-Maghami S et al (2017) Incomplete excision of cervical precancer as a predictor of treatment failure: a systematic review and meta-analysis. Lancet Oncol 18(12):1665–1679. https://doi.org/10.1016/S1470-2045(17)30700-3

Christianson MS, Barker MA, Lindheim SR (2008) Overcoming the challenging cervix: techniques to access the uterine cavity. J Low Genit Tract Dis 12(1):24–31. https://doi.org/10.1097/lgt.0b013e318150676d

Hasegawa K, Torii Y, Kato R, Udagawa Y, Fukasawa I (2016) The problems of cervical conization for postmenopausal patients. Eur J Gynaecol Oncol 37(3):327–331

Maier E, Gieseking F, Lellé RJ (2017) Stenose der Cervix uteri. Praktische Gyn 22:1–6

Martin-Hirsch PL, Paraskevaidis E, Kitchener H (2000) Surgery for cervical intraepithelial neoplasia. Cochrane Database Syst Rev 2:CD001318

Pergialiotis V, Vlachos D-E, Pitsouni E, Perrea D, Vlachos GD (2015) Vaginal misoprostol for overcoming inadequate colposcopies: a meta-analysis of randomized controlled trials. J Low Genit Tract Dis 19(3):257–261. https://doi.org/10.1097/LGT.0000000000000066

Polanco Jacome EC, Maerki J, Chau K, Akerman M, Sajjan S, Klein M et al (2018) Lack of transformation zone in cervical Pap tests, should it be a concern? A quality assurance initiative. Diagn Cytopathol 46(7):584–588. https://doi.org/10.1002/dc.23955

Santesso N, Mustafa RA, Wiercioch W, Kehar R, Gandhi S, Chen Y et al (2016) Systematic reviews and meta-analyses of benefits and harms of cryotherapy, LEEP, and cold knife conization to treat cervical intraepithelial neoplasia. Int J Gynaecol Obstet 132(3):266–271. https://doi.org/10.1016/j.ijgo.2015.07.026

Soutter WP, Butler JS, Tipples M (2006) The role of colposcopy in the follow up of women treated for cervical intraepithelial neoplasia. BJOG 113(5):511–514

Sultana F, English DR, Simpson JA, Canfell K, Gertig DM, Saville M (2014) High-grade cervical abnormalities and cervical cancer in women following a negative Pap smear with and without an endocervical component: a cohort study with 10 years of follow-up. Int J Cancer 135(5):1213–1219. https://doi.org/10.1002/ijc.28756

Thompson V, Marin R (2013) Is colposcopy necessary at twelve months after large loop excision of the transformation zone? A clinical audit. Aust N Z J Obstet Gynaecol 53(6):571–573. https://doi.org/10.1111/ajo.12153

Colposcopy During Pregnancy 10

Contents

If the cervical smear is abnormal during pregnancy, colposcopic triage is crucial to rule out invasive disease. Due to physiologic tissue changes due to pregnancy, colposcopy is particularly demanding. In patients who previously have not had regular cervical screening, a Pap smear and an HPV screening test (≥30 years) should be obtained at the time of the first office visit. If test results suggest CIN2+ disease, colposcopy is required.

Colposcopy with targeted biopsy is feasible at any stage of pregnancy and does not involve an increased risk for the fetus (Hunter et al. 2008). Also, the diagnosis of cervical precancer should not influence obstetrical management, i.e., neither preterm delivery nor cesarean section is required (Flannelly 2010; Henes et al. 2013). However, according to a meta-analysis by Danhof et al. (2015), the presence of CIN, even when not being treated, confers a significant risk of preterm delivery compared to women without CIN. Therefore, it cannot be ruled out that HPV infection and CIN constitute independent risk factors for the pregnant patient apart from any type of surgical intervention of the cervix.

Since HSIL has a low probability of malignant progression within the relatively short time period of pregnancy, surgical treatment of dysplasia should be postponed until after delivery and until pregnancy-related changes have regressed. Thus, the primary objective of colposcopic diagnosis in pregnancy is to rule out invasive disease.

It is important to realize that pregnancy itself is not to be considered a risk factor for malignant transformation of HSIL. Preliminary data presented by Ciavattini et al. (2017) even suggest a less aggressive behavior of preneoplastic cervical lesions in pregnant patients compared to nonpregnant patients. Whereas in nonpregnant women both Ki67 and p16 expression increased significantly with CIN grade, this increase could not be observed in pregnant patients.

R. J. Lellé, V. Küppers, *Colposcopy*, https://doi.org/10.1007/978-3-030-85388-4_10

However, even within a setting where colposcopy is readily and timely available during pregnancy, advanced stage cervical carcinoma still occurs. The overall prognosis for cervical cancer diagnosed during pregnancy is not worse compared to cervical cancer not associated with pregnancy. Even an intentional delay of oncologic treatment until the fetus reaches maturity does not have a negative impact on prognosis (Takushi et al. 2002).

10.1 Pregnancy-Related Changes of the Cervix

Colposcopic evaluation of the cervix is more difficult during pregnancy due to physiological changes. Therefore, the colposcopist has to be familiar with both normal and abnormal colposcopic images in pregnancy.

Due to increased fluid retention within the cervix and subsequent increase of volume, the squamocolumnar junction can be visualized more frequently during pregnancy. If the squamocolumnar junction cannot be seen during the first trimester, it may well be visible on repeat colposcopy a few weeks later.

The further along the pregnancy, the more difficult the colposcopic evaluation becomes. After the 30th week of pregnancy, adequate colposcopic assessment may no longer be possible.

Almost all of the observed changes are due to the increasing level of estrogen during pregnancy and may lead to overdiagnosis of dysplasia and possibly cancer.

As the cervix becomes hypertrophic and edematous, the tissue assumes a bluish hue. In the Anglo-American literature, this is called "Chadwick's sign." In the nineteenth century, Chadwick recognized the bluish discoloration as a pregnancy-related change (Gleichert 1971).

The cervical glandular epithelium is particularly active and prominent during pregnancy. The transformation zone is gradually shifting toward the ectocervix. The gland cells secrete a large amount of cervical mucus, which can complicate colposcopic assessment (Fig. 10.1). The glandular epithelium, which undergoes metaplastic changes, may be prominently vascularized and misinterpreted as suspicious for cancer (Figs. 10.2 and 10.3).

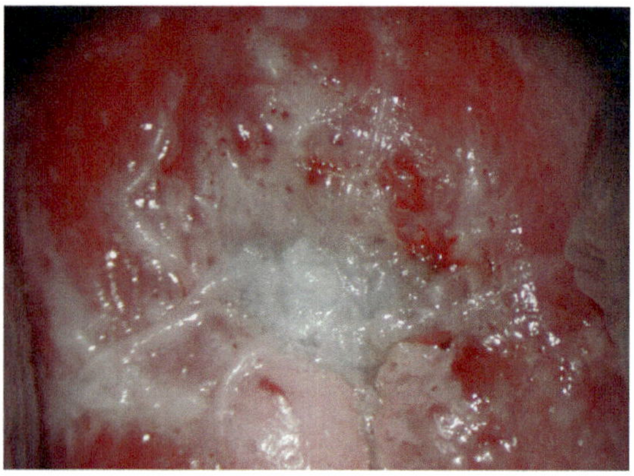

Fig. 10.1 CIN3 in the 35th week of pregnancy. The opaque acetowhite areas are partially obscured by increased mucus secretion

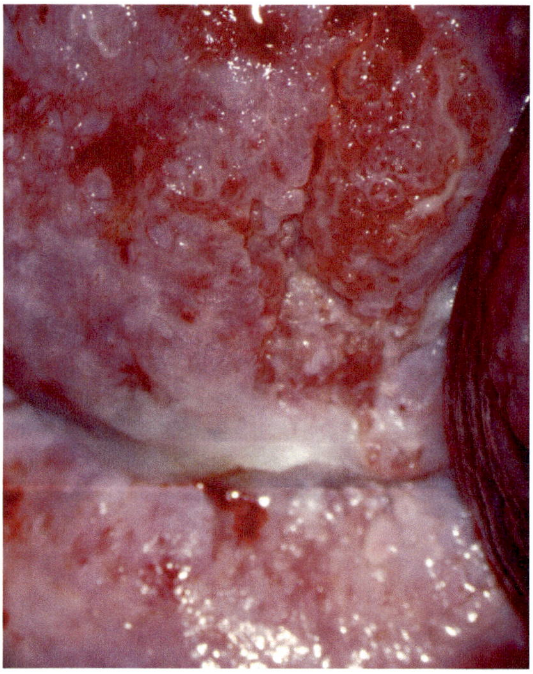

Fig. 10.2 CIN3 in the 31st week of pregnancy. At the anterior (ventral) part of the cervix, the partially transformed glandular epithelium is very prominent and polypous. By colposcopic inspection alone, invasion cannot be ruled out

Stromal cell hypertrophy leads to "pseudopunctation." This should not be confused with the irregular punctation within an acetowhite area that is typically caused by dysplasia (Fig. 10.4).

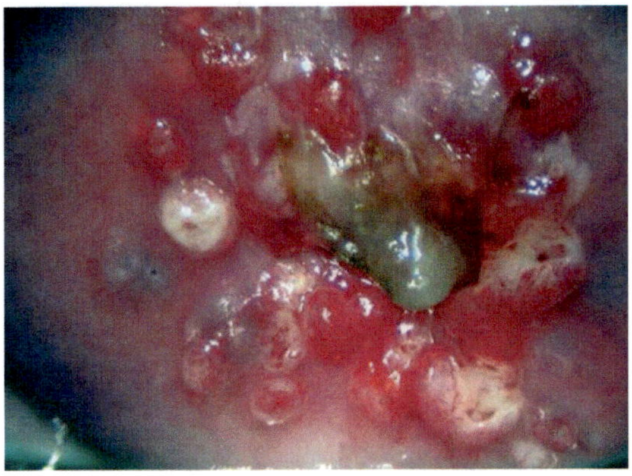

Fig. 10.3 CIN3 in the tenth week of pregnancy. Within the mature transformation zone, the gland openings are surrounded by a coarse-white epithelium (periglandular cuffing) with prominent but not atypical vessels

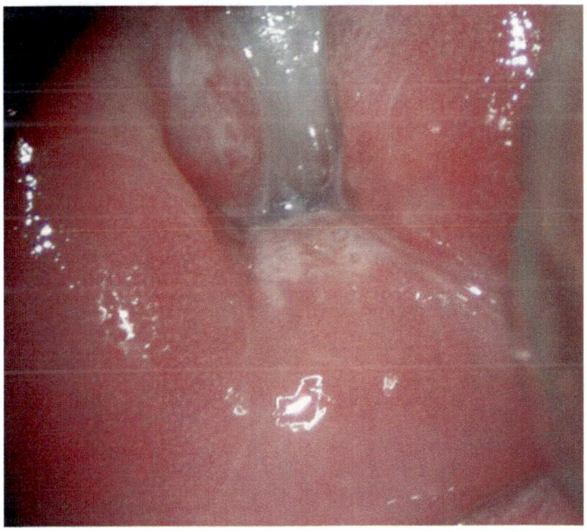

Fig. 10.4 "Pseudo-punctation" of a normal cervix in the 26th week of pregnancy. The punctation is regular, and there is no acetowhite staining

The application of acetic acid causes a more intense white reaction (Figs. 10.5, 10.6, 10.7, 10.8, 10.9, and 10.10). Also, the acetowhite epithelium may be raised above the level of the normal epithelium (Figs. 10.11 and 10.12). Sometimes, the intense acetowhite staining has a "gyrated" appearance (Figs. 10.13 and 10.14). Since the acetowhite reaction is more pronounced in both dysplasia and metaplasia, it may be misinterpreted as major change.

The high glycogen content of the intermediate cells of the squamous epithelium, which are called "navicular cells" by the cytopathologist due to their boat-shaped morphology, leads to a deep chestnut-brown coloration on Schiller's iodine test.

It is relatively common for stromal cells of the cervix to undergo decidualization (decidual transformation). In fact, Schneider and Barnes (1981) identified cervical decidua in 30.8% of pregnant uteri. In one-third of these patients, decidual cells were detected on the cytological smear.

Both the colposcopic appearance (Figs. 10.15, 10.16, 10.17, 10.18, and 10.19) and the cytological features of cervical decidualization may be misdiagnosed as high-grade cervical dysplasia or squamous cell carcinoma (van Diepen et al. 2015). In cases like that, targeted biopsy will provide clarification. Differential diagnosis of decidual polyps protruding from the cervical canal also includes cervical myoma (Fig. 10.20).

Decidual transformation occasionally occurs outside of pregnancy and may also be confused with high-grade dysplasia (Fig. 10.21).

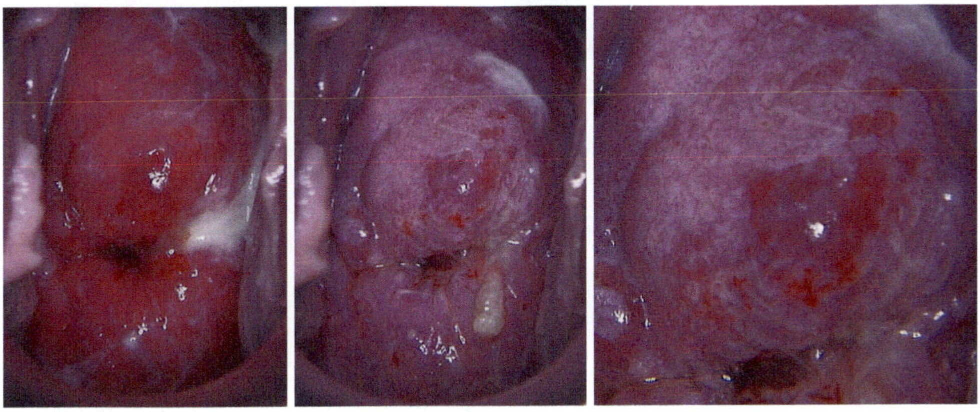

Fig. 10.5 HSIL/CIN2 in the 18th week of pregnancy. The cervix is already enlarged due to physiologic changes in pregnancy. The entire cervix is acetowhite with a slightly irregular mosaic (major change)

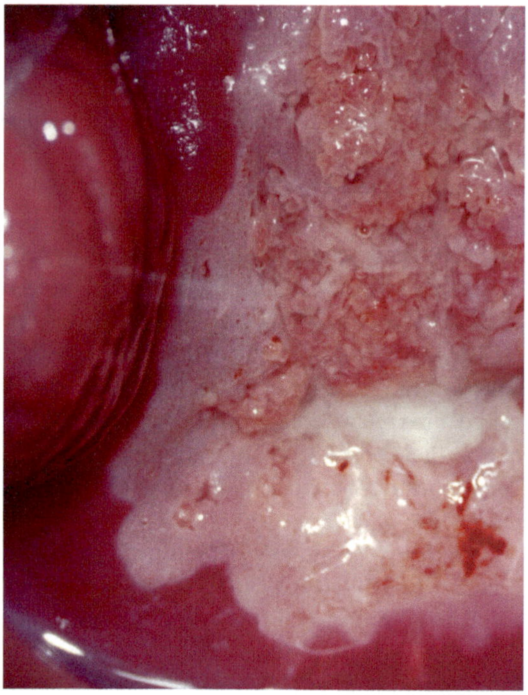

Fig. 10.6 CIN3 in the 22nd week of pregnancy. The acetowhite reaction is very prominent (major change)

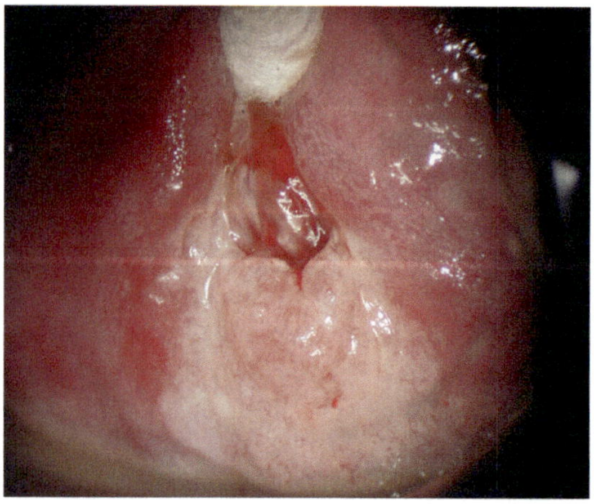

Fig. 10.7 CIN3 in the 24th week of pregnancy. In addition to "pseudo-punctation" anteriorly (ventrally), there is a raised and sharply delimited acetowhite area at the posterior (dorsal) cervix (major change)

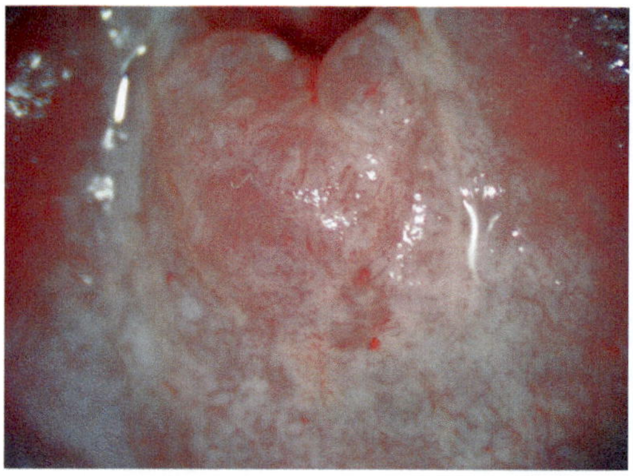

Fig. 10.8 CIN3 in the 24th week of pregnancy (see Fig. 10.7). At higher magnification, an irregular mosaic is visible (major change)

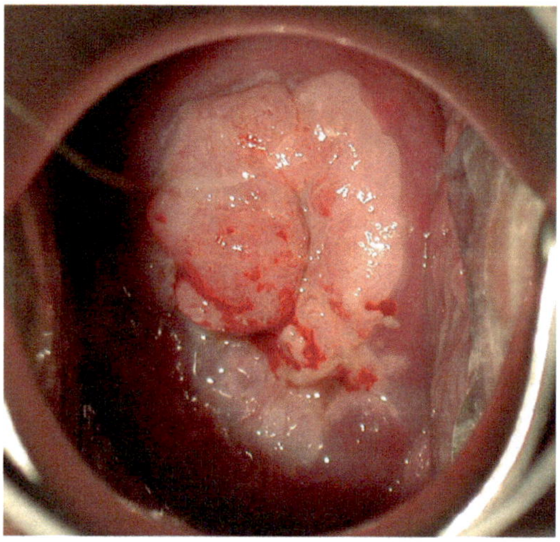

Fig. 10.9 CIN3 in the 21st week of gestation. Almost the entire anterior (ventral) cervix is acetowhite with raised borders (major change)

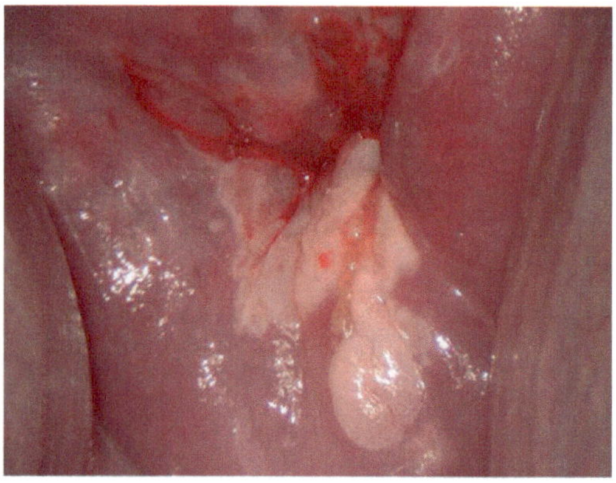

Fig. 10.10 CIN3 in the 27th week of pregnancy. There is intense acetowhite opaque staining with sharp borders and slightly raised epithelium (major change)

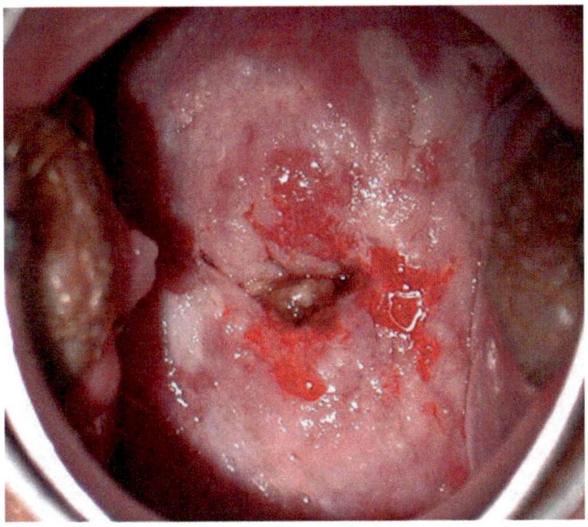

Fig. 10.11 CIN3 in the 25th week of pregnancy. The acetowhite epithelium has an irregular surface. Multiple biopsies should be obtained to rule out invasion

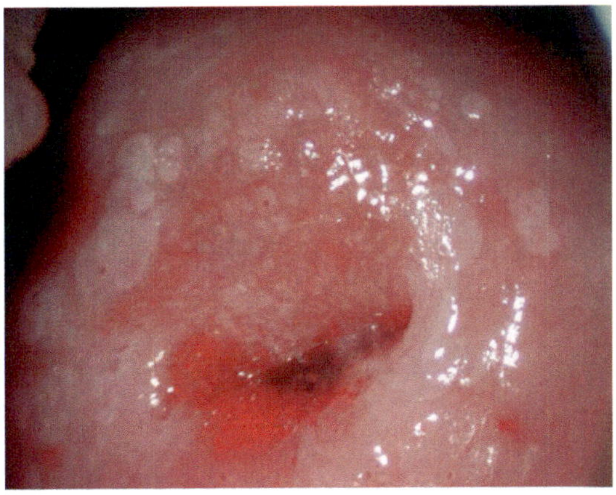

Fig. 10.12 CIN3 in the 8th week of pregnancy. The acetowhite epithelium shows coarse punctation and an irregular mosaic (major change). Also, there are several inner border lesions

In summary, the following pregnancy-related changes of the cervix are observed colposcopically:

- The cervix becomes increasingly hypertrophic due to fluid retention.
- The squamocolumnar junction gradually shifts toward the ectocervix.
- The mucous secretion of the endocervical epithelium increases.
- Partial decidualization (decidual transformation) of the cervix may occur.
- "Pseudo-punctation" may be observed.
- The local blood flow is increased significantly.
- Local blood flow is increased with prominent vessels.
- The acetowhite reaction of both dysplastic epithelium and immature metaplasia is more pronounced.
- Lugol's staining is also more intense as more glycogen is stored.
- Deciduosis occurs frequently and may mimic CIN or cancer.

Occasionally, condylomata acuminata occur during pregnancy. Typical condylomata do not necessarily need to be confirmed by biopsy. In the event of extensive involvement of vulva, vagina, and cervix, cesarean section may be indicated (Fig. 10.22), unless condylomata can be eliminated prior to delivery (CO_2 laser vaporization around the 32nd week of gestation).

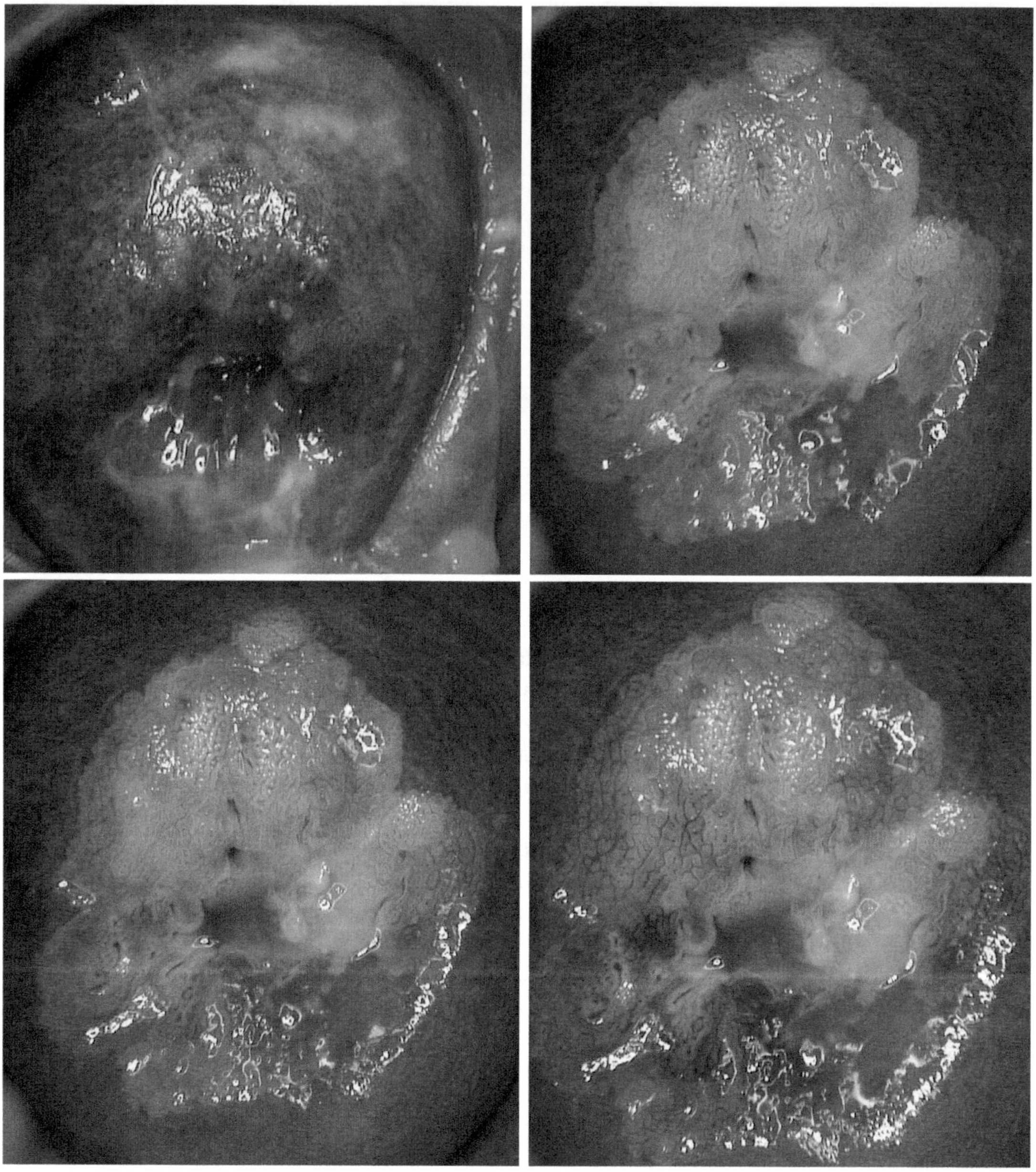

Fig. 10.13 CIN3 in the 16th week of gestation. There is "gyration" of the intensely acetowhite squamous epithelium (major change)

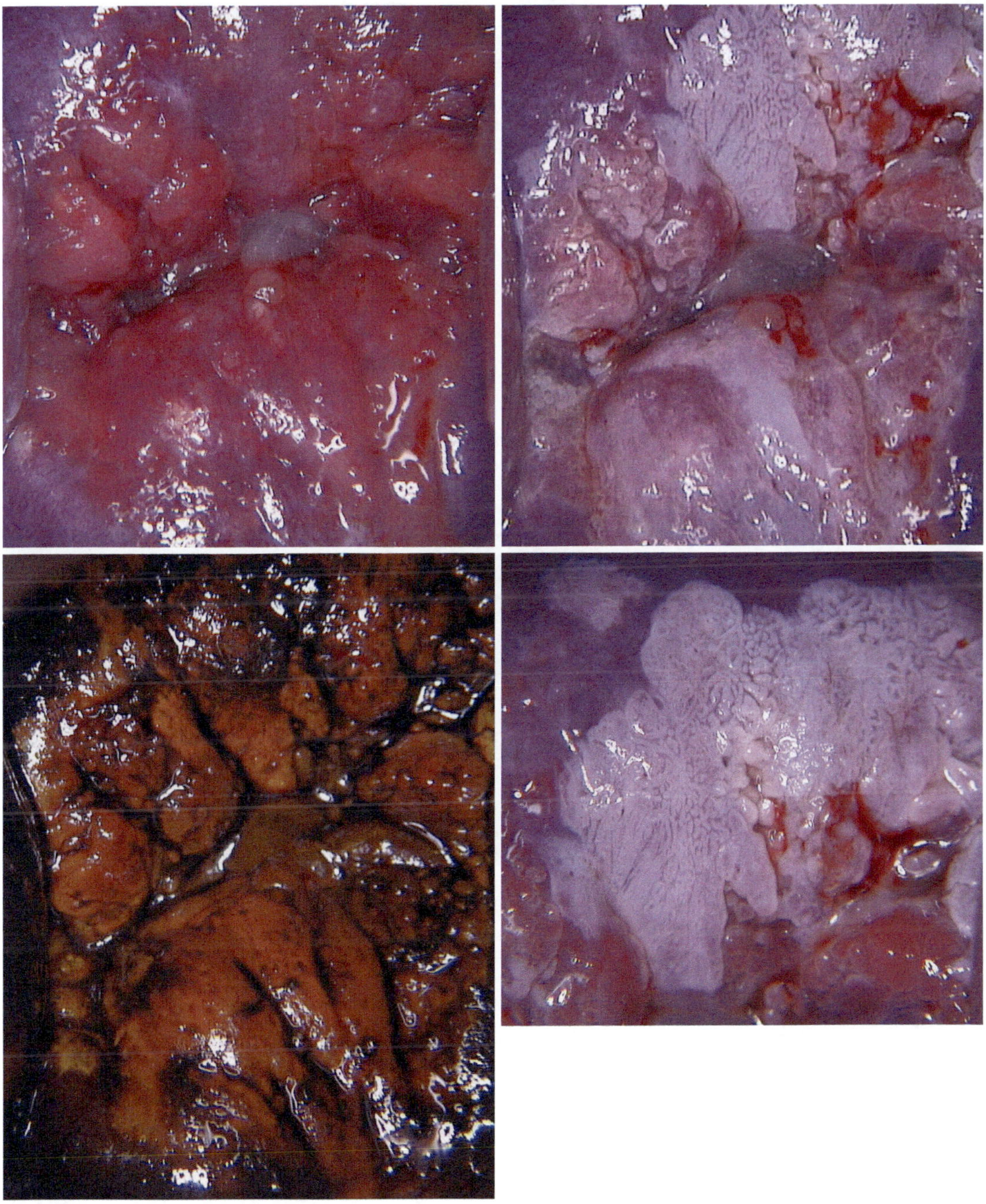

Fig. 10.14 CIN in the 27th week of gestation. The intensely acetowhite area is "gyrated" with a ridge sign at 12 o'clock

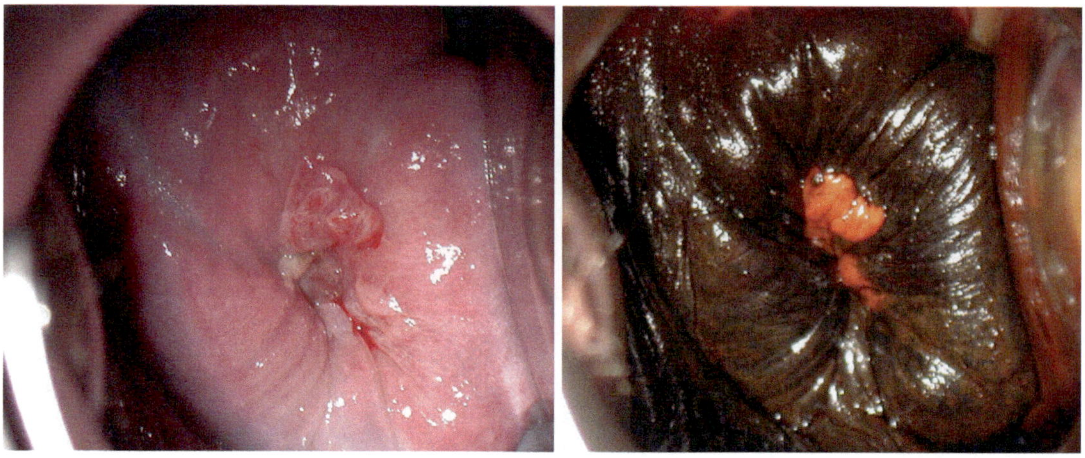

Fig. 10.15 Decidual polyp in the 32nd week of pregnancy. One year ago, the 31-year-old patient underwent cone biopsy for HSIL. There is a considerable tissue defect and scarring. The decidual polyp is Lugol-negative

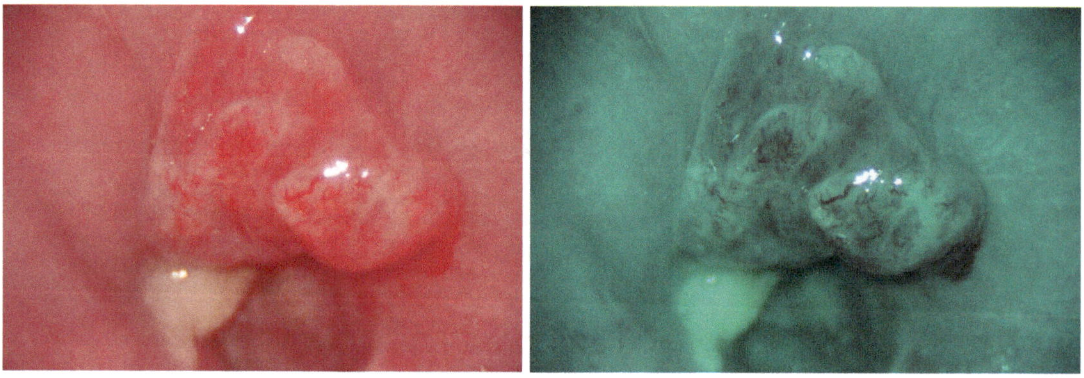

Fig. 10.16 Decidual polyp in the 32nd week of pregnancy (see Fig. 10.15). At 12 o'clock, there is a small exophytic lesion with very small and finely branched blood vessels

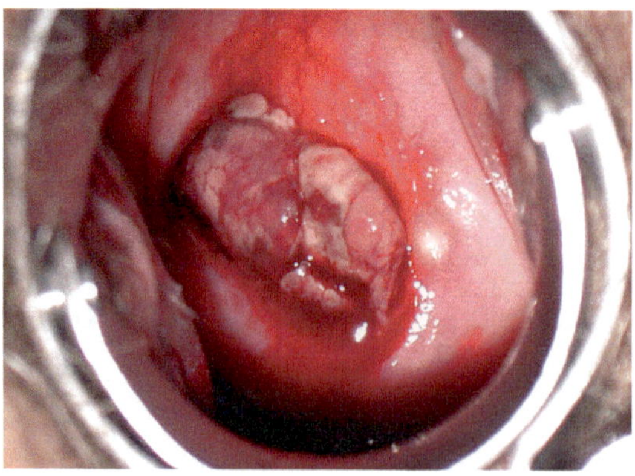

Fig. 10.17 Decidual polyp in the eighth week of pregnancy. Differential diagnosis includes incipient spontaneous abortion and even invasive disease

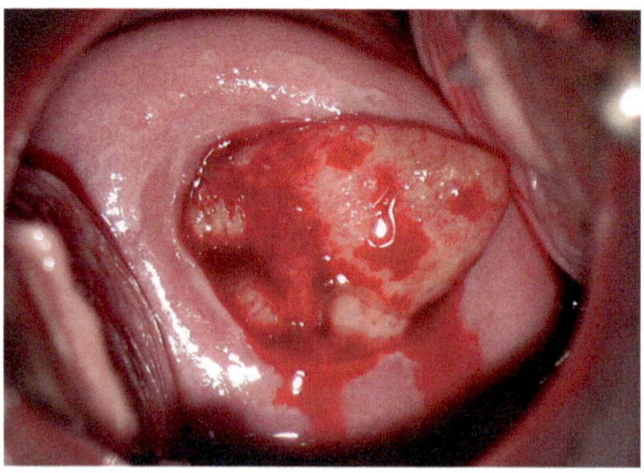

Fig. 10.18 Decidual polyp in the 13th week of pregnancy. If in doubt, biopsy should be performed

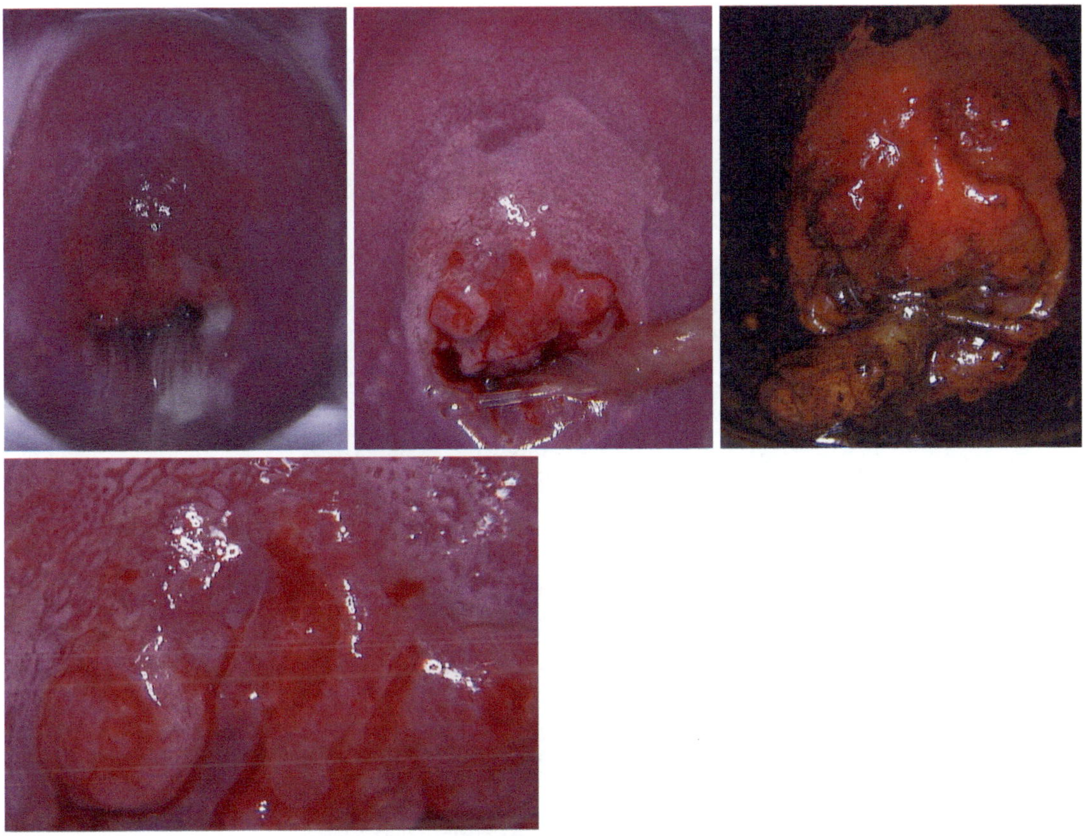

Fig. 10.19 HSIL/CIN2 and deciduosis in the 24th week of pregnancy. At 12 o'clock, there is a typical major change indicating HSIL. Close to the cervical canal, a slightly exophytic lesion is seen that is bleeding on touch. Interestingly, the image prior to application of acetic acid rather clearly suggests deciduosis. If any doubt remains, invasive disease should be ruled out by biopsy

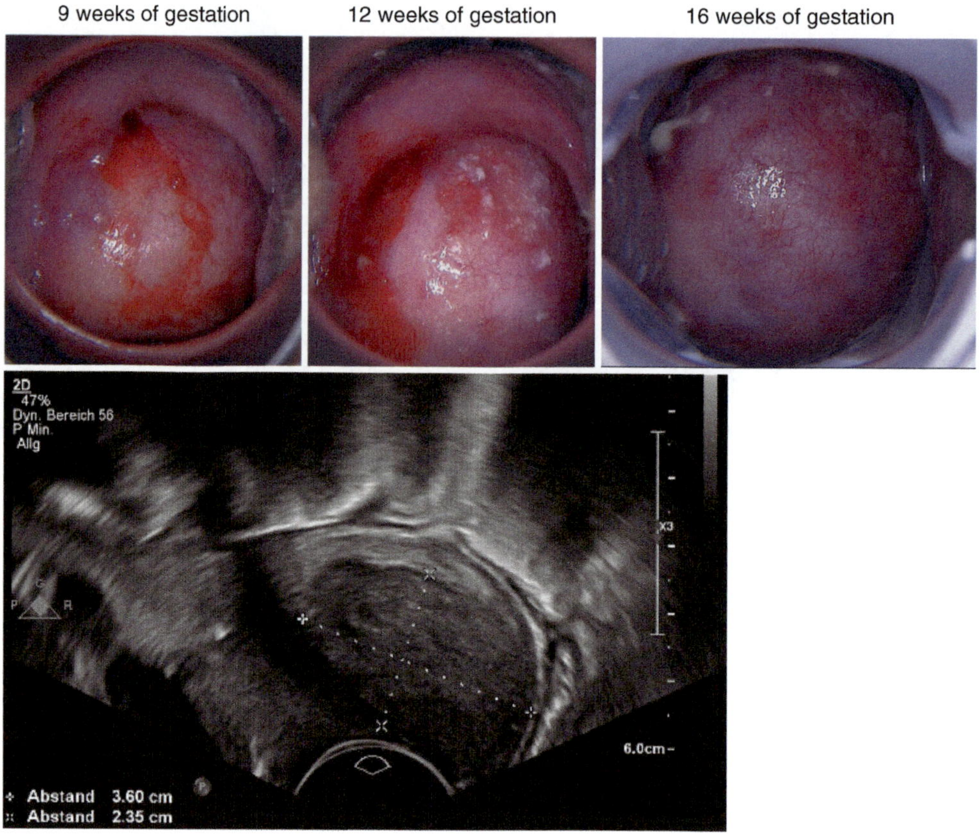

Fig. 10.20 A 34-year-old patient with cervical myoma in pregnancy. The patient has had two previous conizations for HSIL

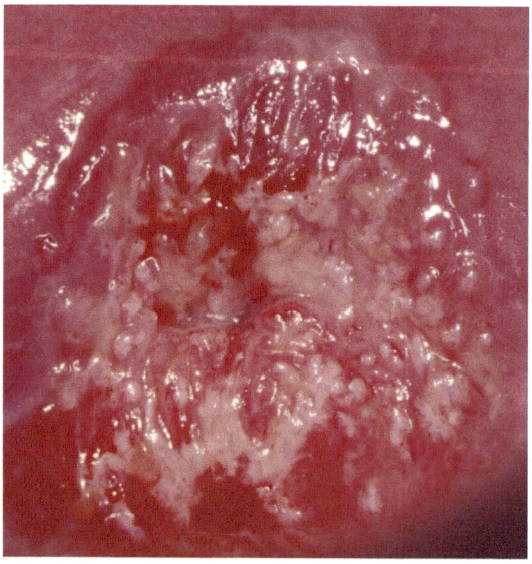

Fig. 10.21 Decidual transformation outside of pregnancy. This can be caused by progestins. The patient uses a NuvaRing® for contraception, which releases the gestagen etonogestrel in addition to ethinylestradiol

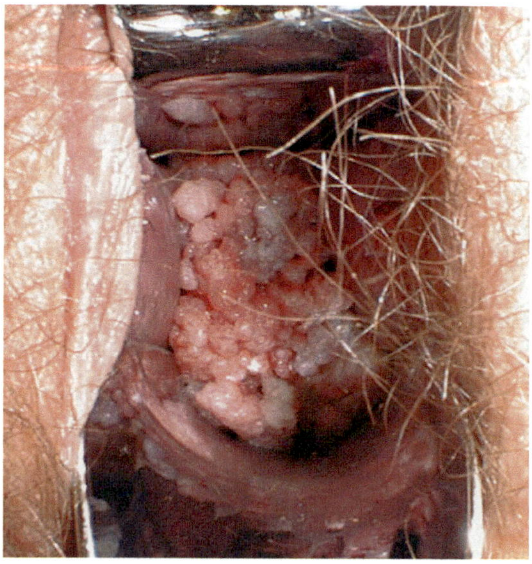

Fig. 10.22 Condylomata acuminata of cervix and vagina in the 33rd week of pregnancy. Due to the extent of warts, cesarean section should be done

10.2 Management of Cervical Dysplasia During Pregnancy

Colposcopic examination during pregnancy does not differ significantly from the nonpregnant patient. However, the blades of the speculum need to be sufficiently wide so that the vaginal walls do not impede inspection of the cervix. By placing a protective cover or condom—as used for the vaginal ultrasound probe—over the speculum and incising its tip, the vaginal walls can be further pushed aside.

Figure 10.23 suggests an algorithm on how to proceed during pregnancy, when the Pap smear is abnormal.

In most cases, a tissue biopsy should be obtained during colposcopy as colposcopic assessment is less reliable due to tissue changes related to pregnancy. Cervical biopsies are feasible at any time of gestation.

Compared to nonpregnant patients, the procedure is less likely to cause discomfort or pain. However, the cervix is much better vascularized, and considerable bleeding from the biopsy site may occur. However, hemostasis can be achieved just as effectively as in nonpregnant patients. It is helpful to apply pressure on the biopsy site immediately after taking the tissue sample using a cotton tip. Then Monsel's solution is applied. If hemostasis is still unsatisfactory, a tampon is loosely inserted into the vagina, and the patient is instructed to remove it after 3–4 h.

In pregnant patients, endocervical curettage is not advisable to avoid injury of the amniotic sac. If the transformation zone is not visible, colposcopy is repeated 6–8 weeks later.

If the diagnosis of dysplasia is confirmed, repeat colposcopies are done depending on both the colposcopic diagnosis and the biopsy result. A high-grade lesion should be reevaluated every 8 weeks.

During pregnancy, any suspicion of invasive disease based on cytopathology and/or colposcopy (Figs. 10.24, 10.25, and 10.26) must be either confirmed or ruled out through targeted biopsy or biopsies.

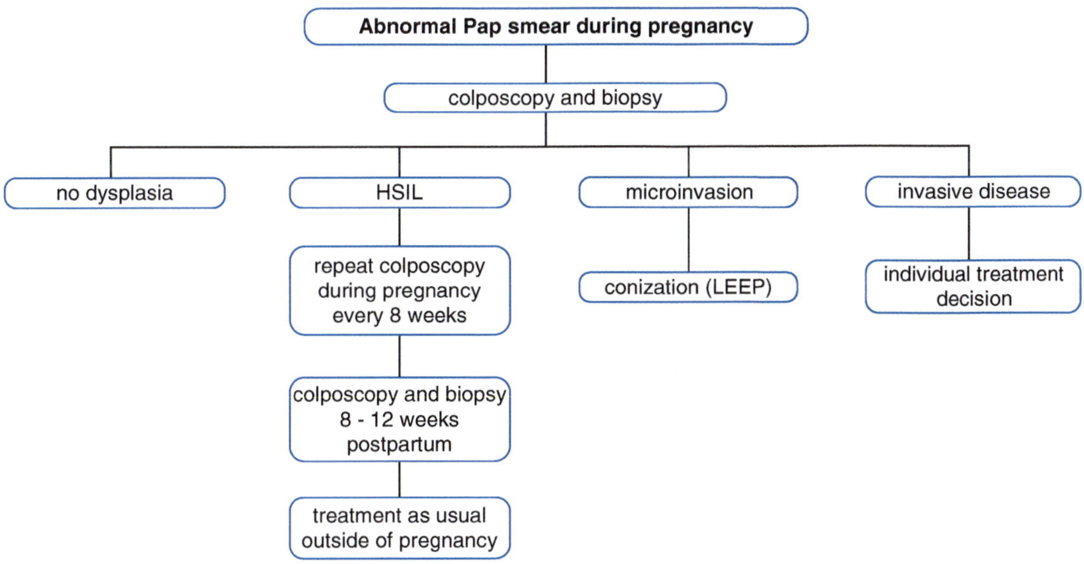

Fig. 10.23 Algorithm for triage of an abnormal Pap smear during pregnancy

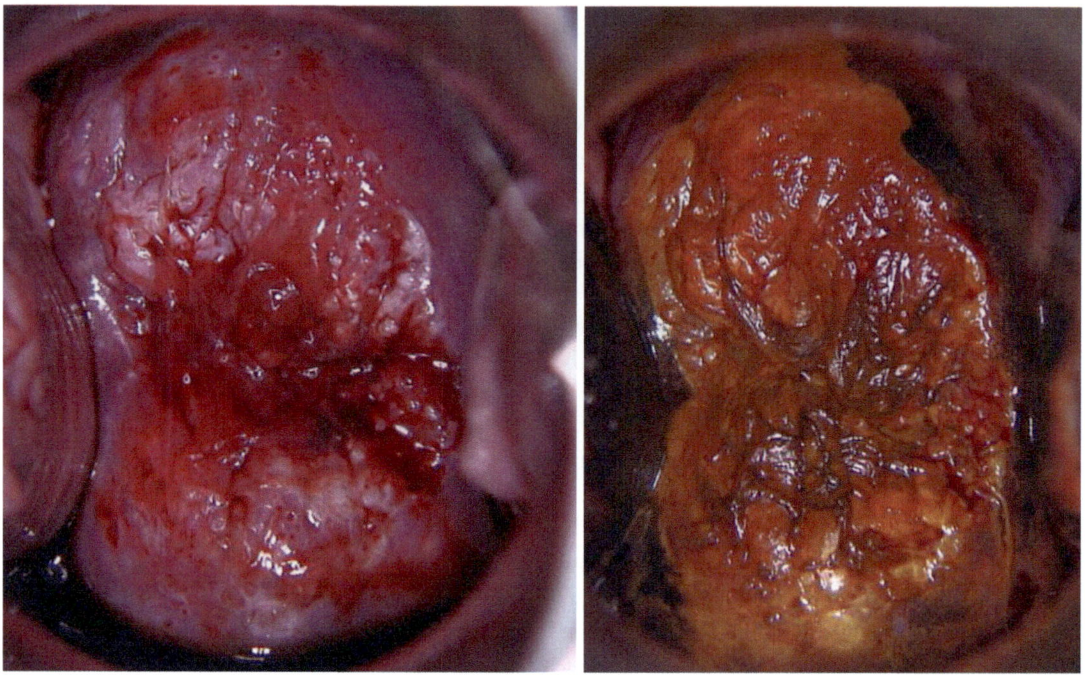

Fig. 10.24 CIN3 in the 23rd week of gestation. The patient is 29 years old. The surface of the large acetowhite and Lugol-negative transformation zone is irregular and bleeding on touch. Invasion should be ruled out by (repeat) biopsy

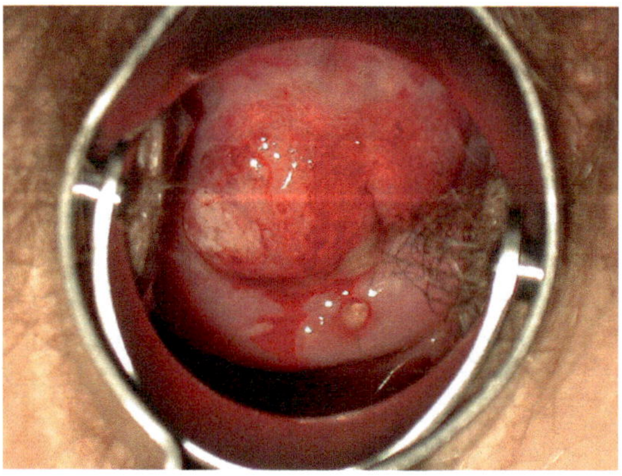

Fig. 10.25 Squamous cell carcinoma in the 11th week of pregnancy. The 36-year-old patient, gravida I, is free of symptoms. The Pap smear had been normal. A biopsy revealed squamous cell carcinoma. The patient opted for termination of the pregnancy with surgical treatment (radical hysterectomy). Histological examination revealed a 3.5 cm poorly differentiated squamous cell carcinoma with lymph-vascular space invasion

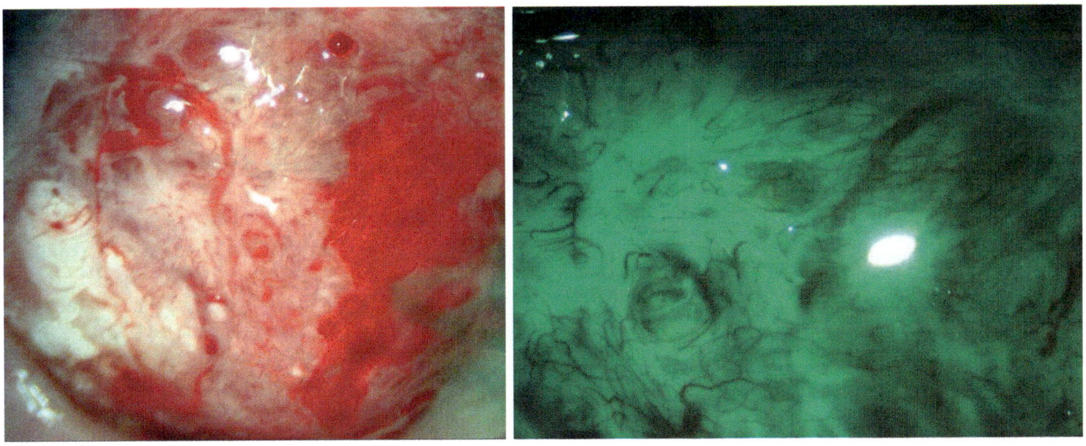

Fig. 10.26 Squamous cell carcinoma in the 11th week of gestation (see Fig. 10.25). Especially when viewed with the green filter, vessels are grossly atypical. Also, there is focal keratinization

10.3 Conization (LEEP) During Pregnancy

Cold-knife conizations or loop resections during pregnancy are usually not indicated for preinvasive disease and should be avoided whenever possible. However, if invasive disease is suspected and the diagnosis cannot be clarified through targeted biopsy, a more comprehensive tissue removal from the cervix may be necessary.

Conization in pregnancy is mainly diagnostic and not therapeutic, as it is usually not possible to obtain free margins due to pregnancy changes.

As an alternative to cold-knife conization, loop resection (LEEP) is also acceptable during pregnancy (Mitsuhashi and Sekiya 2000). First, a cerclage suture is placed but not tied. Then the posterior (dorsal) cervical tissue is removed with an appropriately sized loop followed by removal of the anterior (ventral) tissue. Finally, the cerclage suture is tied. This will significantly reduce bleeding. Finally, the wound surface is coagulated (Fig. 10.27). If hemostasis is still not satisfactory, absorbable sutures are placed.

A meta-analysis by Danhof et al. (2015) came to the conclusion that the risk of preterm delivery is significantly increased by CIN surgery during pregnancy, not however when CIN had been previously treated outside of pregnancy, thus contradicting numerous articles quoted above that demonstrate an increased risk after any type of previous cervical resection for preinvasive disease.

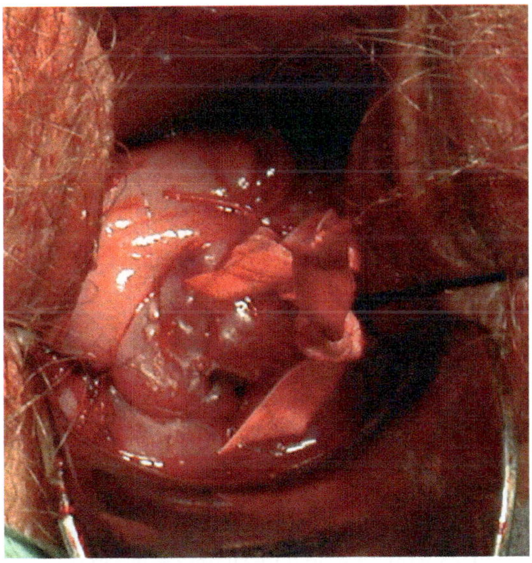

Fig. 10.27 Cervix immediately after conization and cerclage during pregnancy

10.4 Management of HSIL After Delivery

Eight to 12 weeks after delivery, the cervix is reevaluated colposcopically. Any abnormal areas (major or minor change) are biopsied.

Ideally, high-grade preinvasive disease should be confirmed again histopathologically after delivery before surgical treatment is performed, as CIN2 and CIN3 have a tendency to regress after birth, although the majority of patients will eventually have to undergo surgery.

CIN1 lesions have a higher probability of regression during pregnancy than outside of pregnancy (Serati et al. 2008). Yost et al. (1999) reported a high regression rate of 68% for CIN2 lesions and 70% for CIN3, respectively. In this study, CIN diagnosis was based on targeted biopsy during pregnancy. Therefore, results are more reliable than those based on cytopathological evaluation only. In contrast, Henes et al. (2013) found a CIN3/AIS remission rate of only 9.3%.

A likely explanation for spontaneous CIN regression after pregnancy is exfoliation of dysplastic epithelium through the trauma of birth. However, regression rates were identical in patients who undergo cesarean section, with or without laboring (Yost et al. 1999). Schuster et al. (2018) also found that the mode of delivery does not significantly influence the natural history of CIN diagnosed during pregnancy. Spontaneous postpartum regression was documented in 15 out of 40 women who delivered vaginally and in 10 out of 23 women who underwent cesarean section. Therefore, Yost et al. hypothesized that other factors may be responsible such as the resolution of immunosuppression occurring after delivery. Also, smaller size lesions may be completely eliminated by colposcopically guided biopsies, thus giving the impression of spontaneous regression.

As there is always a chance of spontaneous resolution of dysplasia, it is advisable to repeat the entire diagnostic process postpartum and reconfirm CIN2+ disease prior to surgical treatment.

References

Ciavattini A, Sopracordevole F, Di Giuseppe J, Moriconi L, Lucarini G, Mancioli F et al (2017) Cervical intraepithelial neoplasia in pregnancy: interference of pregnancy status with p16 and Ki-67 protein expression. Oncol Lett 13(1):301–306. https://doi.org/10.3892/ol.2016.5441

Danhof NA, Kamphuis EI, Limpens J, van Lonkhuijzen LRCW, Pajkrt E, Mol BWJ (2015) The risk of preterm birth of treated versus untreated cervical intraepithelial neoplasia (CIN): a systematic review and meta-analysis. Eur J Obstet Gynecol Reprod Biol 188:24–33. https://doi.org/10.1016/j.ejogrb.2015.02.033

Flannelly G (2010) The management of women with abnormal cervical cytology in pregnancy. Best Pract Res Clin Obstet Gynaecol 24(1):51–60. https://doi.org/10.1016/j.bpobgyn.2009.07.001

Gleichert JE (1971) Etienne Joseph Jacquemin, discoverer of 'Chadwick's sign'. J Hist Med Allied Sci 26:75–80

Henes M, Neis F, Rall K, Iftner T, Staebler A, Fehm T, Rothmund R (2013) Abnormal cytology during pregnancy--a retrospective analysis of patients in a dysplasia clinic. Anticancer Res 33(2):711–715

Hunter MI, Monk BJ, Tewari KS (2008) Cervical neoplasia in pregnancy. Part 1: screening and management of preinvasive disease. Am J Obstet Gynecol:3–9

Mitsuhashi A, Sekiya S (2000) Loop electrosurgical excision procedure (LEEP) during first trimester of pregnancy. Int J Gynaecol Obstet 71(3):237–239

Schneider V, Barnes LA (1981) Ectopic decidual reaction of the uterine cervix: frequency and cytologic presentation. Acta Cytol 25(6):616–622

Schuster S, Joura E, Kohlberger P (2018) Natural history of squamous intraepithelial lesions in pregnancy and mode of delivery. Anticancer Res 38(4):2439–2442. https://doi.org/10.21873/anticanres.12496

Serati M, Uccella S, Laterza RM, Salvatore S, Beretta P, Riva C, Bolis PF (2008) Natural history of cervical intraepithelial neoplasia during pregnancy. Acta Obstet Gynecol Scand 87(12):1296–1300. https://doi.org/10.1080/00016340802482986

Takushi M, Moromizato H, Sakumoto K, Kanazawa K (2002) Management of invasive carcinoma of the uterine cervix associated with pregnancy: outcome of intentional delay in treatment. Gynecol Oncol 87(2):185–189

van Diepen DA, Hellebrekers B, van Haaften A-M, Natté R (2015) Cervical deciduosis imitating dysplasia. BMJ Case Rep 2015:bcr2015210030. https://doi.org/10.1136/bcr-2015-210030

Yost NP, Santoso JT, McIntire DD, Iliya FA (1999) Postpartum regression rates of antepartum cervical intraepithelial neoplasia II and III lesions. Obstet Gynecol 93(3):359–362

11 Colposcopy of Radiation-Induced Changes

> Following previous pelvic radiation therapy, the colposcopic distinction between tumor recurrence and radiation-induced changes poses a challenge to colposcopy.

Following radiation therapy of the pelvis, teletherapy, and/or brachytherapy of the cervix and vagina, many of the criteria for colposcopic assessment are no longer applicable. Usually, both the acetic acid reaction and the Schiller's test are negative. The irradiated tissue is atrophic and exhibits marked vascular changes (Fig. 11.1). In addition, radiation-induced tissue defects and ulcerations may occur (Figs. 11.2 and 11.3).

For clinical assessment, the patient's history is of crucial importance. A repeat colposcopic exam after an interval of 3 to 4 weeks may also help to differentiate between radiation-induced changes and recurrent malignancy.

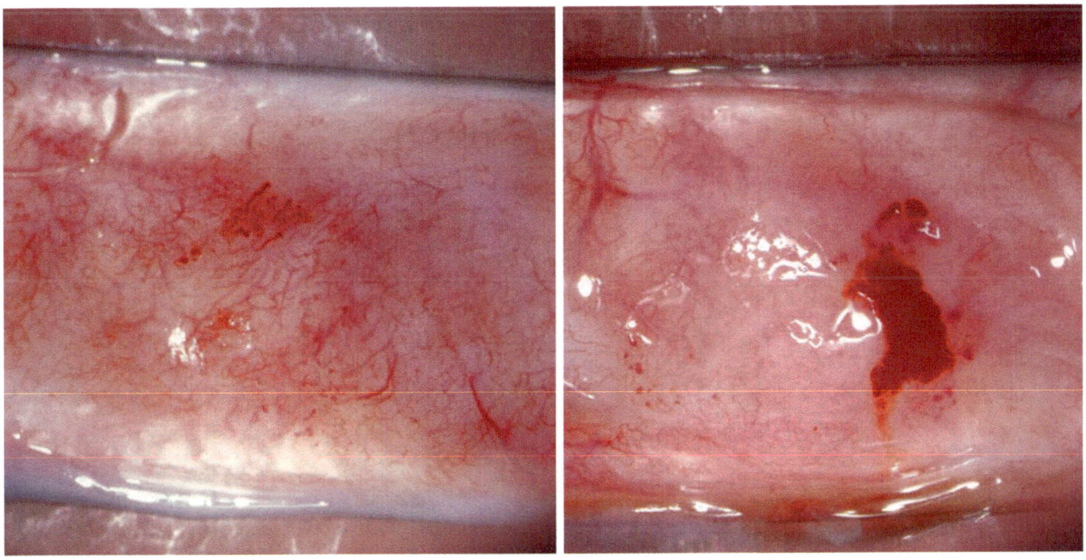

Fig. 11.1 Characteristic vascular changes after radiation therapy. Previously, the 45-year-old patient had undergone radical hysterectomy for cervical carcinoma followed by irradiation of the pelvis. Typical telangiectasia is seen with mucosal bleeding

R. J. Lellé, V. Küppers, *Colposcopy*, https://doi.org/10.1007/978-3-030-85388-4_11

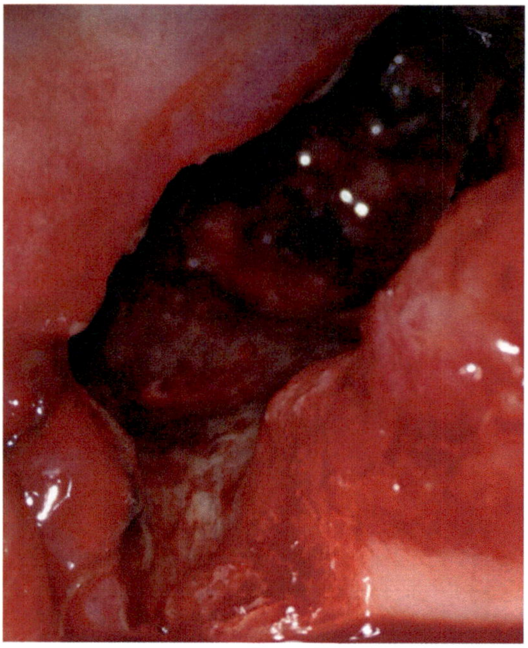

Fig. 11.2 Squamous cell carcinoma of the cervix FIGO stage IIB treated by primary chemoradiation. A large necrotic cavity is seen in the upper vagina due to the decaying tumor tissue

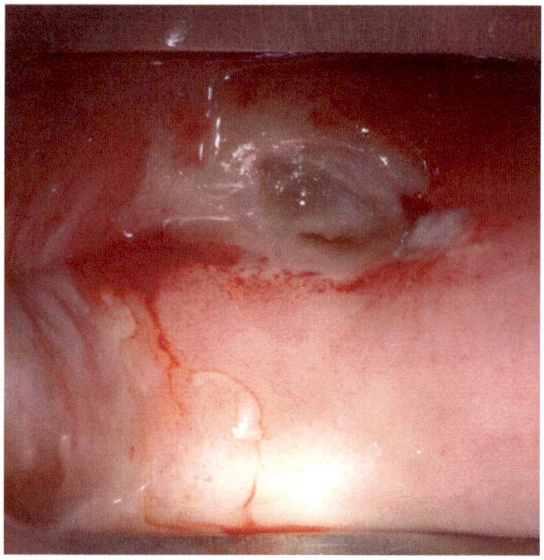

Fig. 11.3 Squamous cell carcinoma of the cervix FIGO stage IIB 6 months after completion of chemoradiation. The mucosa of the upper vagina is atrophic with a small ulcer, which is caused by irradiation and not by persistent or recurrent disease

However, if cancer cannot be ruled out, definite clarification by obtaining one or more biopsies is recommended. Due to radiation-induced atrophy of the vagina, special caution is required to avoid the risk of fistula formation to the bladder or rectum, in case of removing too much tissue.

12 Colposcopy of the Vagina

Contents

> Colposcopy of the vagina is particularly important in order to diagnose high-grade vaginal intraepithelial neoplasia (VAIN1 to 3), which is considered to be the precursor of carcinoma of the vagina in analogy to CIN and cervical cancer.

Compared to colposcopy of the vulva and cervix, inspection of the vagina can be challenging. Without the speculum, only the epithelium up to the hymenal area and the urethral orifice is visible. After insertion of a Cusco speculum for visualization of the cervix, only a limited portion of the lateral vaginal walls is visible. In order to adequately assess the vagina, the speculum must be partially closed, rotated, and retracted while inspecting the vaginal epithelium. While one hand is required to move the speculum, the colposcope must be adjusted and continually refocused with the other hand. The speculum must be moved carefully in order to avoid unnecessary discomfort to the patient.

The entire length of the vagina needs to be inspected. However, vaginal intraepithelial neoplasia is usually located within the upper one-third of the vagina, i.e., close to the vaginal scar after previous hysterectomy. If the cervix has not been removed, special attention is paid to the vaginal tissue directly adjacent to the cervix. After previous hysterectomy, the vaginal scar needs to be unfolded completely and inspected closely.

Vaginal inspection is performed twice: first after application of 5% acetic acid and then after using Lugol's solution.

For the diagnosis of vaginal disease, especially vaginal intraepithelial neoplasia, Schiller's iodine test is crucial to colposcopic assessment, as VAIN may manifest itself as otherwise invisible iodine-negative tissue areas.

Any abnormalities, including iodine-negative areas in the absence of vaginal atrophy, are

R. J. Lellé, V. Küppers, *Colposcopy*, https://doi.org/10.1007/978-3-030-85388-4_12

biopsied. Compared to cervical sampling, most patients do not feel any discomfort when small biopsies are obtained. Usually, no hemostasis is required.

Biopsies should remove the entire epithelial thickness including some of the stromal tissue, in order to detect or exclude invasive diseases. However, in older patients with atrophic vaginal walls and/or prior radiation therapy, deep biopsies should be avoided due to the risk of bladder or bowel injury.

If part of the upper vagina cannot be visualized following hysterectomy, a narrow curette (e.g., Stiefel® curette; see Chap. 7) can be used to obtain tissue material for histopathologic evaluation.

Vaginal tumors are rare and are mostly benign as, for example, Gartner's duct cysts, which develop from embryologic remnants of the Wolffian or mesonephric duct (Fig. 12.1). Gartner's duct cysts are usually diagnosed by chance as there are no symptoms.

Inspection of the vagina should be part of every colposcopic exam of the cervix. However, there are also some special indications for vaginal colposcopy.

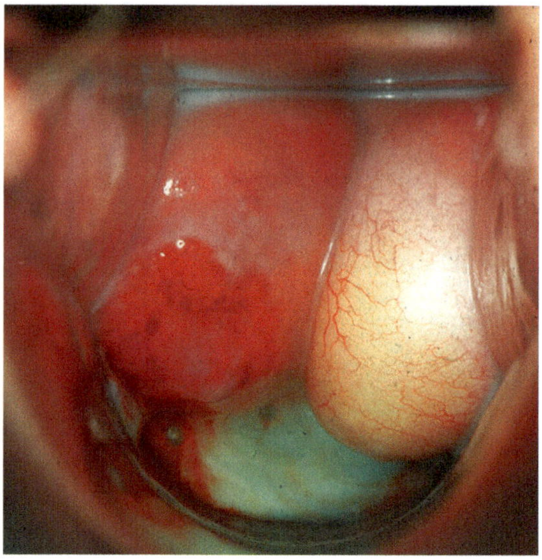

Fig. 12.1 Gartner's duct cyst in the vagina

- **Special Indications for Colposcopy of the Vagina:**
  - Any abnormality seen on routine gynecological examination
  - Abnormal Pap tests after cervical disease has been ruled out colposcopically
  - Abnormal Pap test after treatment for CIN and normal-appearing cervix
  - Abnormal Pap test after hysterectomy, especially after hysterectomy for CIN or cervical carcinoma
  - Abnormal Pap test and/or CIN in immunosuppressed patients (multifocal intraepithelial neoplasia)

- **Colposcopy of the cervix always includes colposcopy of the vagina.**

12.1 Condylomata Acuminata

Condylomata acuminata may be found in the vagina and/or on the cervix (Figs. 12.2 and 12.3). Patients with vaginal condylomata usually do not have any specific symptoms, and the condylomata may be seen when colposcopy is done for HPV-related disease of the cervix or vulva.

Patients with immunosuppressive diseases (HIV) or immunosuppressive treatment (following organ transplants) are prone to multicentric HPV-related diseases including vaginal condylomata acuminata (Fig. 12.2).

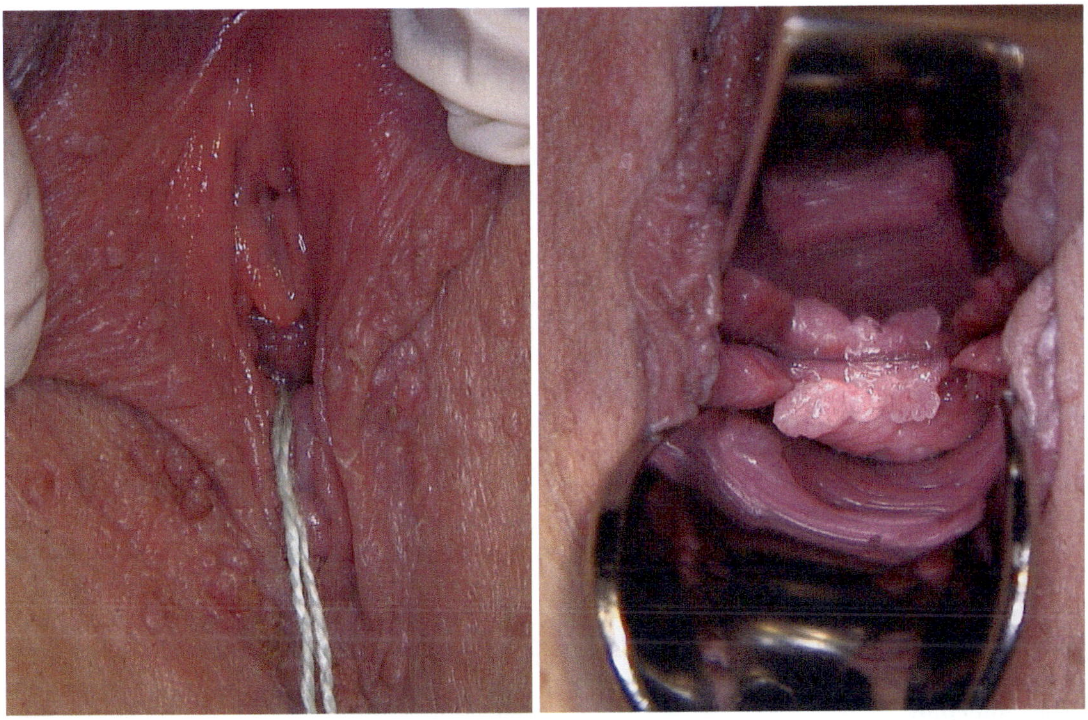

Fig. 12.2 Condylomata acuminata of the vulva and vagina. The patient is 16 years old and has had a renal transplant 8 years previously

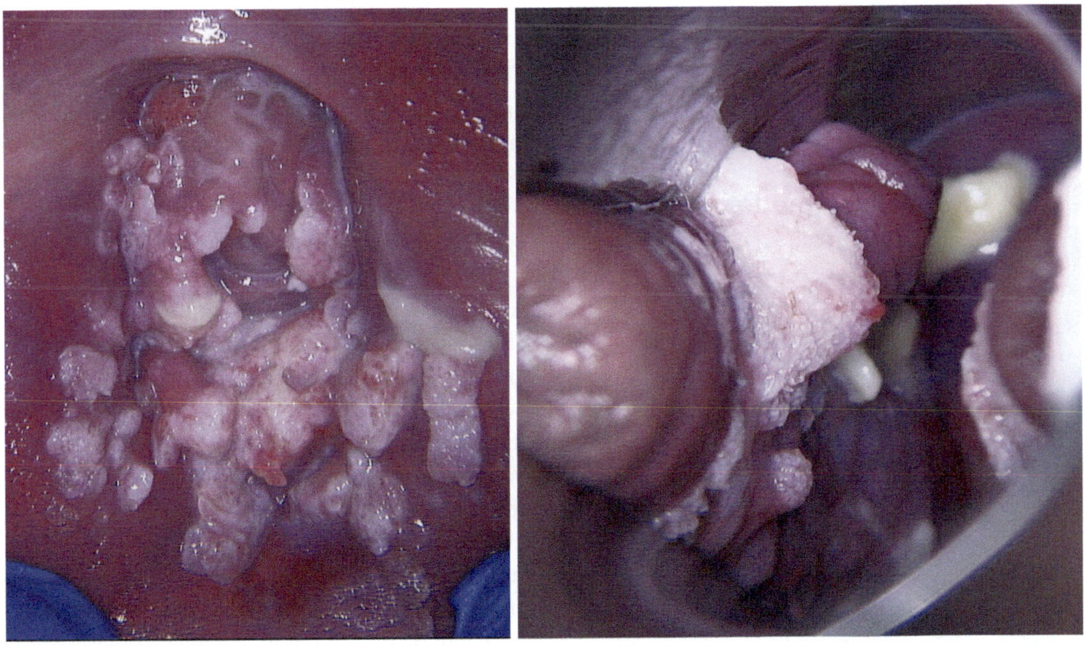

Fig. 12.3 Extensive condylomata acuminata of the vagina and around the urethra in the 34th week of gestation

12.2 Adenoma

Adenomas of the vagina are rare. Embryologically, vaginal adenomas originate from the mesonephric and paramesonephric system. The presence of adenomas of the paramesonephric system is called adenosis vaginae (Fig. 12.4). Adenosis vaginae is derived from the Müller epithelium and, on histopathological examination, is very similar to cervical glands. The pathogenesis of adenosis vaginae is still unknown. Various causes are discussed, including mechanical and chronic inflammatory irritation.

In the United States, adenosis of the vagina had been reported in women whose mothers had been treated with stilbene derivatives such as diethylstilbestrol (DES) during the first trimester of pregnancy. In the United States, DES treatment had been widely used during the 1940s for treatment of women with imminent or habitual spontaneous abortion.

Vaginal adenosis may also occur without DES substitution.

The main symptom of vaginal adenosis is increased vaginal discharge. Some patients complain of dyspareunia and a foreign body sensation.

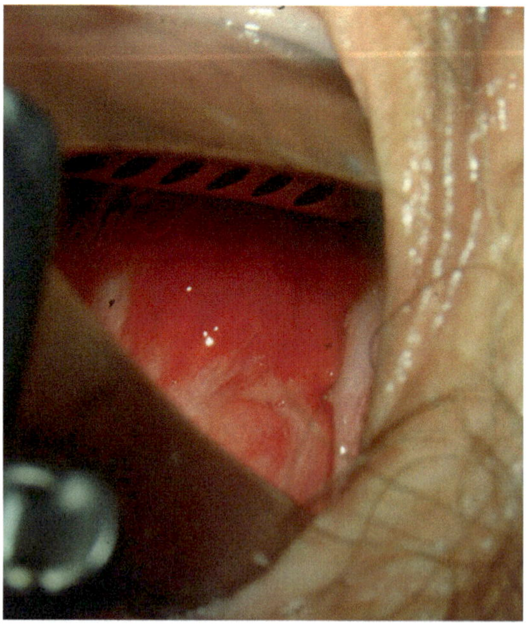

Fig. 12.4 Adenosis vagina

The colposcopic examination reveals small cystic lesions or small reddish areas, usually located in the upper one-third of the vagina. To confirm the colposcopic diagnosis, targeted biopsies from the vagina are obtained. Histopathological examination will clarify the diagnosis and rule out malignancy. Although adenosis of the vagina is not considered to be a premalignant lesion, patients should receive annual follow-up exams (colposcopy and Pap test).

If the patient is free of symptoms and no malignancy is suspected, a wait-and-see strategy is appropriate. In the symptomatic patient, small lesions can be removed by CO_2 laser vaporization, electrosurgery, or cold-knife excision after biopsies have been obtained. If a large area of the vagina is involved, an individual decision has to be made depending on the symptoms and the needs of the patient. Rarely, partial or total colpectomy will be necessary.

Malignant transformation should be suspected when a bloody discharge or overt vaginal bleeding occurs.

12.3 Vaginal Intraepithelial Neoplasia (VAIN)

The colposcopic diagnosis of vaginal intraepithelial neoplasia (VAIN) is of great clinical importance and will therefore be discussed in detail.

12.3.1 Pathogenesis of VAIN

Analogous to cervical intraepithelial neoplasia of the cervix (CIN), premalignant changes of the squamous epithelium of the vagina are called "vaginal intraepithelial neoplasia" or VAIN (Fig. 12.5). The histopathological appearance of VAIN and CIN is very similar, and VAIN is also an HPV-related disease.

According to Srodon et al. (2006), the distribution of HPV types is very similar to distribution of HPV in CIN, suggesting a close relationship between the two diseases, whereas vulvar precursors show a different HPV distribution pattern. Furthermore, VAIN may occur synchronously or metachronously in multicentric lower genital tract disease including involvement of cervix,

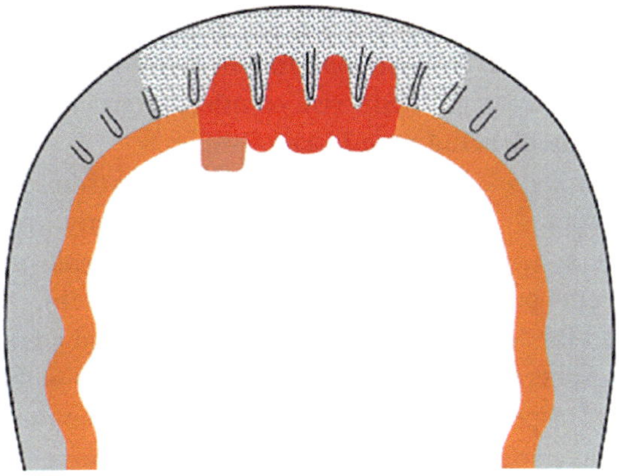

Fig. 12.5 Vaginal intraepithelial neoplasia (VAIN) analogous to the depictions of CIN (Chap. 3)

vagina, vulva, and anus (Hampl et al. 2007). Hampl et al. (2007) detected HPV 16 DNA in 7 out of 11 high-grade VAIN lesions. This suggests that the widespread use of the prophylactic HPV vaccine will also help prevent vaginal dysplasia.

As with cervical dysplasia, VAIN is subdivided into three grades: low-grade (VAIN1), intermediate grade (VAIN2), and high-grade (VAIN3) disease. VAIN2 and VAIN3 are called "high-grade squamous intraepithelial lesions" (HSIL), again in analogy to HSIL of the cervix.

VAIN3 is considered to be a direct precursor of squamous cell carcinoma of the vagina, whereas VAIN1 and VAIN2 are less likely to develop into cancer. However, there are not sufficient data to reliably support these assumptions.

Diakomanolis et al. (2002) observed an average age of onset for VAIN1 and VAIN2 of 44.5 and 47.8 years, respectively, whereas the age of onset in VAIN3 patients was significantly higher: 61.8 years. This suggests that the biological characteristics of high-grade vaginal dysplasia or VAIN3 differ fundamentally from those of VAIN1 and VAIN2.

In 1981, Woodruff (1981) still maintained that vaginal intraepithelial neoplasia is very rare, even less common than invasive squamous cell carcinoma of the vagina. Especially, VAIN without previous CIN had been observed very rarely at that time. To date, there are still no reliable epidemiological data on the frequency of VAIN. However, due to the widespread use of Pap smear screening, even in women whose uterus has been removed, vaginal intraepithelial neoplasia is more likely to be diagnosed.

Vaginal dysplasia is frequently associated with cervical dysplasia (CIN), occurring either simultaneously or following CIN treatment by conization or hysterectomy.

The routine use of the Pap test after hysterectomy for benign disease is not necessary.

In a group of women who were 50 years or older and had undergone hysterectomy, Fox et al. (1999) found that the likelihood of an abnormal Pap test was ten times lower than in women who still had a uterus.

Similarly to cervical intraepithelial neoplasia, the etiology of vaginal intraepithelial neoplasia is HPV-associated. However, following the HPV high-risk infection, vaginal intraepithelial neoplasia develops less frequently than its cervical counterpart. As the cervical transformation zone is the predilection site for CIN, a vaginal transformation zone occurs only in women who had been exposed to diethylstilboestrol. Therefore, de novo formation within the area of the original squamous epithelium must be assumed. This may also explain the longer time interval between HPV infection and the development of vaginal dysplasia.

From a clinical point of view, high-grade VAIN, like high-grade CIN, may ultimately develop into vaginal cancer. In the immunocompetent patient, this is less likely than in CIN3 and cervical cancer. However, data on the cancer risk of VAIN is limited. Aho et al. (1991) presented a clinical follow-up of 23 patients who did not undergo treatment. Half of these women also had cervical or vulvar dysplasia. In two patients (9%), invasive carcinoma developed within the 3-year observation period. In three patients (13%), the dysplastic changes of the vagina persisted, and in 18 patients (78%), spontaneous regression occurred.

Rome and England (2000) observed progression to invasive carcinoma after 1–14 years in 8 out of 100 patients with VAIN3. Two of these eight patients had not undergone treatment for VAIN. For the remaining six patients, various surgical treatment modalities had been used previously.

As long as the cancer risk of vaginal intraepithelial neoplasia is unknown, VAIN3 and possibly VAIN2 must be regarded as a precursor to vaginal carcinoma. Early detection of VAIN3 by cytological screening in certain risk groups, its verification by colposcopic examination, and the subsequent treatment of

epithelial dysplasia may prevent development of vaginal carcinoma.

The following four clinical scenarios can be differentiated in the diagnosis and therapy of VAIN:

- VAIN with existing cervix with or without simultaneous CIN
- VAIN following hysterectomy for the treatment of (recurrent) CIN
- VAIN following hysterectomy in women with no known history of CIN
- VAIN in immunosuppressed patients

12.3.2 VAIN with Existing Cervix with or without Simultaneous CIN

When colposcopic triage of an abnormal Pap test and/or positive HPV test is focused solely on the cervix, there is a risk of overlooking simultaneous VAIN. A Pap test obtained directly from the ectocervix and the cervical canal may show dysplastic cells, if VAIN is present in the absence of CIN, since the vaginal epithelium of the upper third of the vagina, the most common site of vaginal dysplasia, is in direct contact with the ectocervix. If no abnormality is detected colposcopically in patients with a Pap test suggesting HSIL, a thorough evaluation of the vagina is required.

The risk of underlying VAIN instead of CIN in patients with an abnormal Pap smear result is one of several reasons why patients should not undergo cervical surgery for dysplasia without proper preoperative colposcopic evaluation of the cervix.

12.3.3 VAIN Following Hysterectomy

Vaginal intraepithelial neoplasia is most commonly observed when the uterus has already been removed. According to the data from Rome and England (2000), this has been the case in 55% of VAIN patients.

Removal of the uterus for the treatment of recurrent cervical dysplasia is considered to be an acceptable therapeutic option, often requested by the patient herself. However, there is a significant risk of subsequent vaginal intraepithelial neoplasia.

Das et al. (2005) presented data from 33 patients who underwent hysterectomy for persistent or recurrent cervical dysplasia. Four patients (12%) subsequently developed VAIN. Schockaert et al. (2008) performed a retrospective analysis on women with CIN2+ without a previous history of VAIN. Hysterectomy was performed within 6 months of CIN diagnosis. The incidence rate of subsequent VAIN2+ was 7.4%. This included two patients with carcinoma of the vagina.

Obviously, HPV DNA is still present within the vagina following hysterectomy. Schneider et al. (1987) identified viral DNA in one-third of patients who had undergone hysterectomy for either cervical carcinoma, CIN, or other types of anogenital carcinoma.

If the Pap test is still abnormal or abnormal again following hysterectomy for CIN, it is a particularly frustrating situation for the patient as well as the attending doctor.

Overall, hysterectomy should not be considered a standard treatment option for CIN, not even for recurrent CIN, and the procedure's limitations have to be discussed with the patient.

To avoid overlooking preexisting VAIN prior to hysterectomy for recurrent cervical dysplasia, careful colposcopic evaluation of the vagina is required. Scarring of the upper vagina resulting from hysterectomy further complicates diagnosis and management of VAIN as the dysplastic epithelium may be difficult to reach.

VAIN may also occur in patients without a history of cervical dysplasia, who underwent hysterectomy for benign conditions. Schneider et al. (1987) identified HPV in the vagina of 62 out of 442 women (14%) who had undergone hysterectomy for reasons other than neoplasia. Rome and England (2000) identified VAIN in 18% of patients when hysterectomy was not done due to CIN but due to benign conditions such as myomas. On average, VAIN was diagnosed 15 years after hysterectomy for nonneoplastic conditions.

12.3.4 VAIN and Immunosuppression

Immunosuppressed patients have a much higher risk to develop vaginal intraepithelial neoplasia regardless of the cause of immunosuppression (HIV infection or medication after transplant surgery) (Figs. 12.7 and 12.8). VAIN may occur more frequently in patients whether they have undergone hysterectomy or not.

The risk of multicentric anogenital HPV-related neoplasia is significantly higher in immunosuppressed patients. This needs to be kept in mind when colposcopy is done in the case of suspected cervical and/or vulva disease. Also, VAIN may affect not only the upper vaginal one-third but also the middle and lower third of the vagina.

As with cervical dysplasia, these patients are more likely to develop high-grade disease and possibly squamous cell carcinoma.

12.3.5 Colposcopic Appearance of VAIN

In vaginal intraepithelial neoplasia, regardless of its grading and extent, patients are free of symptoms. The diagnosis is suspected when a Pap smear from the vagina following hysterectomy shows HSIL disease. VAIN is then confirmed colposcopically.

In most patients, only the upper one-third of the vagina is affected. The colposcopic appearance of VAIN may be rather inconspicuous (Figs. 12.6 and 12.7). Sometimes, whitish

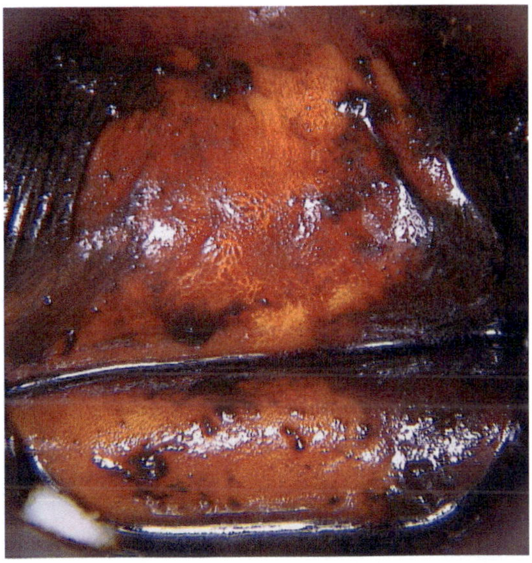

Fig. 12.7 VAIN3 3 years after hysterectomy for uterine prolapse. The 57-year-old patient did not have a history of cervical dysplasia. However, she suffers from Crohn's disease and is treated with immunosuppressive medication. The Lugol-negative epithelium of the upper vaginal pole is the only colposcopic manifestation of VAIN3

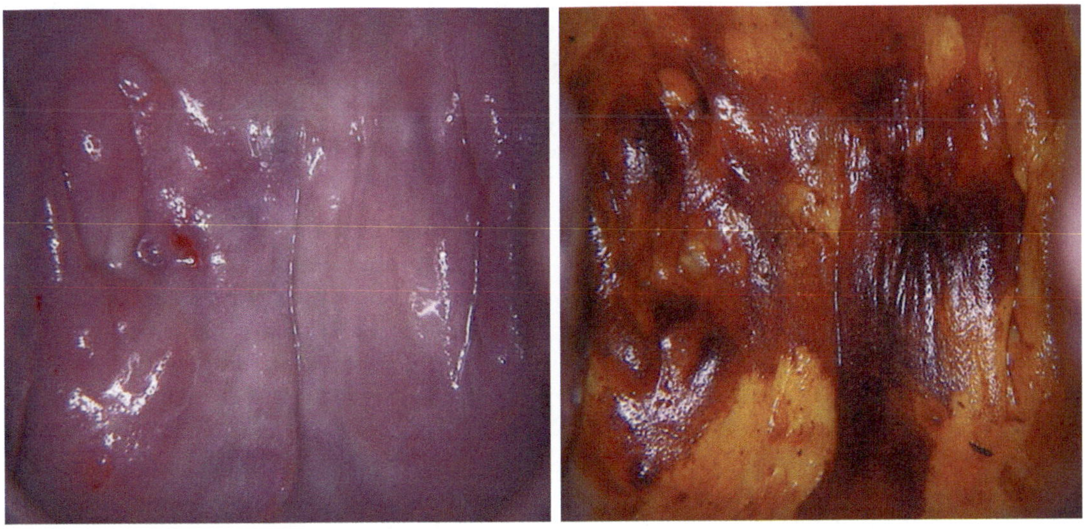

Fig. 12.6 VAIN3 in a 34-year-old patient 6 months after hysterectomy for HSIL of the cervix

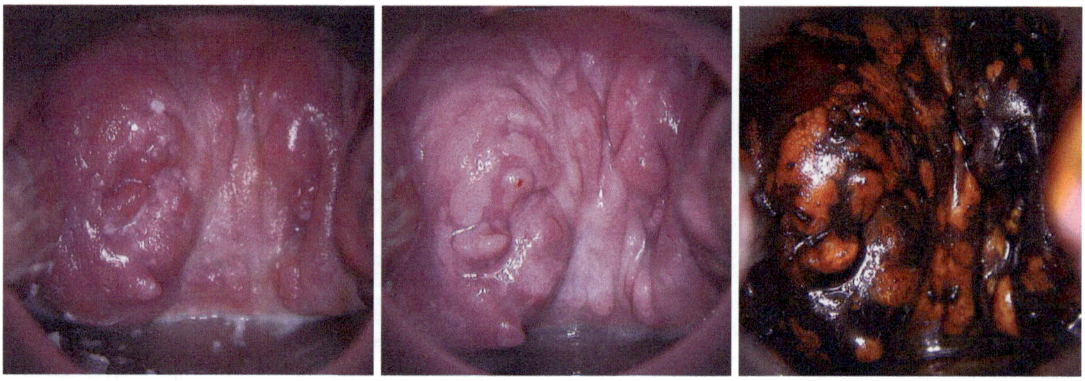

Fig. 12.8 Recurrent HSIL/VAIN2 of a 49-year-old patient with multiple sclerosis. Vaginal hysterectomy had been done 3 years ago for CIN3. The patient already underwent two previous treatment attempts (LEEP and CO_2 laser vaporization). Multiple acetowhite and Lugol-negative areas are seen at the upper vaginal pole

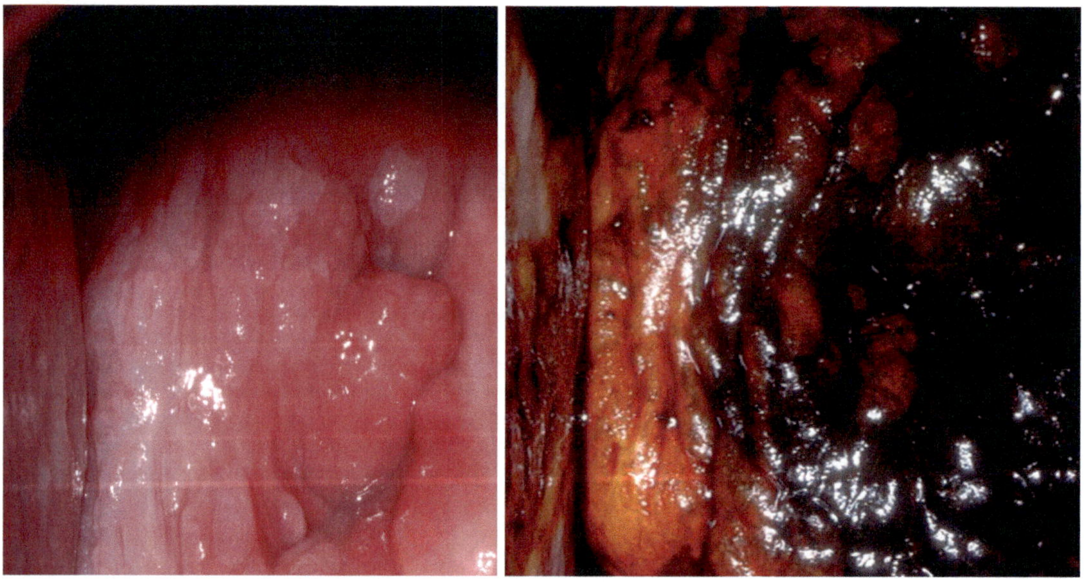

Fig. 12.9 VAIN3 in a 52-year-old patient 16 years after hysterectomy for uterine myomas. The patient does not have a previous history of CIN. Multiple acetowhite lesions are seen that are outlined sharply after applying Lugol's solution

areas and/or tissue abrasions (rag sign) can be seen, when the 5% acetic acid solution is applied. These acetowhite lesions may resemble flat condylomata and remain negative on Schiller's test (Figs. 12.8, 12.9, and 12.10). Discrete differences in color compared to the surrounding tissue and/or a slightly irregular surface may also be seen.

However, in most patients, the only defining colposcopic feature of VAIN are iodine-negative areas with sharp borders. As Schiller's test is crucial for the colposcopic diagnosis of VAIN, atrophic vaginal epithelium should be topically treated with estrogen cream or suppositories prior to colposcopy.

Atypical vessels are rarely found in the vagina. If present, they may indicate high-grade dysplasia (VAIN3) or even carcinoma. Occasionally, an irregular surface, leukoplakia, erythema, and erosion or ulceration are present (Figs. 12.11 and 12.12). In this case, biopsies are mandatory to rule out vaginal carcinoma.

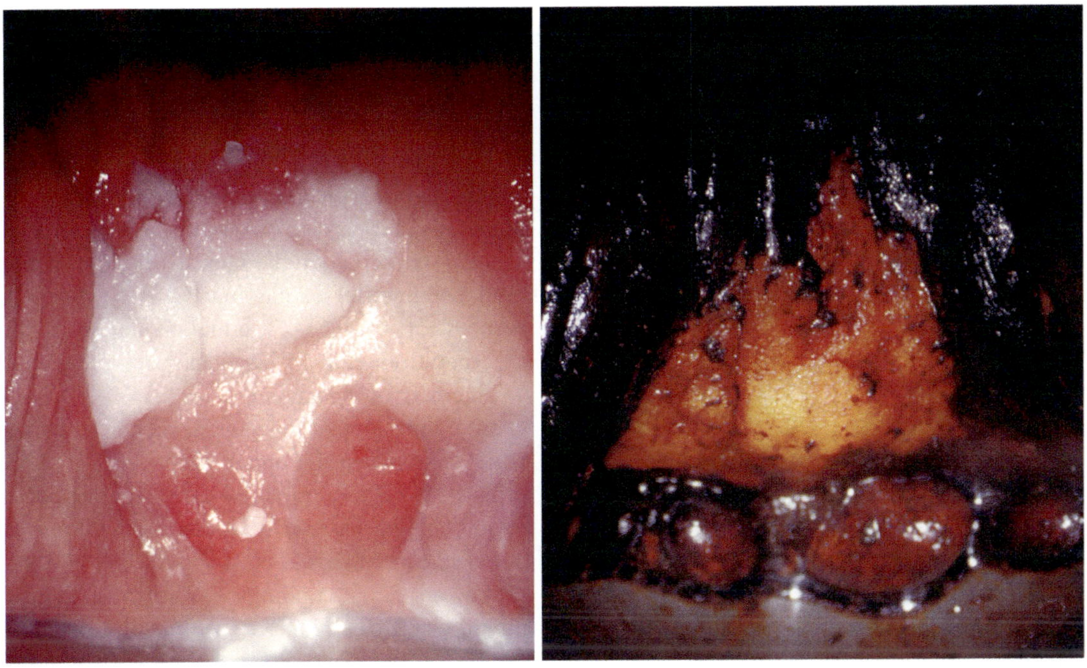

Fig. 12.10 VAIN3 with leukoplakia/hyperkeratosis. The 51-year-old patient had her uterus removed 14 years previously. Now, HSIL was suspected on the Pap test, and biopsy revealed VAIN3

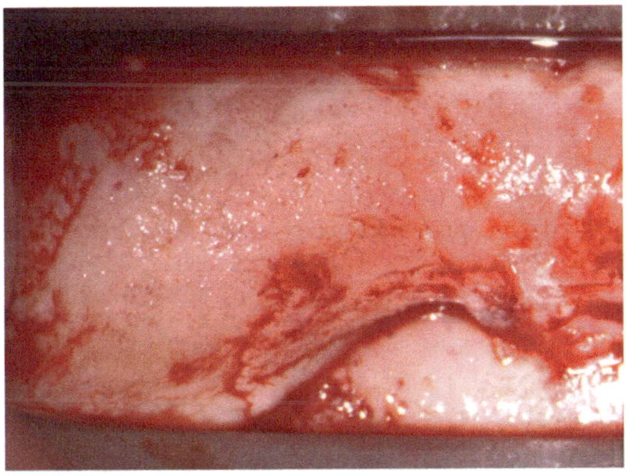

Fig. 12.11 VAIN3 with severe atrophy 5 months after hysterectomy for squamous cell carcinoma. The patient is 80 years old

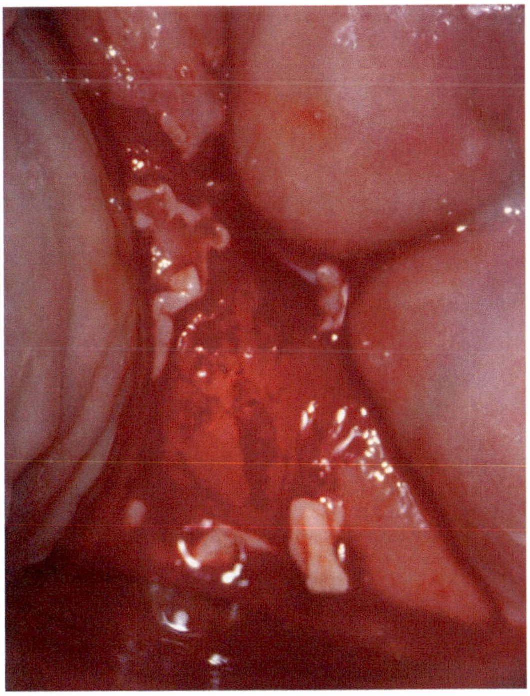

Fig. 12.12 VAIN3 with erosions (rag sign). The 40-year-old patient underwent cone biopsy twice for recurrent cervical dysplasia, and ultimately hysterectomy

On the other hand, colposcopic findings consisting of Lugol-negative areas only with sharp borders do not necessarily indicate low-grade disease. In fact, the distinction between minor and major changes as defined for the colposcopic appearance of low- and high-grade cervical intraepithelial neoplasia (CIN) does not apply to the vagina.

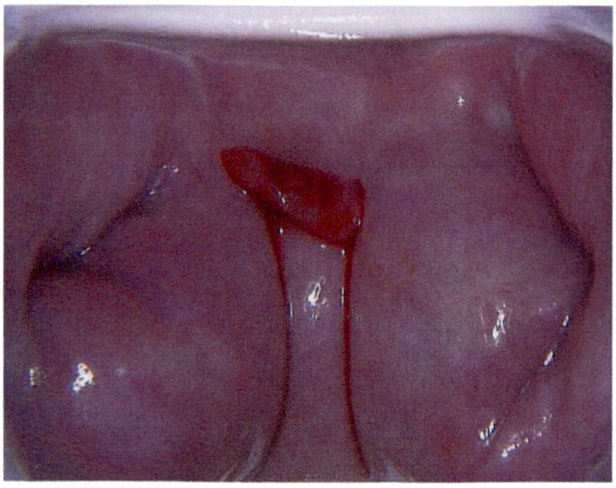

Fig. 12.13 Vaginal vault granulation tissue. The 71-year-old patient underwent vaginal hysterectomy 25 years previously for uterine myomas. The granulation tissue developed following CO_2 laser vaporization for HSIL/VAIN

Primary vaginal carcinomas are almost always squamous cell carcinomas, while adenocarcinomas are more likely to be metastases, most often from endometrial carcinoma. Overall, the colposcopic appearance of vaginal carcinoma is not different from that of cervical carcinoma with involvement of the vagina.

Benign lesions of the vagina, such as granulation tissue within the upper vagina (Figs. 12.13 and 12.14) or tubal prolapse after recent hysterectomy, may occasionally be confused with invasive disease and should be biopsied.

All abnormal findings within the vagina should usually be biopsied, as the appearance of vaginal lesions correlates poorly with histological findings when compared to colposcopic diagnosis of the cervix.

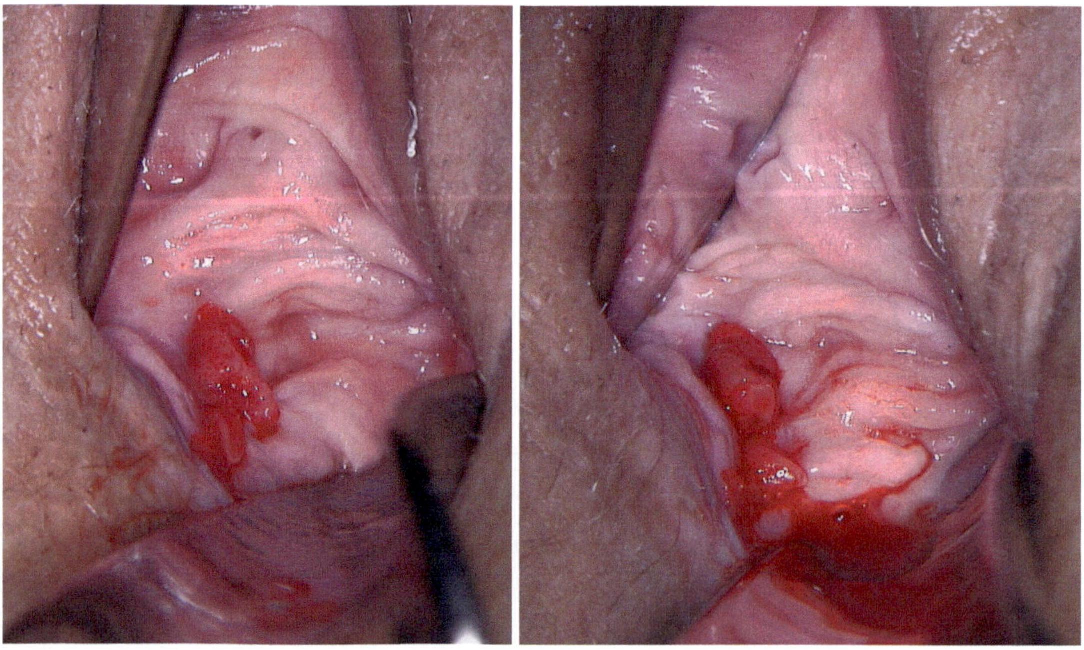

Fig. 12.14 Granulation tissue in the upper third of the vagina. The 36-year-old patient had an episiotomy 5 months previously

12.3.6 Treatment Options for VAIN

There is no treatment of choice for VAIN. Several treatment options are available:

- Wait and see
- Partial or total colpectomy and laser-skinning colpectomy
- Cryosurgery
- CO_2 laser vaporization
- Topical and systemic drug treatment
- Radiation therapy

Which treatment method or which combination of treatment options are appropriate depends on several factors. The number of lesions, their location and grade, previous treatments for VAIN, immunosuppressive disorders, sexual activity, all of these factors play a role in the choice of treatment. The patient should be informed from the outset that recurrences must be expected in about one-third of patients (Frega et al. 2013). Nevertheless, radical procedures as those used to treat invasive cancer are usually not appropriate, as the cancer risk of VAIN is still not known exactly and may be relatively low.

12.3.6.1 Wait and See

In low-grade vaginal dysplasias, especially in women under the age of 40, there is no need for treatment. Colposcopic evaluation should be repeated every 6 months including a Pap smear. VAIN3 is usually treated, whereas VAIN2 is either followed or also treated depending on the individual circumstances and the patient's preferences.

12.3.6.2 Partial or Total Colpectomy and Laser-Skinning Colpectomy

About 80% of VAIN lesions are located in the upper one-third of the vagina (Diakomanolis et al. 2002). Indermaur et al. (2005) consider partial colpectomy to be the treatment of choice for VAIN3, especially when previous hysterectomy has been performed for cervical intraepithelial neoplasia or invasive cervical carcinoma. 52 out of 105 patients treated by partial colpectomy were followed for an average of 25 months. The recurrence rate was only 12%. However, in 13 patients (12%), invasive carcinoma was discovered within the colpectomy specimen.

The occurrence of occult VAIN lesions within the hysterectomy scar also favors surgical excision, as these lesions may not be adequately treated by CO_2 laser vaporization alone.

Partial colpectomy offers the advantage of an accurate histopathological diagnosis and the detection of clinically occult invasive disease. However, partial colpectomy may also lead to shortening of the vagina resulting in dyspareunia.

For small lesions, loop electrosurgical resection may be a treatment option (Patsner 1993). However, Powell and Asbery (2000) strongly advise against it, as a patient subsequently developed bowel perforation and peritonitis.

Although total colpectomy is rarely indicated for the treatment of preinvasive disease, laser-skinning colpectomy as suggested by Luyten et al. (2014) may be a suitable alternative. Luyten et al. performed partial or total laser-skinning colpectomy on 33 heavily pretreated patients with high-grade VAIN covering between 20 and 100% of the vaginal surface. The vaginal wall was resected using the CO_2 laser under colposcopic guidance. VAIN lesions were removed in one piece to a depth of 2–3 mm within the lamina vasorum. Hysterectomy scars were resected to a depth of 5–10 mm. Patients were then treated with a topical anesthetic followed by estrogen cream and the use of a vaginal dilator. Ten patients were diagnosed with invasive disease, which was microinvasive in nine patients. For 23 patients who were followed for 12 months or more, the overall cure rate was 87%. In two patients, moderate shortening of the vagina occurred, whereas another two patients required vaginal reconstructive surgery.

12.3.6.3 Cryosurgery

Cryoprobes suitable for the treatment of small foci of VAIN are available. However, several limitations for cryosurgery of VAIN exist. Most importantly, invasive disease cannot be ruled out. Furthermore, cryosurgery is not suitable, if there is post-hysterectomy scarring of the upper vaginal vault. A major disadvantage is the lack of control of the depth of penetration as well as the amount of tissue destroyed by cryotherapy.

Although numerous articles on the effectiveness and the potential side effects of cryosurgery for cervical lesions exist, no such information is available for VAIN.

12.3.6.4 CO_2 Laser Vaporization

Despite its high relapse rate, CO_2 laser vaporization is still the primary treatment option for a first-time manifestation of VAIN without any suspicion of invasive disease (Fig. 12.15).

The depth of penetration of the CO_2 laser beam can be accurately controlled by:

- Adjustment of power (wattage)
- Focusing and defocusing of the laser beam
- Duration of contact between laser beam and tissue

Benedet et al. (1992) carried out systematic measurements on histological specimens and came to the conclusion that a penetration depth of 1.5 mm is sufficient.

Based on a literature review by Indermaur et al. (2005), the effectiveness of CO_2 laser vaporization for treatment of VAIN is 70% (50–100%).

A retrospective analysis of 65 patients was done by Jentschke et al. (2015). The mean age was 61 years. 55% of lesion were located in the upper third of the vagina with 42% being multifocal. Two-thirds of patients had had a previous hysterectomy for cervical dysplasia. Most patients were treated by CO_2 laser vaporization. Relapse rate was as high as 57%. Four patients were diagnosed with vaginal cancer either in connection with VAIN3 at the time of initial diagnosis (three patients) or during follow-up (one patient, 22 months after first laser treatment).

The risk of relapse after laser treatment was associated with a positive HPV high-risk test result on the HC2 test.

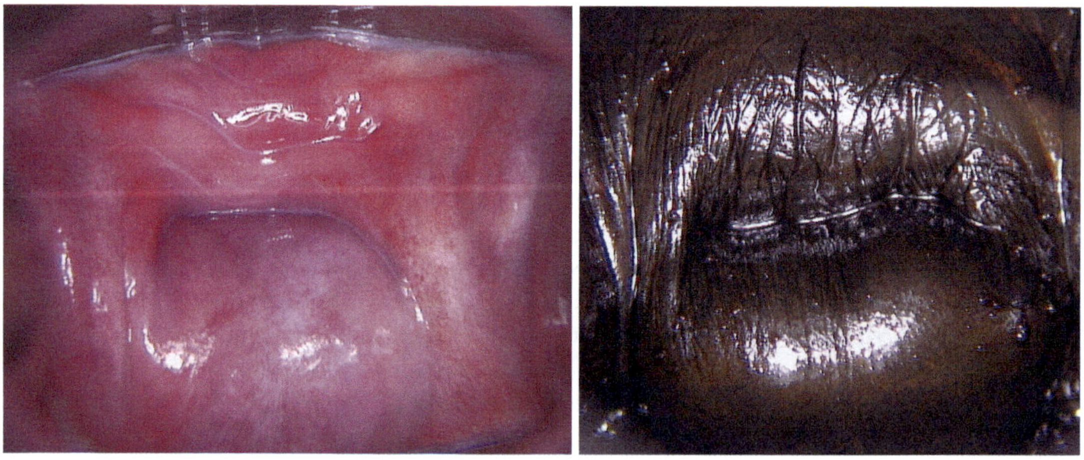

Fig. 12.15 Successful CO_2 laser vaporization for VAIN. The 79-year-old patient underwent vaginal hysterectomy 2 years previously for cervical dysplasia. The entire vaginal vault is Lugol-positive. The hysterectomy scar mimics a cervix

12.3.6.5 Topical and Systemic Drug Treatment

A 5% 5-fluorouracil cream may be used for topical treatment of VAIN, and 1.5 to 2.0 g are inserted into the vagina for a duration of 5 to 7 consecutive days. The mucosa of the vulva is protected from local irritation by a zinc oxide ointment. After 12 weeks, the therapeutic effect is evaluated. Indermaur et al. (2005) reported recurrence rates between 7 and 59%.

A 5-fluorouracil cream has considerable side effects. Frequently, patients complain of burning pain. Also, ulcerations of the vaginal mucosa may occur.

Although not officially approved for treatment of VAIN, imiquimod (Aldara®) may be used. Imiquimod is an immunomodulator that has shown its effectiveness for the treatment of condylomata acuminata, basalioma, and also HSIL of the vulva. Whereas topical imiquimod treatment has been studied extensively for treatment of HSIL of the vulva, data are scarce for both CIN and VAIN (de Witte et al. 2015).

Haidopoulos et al. (2005) treated seven patients with severe vaginal dysplasia with topical imiquimod and achieved responses in five patients. However, the HP virus was not eliminated. In two cases, VAIN1 persisted.

In a prospective randomized trial comparing different treatment modalities for VAIN (Tainio et al. 2016), topical imiquimod treatment was as effective as laser surgery with a histological regression rate of 80% (n = 8/10). Furthermore, HPV clearance was significantly higher in the imiquimod arm than in the laser arm: 63% versus 11%, respectively. Patients administered imiquimod themselves, and 12.5 mg suppositories were manufactured by a collaborating pharmacy. Treatment took 8 weeks with a total of 14 doses.

In another trial (Daayana et al. 2010), imiquimod was injected. In this phase II trial, complete response was 63% at week 52 posttreatment with an HPV clearance rate of 36%.

In 2017, Tranoulis et al. (2017) did a meta-analysis on imiquimod use for VAIN and identified six articles including a total of 94 patients. The complete response rate was 76.5% with an HPV clearance rate of 52.5%.

Several experimental therapeutic HPV vaccines have been tried on VAIN patients with limited success. Data on a potential reduction of the risk of recurrence following vaccination with one of the available prophylactic vaccines are not available (Bryan et al. 2019).

12.3.6.6 Radiation Therapy

Radiotherapy is the treatment of choice for invasive squamous cell carcinoma of the vagina. Graham et al. (2007) treated 22 patients with recurrent VAIN aged 37–70 years (median 56 years) with a brachytherapy dose of 48 Gy. The median follow-up time was 77 months. The cure rate was high: Only three patients relapsed. However, two of these patients had developed invasive disease.

The local side effects of radiation treatment are a major concern. Although no immediate toxicity occurred in the patients treated by Graham et al. (2007), there were ulcerations or stenosis of the vagina in five patients.

Therefore, routine treatment of recurrent VAIN3 by radiation therapy is not indicated due to the possibility of significant side effects.

12.4 Vaginal Carcinoma

Primary squamous cell carcinoma of the vagina is a rare tumor entity. It is likely that high-grade vaginal dysplasia (VAIN3) is the precursor. Peters et al. (1985) reported six cases in which a "microcarcinoma" of the vagina with a depth of invasion of up to 2.5 mm was diagnosed. In all of these patients, the invasive cancer was located within a precursor lesion. At this early stage of the disease, the survival rate was 100%. However, according to Schäfer et al. (1997), only 43% of tumors are diagnosed as stage I disease. FIGO staging of carcinoma of the vagina is shown in Table 12.1.

For most patients, combined radiation (teletherapy and brachytherapy) is the treatment of choice. Colpectomy may only be suitable for patients with microinvasive disease, i.e., with a depth of invasion of less than 2.5 mm as defined by Peters et al. (1985).

Table 12.1 FIGO staging of carcinoma of the vagina based on the staging of cervical carcinoma

FIGO stage	
0	Vaginal intraepithelial neoplasia grade 3 (VAIN3), "carcinoma in situ"
I	Carcinoma is confined to the vaginal wall
II	Carcinoma infiltrates the subvaginal tissue but does not reach the pelvic wall
III	Carcinoma extends to the pelvic wall
IV	Carcinoma extends beyond the pelvis or infiltrates the mucosa of the urinary bladder or rectum (Bullous edema alone does not justify assignment to stage IV)
IVA	The tumor invades the mucosa of the urinary bladder and/or rectum and/or spreads beyond the pelvis
IVB	Distant metastases

The 5-year survival rate of patients with vaginal cancer after primary radiation therapy is 41% (Schäfer et al. 1997) with a survival rate of 62% for stage I patients.

12.5 Vaginal Metastases

When adenocarcinoma is diagnosed within the vagina, it is most likely a metastasis originating, for example, from carcinoma of the endometrium or colon. In patients with previous endometrial cancer, the vagina is the most common site of recurrence (Figs. 12.16 and 12.17).

Occasionally, vaginal manifestations of advanced ovarian cancer are found. Whereas primary high grade serous ovarian cancer usually does not penetrate the vaginal wall, recurrent tumors may occasionally be seen at the vaginal cuff after previous hysterectomy (Fig. 12.18).

All abnormal findings of the vagina should be biopsied with the exception of suspected gestational trophoblastic neoplasia (GTN), as hemostasis may be difficult to achieve. In all other instances, bleeding can be controlled by a vaginal tampon.

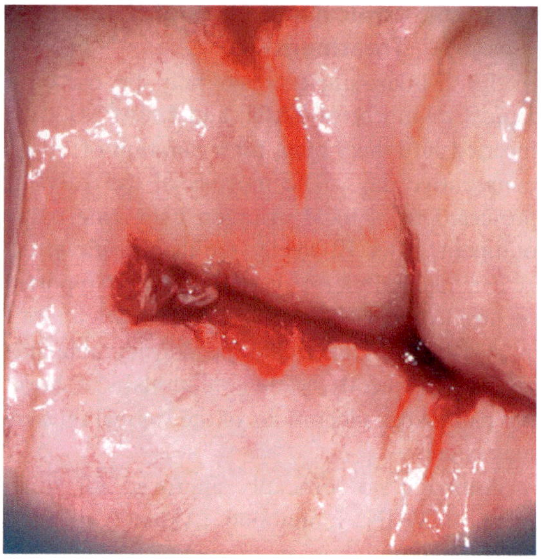

Fig. 12.16 Vaginal recurrence 14 months after treatment for endometrial cancer. The 77-year-old patient underwent hysterectomy for endometrial carcinoma FIGO stage Ic G2 with subsequent radiation therapy. The vaginal vault is retracted and vaguely resembles the ectocervix with a small amount of soft tumor tissue protruding

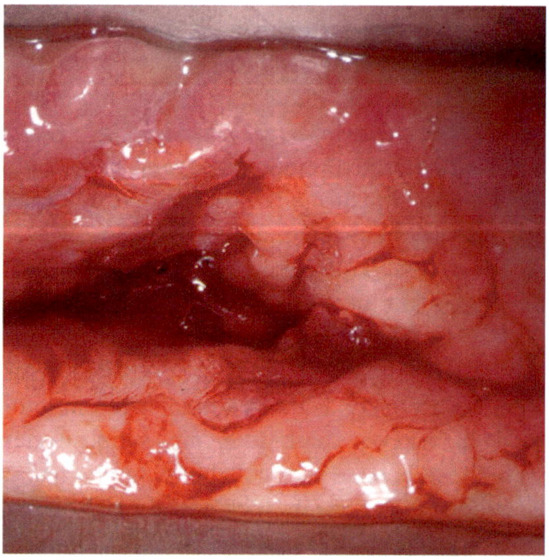

Fig. 12.17 Vaginal recurrence of endometrial carcinoma. The 78-year-old patient underwent hysterectomy 20 months previously for FIGO stage Ic G2 disease. The upper vaginal pole is retracted and bleeding

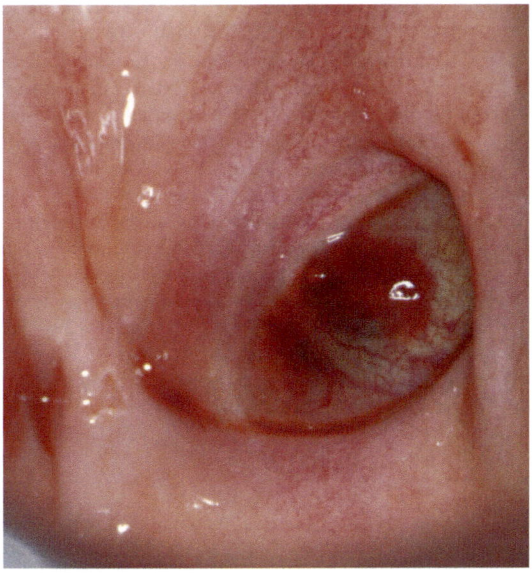

Fig. 12.18 Vaginal metastasis from ovarian carcinoma. Three years earlier, the 50-year-old patient underwent treatment for high grade serous carcinoma of the ovary. As part of the primary tumor surgery, hysterectomy had been performed. Now, the patient complained for vaginal bleeding

References

Aho M, Vesterinen E, Meyer B, Purola E, Paavonen J (1991) Natural history of vaginal intraepithelial neoplasia. Cancer 68(1):195–197

Benedet JL, Wilson PS, Matisic JP (1992) Epidermal thickness measurements in vaginal intraepithelial neoplasia. A basis for optimal CO2 laser vaporization. J Reprod Med 37(9):809–812

Bryan S, Barbara C, Thomas J, Olaitan A (2019) HPV vaccine in the treatment of usual type vulval and vaginal intraepithelial neoplasia: a systematic review. BMC Womens Health 19(1):3. https://doi.org/10.1186/s12905-018-0707-9

Daayana S, Elkord E, Winters U, Pawlita M, Roden R, Stern PL, Kitchener HC (2010) Phase II trial of imiquimod and HPV therapeutic vaccination in patients with vulval intraepithelial neoplasia. Br J Cancer 102(7):1129–1136. https://doi.org/10.1038/sj.bjc.6605611

Das N, Naik R, Jackson S, De Barros Lopes A, Monaghan JM, Godfrey KA, Hatem MH (2005) Recurrent smear abnormalities where repeat loop treatment is not possible: is hysterectomy the answer? Gynecol Oncol 97(3):751–754. https://doi.org/10.1016/j.ygyno.2005.01.003

de Witte CJ, van de Sande AJM, van Beekhuizen HJ, Koeneman MM, Kruse AJ, Gerestein CG (2015) Imiquimod in cervical, vaginal and vulvar intraepithelial neoplasia: a review. Gynecol Oncol 139(2):377–384. https://doi.org/10.1016/j.ygyno.2015.08.018

Diakomanolis E, Stefanidis K, Rodolakis A, Haidopoulos D, Sindos M, Chatzipappas I, Michalas S (2002) Vaginal intraepithelial neoplasia: report of 102 cases. Eur J Gynaecol Oncol 23(5):457–459

Fox J, Remington P, Layde P, Klein G (1999) The effect of hysterectomy on the risk of an abnormal screening Papanicolaou test result. Am J Obstet Gynecol 180(5):1104–1109

Frega A, Sopracordevole F, Assorgi C, Lombardi DV, Catalano A et al (2013) Vaginal intraepithelial neoplasia: a therapeutical dilemma. Anticancer Res 33(1):29–38

Graham K, Wright K, Cadwallader B, Reed NS, Symonds RP (2007) 20-year retrospective review of medium dose rate intracavitary brachytherapy in VAIN3. Gynecol Oncol 106(1):105–111. https://doi.org/10.1016/j.ygyno.2007.03.005

Haidopoulos D, Diakomanolis E, Rodolakis A, Voulgaris Z, Vlachos G, Intsaklis A (2005) Can local application of imiquimod cream be an alternative mode of therapy for patients with high-grade intraepithelial lesions of the vagina? Int J Gynecol Cancer 15(5):898–902. https://doi.org/10.1111/j.1525-1438.2005.00152.x

Hampl M, Wentzensen N, Vinokurova S, von Knebel Doeberitz M, Poremba C, Bender HG, Kueppers V (2007) Comprehensive analysis of 130 multicentric intraepithelial female lower genital tract lesions by HPV typing and p16 expression profile. J Cancer Res Clin Oncol 133(4):235–245. https://doi.org/10.1007/s00432-006-0162-0

Indermaur MD, Martino MA, Fiorica JV, Roberts WS, Hoffman MS (2005) Upper vaginectomy for the treatment of vaginal intraepithelial neoplasia. Am J Obstet Gynecol 193(2):571–577. https://doi.org/10.1016/j.ajog.2005.03.055

Jentschke M, Hoffmeister V, Soergel P, Hillemanns P (2015) Clinical presentation, treatment and outcome of vaginal intraepithelial neoplasia. Arch Gynecol Obstet 293(2):415–419. https://doi.org/10.1007/s00404-015-3835-6

Luyten A, Hastor H, Vasileva T, Zander M, Petry KU (2014) Laser-skinning colpectomy for extended vaginal intraepithelial neoplasia and microinvasive cancer. Gynecol Oncol 135(2):217–222. https://doi.org/10.1016/j.ygyno.2014.08.019

Patsner B (1993) Treatment of vaginal dysplasia with loop excision: report of five cases. Am J Obstet Gynecol 169(1):179–180

Peters WA, Kumar NB, Morley GW (1985) Microinvasive carcinoma of the vagina: a distinct clinical entity? Am J Obstet Gynecol 153(5):505–507

Powell JL, Asbery DS (2000) Treatment of vaginal dysplasia: just a simple loop electrosurgical excision procedure? Am J Obstet Gynecol 182(3):731–732

Rome RM, England PG (2000) Management of vaginal intraepithelial neoplasia: a series of 132 cases with long-term follow-up. Int J Gynecol Cancer 10(5):382–390

Schäfer U, Micke O, Prott FJ, Kugler R, Neff A, Willich N (1997) The results of primary radiotherapy in vaginal carcinoma. Strahlenther Onkol 173(5):272–280

Schneider A, De-Villiers EM, Schneider V (1987) Multifocal squamous neoplasia of the female genital tract: significance of human papillomavirus infection of the vagina after hysterectomy. Obstet Gynecol 70(3): 294–298

Schockaert S, Poppe W, Arbyn M, Verguts T, Verguts J (2008) Incidence of vaginal intraepithelial neoplasia after hysterectomy for cervical intraepithelial neoplasia: a retrospective study. Am J Obstet Gynecol 199(2):113. https://doi.org/10.1016/j.ajog.2008.02.026

Srodon M, Stoler MH, Baber GB, Kurman RJ (2006) The distribution of low and high-risk HPV types in vulvar and vaginal intraepithelial neoplasia (VIN and VaIN). Am J Surg Pathol 30(12):1513–1518. https://doi.org/10.1097/01.pas.0000213291.96401.48

Tainio K, Jakobsson M, Louvanto K, Kalliala I, Paavonen J, Nieminen P, Riska A (2016) Randomised trial on treatment of vaginal intraepithelial neoplasia-Imiquimod, laser vaporisation and expectant management. Int J Cancer 139(10):2353–2358. https://doi.org/10.1002/ijc.30275

Tranoulis A, Laios A, Mitsopoulos V, Lutchman-Singh K, Thomakos N (2017) Efficacy of 5% imiquimod for the treatment of Vaginal intraepithelial neoplasia-A systematic review of the literature and a meta-analysis. Eur J Obstet Gynecol Reprod Biol 218:129–136. https://doi.org/10.1016/j.ejogrb.2017.09.020

Woodruff JD (1981) Carcinoma in situ of the vagina. Clin Obstet Gynecol 24(2):485–501

Colposcopy of the Vulva

13

Contents

Several disease of the vulva can be diagnosed visually. The colposcope may help to further improve the sensitivity as well as the specificity of vulvar diagnosis.

13.1 Anatomy of the Vulva

For the recognition and assessment of pathological changes of the vulva, knowledge of the normal anatomy is of fundamental importance.

The basic anatomy of the vulva encompasses the following components (Fig. 13.1):

- Mons veneris
- Labium majus and minus
- Glans and prepuce of clitoris
- Urethral orifice
- Hymen
- Vestibule of the vagina
- Posterior commissure (fourchette)

Within the vestibule of the vagina the following orifices are located:

- The urethral orifice
- Skene's ducts (lateral to the urethra)
- Bartholin's ducts

The labia majora correspond to the scrotum of the male. They are connected ventrally and form the mons veneris, which covers the symphysis. Posteriorly, the labia majora come together to form the perineum. The lateral aspect of the labia majora contains numerous hair follicles and apocrine sweat glands, while the sebaceous glands are predominantly located in the medial aspect.

R. J. Lellé, V. Küppers, *Colposcopy*, https://doi.org/10.1007/978-3-030-85388-4_13

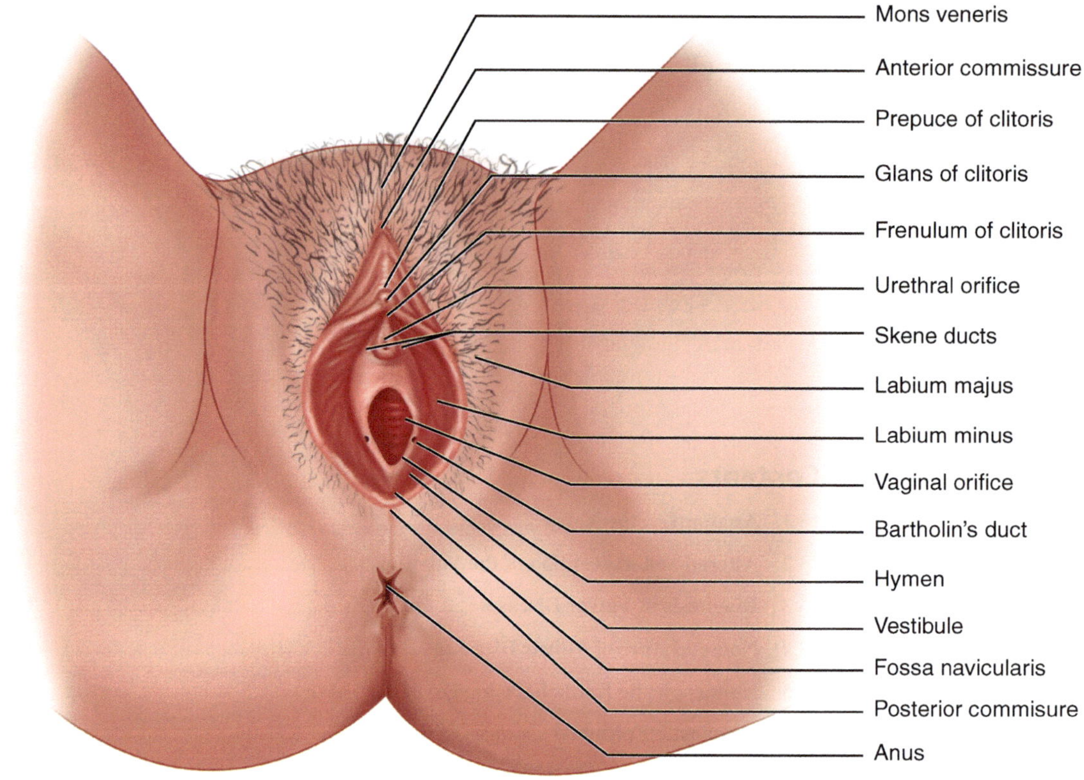

Fig. 13.1 Basic anatomy of the vulva

The labia minora are two thin highly vascular skinfolds that are covered by the labia majora. The lateral aspects of the labia minora contain sebaceous glands. These may become visible as small yellowish papules when the skin is stretched. The labia minora have neither hair follicles nor adipose tissue. Anteriorly, the labia minora become the prepuce of the clitoris. Posteriorly, they form the posterior commissure, also called the posterior fourchette.

The clitoris corresponds to the male penis. As a result of its dense nerve supply from the main branches of the pudendal nerve, the clitoris is particularly sensitive.

During life phases, physiological changes of the appearance of the vulva occur. The different stages of physical maturity have been described by Marshall and Tanner (1969). During puberty, the labia enlarge, and there is increased vulvar pigmentation. With sexual maturity, the hormonal cycle will also affect the vulva. Especially the epithelium of the vagina as well as the epithelium on the medial aspect of the labia minora is subject to changes of the estrogen level during the menstrual cycle. Vascular changes, which are caused by the influence of progestins during the second half of the menstrual cycle, lead to an increased fragility of the dermal vessels. The drop in hormonal secretion during menopause causes atrophic changes of the vulva. These changes are particularly obvious on the labia minora and majora as well as on the clitoris.

13.2 Altered Self-Perception of the Vulva

Vulvar anatomy is quite variable. Of course, the "perfect vulva" does not exist. However, self-perception may be distorted through media influence and especially the Internet (Clerico et al. 2017).

Kreklau et al. (2018) tried to define "the normal vulva" through systematic measurements of 657 women 15–84 years old who frequented the Cantonal Hospital Lucerne, Switzerland. Not surprisingly, there are considerable variations. For example, the (left) labium minor was found to be between 5 and 100 mm in length with an average length of 43 mm (Table 13.1).

Table 13.1 Genital measurements from 657 women aged 15–84 years (Kreklau et al. 2018)

	Mean (in mm)	Standard deviation	Minimum (in mm)	Maximum (in mm)
Width of clitoris	4.62	2.538	1	22
Length of clitoris	6.89	4.965	0.5	34
Distance clitoris—urethra	22.63	7.661	3	65
Introitus opening	27.91	10.36	6	75
Length of perineum	21.34	8.544	3	55
Length of labia majora (right)	79.71	15.25	12	180
Length of labia majora (left)	79.99	15.44	20	180
Length of labia minora (right)	42.1	16.35	6	100
Length of labia minora (left)	42.97	16.29	5	100
Width of labia minora (right)	13.4	7.875	2	61
Width of labia minora (left)	14.15	7.643	1	42

Occasionally, the desire for a "correction" of the labia minora is expressed by a patient. In most cases, patients desire that the labia minora shall be reduced in size. According to Borkenhagen et al. (2009), the perceptions of these patients are very much influenced by depictions of intimate areas in the media. Only rarely do objective medical reasons exist for this kind of plastic surgery.

In Western civilization, it has become increasingly common for younger women to regularly remove the pubic hair. In a survey from Germany, where pubic shaving is uncommon within the older generation, Matthiesen and Mainka (2011) interviewed 160 female and male adolescents between the ages of 16 and 19. About 94% of the girls and 81% of the boys said that they completely or partially remove their pubic hair. Sexually active adolescents more frequently practice pubic shaving compared to sexually non-active respondents. Obviously, experiences from watching pornography do not influence the frequency of pubic shaving. Considerations of personal hygiene are the main reasons given for pubic shaving: Someone who does not remove his/her pubic hair is considered to be unkempt.

Intimate jewelry, especially piercing of the labia or clitoris, is increasingly common, although it has a centuries-old tradition. Through intimate piercing, women expect a greater attractiveness and increased sexual pleasure, especially through clitoral piercing (Fig. 13.2).

The prevalence of genital piercing seems to be relatively low so far. According to a British study (Bone et al. 2008), 14.6% of all adult women had piercings at sites other than the earlobe. However, the prevalence in the genital area was only 0.3%.

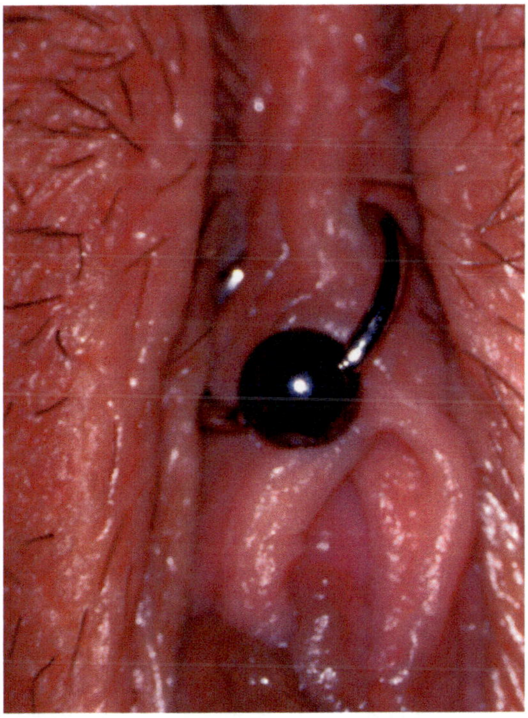

Fig. 13.2 Clitoris jewelry with piercing of the corpus clitoridis

Genital piercing is associated with a high complication rate. In the study by Bone et al. (2008), swelling, infections, or hemorrhage were reported in 45% of the 16- to 24-year-olds.

From a medical point of view, pubic shaving as well as an increased self-perception of the female genitalia may offer an opportunity for the early detection of vulvar lesions, especially of premalignant and malignant nature.

Prior to electrosurgical procedures (LEEP), metal rings or beads have to be removed.

13.3 Diagnosis of Vulvar Diseases

Meticulous inspection of the vulva, preferably with the help of the colposcope, is the basis for the diagnosis of the huge variety of dermatological and infectious diseases of the vulva, as well as for the early detection of vulvar cancer and its precursors.

Compared to cytopathology of the cervix, vulvar cytology is often more ambiguous and difficult to interpret.

Therefore, any vulvar abnormalities, especially persistent pigmented and nonpigmented hyperkeratotic lesions and/or ulcerations, should be biopsied to rule out preneoplasia or cancer of the vulva. Small tissue samples are obtained under local anesthesia as part of the colposcopic workup.

The differential diagnostic assessment of ulcerations and circumscribed hyperkeratosis in patients with lichen sclerosus or squamous hyperplasia of the vulva is particularly difficult. Although these diseases are not considered to be precancerous lesions, the probability of preneoplasia or vulvar carcinoma is increased.

Tissue sampling as an office procedure is usually well tolerated. Ideally, the skin is anesthetized by a 4% lidocaine cream 20–30 min prior to injection of the local anesthetic, which is painless if a thin 30 G needle is used. A punch biopsy technique is recommended (Fig. 13.3). If the diameter of the punch is small (3–4 mm), no suture is needed, and hemostasis is achieved by direct pressure to the biopsy site. Alternatively, a small amount of Monsel's solution is applied.

If a larger punch is used (5–6 mm), the wound is closed with a single absorbable suture. The tissue cylinder is placed in formalin solution and can be oriented by the pathologist.

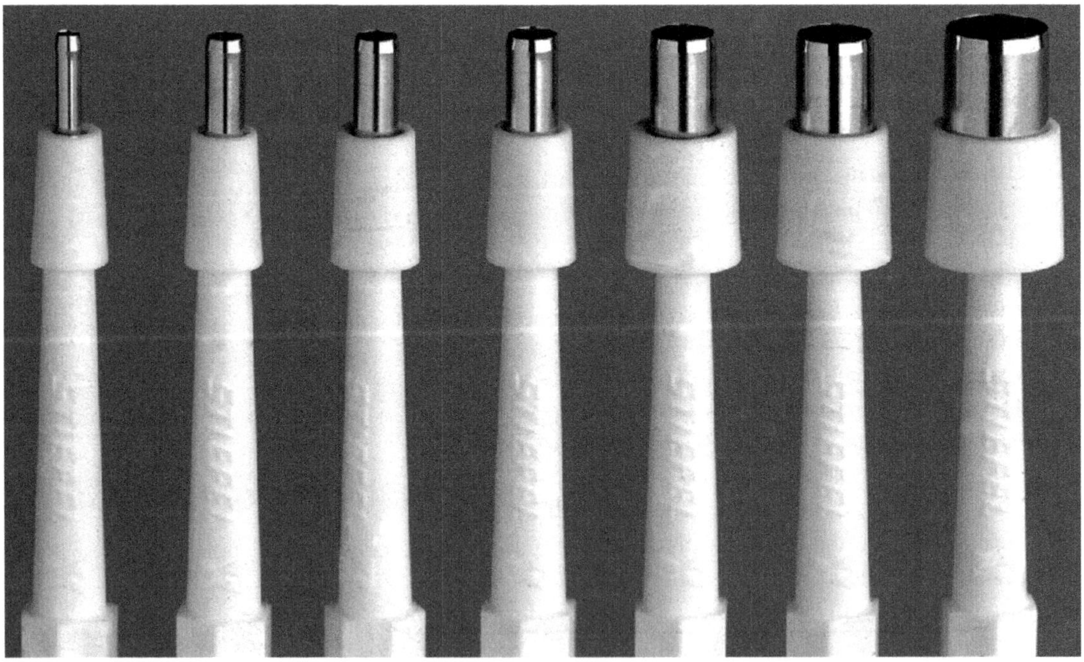

Fig. 13.3 Disposable instruments of different sizes for punch biopsy of the vulva (Stiefel GmbH, Germany)

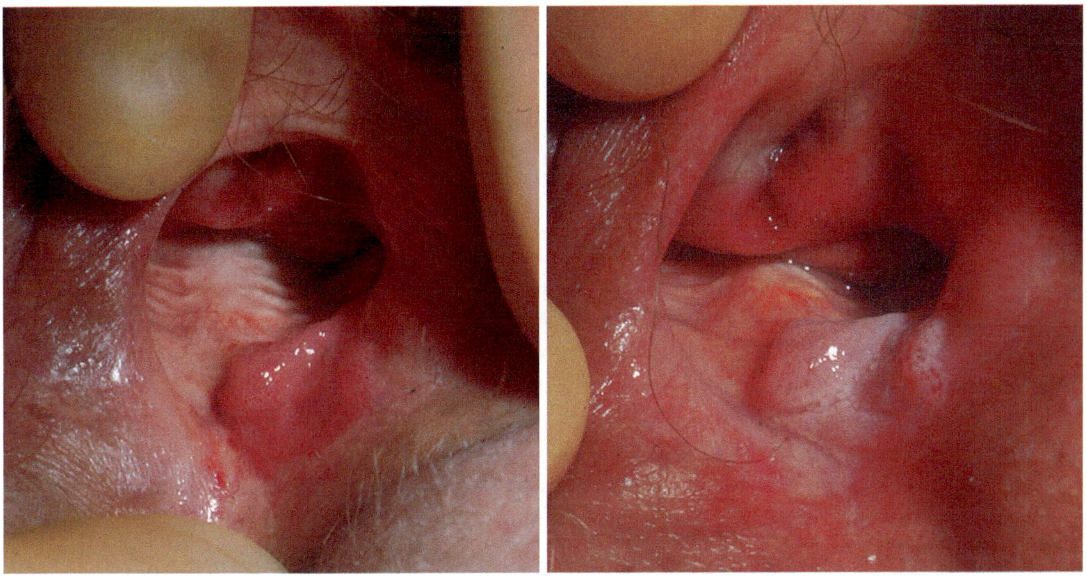

Fig. 13.4 HSIL of the introitus vulvae before (left) and after (right) application of 5% acetic acid. A coarse mosaic with irregular punctation is seen

Staining of the vulva with a 4–5% acetic acid solution may be helpful to evaluate lesions located within the non-keratinizing areas of the vulva (Fig.13.4). However, the keratinizing epithelium reacts differently to the vinegar solution and may lead to unspecific acetowhite staining.

Routine screening for HPV DNA does not improve the early detection of vulvar preneoplasia.

13.4 Nomenclature of Vulvar Diseases

In addition to infectious diseases caused by candida, trichomonas, or herpesvirus that are frequently diagnosed, there is a wide range of diseases that occur less frequently and may be associated with considerable morbidity. These patients should be referred to a dermatologist or a gynecologist specializing in vulvar diseases. These patients require an often time-consuming workup including a detailed history, a general as well as a gynecological examination, colposcopic evaluation, and, in many cases, histological clarification of the findings as described above.

An internationally recognized classification of vulvar disease has been created by the International Society for the Study of Vulvovaginal Disease (ISSVD) (ISSVD1989). Non-neoplastic epithelial changes are distinguished from neoplastic changes.

In particular, the classification of neoplastic epithelial changes of the vulva is crucial and has been updated regularly by the ISSVD. In 2007 (Heller 2007), the classification "VIN1, VIN2, and VIN3" was dropped since "VIN1" does not present a risk of progression to carcinoma. On the other hand, VIN2 and VIN3, which may be difficult to differentiate histologically, are not distinguished anymore and called "VIN."

In the following chapters, the most common vulvar diseases are described.

In 2016, the *ISSVD classification* was modified again (Bornstein et al. 2016), and three distinct entities are defined:

1. LSIL = Low-grade squamous intraepithelial lesion (vulvar LSIL, flat condyloma, HPV effects)
2. HSIL = High-grade squamous intraepithelial lesion (vulvar HSIL, VIN usual type)
3. DVIN = Differentiated-type vulvar intraepithelial neoplasia

Although the ISSVD terminology can be regarded as the gold standard from a clinician's point of view, there is the *WHO classification* of tumors to consider which is used as a reference by pathologists worldwide and which was last updated 2020 (WHO Classification of Tumours Editorial Board 2020). However, the WHO classification differs only slightly from the ISSVD classification. The following two entities are defined:

1. Squamous intraepithelial lesions, HPV-associated
2. Vulvar intraepithelial neoplasia, HPV-independent

For the first entity, the following terminology is considered "acceptable": low-grade squamous intraepithelial lesion (VIN1), high-grade intraepithelial lesion (VIN2), high-grade intraepithelial lesion (VIN3), VIN2 or 3 of usual type. For the second entity, "differentiated VIN" is listed as "acceptable."

13.5 Nonneoplastic Epithelial Changes of the Vulva

Nonneoplastic epithelial changes of the vulva encompass a large variety of diseases and dermatologic changes that need to be distinguished from neoplastic epithelial changes.

Due to the large number of possible diagnoses, the ISSVD, so far, has not achieved an adequate and clinically oriented classification of these diseases, which takes into account the patients' symptoms and the different dermatological conditions.

The most common dermatological diagnoses encountered by the gynecologist are lichen sclerosus and lichen planus.

13.5.1 Lichen Sclerosus

The etiology of anogenital lichen sclerosus is unknown (Powell and Wojnarowska 1999; Murphy 2010). In advanced lichen sclerosus, a complete loss of the small labia (Fig. 13.5) and stenosis of the vaginal opening (Fig. 13.6) are observed. The vagina itself is not affected.

Lichen sclerosus may occur independently from hormonal influences at any age including childhood. Porcelain-white skin and circumscribed hyperkeratosis are typical of lichen sclerosus (Fig. 13.7). These changes may remain asymptomatic or may be associated with pruritus and/or a burning discomfort or pain. Vaginal stenosis and injuries to the labia minora and the posterior fourchette often result in dyspareunia. If the perianal area is involved (Fig. 13.8), defecation may lead to painful skin tears. Synechiae typically involve the labia minora and the subclitoral region (Figs. 13.9 and 13.10).

Children and adolescents may also be affected by lichen sclerosus (Figs. 13.11 and 13.12).

Whether lichen sclerosus is to be regarded as a precancerous condition or not is discussed controversially. However, it is important to note that the incidence of carcinoma in vulvar lichen sclerosus is significantly higher (4–7%) than in patients without lichen sclerosus (Bleeker et al. 2016; Buckley and Fox 1988) (Fig. 13.13).

According to a large epidemiologic study from the Netherlands (Bleeker et al. 2016), which

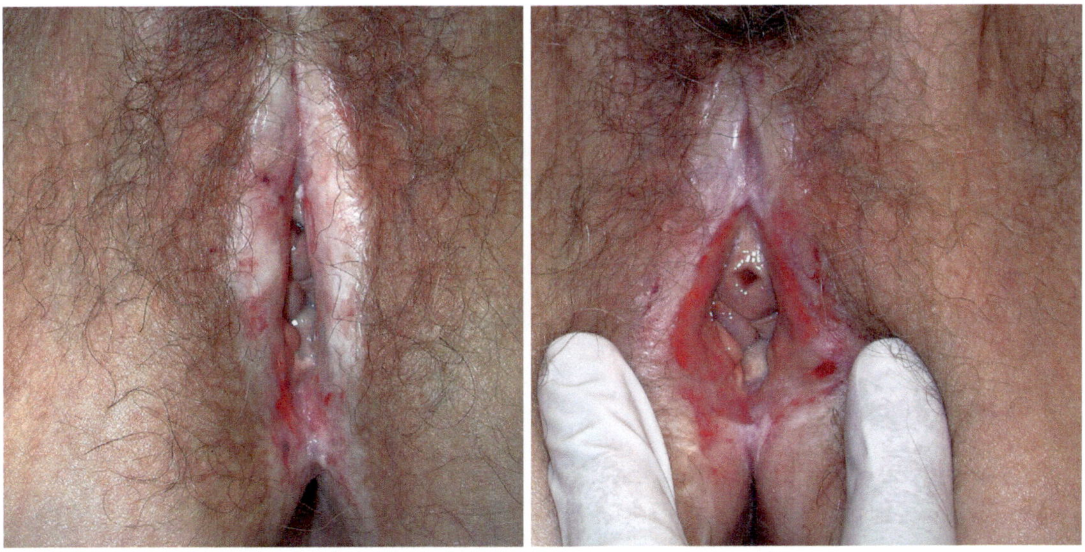

Fig. 13.5 Advanced lichen sclerosus of the vulva. The 53-year-old woman had itching, a burning sensation, and pain for about 30 years. The labia minora have disappeared. There is severe atrophy of the clitoral region also. The white color is due to hyperkeratosis. The overall picture gives the impression of previous vulvectomy

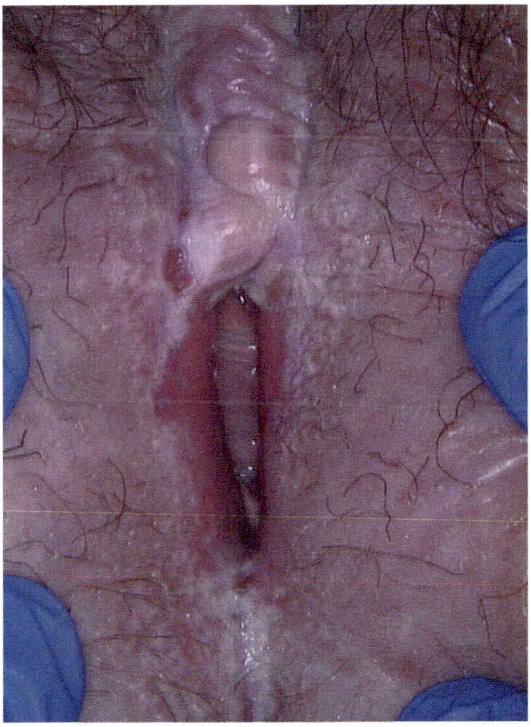

Fig. 13.6 Lichen sclerosus of the vulva (68 years). Vulvar atrophy has led to skin contraction around the introitus

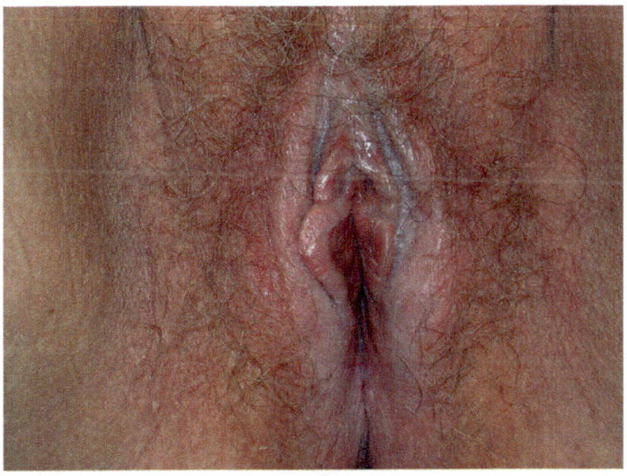

Fig. 13.7 Lichen sclerosus of the vulva. The 71-year-old patient has been complaining of itching for about 17 years. There is only minor atrophy and discrete hyperkeratosis

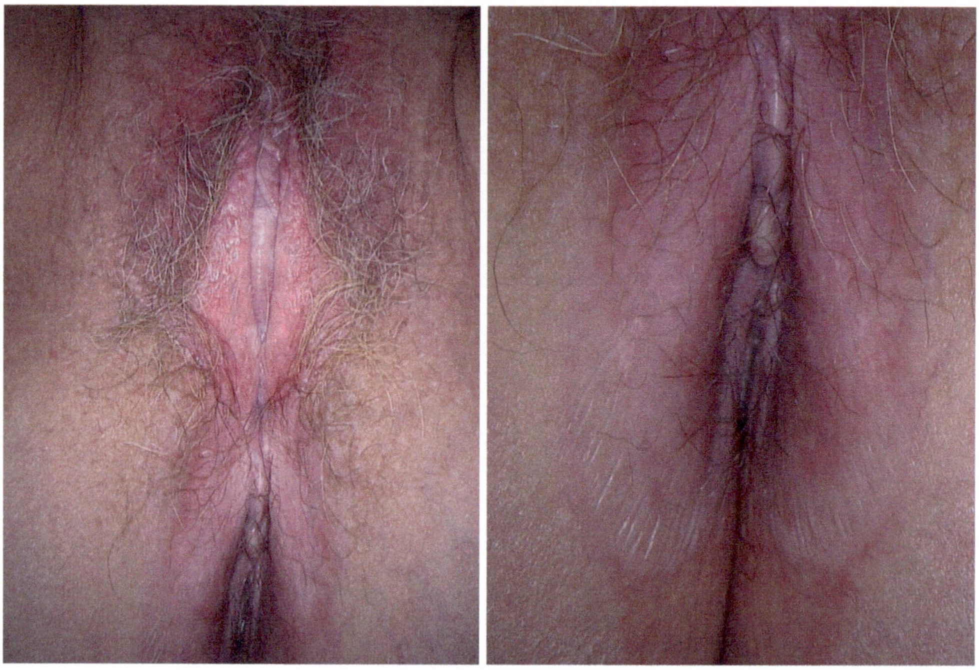

Fig. 13.8 Lichen sclerosus of the vulva and perianal region (71 years). Frequently, the perianal skin is also affected ("figure of eight")

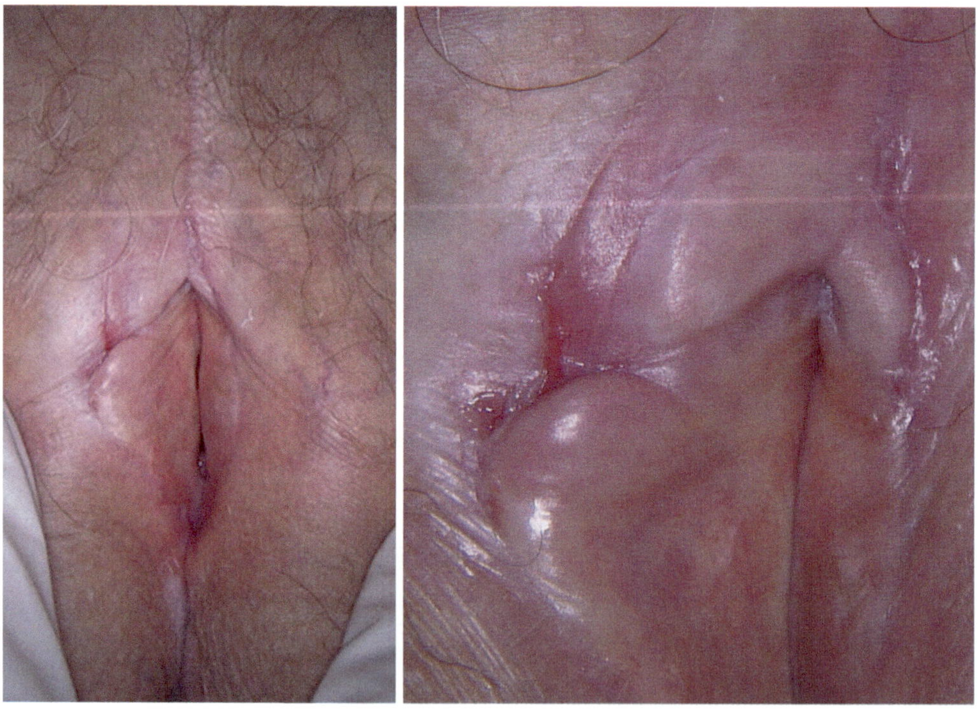

Fig. 13.9 Lichen sclerosus of the vulva (74 years). The labia minora are only partially visible due to atrophy and synechiae. There is a painful rhagade close to the right labium minus

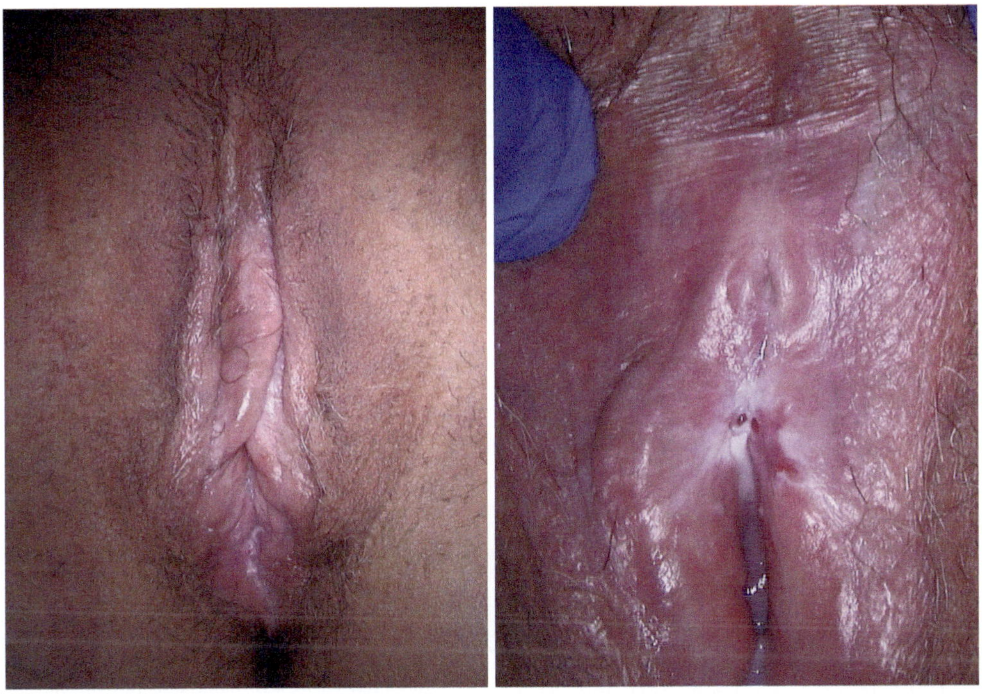

Fig. 13.10 Lichen sclerosus of the vulva. The 53-year-old patient has a history of lichen sclerosus for more than 20 years. Underneath the clitoris, there is a characteristic synechia as well as prominent hyperkeratosis

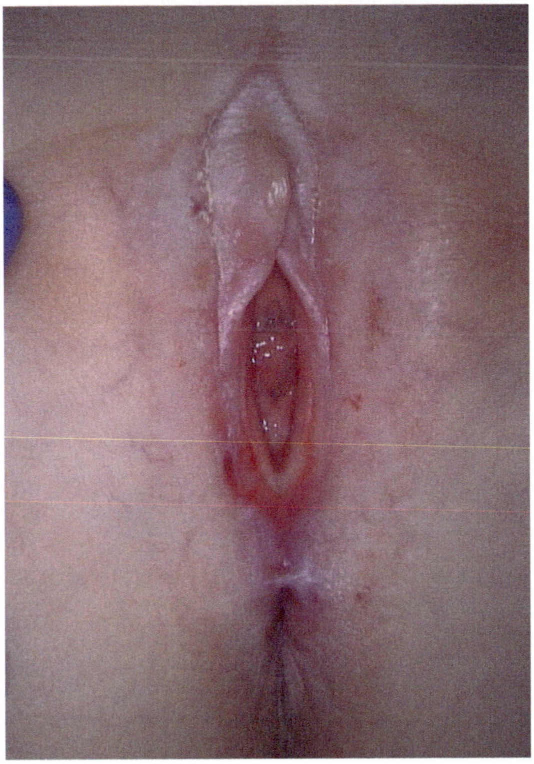

Fig. 13.11 Lichen sclerosus of the vulva in a 5-year-old girl

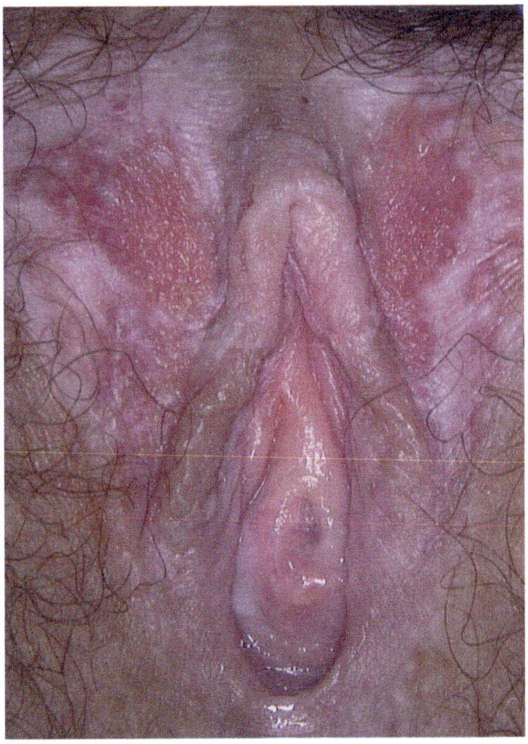

Fig. 13.12 Lichen sclerosus of the vulva. The patient is only 16 years old. Mostly the anterior (ventral) vulva is affected with prominent hyperkeratosis

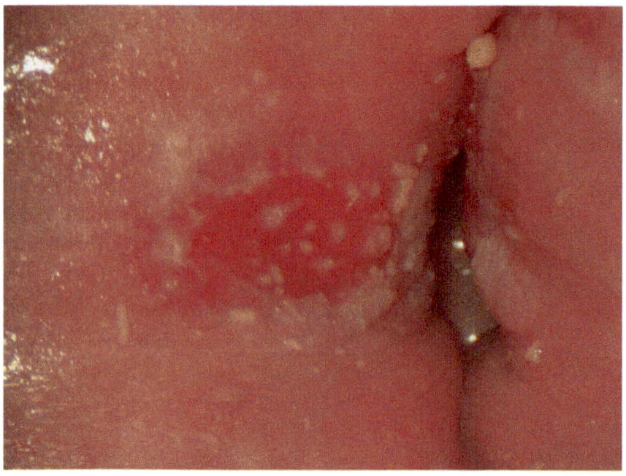

Fig. 13.13 Lichen sclerosus with vulvar carcinoma. Biopsy from the erythroplakia on the right side of the introitus reveals moderately differentiated keratinizing squamous cell carcinoma

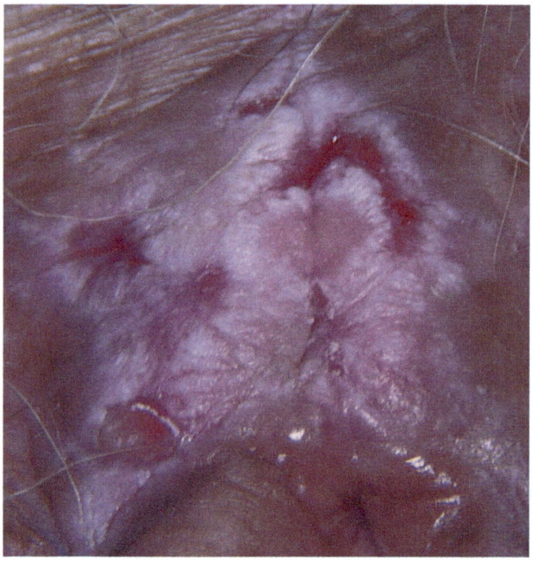

Fig. 13.14 Lichen sclerosus of the vulva (75 years). In the area of the clitoris, several skin defects are seen within an area of hyperkeratosis. These defects are probably due to scratching. However, malignant transformation has to be ruled out

included more than 3000 women over a 20-year period, the incidence of lichen sclerosus has been rising significantly over the last decades with an almost 100% increase between 1991 and 2011. The median age at first diagnosis was 59.8 years with a cumulative incidence of squamous cell carcinoma of the vulva of 6.7%. Age ≥70 years and concomitant vulvar intraepithelial neoplasia were identified as risk factors for the development of invasive disease.

The Finnish Hospital Discharge Registry listed 7616 patients with a diagnosis of lichen sclerosus of the vulva between 1971 and 2012 (Halonen et al. 2017). Within the follow-up period until 2014, 812 cancers were diagnosed with an increased risk of cancer of the vulva (182 cases; standard incidence rate 33.6) and the vagina (4 cases; standard incidence rate 3.69). Interestingly, the risk of cervical cancer and lung cancer was significantly decreased in lichen sclerosus patients.

The diagnosis of lichen sclerosus is usually made visually, i.e., by inspection and colposcopic examination. No routine histopathologic evaluation is required. If skin defects and hyperkeratosis persist, biopsies should be obtained to rule out preneoplasia or neoplasia (Figs. 13.14, 13.15, and 13.16).

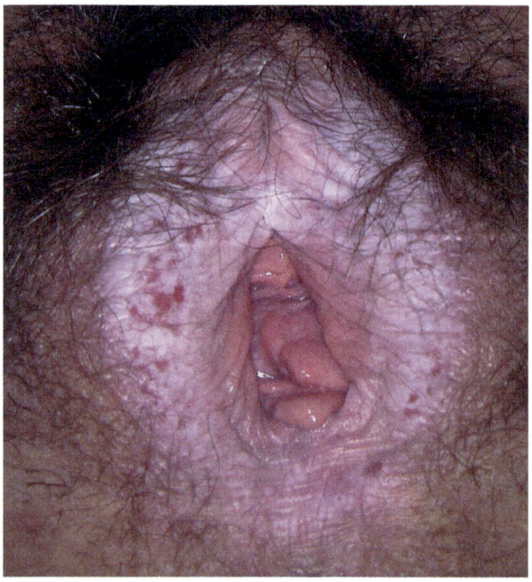

Fig. 13.15 Lichen sclerosus of the vulva (79 years) with total vulvar atrophy, diffuse leukoplakia, and skin defects on the right

The gold standard for treatment especially in women remains potent to very potent topical steroids (Kirtschig et al. 2015). The treatment of choice is the application of class I corticosteroids such as clobetasol propionate. Mometasone furoate has also proven to be effective.

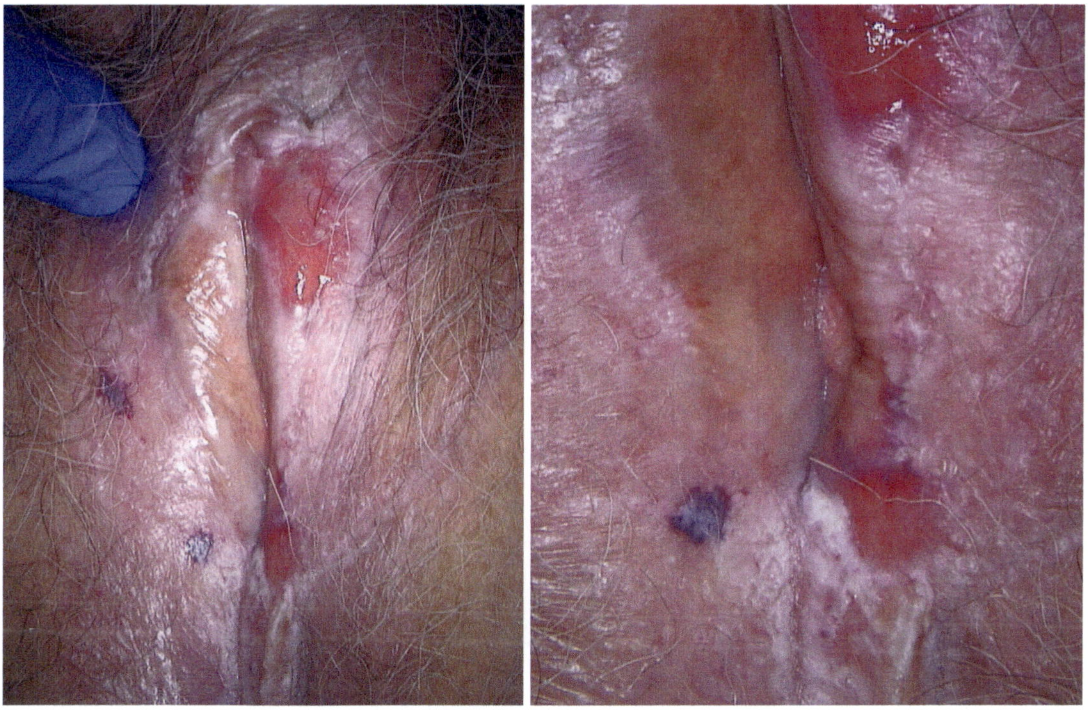

Fig. 13.16 Lichen sclerosus of the vulva (79 years). There are areas of subepidermal bleeding as well as superficial skin defects, from which biopsies should be obtained

In recent years, maintenance therapy has been recommended with the long-term application of the corticosteroid ointment one to three times per week. Lee et al. (2015) performed a prospective longitudinal cohort study on 507 women with biopsy-proven lichen sclerosus over a 6-year period. Patients received preventive topical corticosteroids in order to normalize both skin color and skin texture. The long-term outcomes of compliant and noncompliant patients was compared. Long-term use of topical steroids indeed altered the course of disease with a significant improvement of symptom control, reduction of scarring, and even the occurrence of invasive disease. None of the 350 compliant patients developed vulvar cancer compared to 7 out of 150 partially compliant patients ($p < 0.001$). Only minimal corticoid side effects were observed.

Topical hormones, for example, estrogen, have not been proven to be effective for the treatment of lichen sclerosus. The use of a 2% testosterone propionate cream has been discouraged for many years due to a lack of efficacy and due to the virilizing effects after long-term use (Fig. 13.17).

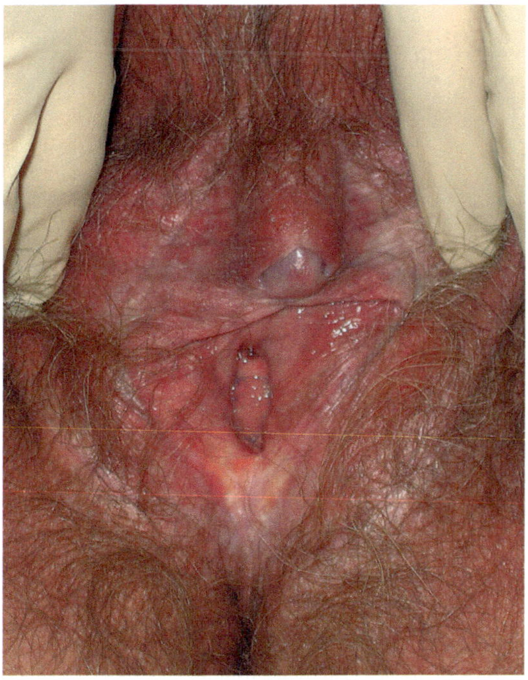

Fig. 13.17 Hypertrophy of the clitoris. The use of a testosterone ointment over a period of 10 years for the treatment of lichen sclerosis has led to clitoral hypertrophy

13.5.2 Lichen Ruber Planus

The erosive manifestation of lichen planus or lichen ruber planus typically causes skin defects of the vulva (Fig. 13.18) and vagina (Fig. 13.19), as well as of the mucous membrane of the mouth (Fig. 13.20). The scalp may also be affected and lead to alopecia (Fig. 13.21). In addition to epithelial defects, there are less obvious reticulate white or purple papules or plaques.

Patients frequently complain of pain and burning sensations, dyspareunia, and postcoital bleeding. In most patients, these changes will also spread to the vagina in the course of time. Adhesions of the vulva and vagina may develop. Sometimes, the cervix is not visible anymore due to stenosis of the upper one-third of the vagina.

Pain within the oral cavity is rarely reported at first presentation but may occur later in the course of the disease. Skin lesions may also be found on the inside of the wrist and anterior aspect of the shin: purple polygonal papules and pruriginous plaques.

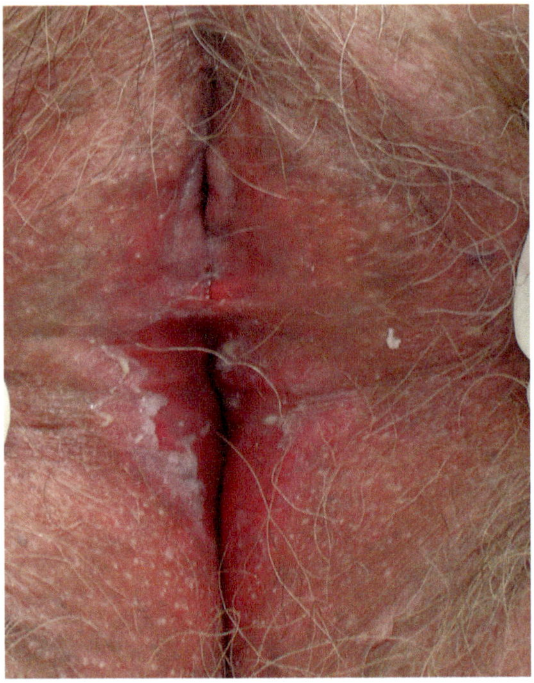

Fig. 13.18 Lichen planus of the vulva (66 years). The diagnosis was established by biopsy of the oral mucosa

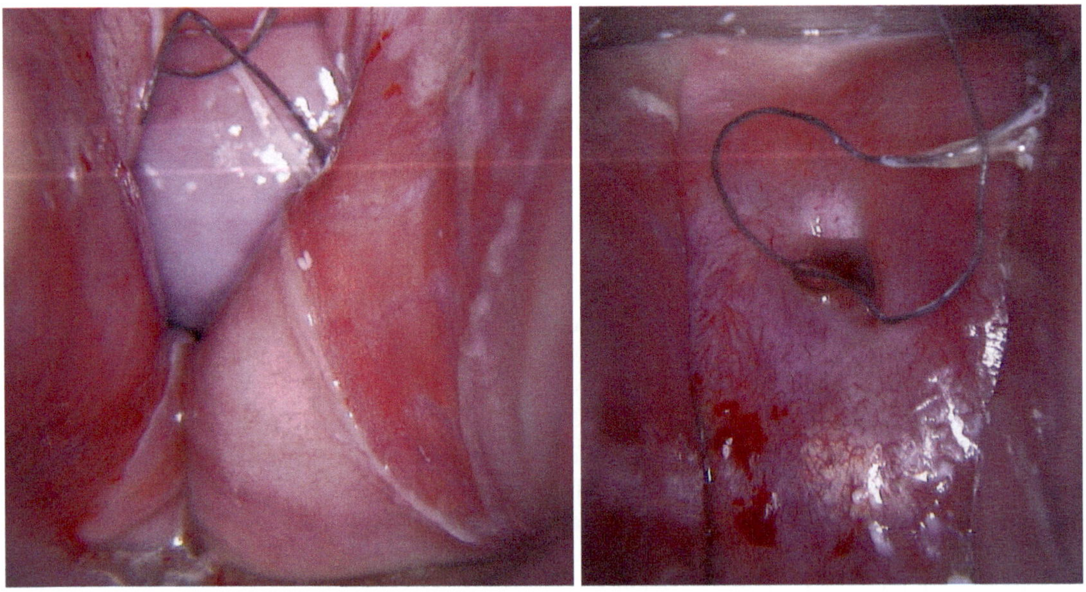

Fig. 13.19 Lichen ruber involving the upper one-third of the vagina and the cervix. The 41-year-old patient has been effectively treated with pimecrolimus

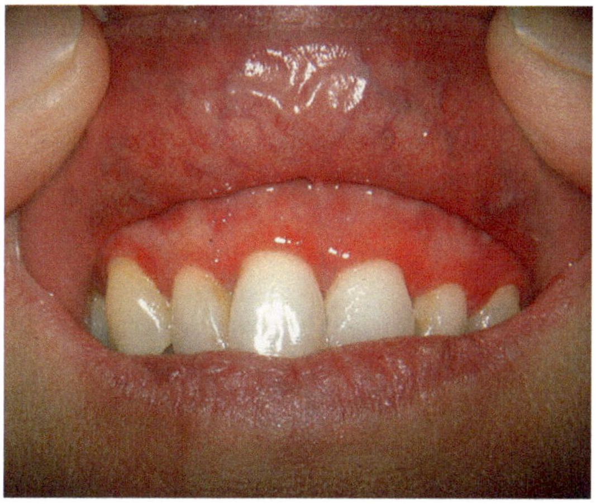

Fig. 13.20 Lichen planus of the gingiva. The vulvar changes from lichen planus were undiagnosed over a period of 3 years. Eventually, the dentist made the correct diagnosis

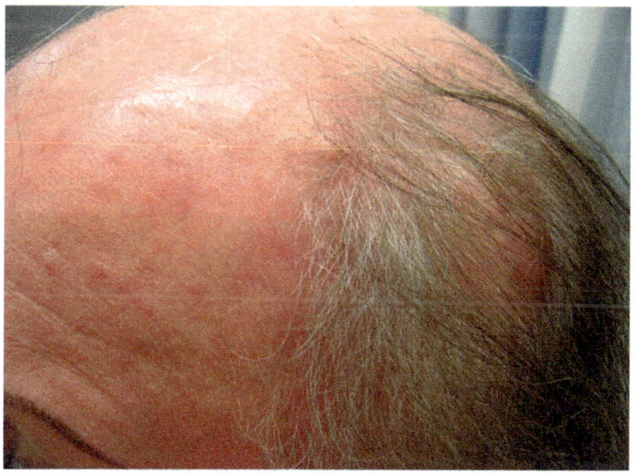

Fig. 13.21 Lichen planus. Involvement of the scalp has led to alopecia

The diagnosis of lichen planus is primarily made visually by inspection and colposcopic examination. It may be confirmed by biopsy.

Lichen planus is treated with topical steroids. When the vagina is involved, foam preparations of corticosteroids as used for treatment of inflammatory bowel diseases are useful. In some patients, symptoms may be controlled by topical tacrolimus or pimecrolimus (Fig. 13.19).

According to Halonen et al. (2018), lichen ruber planus increases the cancer risk significantly for the following locations: lip, tongue, oral cavity, esophagus, larynx, and vulva. For vulvar cancer, the standard incidence rate (ratio of observed to expected number of cancers) was 1.99.

13.6 Neoplastic Epithelial Changes of the Vulva

Although visual diagnosis of the vulva is possible, it is not uncommon for vulvar carcinoma to be diagnosed at an advanced stage. Older women may postpone the visit to the gynecologist, and invasive disease may have persisted for years and may be well advanced. Also, the clinical picture of preneoplasia (HSIL and DVIN) shows a greater variety than, for example, high-grade cervical intraepithelial neoplasia. Thus, neoplastic changes of the vulva may initially not be recognized as such.

Misdiagnosis of vulvar cancer leads to a delay of treatment. This is particularly relevant, as in advanced stages of vulvar cancer, extensive surgical procedures are required, leading to significant morbidity with a high psychological burden (Andersen and Hacker 1983). Therefore, the early recognition and correct diagnosis of vulvar cancer precursors is of special importance. Usually, vulvar biopsy is indicated.

Among the neoplastic epithelial changes of the vulva, HPV-associated diseases are particularly important. Many patients do not complain of symptoms, including those with condylomata acuminata, which may be diagnosed on routine gynecological examination.

Also, HSIL and DVIN patients as well as patients with Paget's disease of the vulva may not experience symptoms. Melanoma is usually completely asymptomatic.

13.6.1 Condylomata Acuminata

Condylomata acuminata are the most common benign tumors of the anogenital area. These benign warts are caused by human papillomaviruses (HPV) and thus are the most common HPV-associated disease as well as the most common sexually transmitted disease among women and men.

Of the more than 100 different genotypes of the HPV family, over 30 types may affect the anogenital area. Most HPV infections are asymptomatic or subclinical.

However, more than 90% of all condylomata acuminata manifestations are associated with the presence of HPV low risk types 6 and 11.

Transmission of HPV occurs through sexual intercourse and other intimate contact. During delivery, HPV can be transmitted within the birth canal from the mother to the newborn. Subsequently, the child may develop genitourinary warts, and and in rare cases laryngeal papilloma. If condylomata acuminata occur in childhood (Fig. 13.22), sexual abuse should be ruled out.

The incubation period of genitourinary warts is variable and takes between 4 weeks up to several months. The most important independent risk factor for condylomata acuminata infection is the number of sexual partners. Condylomata acuminata are frequently asymptomatic (Fig. 13.23). Rare accompanying symptoms are pruritus vulvae, burning, and vaginal discharge. Condylomata acuminata can persist for months and years. Spontaneous healing of warts occurs in up to 30% of patients.

Diagnosis is made by visual inspection with the aid of a colposcope. Application of a 3% solu-

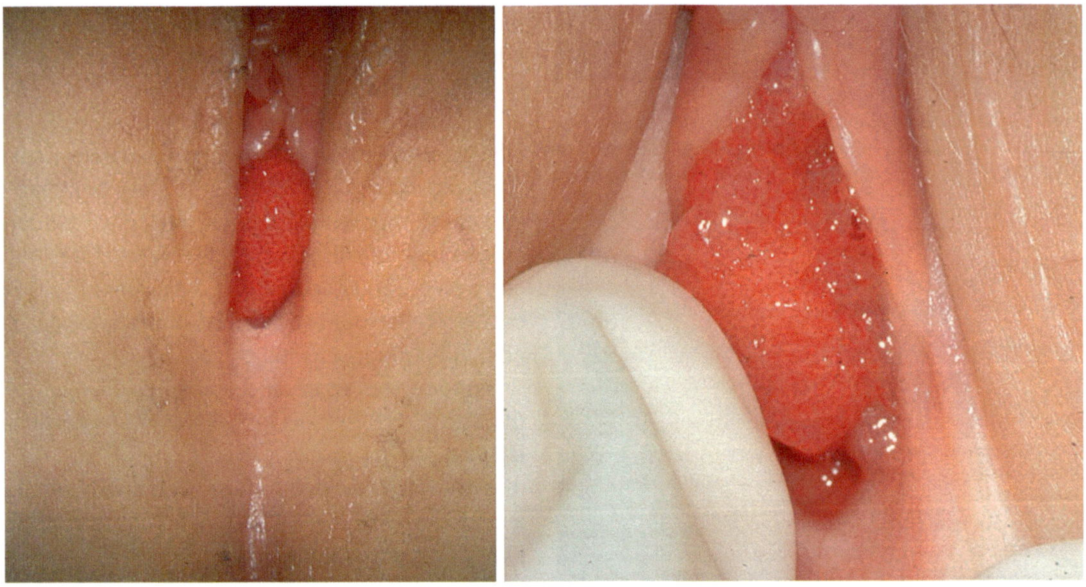

Fig. 13.22 Condylomata acuminata in an 11-year-old girl without evidence of sexual abuse

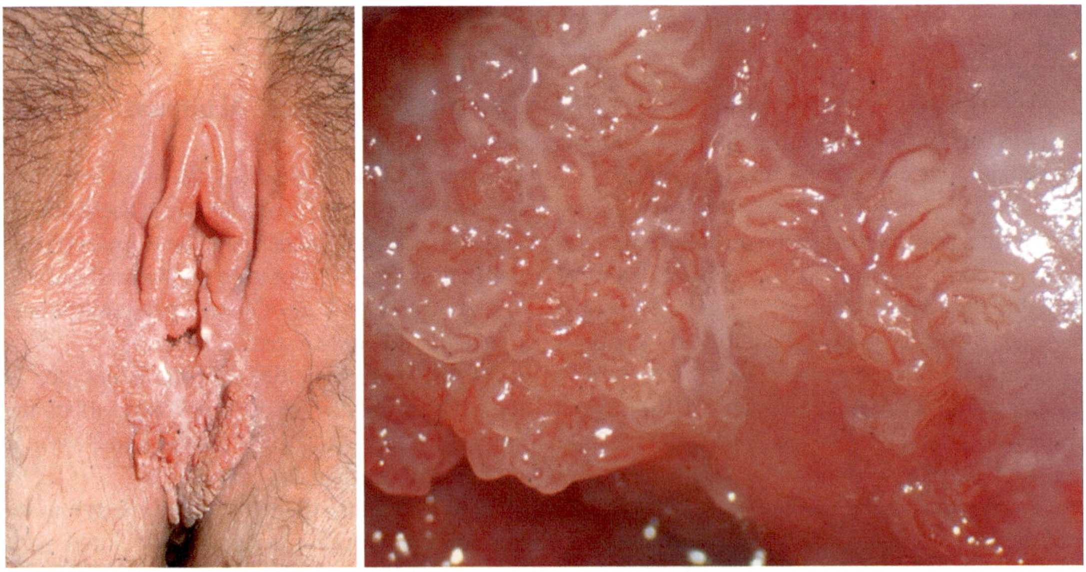

Fig. 13.23 Condylomata acuminata of the perineum and the cervix uteri (right)

tion of acetic acid may be helpful. Due to the frequent occurrence of condylomata in association with intraepithelial neoplasms, a speculum exam with colposcopic examination of vagina and cervix is required (Fig. 13.24).

Condylomata acuminata are usually multifocal. When the warts are located close to the urethra, intraurethral condyloma need to be ruled out by urethroscopy. When located in the perianal and anal area, a proctoscopic exam is indicated.

As stated above, visual diagnosis is usually sufficient. Whenever the diagnosis is in doubt (Fig. 13.25) or when condylomata are recurring frequently, histopathologic evaluation is required (Buckley and Fox 1988).

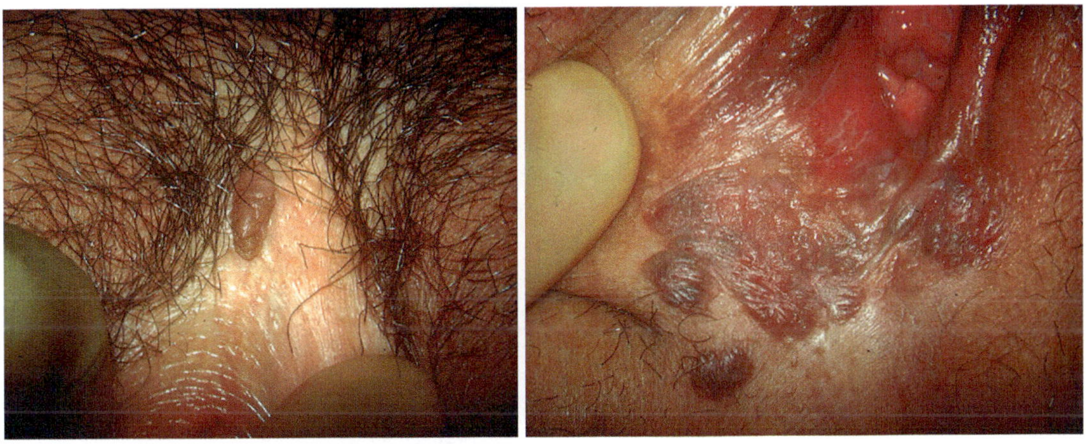

Fig. 13.24 Condylomata acuminata in association with HSIL of the vulva. There is a small condyloma at the anterior fourchette (left) and HSIL of the vulva at the posterior commissure

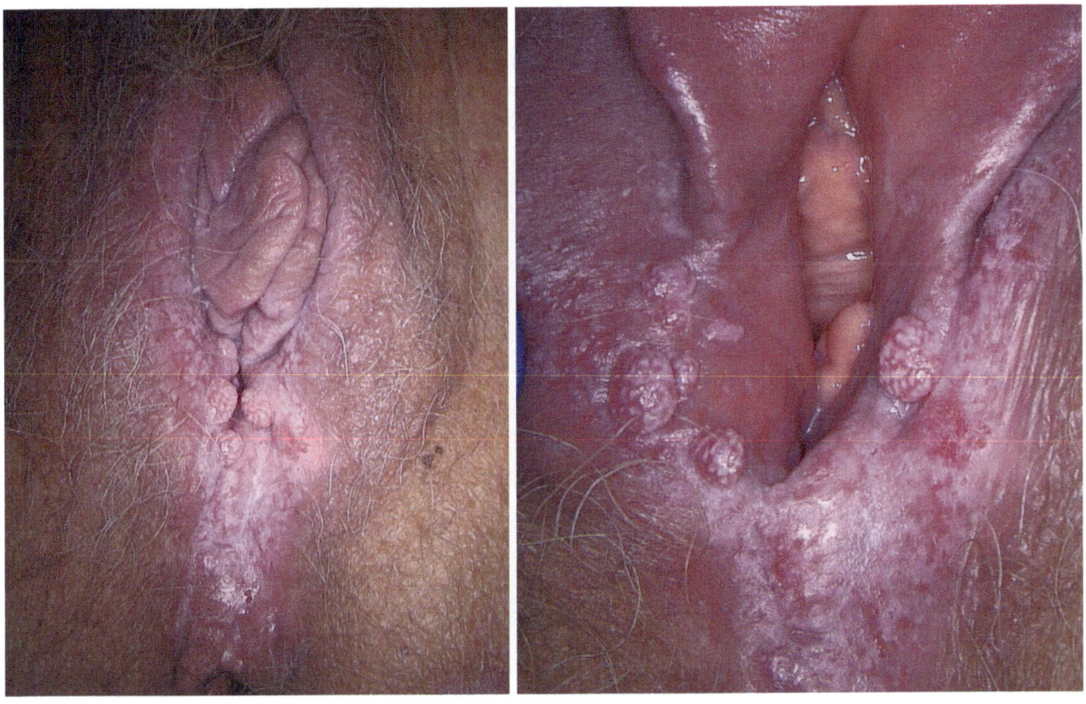

Fig. 13.25 Lichen sclerosus and recurrent condylomata acuminata (55 years). Due to the unusual appearance of these lesions, biopsy is recommended

Condylomata acuminata must not be confused with intraepithelial neoplasia of the vulva (VIN) (Fig. 13.26). Also, micropapillomatosis labialis vulvae (Figs. 13.27 and 13.28), which does not need treatment, must not be misinterpreted as condylomata.

When the diagnosis of condylomata acuminata has been established, several treatment options are available, either medical or surgical.

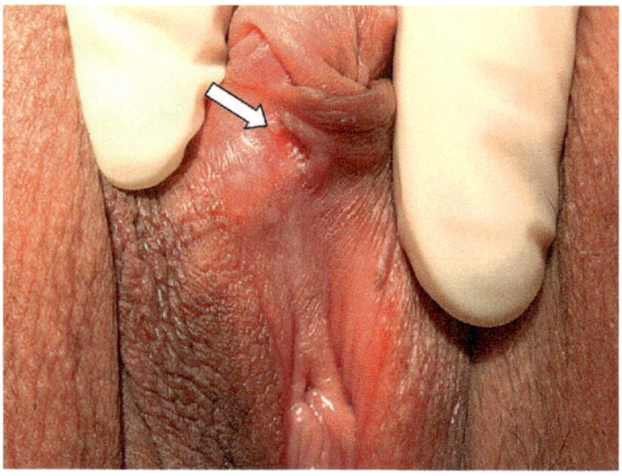

Fig. 13.26 Differential diagnosis of condylomata acuminata versus HSIL/vulva versus invasive carcinoma. On the inside of the left labium minus, the 41-year-old patient had several lesions reminiscent of condylomata acuminata, however with dark pigmentation. Biopsy revealed HSIL of the vulva with evidence of HPV 16. Just below the clitoris, a very small tissue defect is seen (arrow), which is due to HSIL of the vulva with microcarcinoma (depth of invasion less than 1 mm)

In the case of extensive condylomata manifestation, laser therapy under colposcopic guidance is recommended. Alternatively, electrosurgical methods are used. However, scarring may occur, whereas with the CO_2 laser, the best cosmetic result is achieved. Treatment is done under local or general anesthesia.

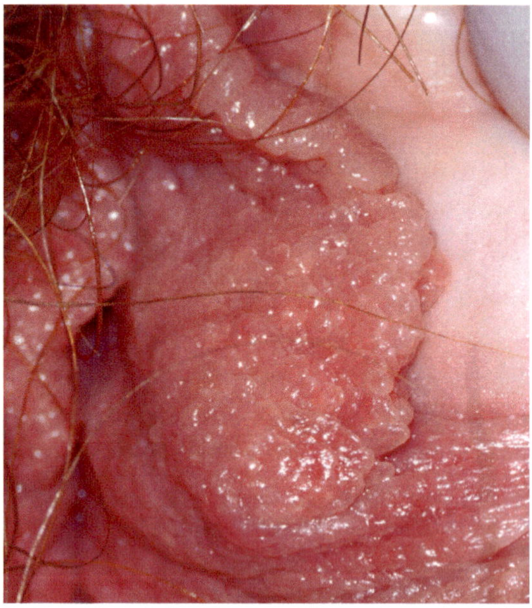

Fig. 13.27 Micropapillomatosis labialis. These changes are unrelated to HPV and may not be confused with condylomata acuminata

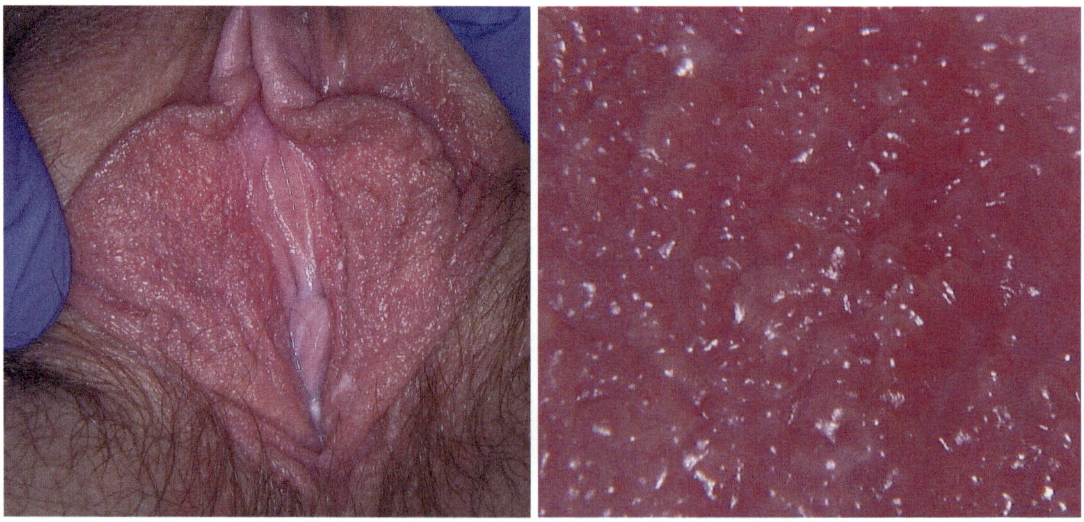

Fig. 13.28 Vestibular papillomatosis (hirsuties papillaris, micropapillomatosis) of a 21-year-old patient presenting with vulvodynia. Papillomatosis is a benign condition that is not HPV-related and should not be treated

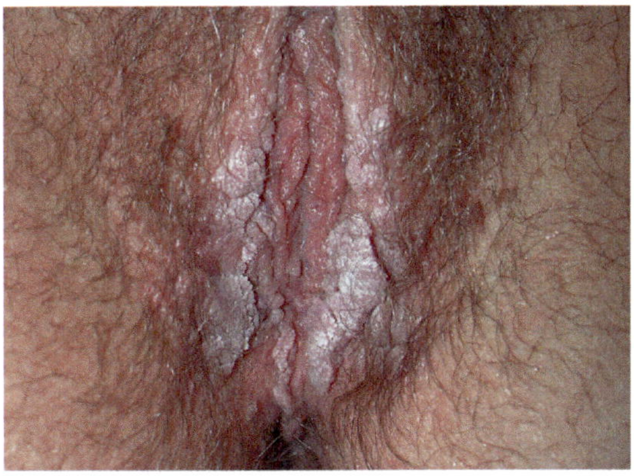

Fig. 13.29 Condylomata acuminata of the vulva (21 years). This extensive manifestation had been treated effectively with imiquimod cream

In the past, condylomata have been treated with topical podophyllin. However, the use of podophyllin is no longer recommended because of its poor treatment effect and its considerable toxicity (Lacey et al. 2003, by Krogh et al. 2000).

Instead, podophyllotoxin as a 0.5% solution or as a 0.15% cream is used. Unlike podophyllin, podophyllotoxin can be applied by the patient herself.

In recent years, topical imiquimod (5%), an immune response modifier, has become the treatment of choice (Fig. 13.29). In addition, Veregen®, a cream made from green tea extract, which has antioxidant properties, has also proven to be effective (Bhatia 2012).

Trichloroacetic acid (TCA), which may be used in concentrations of 70% or 85%, causes cell necrosis when applied to the skin. It is the only drug that can be used for treatment of external genital warts during pregnancy.

TCA is applied in the doctor's office using a cotton swab. Patients often complain of a burning discomfort during treatment. Only very small quantities should be applied.

Extensive involvement of the vulva, vagina, and cervix uteri during pregnancy is particularly difficult to treat. In addition to the risk of birth canal injury during delivery, the risk of peripartum HPV infection should be taken into account. However, regardless of whether the condylomata are removed during pregnancy or not, the risk for the child seems to be low (Watts et al. 1998). Despite the low infection risk for the child, most patients opt for primary cesarean section to avoid the risk of infection.

Spontaneous delivery is preferable if the warts can be removed by CO_2 laser surgery by the 34th week of gestation.

13.6.2 Vulvar Intraepithelial Neoplasia (VIN)/HSIL of the Vulva

In the following chapter, both the WHO nomenclature (VIN) as well as the ISSVD terminology (HSIL of the vulva) are used.

Analogous to high-grade cervical intraepithelial neoplasia (CIN2/CIN3), vulvar intraepithelial neoplasia (VIN) is considered a precancerous lesion. As far as can be determined by retrospective studies, the risk of cancer does not appear to be high. In a survey of 303 patients (Wallbillich et al. 2012), seven patients (2.3%) developed invasive carcinoma after a median interval of 109 months (12–327 months). A major challenge for management of vulvar intraepithelial neoplasia is the high rate of recurrence, which was as high as 28.7% in the study quoted above.

Smokers were significantly more likely to suffer recurrences. Obviously, smoking is also a risk factor for the development of VIN. Forty percent of those affected were active smokers, and 26% had smoked in the past.

The clinical appearance of VIN is quite variable. Papillary or pigmented lesions of a condylomatous character are often referred to as "bowenoid papulosis" (Fig. 13.30).

Other characteristic manifestations of VIN are nonpigmented, slightly raised, partially papillary, or hyperkeratotic (Figs. 13.31, 13.32, and 13.33). Occasionally, large erythematous lesions are seen (Fig. 13.34). This used to be called "erythroplasia de Queyrat." According to the official nomenclature of the vulva, it is referred to as HSIL of the vulva or VIN.

Occasionally, basal cell carcinoma of the vulva is seen, which may be difficult to differentiate visually from VIN (Figs. 13.35 and 13.36).

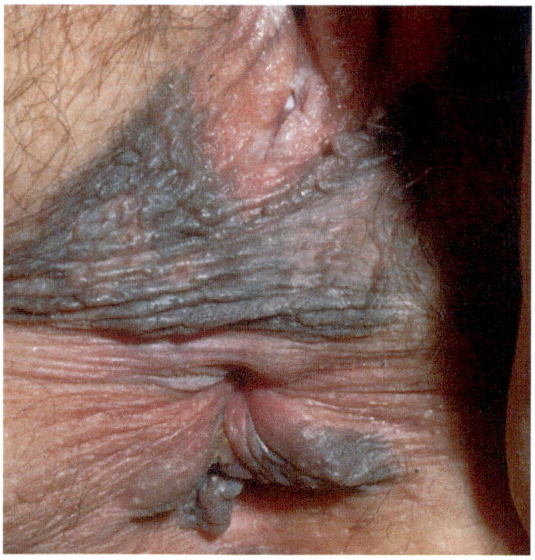

Fig. 13.30 HSIL of the vulva as well as AIN

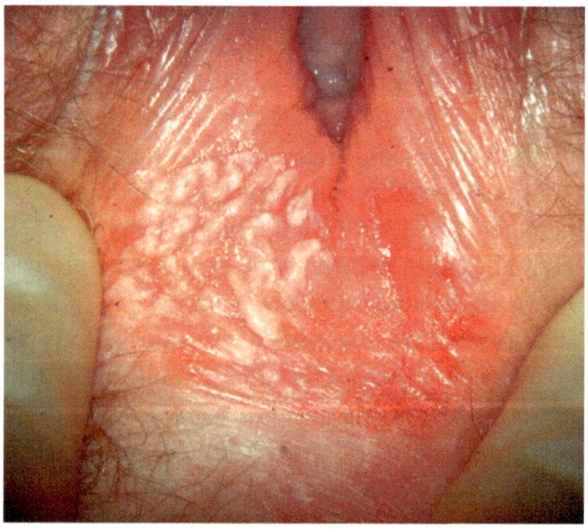

Fig. 13.31 HSIL of the vulva. The clinical picture is not necessarily typical of HSIL of the vulva and illustrates its high variability

VIN may be multifocal (Fig. 13.37). Intraepithelial neoplasia may also affect the perianal and anal skin. Also, simultaneous cervical intraepithelial dysplasia may occur. Other HPV-related changes such as condylomata acuminata may also be present.

In recent years, an increasing number of young women with both intraepithelial and invasive lesions are seen, which are predominantly located in the midline between clitoris and urethra. Therefore, any persistent abnormalities, especially erosions or ulcerations, need to be biopsied to avoid any delay of treatment in the case of malignant disease.

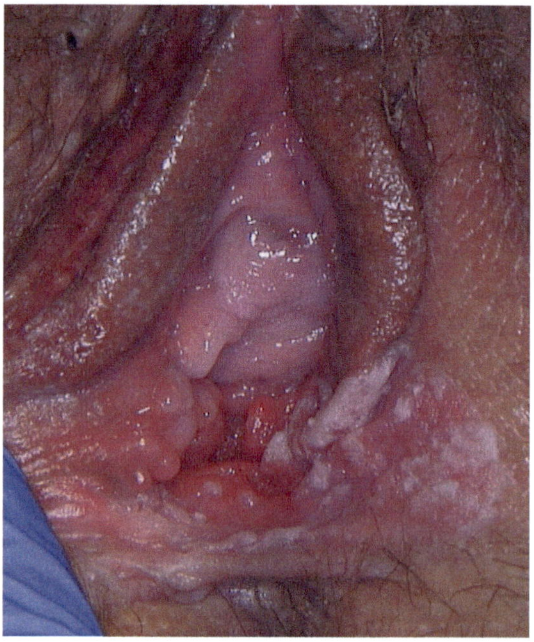

Fig. 13.32 HSIL of the vulva (36 years). The hyperkeratotic lesions are extending onto the vagina

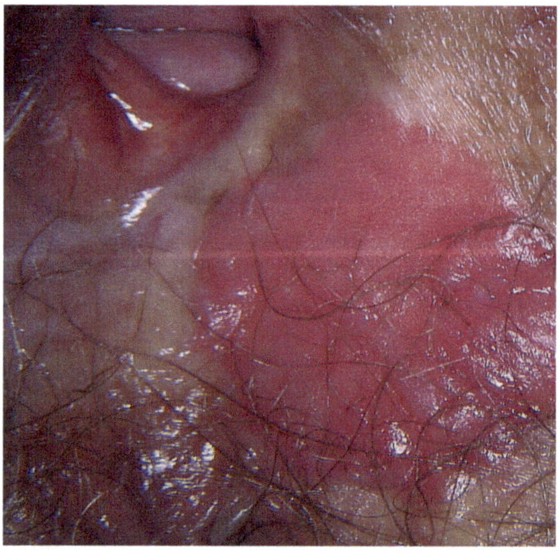

Fig. 13.33 Recurrent HSIL of the vulva (61 years). The patient has had three previous CO_2 laser surgeries

Usually, vulvar intraepithelial dysplasia is treated by surgery (CO_2 laser resection and/or vaporization).

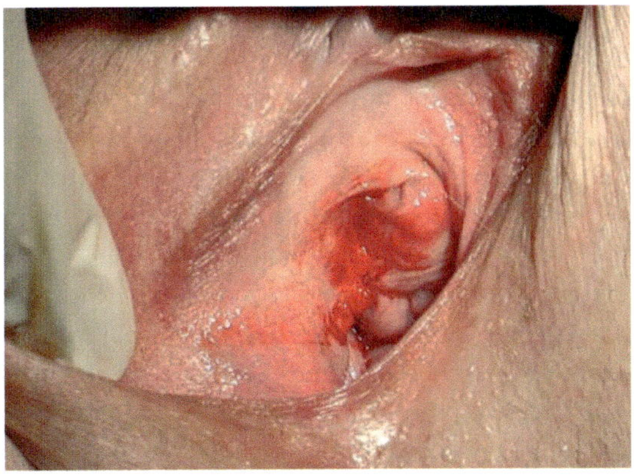

Fig. 13.34 HSIL of the vulva as erythroplakia of the mucosa (formerly "erythroplasia de Queyrat")

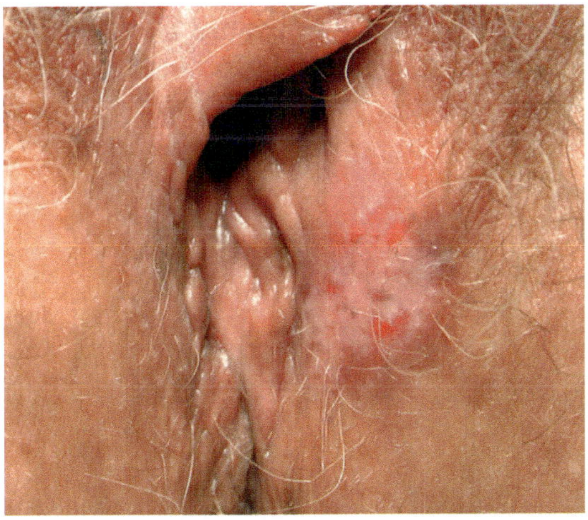

Fig. 13.35 Basalioma of the vulva

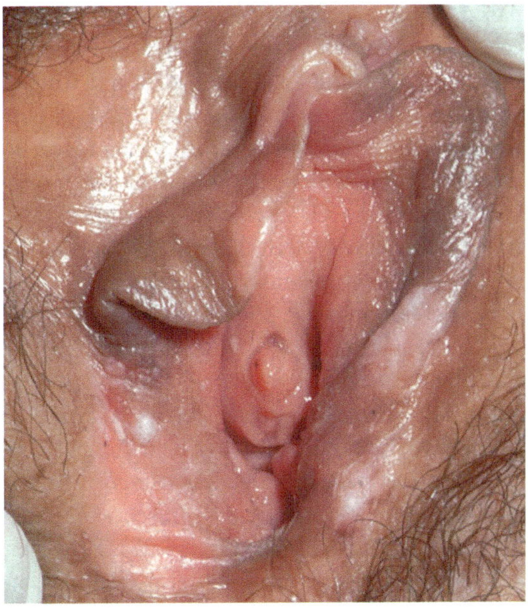

Fig. 13.37 Multifocal HSIL of the vulva with hyperkeratosis

Other treatment options are limited. Attempts have been made to develop a therapeutic HPV vaccine to treat VIN (Kenter et al. 2009). Also, imiquimod, which is used for topical condylomata acuminata treatment, has been used successfully to treat recurrent VIN (Terlou et al. 2011; van Seters et al. 2008).

CO_2laser vaporization is the treatment of choice for vulvar intraepithelial neoplasia. Com-

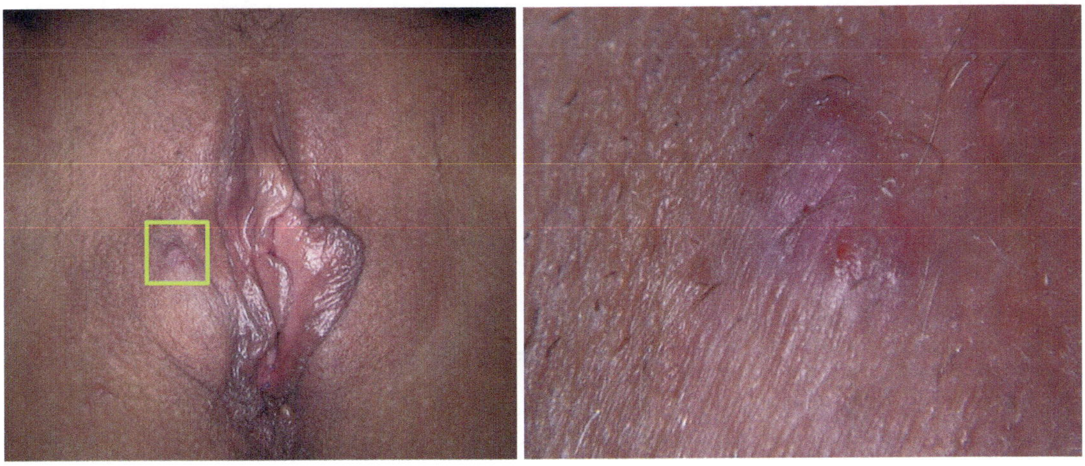

Fig. 13.36 Basalioma of the vulva

pared to other treatment modalities such as cold-knife excision or electrosurgical resection or coagulation, the CO_2 laser does not lead to scarring or mutilation of the vulva. This is particularly important if lesions are located close to the clitoris and/or close to the anal canal.

The focused CO_2 laser beam can be used to superficially excise the skin, if the area to be treated is not too extensive. As VIN, by definition, is not an invasive condition, no safety margins are required.

Colombo-Benkmann et al. (2008) use an ultrasound scalpel (Harmonic Scalpel, Ethicon, Norderstedt) for the removal of anal and perianal condylomata and report good cosmetic results. The procedure is suitable for the resection of anal intraepithelial neoplasias (Fig. 13.38). However, no data are available on long-term results compared to CO_2 laser surgery.

13.6.3 Paget's Disease

The vulva is the most common site of extramammary Paget's disease. On histopathological examination, large adenoid cells are found within the squamous epithelium as well as in the area of the skin appendages (Londero et al. 2013). The skin changes often start within the hairy parts of the vulva. The skin of the anal area may also be affected. Unlike VIN, Paget's disease of the vulva is more likely to affect postmenopausal women.

Paget's disease of the vulva presents as sharply demarcated, reddish areas with small islands of white epithelium due to hyperkeratosis (Figs. 13.39 and 13.40). Small manifestation of Paget's disease is often misinterpreted as eczema (Fig. 13.41), large areas as fungal infection.

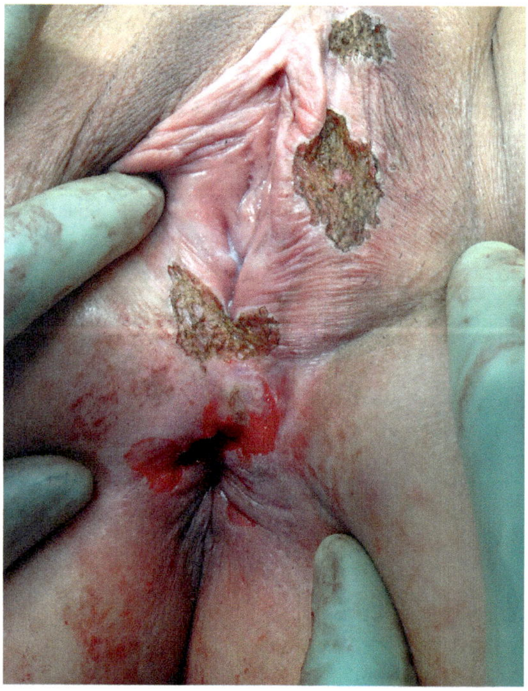

Fig. 13.38 Ablation of anal and perianal intraepithelial neoplasia using an ultrasound scalpel (Harmonic Scalpel, Ethicon, Norderstedt, Germany). Vulvar condylomata were treated by CO_2 laser vaporization

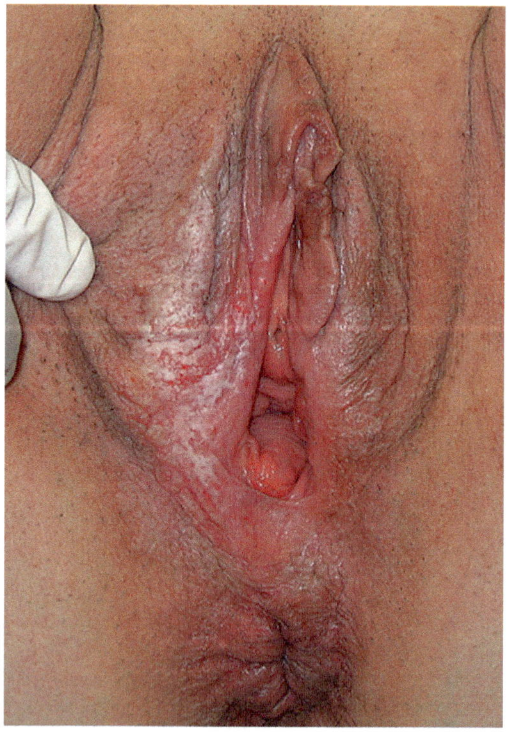

Fig. 13.39 Paget's disease of the vulva. For the past five years, the 69-year-old woman has had a persistent pruritus on the right side of the vulva

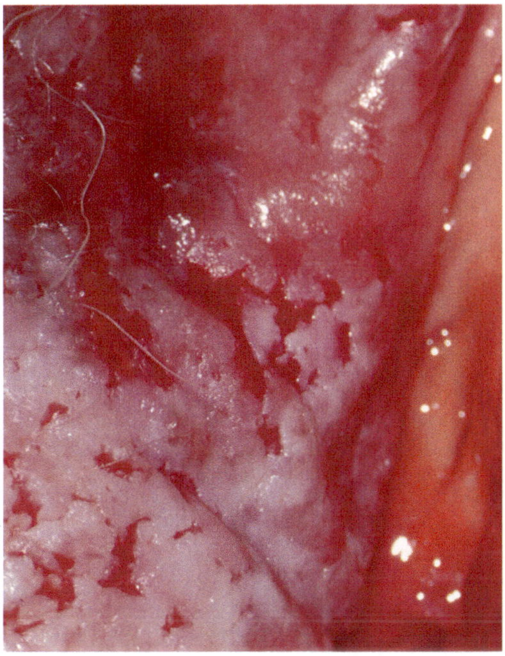

Fig. 13.40 Paget's disease of the vulva. A 15-fold colposcopic magnification shows the reddish color with island-like areas of hyperkeratosis

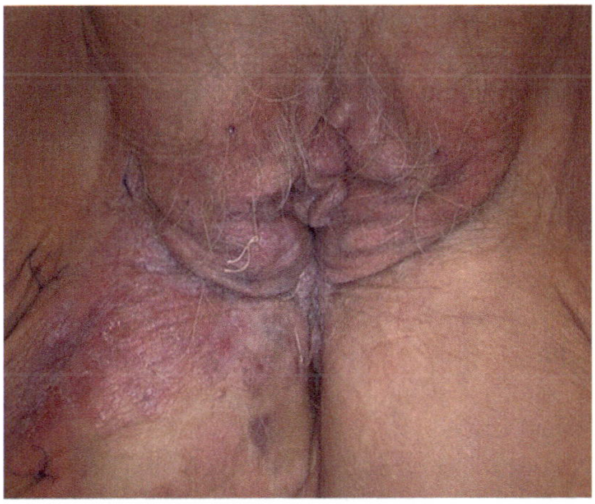

Fig. 13.41 Paget's disease of the vulva (77 years). The involved epidermis has an eczema-like appearance

Up to one-third of patients with Paget's disease of the vulva have adenocarcinoma elsewhere.

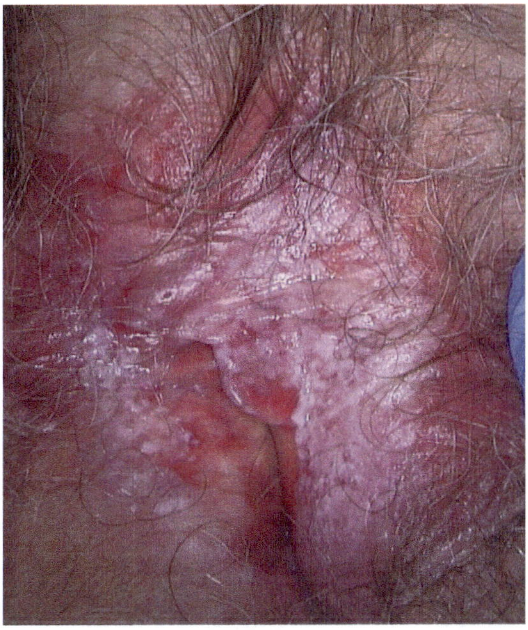

Fig. 13.42 Recurrent Paget's disease of the vulva. The 75-year-old patient had been diagnosed 12 years previously

Paget's disease of the vulva is treated surgically. Thus, invasive disease can be ruled out. Unfortunately, even wide resection margins are often not free of disease, and recurrences occur frequently (Figs. 13.42 and 13.43). Therefore, ultraradical resections should be avoided. Recurrent disease is then treated with the immune response modifier imiquimod. Intermittent application of imiquimod is a highly effective treatment option for recurrent Paget's disease (Bertozzi et al. 2009; Londero et al. 2013; Luyten et al. 2006, 2014). A retrospective study of 21 women treated with imiquimod for primary or recurrent disease (Luyten et al. 2014) showed a 81.0% response rate with 11 patients (52.4%) achieving a complete response. No patients with progressive disease were observed. Thus, conservative treatment with imiquimod may help to avoid mutilating surgery.

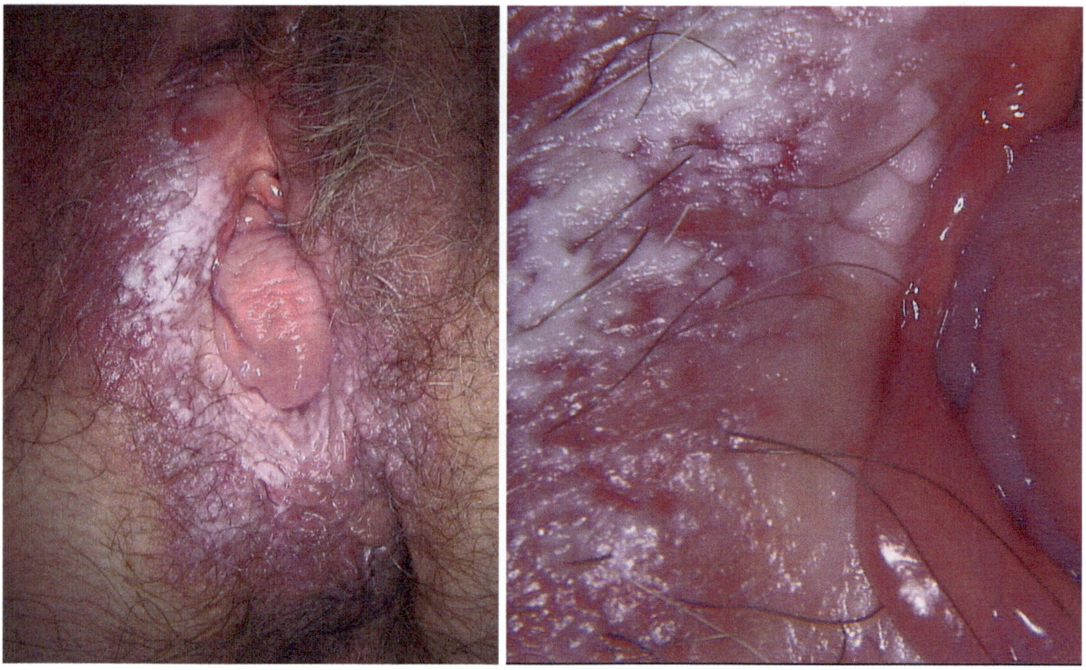

Fig. 13.43 Recurrent Paget's disease of the vulva. The 80-year-old patient had been treated with local resection as well as imiquimod cream

13.6.4 Carcinoma of the Vulva

The epidemiology of vulvar cancer has changed significantly in recent decades. The incidence of both preinvasive as well as invasive lesions has increased. Also, carcinoma of the vulva is increasingly common in younger women, mostly as so-called midline vulvar carcinomas (Hampl et al. 2008).

These midline carcinomas are typically located close to or in between clitoris and urethra (Figs. 13.44, 13.45, 13.46, 13.47, 13.48, 13.49, 13.50). So far, it has not been possible to assign a specific biomolecular profile to such midline carcinomas (Reuschenbach et al. 2013). Surprisingly, there is no association with HPV infection.

The symptoms of patients with squamous cell carcinoma of the vulva are nonspecific. Typical early symptoms, which may point to the correct diagnosis, do not exist. Some patients complain of itching and/or pain or soreness of the vulva at the time of diagnosis. Many patients will state that these symptoms have persisted for years. Less commonly, patients will complain of occasional bleeding or the appearance of nodules. However, early stage vulvar cancer will not cause any symptoms at all (Fig. 13.51).

It is not unusual that the diagnosis of vulvar cancer is delayed considerably (Fig. 13.52). Patients frequently ignore initial symptoms. The doctor might also misdiagnose early stage invasive disease and recommend some kind of symptomatic topical treatment (Figs. 13.53 and 13.54).

When carcinoma of the vulva is suspected, visual inspection with the aid of the colposcope is done. The vulva itself as well as the perineum including the perianal and anal area are examined. To rule out multicentric HPV-related disease, colposcopic examination of the vagina and cervix is performed routinely.

Large exophytic and/or necrotic tumor masses, which are sometimes seen in older patients, still need to be biopsied to confirm the clinical diagnosis. One or several biopsies are taken from the margins of the tumor to unequivocally establish the diagnosis of invasive disease. Necrotic tumor areas are not suitable for biopsy.

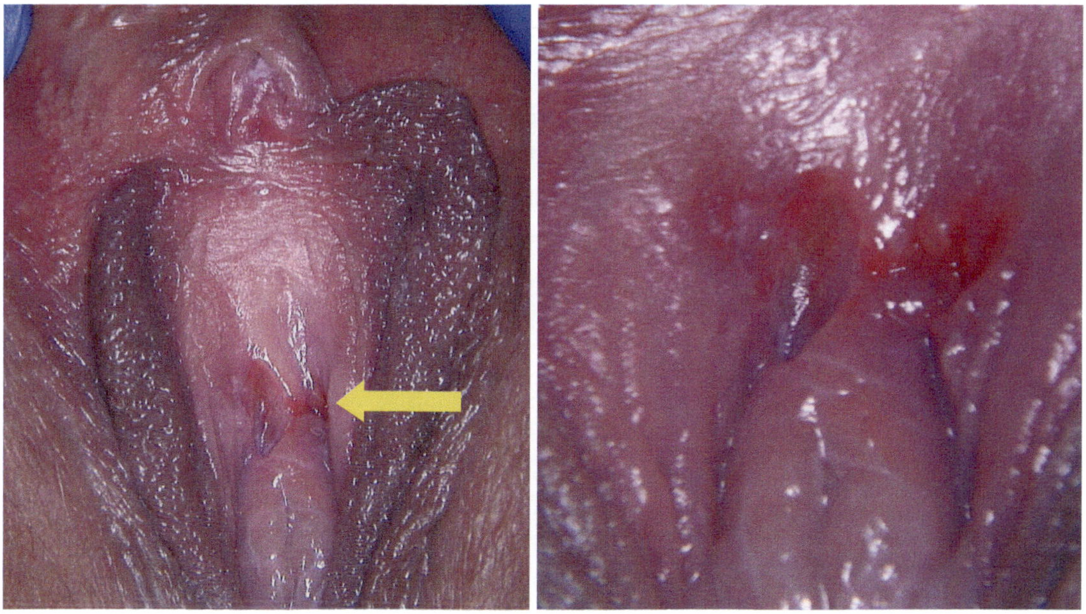

Fig. 13.44 Carcinoma of the vulva close to the urethra (30 years)

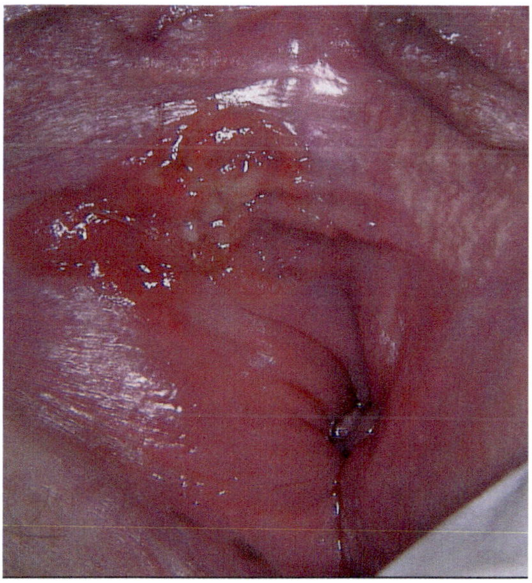

Fig. 13.45 Carcinoma of the vulva (38 years). The cancer is located directly at the clitoris

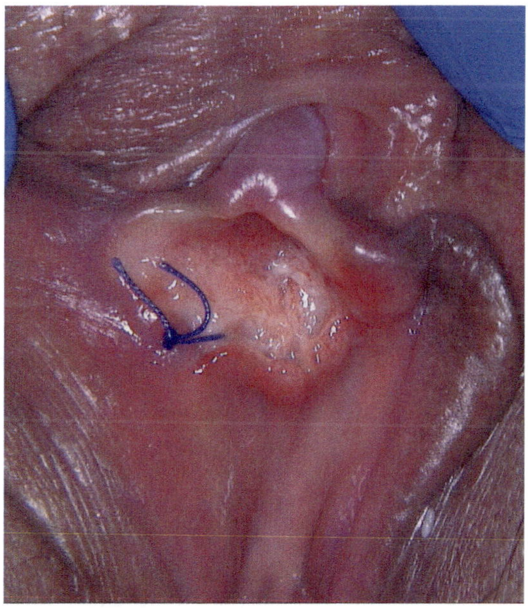

Fig. 13.46 Carcinoma of the vulva (59 years). The patient described a burning sensation starting 7 months previously. The tumor is very close to the glans clitoridis

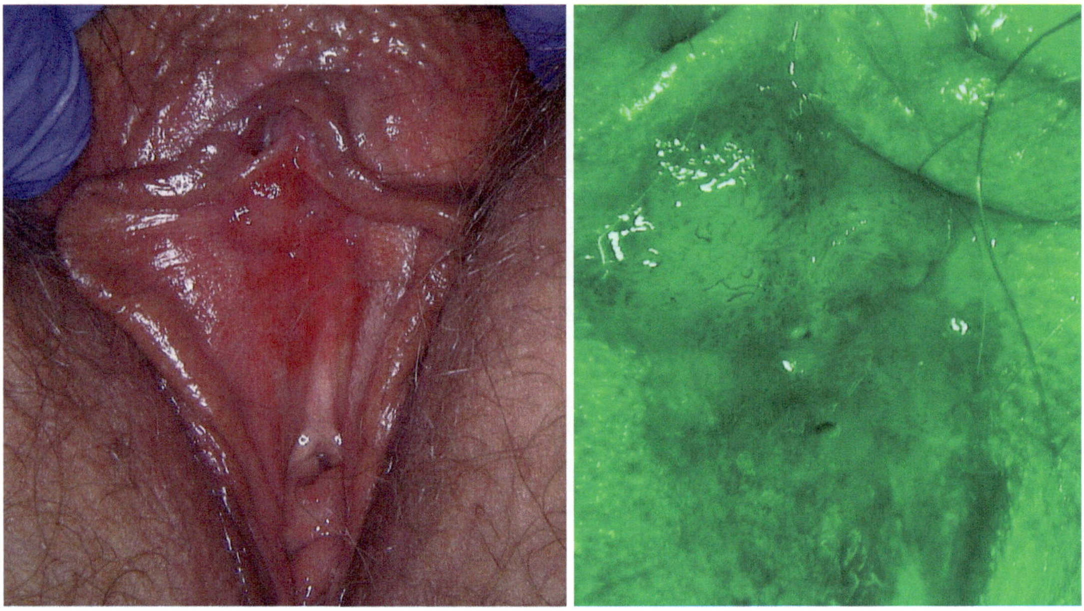

Fig. 13.47 Microcarcinoma of the anterior (ventral) vulva (59 years) with atypical vessels

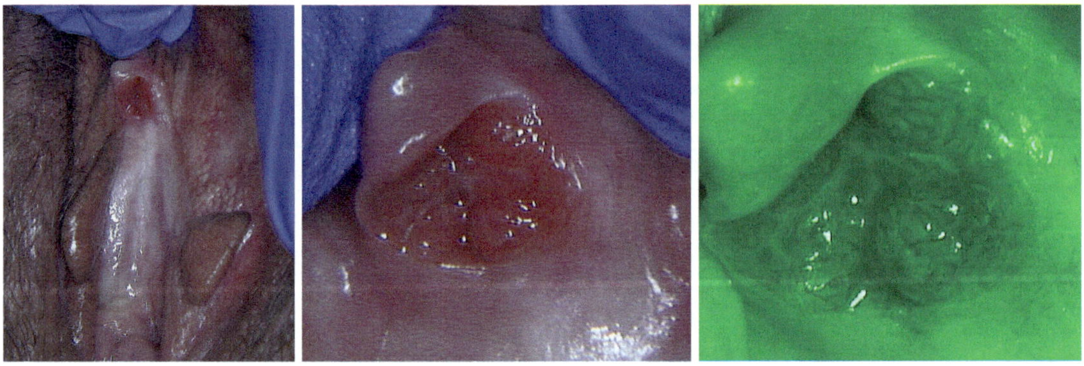

Fig. 13.48 Carcinoma of the glans clitoridis. The 33-year-old patient had been treated previously for HSIL of the vulva

Smaller tumors of less than 2 cm in diameter can be excised entirely. Depending on the location of the lesion, for example, close to the posterior fourchette, this may be done under local anesthesia.

If the examination of the vulva is particularly uncomfortable or if multiple biopsies are required ("mapping"), general anesthesia should be considered.

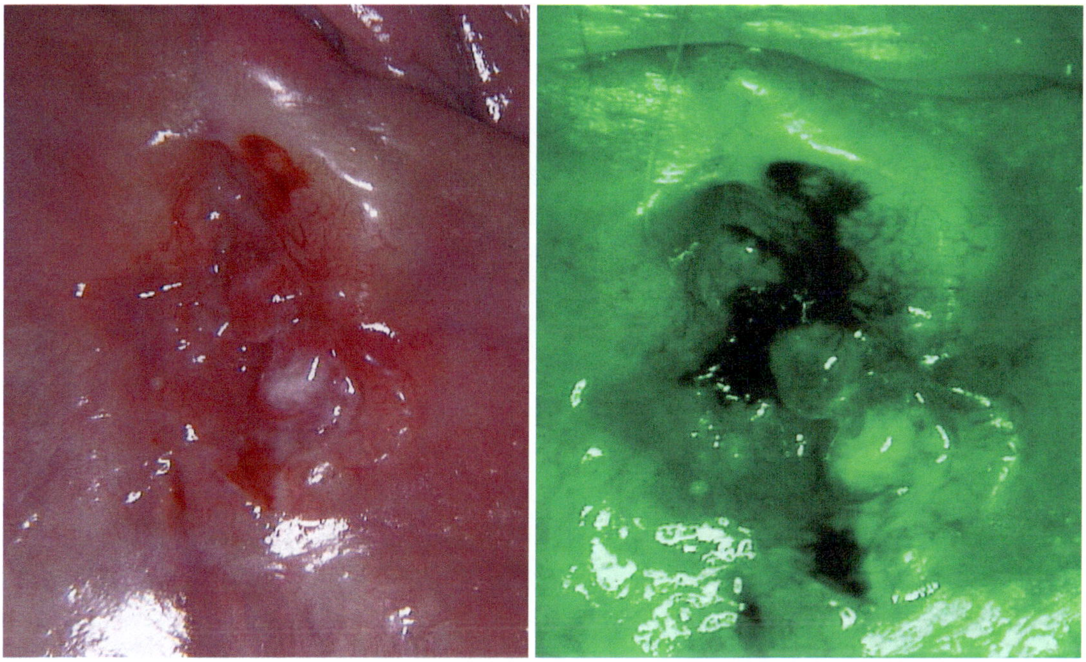

Fig. 13.49 Carcinoma of the vulva with involvement of the clitoris (56 years)

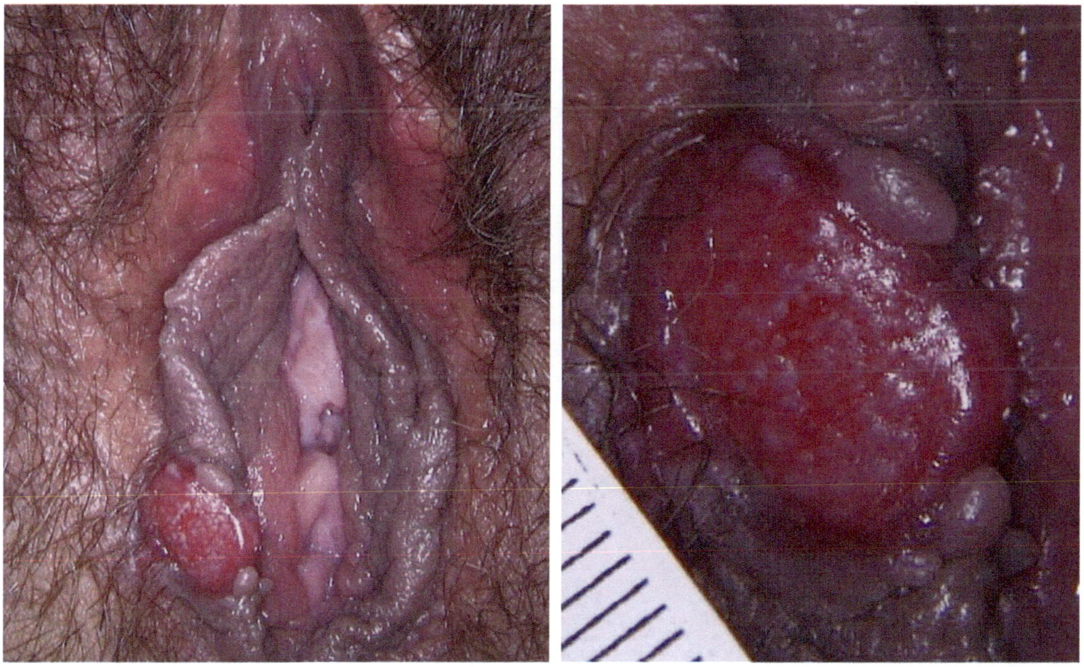

Fig. 13.50 Carcinoma of the vulva (39 years). In contrast to the frequent midline vulvar cancer in young women, the right dorsal labium is involved, which nowadays must be considered an unusual localization for this young patient

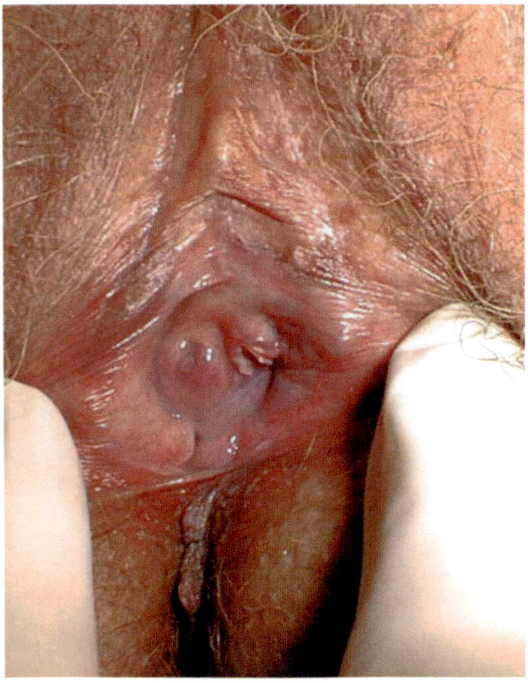

Fig. 13.51 Carcinoma of the vulva close to the urethra (68 years). The lesion had been detected during a routine gynecological exam

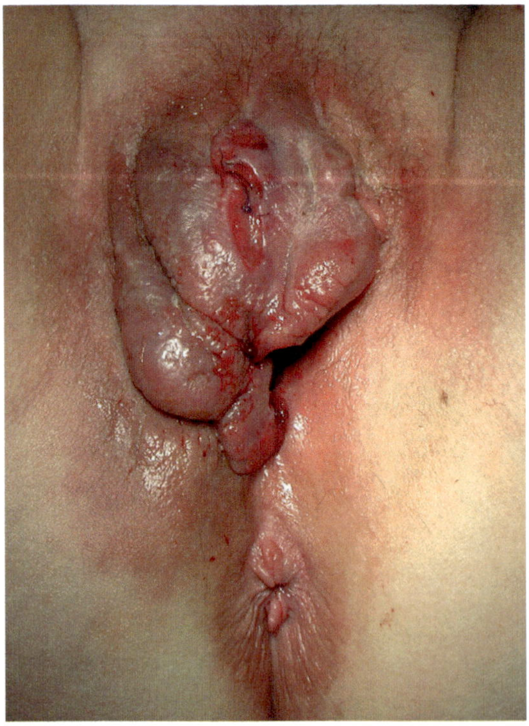

Fig. 13.52 Advanced carcinoma of the vulva. In addition to the exophytic tumor mass, the sphincter is also involved

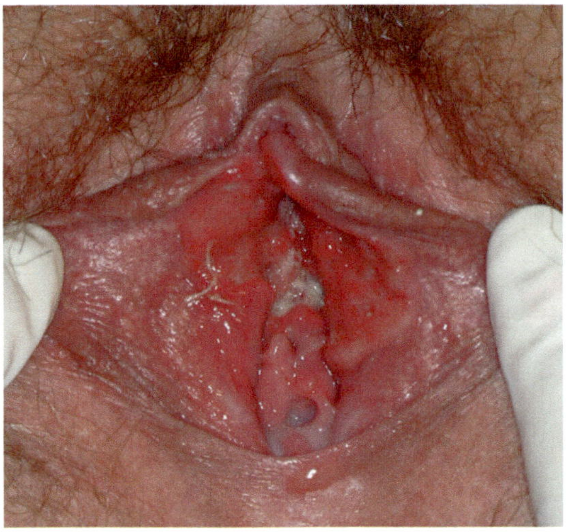

Fig. 13.53 Advanced midline vulvar carcinoma in an 18-year-old patient. Symptoms started 6 months previously and were initially misinterpreted as candida infection. The poorly differentiated squamous cell carcinoma has a diameter of 4 cm

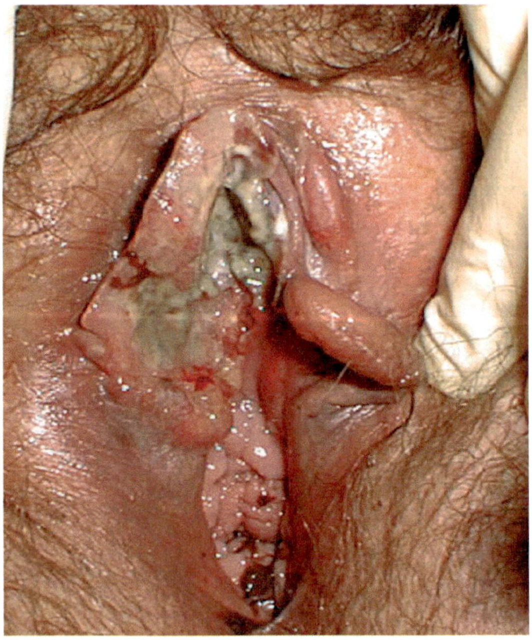

Fig. 13.54 Advanced midline carcinoma of the vulva. The 39-year-old patient had been treated for infection for the duration of 1 year. At the time of cancer diagnosis, the poorly differentiated squamous cell carcinoma was far advanced with lymph-vascular and vascular space involvement and bilateral inguinal lymph node metastases

13.6.5 Malignant Melanoma

Pigmented lesions of the vulva are detected frequently on colposcopic examination. Usually, these pigmentations are harmless, such as vulvar melanosis. Occasionally, localized hyperpigmentations may occur after infectious diseases. Only about 2% of pigmented vulvar lesions are nevi.

Melanocytic nevi of the vulva should be examined with great care to rule out malignant melanoma.

Subsequent to squamous cell carcinoma, malignant melanoma is the second most common malignant tumor of the vulva. The pathogenesis of vulvar melanoma is unclear. The role of human papillomavirus is unproven. Interestingly, several sequencing studies show a distinct pattern of mutations, which is different from melanomas other than of the female genital tract, so that gynecologic melanomas may be a distinct subtype, and targeted therapy trials should be designed specifically for vulvar and vaginal melanoma (Gadducci et al. 2018). For example, vulvar melanomas may carry c-KIT, NRAS, or BRAF mutations, which are amenable to targeted treatment regimens.

Early diagnosis of melanoma is crucial as the overall prognosis is highly dependent on the initial depth of invasion. Unfortunately, vulvar melanomas are usually diagnosed at an advanced stage (Figs. 13.55 and 13.56). In fact, late diagnosis is more frequent when the tumor is located on the vulva compared to other tumor sites.

The so-called dysplastic nevus (also: dysplastic melanocytic nevus, atypical nevus, Clark's nevus) may occur both sporadically and in patients with melanoma. These nevi may exhibit irregular borders, asymmetry, and pronounced or less pronounced pigmentation. Patients with dysplastic nevi have an increased risk of developing malignant melanoma, and nevi should be excised.

Small lesions are removed in their entirety. From large lesions, one or more biopsies are obtained. Contrary to previous believes, incisional biopsy does not worsen the prognosis of melanoma (Pflugfelder et al. 2010). However, a retrospective study of histopathological records by Sharma et al. (2016) came to the conclusion that excisional biopsy remains the gold standard for management of melanoma, as incisional biopsy appears to underestimate the extent of

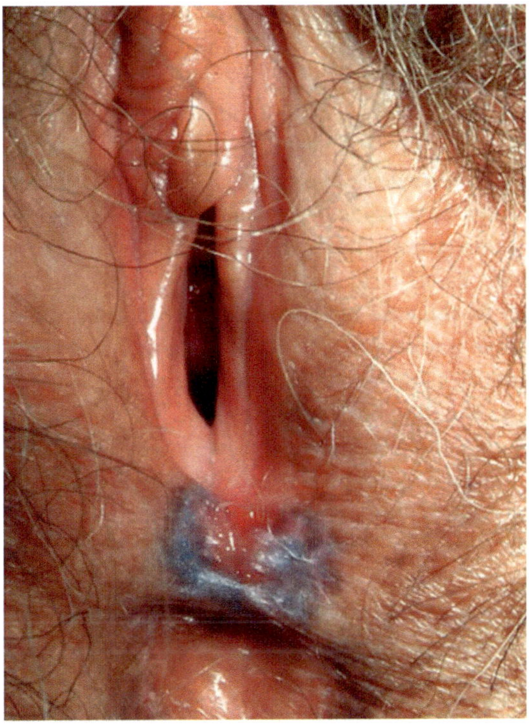

Fig. 13.55 Vulvar melanoma with irregular hyperpigmentation

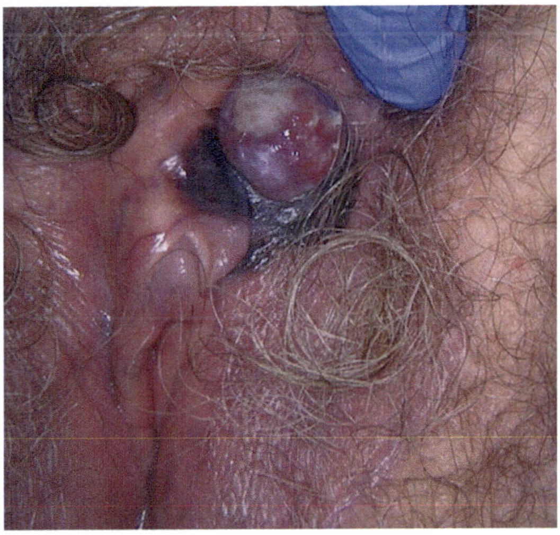

Fig. 13.56 Malignant melanoma of the vulva (82 years)

the disease. Both the Breslow thickness and the Clark's level were significantly higher in excision biopsies compared to specimens from an incisional biopsy. Mitotic rates were also consistently higher in excisional specimens.

Nevertheless, Sharma et al. concede that incisional biopsy is still acceptable if the suspicious lesion is fairly large and is located in a cosmetically sensitive area of the body.

In the case of suspected vulvar melanoma, close proximity to the clitoris and/or urethra justifies incisional biopsy to confirm or rule out the diagnosis of melanoma.

Patients with malignant melanoma are treated in close collaboration with a dermatologic oncologist, as medical and surgical treatment options differ significantly from those available for patients with squamous cell carcinoma of the vulva.

Prognosis of melanoma of the vulva is very poor with a 5-year survival rate of 37–50% (Gadducci et al. 2018).

13.6.6 Follow-Up

For patients with previous HSIL of the vulva, the first follow-up exam should be after 8–12 weeks. The vulva as well as the entire lower genital tract should be carefully examined again, as HSIL of the vulva is frequently multicentric with involvement of the cervix and vagina. This is especially true for patients with reduced immune defense.

During the following 2 years, both patients with carcinoma of the vulva as well as high-risk HSIL patients should be seen by the gynecologist every 3 months. All abnormal findings of the vulva should be biopsied. If there is no recurrence within the first 2 years, half-year intervals are recommended until the end of the fifth year.

References

Andersen BL, Hacker NF (1983) Psychosexual adjustment after vulvar surgery. Obstet Gynecol 62(4): 457–462

Bertozzi S, Londero AP, Fruscalzo A, Marchesoni D, Lellé RJ (2009) Paget disease of the vulva: resolution after local treatment with imiquimod–report of a case and review of the literature. Gynakol Geburtshilfliche Rundsch 49(4):326–330. https://doi.org/10.1159/000301110

Bhatia N (2012) Overview of HPV-related dermatoses and applications of sinecatechins ointment. Curr Derm Rep 1:161–167

Bleeker MCG, Visser PJ, Overbeek LIH, van Beurden M, Berkhof J (2016) Lichen sclerosus: incidence and risk of vulvar squamous cell carcinoma. Cancer Epidemiol Biomark Prev 25(8):1224–1230. https://doi.org/10.1158/1055-9965.EPI-16-0019

Bone A, Ncube F, Nichols T, Noah ND (2008) Body piercing in England: a survey of piercing at sites other than earlobe. BMJ 336(7658):1426–1428. https://doi.org/10.1136/bmj.39580.497176.25

Borkenhagen A, Brähler E, Kentenich H (2009) Intimchirurgie - ein gefährlicher Trend. Dtsch Arztebl 106(11):500–502

Bornstein J, Bogliatto F, Haefner HK, Stockdale CK, Preti M, Bohl TG, Reutter J (2016) The 2015 International Society for the Study of Vulvovaginal Disease (ISSVD) terminology of vulvar squamous intraepithelial lesions. Obstet Gynecol 127(2):264–268. https://doi.org/10.1097/AOG.0000000000001285

Buckley CH, Fox H (1988) Epithelial tumours of the vulva. In: Ridley CM (ed) The vulva. Churchill Livingstone, Edinburg, p 287

Clerico C, Lari A, Mojallal A, Boucher F (2017) Anatomy and aesthetics of the labia minora: the ideal vulva? Aesthet Plast Surg 41(3):714–719. https://doi.org/10.1007/s00266-017-0831-1

Colombo-Benkmann M, Tubergen D, Buchweitz O, Senninger N (2008) Ultrasonic technology: a new treatment option for anal condylomata acuminata. Dis Colon Rectum 51(11):1681–1685. https://doi.org/10.1007/s10350-008-9311-7

Gadducci A, Carinelli S, Guerrieri ME, Aletti GD (2018) Melanoma of the lower genital tract: prognostic factors and treatment modalities. Gynecol Oncol 150(1):180–189. https://doi.org/10.1016/j.ygyno.2018.04.562

Halonen P, Jakobsson M, Heikinheimo O, Riska A, Gissler M, Pukkala E (2017) Lichen sclerosus and risk of cancer. Int J Cancer 140(9):1998–2002. https://doi.org/10.1002/ijc.30621

Halonen P, Jakobsson M, Heikinheimo O, Riska A, Gissler M, Pukkala E (2018) Cancer risk of Lichen planus: a cohort study of 13,100 women in Finland. Int J Cancer 142(1):18–22. https://doi.org/10.1002/ijc.31025

Hampl M, Deckers-Figiel S, Hampl JA, Rein D, Bender HG (2008) New aspects of vulvar cancer: changes in localization and age of onset. Gynecol Oncol 109(3):340–345. https://doi.org/10.1016/j.ygyno.2008.01.041

Heller DS (2007) Report of a new ISSVD classification of VIN. J Low Genit Tract Dis 11(1):46–47. https://doi.org/10.1097/01.lgt.0000236969.27502.71

ISSVD (1989) Report of the ISSVD terminology commission: proc. VIII. world congress, Stockholm, Sweden. J Reprod Med 31:973–975

Kenter GG, Welters MJ, Valentijn AR, Lowik MJ, Berends-van der Meer DM, Vloon AP et al (2009) Vaccination against HPV-16 oncoproteins for vulvar intraepithelial neoplasia. N Engl J Med 361(19):1838–1847. https://doi.org/10.1056/NEJMoa0810097

Kirtschig G, Becker K, Günthert A, Jasaitiene D, Cooper S, Chi CC et al (2015) Evidence-based (S3) guideline on (anogenital) Lichen sclerosus. J Eur Acad Dermatol Venereol 29(10):1–43. https://doi.org/10.1111/jdv.13136

Kreklau A, Vâz I, Oehme F, Strub F, Brechbühl R, Christmann C, Günthert A (2018) Measurements of a "normal vulva" in women aged 15-84: a cross-sectional prospective single-centre study. BJOG 125(13):1656–1661. https://doi.org/10.1111/1471-0528.15387

Krogh G, Lacey CJ, Gross G, Barrasso R, Schneider A (2000) European course on HPV associated pathology: guidelines for primary care physicians for the diagnosis and management of anogenital warts. Sex Transm Infect 76(3):162–168

Lacey CJ, Goodall RL, Tennvall GR, Maw R, Kinghorn GR, Fisk PG et al (2003) Randomised controlled trial and economic evaluation of podophyllotoxin solution, podophyllotoxin cream, and podophyllin in the treatment of genital warts. Sex Transm Infect 79(4):270–275

Lee A, Bradford J, Fischer G (2015) Long-term management of adult vulvar lichen sclerosus: a prospective cohort study of 507 women. JAMA Dermatol 151(10):1061–1067. https://doi.org/10.1001/jamadermatol.2015.0643

Londero AP, Bertozzi S, Salvador S, Fruscalzo A, Aietti D, Grassi T et al (2013) A review of extramammary Paget's disease: clinical presentation, diagnosis, management and prognosis. J Med Med Sci 4:134–148

Luyten A, Brummer O, Kuhnle H, Kreipe HH, Reinecke-Luthge A, Petry KU (2006) Neue Optionen bei der Therapie des Morbus Paget der Vulva. Geburtshilfe Frauenheilkd 66:1–6

Luyten A, Sorgel P, Clad A, Gieseking F, Maass-Poppenhusen K, Lellé RJ et al (2014) Treatment of extramammary Paget disease of the vulva with imiquimod: a retrospective, multicenter study by the German Colposcopy Network. J Am Acad Dermatol 70(4):644–650. https://doi.org/10.1016/j.jaad.2013.12.008

Marshall WA, Tanner JM (1969) Variations in pattern of pubertal changes in girls. Arch Dis Child 44(235):291–303

Matthiesen S, Mainka J (2011) Intimrasur als neue Körpernorm bei Jugendlichen. BZgA Forum 3:25–29

Murphy R (2010) Lichen sclerosus. Dermatol Clin 28(4):707–715. https://doi.org/10.1016/j.det.2010.07.006

Pflugfelder A, Weide B, Eigentler TK, Forschner A, Leiter U, Held L et al (2010) Incisional biopsy and melanoma prognosis: facts and controversies. Clin Dermatol 28(3):316–318. https://doi.org/10.1016/j.clindermatol.2009.06.013

Powell JJ, Wojnarowska F (1999) Lichen sclerosus. Lancet 353(9166):1777–1783

Reuschenbach M, Roos J, Panayotopoulos D, Baldus S, Schnurch HG, Berger A et al (2013) Characterization of squamous cell cancers of the vulvar anterior fourchette by human papillomavirus, p16INK4a, and p53. J Low Genit Tract Dis 17(3):289–297

Sharma KS, Lim P, Brotherston MT (2016) Excision versus incision biopsy in the management of malignant melanoma. J Dermatolog Treat 27(1):88–90. https://doi.org/10.3109/09546634.2015.1034083

Terlou A, van Seters M, Ewing PC, Aaronson NK, Gundy CM, Heijmans-Antonissen C et al (2011) Treatment of vulvar intraepithelial neoplasia with topical imiquimod: seven years median follow-up of a randomized clinical trial. Gynecol Oncol 121(1):157–162. https://doi.org/10.1016/j.ygyno.2010.12.340

van Seters M, van Beurden M, Kate FJ, Beckmann I, Ewing PC, Eijkemans MJ et al (2008) Treatment of vulvar intraepithelial neoplasia with topical imiquimod. N Engl J Med 358(14):1465–1473. https://doi.org/10.1056/NEJMoa072685

Wallbillich JJ, Rhodes HE, Milbourne AM, Munsell MF, Frumovitz M, Brown J et al (2012) Vulvar intraepithelial neoplasia (VIN 2/3): comparing clinical outcomes and evaluating risk factors for recurrence. Gynecol Oncol 127(2):312–315. https://doi.org/10.1016/j.ygyno.2012.07.118

Watts DH, Koutsky LA, Holmes KK, Goldman D, Kuypers J, Kiviat NB, Galloway DA (1998) Low risk of perinatal transmission of human papillomavirus: results from a prospective cohort study. Am J Obstet Gynecol 178(2):365–373

WHO Classification of Tumours Editorial Board (2020) Female genital tumours. IARC Press, Lyon

The Immunocompromised Patient 14

Contents

> Patients with reduced immunological defenses either due to disease (HIV infection) or immunosuppressive medication (e.g. following organ transplantation) are more susceptible to HPV-related diseases. Therefore, this group of patients requires special attention within a colposcopy clinic.

Immunocompromised or immunosuppressed patients are more likely to develop HPV-related diseases and undergo faster progression of these diseases. Therefore, these patients need to be monitored more closely within a colposcopy clinic.

The two most frequent conditions that cause a weakening of the immune system are long-term immunosuppressive medication following organ transplantation (see scenario 18.3.2) or due to other diseases (inflammatory bowel diseases, severe rheumatic disorders, etc.).

14.1 The Relationship Between HIV and HPV

Patients infected by the human immunodeficiency virus (HIV) are especially prone to HPV-related problems (see scenario 18.1.18). Interaction between HPV and HIV infection is complex and not completely understood (Reusser et al. 2015). HIV causes breakdown of the epithelial barrier, thus increasing the susceptibility to HPV infection. Conversely, HPV infection increases the likelihood of subsequent HIV acquisition.

Vaginal candida infections and ascending bacterial infections of the lower genital tract, which may lead to pelvic inflammatory disease, are frequently observed in HIV seropositive patients. In addition, HIV-infected women are at an increased risk for viral infections such as herpes simplex, cytomegalovirus (CMV), or human papillomaviruses of the low and high risk type due to their weakened defense system. Thus, genital warts (condylomata acuminata) caused by HPV types 6 and 11 occur more frequently than in the average population. Also, HPV high risk types are more likely to lead to persistent infections and eventu-

R. J. Lellé, V. Küppers, *Colposcopy*, https://doi.org/10.1007/978-3-030-85388-4_14

ally to intraepithelial neoplasia and possibly to cancer of the lower genital tract.

In young women, prevalence of HPV infection is estimated to be 20–50%, whereas HPV DNA may be up to three times more common in HIV seropositive women compared to HIV-seronegative women (Palefsky et al. 1999). In addition, there is an increased risk of persistent HPV infection.

HIV seropositive women will develop HPV-associated changes, such as condylomata acuminata or intraepithelial neoplasia, five times more frequently (Mandelblatt et al. 1992; Williams et al. 1994; Vermund et al. 1991).

These observations suggest that both HIV infection and HIV-associated immunosuppression promote infection with HPV. The risk of HPV-associated lesions of the lower genital tract, especially of the cervix, is significantly increased (Boshoff and Weiss 2002).

This has been known for a long time. In 1997, Sun et al. (1997) found a prevalence of HPV infections of 31% in young HIV-seronegative women at baseline. After four consecutive examinations, a total of 62% were positive. In contrast, HIV seropositive women were at significantly higher risk: at the initial examination, 56% were HPV positive. The lower the number of CD4+ T-lymphocytes in the peripheral blood, the higher the cumulative proportion of HPV positive patients: with a cell count of >500 CD4+ T-lymphocytes/μl, the cumulative prevalence was 74%, at a cell count of <500 CD4+ T-lymphocytes/μl it was 95%.

Persistent infection was detected in 4% of HIV-seronegative women, and in 24% of HIV positive women. In 20% of cases, there was persistent infection with high risk HPV. Again, a correlation with the number of CD+ cells could be shown (Johnson et al. 1992).

In a screening study conducted in Dar-es-salaam, Tanzania, where the prevalence of HIV is particularly high, 12.9% of women with HIV infection were VIA positive (see Chap. 18) compared to only 3.4% of HIV negative women (Baldur-Felskov et al. 2019). The odds ratio was calculated as 4.26 for HIV infection and VIA positivity.

Compared to women without HIV infection, HIV positive patients are four times more likely to be infected with HPV (Boshoff and Weiss 2002; Kuhn et al. 1999) and to develop a persistent infection. This persistent infection, in turn, causes an approximately fivefold higher prevalence of cervical intraepithelial dysplasia in HIV positive women (11–49%).

The incidence of intraepithelial neoplasia appears to be unaffected by antiretroviral therapy. Although highly active antiretroviral therapy (HAART) reduces the incidence of HIV related disease such as Kaposi sarcoma and non-Hodgkin-lymphoma, it does not protect from HPV-related precancers or cancers (Reusser et al. 2015). Severely immunosuppressed women relapse more quickly, and spontaneous regression of mild dysplasia is less common (Del Mistro and Chieco Bianchi 2001).

In addition to the increased rate of HPV-related precursors, the occurrence of cervical cancer in women with AIDS is 5–15 times higher in Europe and the USA (Serraino et al. 1999; Frisch et al. 2000). Therefore, invasive cervical carcinoma is considered to be one of the diseases that define the acquired immunodeficiency syndrome (AIDS) caused by HIV infection (Petry et al. 1994; Petry et al. 1996).

Reimers et al. (2010) came to the conclusion that CIN in an HIV-infected patient ultimately cannot be cured. Thus, patients with HIV need to be counseled that a permanent elimination of CIN will not be possible.

The rate of condylomata as well as vulvar and anal intraepithelial neoplasia appears to be four times higher (Chiasson et al. 1997), with a prevalence of 6–37% (Spitzer 1999). Special attention must be paid to possible multicentric involvement of the cervix, vagina, vulva, and anus. Thorough colposcopic examination of the entire lower genital tract in HPV positive HIV-infected women is therefore essential (Fig. 14.1).

The relative risk of developing vulvar or vaginal carcinoma is six times higher for HIV positive than for HIV negative women (Frisch et al. 2000). The rate of intraepithelial neoplasia of the anus as well as anal carcinoma is also markedly increased for these patients due to HPV infection of the anal canal (Palefsky et al. 2001).

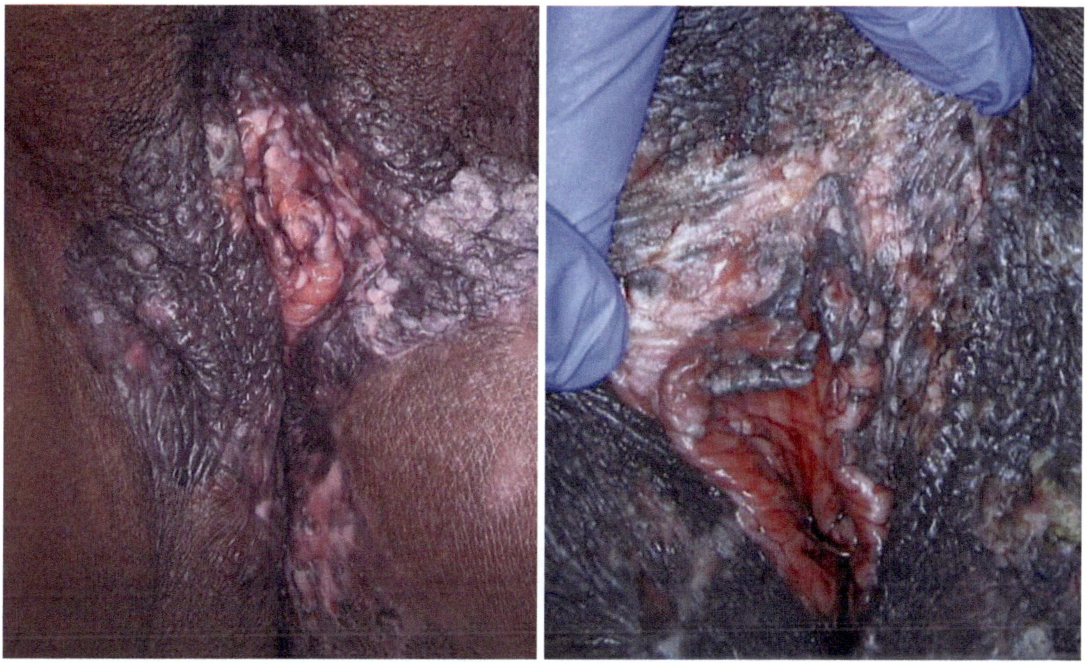

Fig. 14.1 Extensive HSIL of the vulva in an HIV positive patient. The patient is 38 years old and has been diagnosed with HIV infection 12 years previously. She subsequently developed recurrent/persistent HSIL of the cervix, vagina, and vulva. Repeatedly, superficially invasive vulvar lesions have been removed. Unfortunately, no definitive cure exists due to the impaired immune system

14.2 Management of the Immunocompromised Patient

The treatment of HPV-associated changes of the lower genital tract is done either medically or surgically, depending on the disease. The choice of therapy in HIV positive women is based not only on the gynecological findings, but also on the current CDC stage of HIV infection. In the presence of AIDS-defining diseases, an individual treatment decision must be made depending on the overall condition of the patient.

Whereas Lacey (2019) points out that HPV vaccination may be either not effective at all or less effective in patients with HIV infection, Garland and a panel of experts in the field of HPV vaccination (Garland et al. 2017) clearly state: *"Prophylactic HPV sub-unit vaccines are safe and immunogenic in immunocompromised people and it is strongly recommended that vaccination occur according to national guidelines. When delivered to immunocompromised populations, HPV vaccines should be given as a 3-dose regimen."* The authors point out that the resulting antibody titers are frequently lower than those in immunocompetent patients. However, the clinical relevance of this is still unclear as there are not yet enough efficacy data available.

HPV Infections in HIV-Infected Women and Otherwise Immunocompromised Patients

- HIV-infected women are at high risk for persistent HPV infection.
- Infection with viruses of the low risk group predisposes to the development of condylomata of the vulva, cervix, vagina, and anus. Also, the recurrence rate is four to five times higher, regardless of the type of therapy.

- In the case of persistent high risk HPV infection, there is a significantly higher risk of developing preneoplastic disease of the cervix, vagina, vulva, and anus. Multicentric manifestations are common. The risk for carcinoma of the cervix is also increased.

Therefore, HIV-infected women should be followed in the colposcopy clinic every 6–12 months. HPV vaccination should be considered.

References

Baldur-Felskov B, Mwaiselage J, Faber MT, Kjaerem M, la Cour de CD, Munk C et al (2019) Factors associated with a cervical high-grade lesion on cytology or a positive visual inspection with acetic acid among more than 3300 Tanzanian women. Trop Med Int Health 24(2):229–237. https://doi.org/10.1111/tmi.13184

Boshoff C, Weiss R (2002) AIDS-related malignancies. Nat Rev Cancer 2(5):373–382. https://doi.org/10.1038/nrc797

Chiasson MA, Ellerbrock TV, Bush TJ, Sun XW, Wright TC Jr (1997) Increased prevalence of vulvovaginal condyloma and vulvar intraepithelial neoplasia in women infected with the human immunodeficiency virus. Obstet Gynecol 89(5 Pt 1):690–694

Del Mistro A, Chieco Bianchi L (2001) HPV-related neoplasias in HIV-infected individuals. Eur J Cancer 37(10):1227–1235. http://doi.org/S0959-8049(01)00107-1

Frisch M, Biggar RJ, Goedert JJ (2000) Human papillomavirus-associated cancers in patients with human immunodeficiency virus infection and acquired immunodeficiency syndrome. J Natl Cancer Inst 92(18):1500–1510

Garland SM, Brotherton JML, Moscicki AB, Kaufmann AM, Stanley M, Bhatla N et al (2017) HPV vaccination of immunocompromised hosts. Papillomavirus Res 4:35–38. https://doi.org/10.1016/j.pvr.2017.06.002

Johnson JC, Burnett AF, Willet GD, Young MA, Doniger J (1992) High frequency of latent and clinical human papillomavirus cervical infections in immunocompromised human immunodeficiency virus-infected women. Obstet Gynecol 79(3):321–327

Kuhn L, Sun XW, Wright TC Jr (1999) Human immunodeficiency virus infection and female lower genital tract malignancy. Curr Opin Obstet Gynecol 11(1):35–39

Lacey CJ (2019) HPV vaccination in HIV infection. Papillomavirus Res 8:100174. https://doi.org/10.1016/j.pvr.2019.100174

Mandelblatt JS, Fahs M, Garibaldi K, Senie RT, Peterson HB (1992) Association between HIV infection and cervical neoplasia: implications for clinical care of women at risk for both conditions. AIDS 6(2):173–178

Palefsky JM, Minkoff H, Kalish LA, Levine A, Sacks HS, Garcia P et al (1999) Cervicovaginal human papillomavirus infection in human immunodeficiency virus-1 (HIV)-positive and high-risk HIV-negative women. J Natl Cancer Inst 91(3):226–236

Palefsky JM, Holly EA, Ralston ML, Da Costa M, Greenblatt RM (2001) Prevalence and risk factors for anal human papillomavirus infection in human immunodeficiency virus (HIV)-positive and high-risk HIV-negative women. J Infect Dis 183(3):383–391

Petry KU, Scheffel D, Bode U, Gabrysiak T, Kochel H, Kupsch E et al (1994) Cellular immunodeficiency enhances the progression of human papillomavirus-associated cervical lesions. Int J Cancer 57(6):836–840

Petry KU, Kochel H, Bode U, Schedel I, Niesert S, Glaubitz M et al (1996) Human papillomavirus is associated with the frequent detection of warty and basaloid high-grade neoplasia of the vulva and cervical neoplasia among immunocompromised women. Gynecol Oncol 60(1):30–34

Reimers LL, Sotardi S, Daniel D, Chiu LG, Van Arsdale A, Wieland DL et al (2010) Outcomes after an excisional procedure for cervical intraepithelial neoplasia in HIV-infected women. Gynecol Oncol 119(1):92–97. https://doi.org/10.1016/j.ygyno.2010.06.012

Reusser NM, Downing C, Guidry J, Tyring SK (2015) HPV carcinomas in immunocompromised patients. J Clin Med 4(2):260–281. https://doi.org/10.3390/jcm4020260

Serraino D, Carrieri P, Pradier C, Bidoli E, Dorrucci M, Ghetti E et al (1999) Risk of invasive cervical cancer among women with, or at risk for, HIV infection. Int J Cancer 82(3):334–337. https://doi.org/10.1002/(SICI)1097-0215(19990730)82:3<334::AID-IJC5>3.0.CO;2-C

Spitzer M (1999) Lower genital tract intraepithelial neoplasia in HIV-infected women: guidelines for evaluation and management. Obstet Gynecol Surv 54(2):131–137

Sun XW, Kuhn L, Ellerbrock TV, Chiasson MA, Bush TJ, Wright TC Jr (1997) Human papillomavirus infection in women infected with the human immunodeficiency virus. N Engl J Med 337(19):1343–1349

Vermund SH, Kelley KF, Klein RS, Feingold AR, Schreiber K, Munk G, Burk RD (1991) High risk of human papillomavirus infection and cervical squamous intraepithelial lesions among women with symptomatic human immunodeficiency virus infection. Am J Obstet Gynecol 165(2):392–400. http://doi.org/0002-9378(91)90101-V

Williams AB, Darragh TM, Vranizan K, Ochia C, Moss AR, Palefsky JM (1994) Anal and cervical human papillomavirus infection and risk of anal and cervical epithelial abnormalities in human immunodeficiency virus-infected women. Obstet Gynecol 83(2):205–211

15 HPV Vaccination

Contents

Vaccines against HPV are able to prevent HPV-induced precancerous lesions of the lower female genital tract as well as other HPV-related cancers, both in women and men. Ultimately, this has the potential to lead to worldwide elimination of cervical cancer. However, for the foreseeable future, HPV vaccination needs to be complemented by secondary screening. As the incidence of HPV-related disease decreases, screening triage strategies need to be adapted in order to maintain a high level of effectiveness.

As early as 1974, Harald zur Hausen from the German Cancer Research Center in Heidelberg hypothesized that HP viruses play an important role in the development of cervical carcinoma. With zur Hausen's work as well as others, the foundation for the development of HPV vaccination was laid (zur Hausen 2009). In 2008, Harald zur Hausen was awarded the Nobel Prize for Medicine.

Colposcopic diagnosis is part of a strategy for the secondary prevention of cervical carcinoma. Although cervical cytology and colposcopy can detect precancerous lesions and thus prevent the development of cervical cancer in a large number of women, diagnostic and therapeutic efforts do not begin until an HPV-related disease has already manifested itself.

With the approval of two HPV vaccines, Gardasil® and Cervarix® in the years 2006 and 2007, respectively, as well as the nonavalent vaccine Gardasil 9® (2015 in Europe and 2018 in the USA), an additional instrument for the prevention of HPV-related disease is available. Real-life data obtained from the first two vaccines have proven an outstanding level of effectiveness.

R. J. Lellé, V. Küppers, *Colposcopy*, https://doi.org/10.1007/978-3-030-85388-4_15

These vaccines produce antibodies against human papillomaviruses, which will prevent infection on initial contact with the virus. However, an already existing infection cannot be eliminated, as the vaccination mechanism is exclusively prophylactic.

According to Strasser (1978), the current HPV vaccine, which exclusively serves to prevent HPV infection, represents primordial prevention, whereas the prevention of the development of HPV-related disease, which would be called primary prevention, is not possible with the vaccines available today. Instead, therapeutic vaccines are needed to make primary prevention possible.

According to Bruni et al. (2021), 107 WHO member states (55%) have introduced HPV vaccination, and the average performance coverage for the first and the final dose was 67% and 53%, respectively.

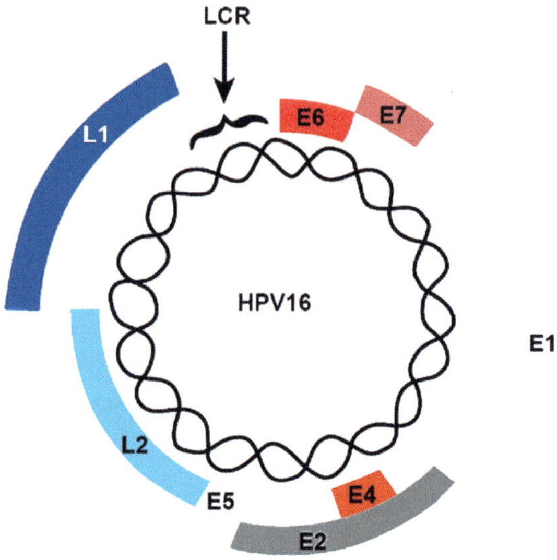

Fig. 15.1 The HPV 16 genome

Table 15.1 Role of the viral proteins of the HPV 16 genome

Protein	Function
L1	Primary structural protein which is able to form the so-called capsomeres, which assemble into virus-like particles (VLP)
L2	Secondary structural protein that can attach to the virus DNA
E6	Interferes with the tumor suppressor p53
E7	Inactivates the retinoblastoma tumor suppressor protein Rb

15.1 Structure of the HP Virus

In order to understand the mode of action of HPV vaccines, a basic knowledge of the structure of the HP virus is required. The following statements refer to HPV type 16, the most common high risk papilloma virus.

The HPV genome consists of a DNA double helix comprising approximately 7900 base pairs (Fig. 15.1). In addition to a so-called control region (LCR = "long control region," regulation of HPV gene expression), the information for the synthesis of a total of ten proteins is encoded. These are classified into early (E1 to E8) and late (L1 and L2) proteins, which refers to the time of protein synthesis within the viral replication cycle. The L proteins, and especially L1, are the structural proteins of the virus. L1 encodes pentagonal capsid proteins that automatically align to form the "virus-like particles" (VLP) which are used for vaccine production (Table 15.1).

Of the early proteins, E6 and E7 confer the ability of HP viruses to transform epidermal cells. E6 and E7 are therefore referred to as oncoproteins, and the respective viruses are called "HPV high-risk types."

15.2 Development of Prophylactic Vaccination

For the production of prophylactic vaccines, virus-like particles (VLP) are assembled out of L1 proteins. The resulting virus-like particles (L1 VLP) will stimulate the formation of specific antibodies. This principle has been implemented in all three vaccines developed so far.

Prophylactic vaccination is not to be confused with therapeutic vaccination, which is still under development. The goal of therapeutic vaccines would be primary prevention, i.e. the regression of HPV-related precancer. This may be achieved by the activation of specific T cells that can attack and destroy HPV infected dysplastic cells.

In a clinical study by Kaufmann et al. (2007), a so-called chimeric virus-like particle (CVLP) was used, which consists of the capsid protein L1 and the oncoprotein E7. Thirty-six patients diagnosed with HSIL (CIN2 or CIN3) were treated and results were compared with a placebo group. L1- and E7-specific cytotoxic T lymphocytes could be induced by the vaccine. In 39% of vaccinated and 25% of non-vaccinated women, HSIL regressed, either back to normal or to low grade dysplasia. However, the difference between the two groups did not reach the level of statistical significance.

To date, no therapeutic HPV vaccine has been successfully tested and approved, whereas prophylactic vaccine development has been highly successful and led to clinical approval after a short period of time.

Hildesheim et al. (2007) studied the effect of prophylactic vaccines (both Gardasil® and Cervarix®) on 18- to 25-year-old women who already were positive for HPV (high-risk positive in the hybrid capture II test) at the time of vaccination. Compared to a control group, no significant reduction after 6 and 12 months, respectively, could be found. The authors concluded that HPV vaccination cannot accelerate clearance of the virus and that it should not be used to treat HPV infection.

Prophylactic vaccines based on the L1 VLP principle are type-specific. Thus, a vaccine must be produced for each individual HPV type. Naturally, the focus was initially on the most common HPV types. HPV 16 and 18 are associated with 75% of all cervical carcinomas in Europe. Also, there is cross-reactivity and cross-protection against phylogenetically related HPV types. The genetic structure of HPV 16 is very similar to that of HPV 31 as is HPV 18 to HPV 45. The resulting cross-protection suggests that the efficacy of a vaccine directed against HPV 16 and 18 alone would be even higher. For Cervarix®, the additional effect through cross-protection is estimated to be 5.1% (Schneider et al. 2007).

The Gardasil® vaccine is also targeted against the two most common low-risk types HPV 6 and 11, which cause genital warts (condylomata acuminata).

In 2015, Joura et al. (2015) introduced the nonavalent HPV vaccine Gardasil 9®, which is directed not only against HPV types 6, 11, 16, and 18 (Gardasil®) but also against five additional HPV high-risk types, i.e. HPV 31, 33, 45, 52, and 58. A study with 14,215 participants who received either Gardasil® or Gardasil 9® showed a similar antibody response. Side-effects related to the injection site were more common in patients who received Gardasil 9® injections, most likely due to the higher concentration of the adjuvant amorphous aluminum hydroxyphosphate sulfate in the vaccine. Indeed, Gardasil 9® is able to prevent HPV-related disease caused by the five additional HPV types.

Based on these results, there is the expectation that the HPV-related disease burden will be even more effectively reduced by the nonavalent vaccine. Therefore, Gardasil 9® is the HPV vaccine of choice and should preferably be used when available.

The prophylactic vaccine is given as three intra-muscular injections, which are administered within half a year. In children and adolescents between the age of 9 and 14 years, two injections are considered sufficient due to the higher vaccine titers that are achieved in this age group. Further studies will show whether a single vaccine dose might also be adequate (Stanley and Dull 2018).

Although it is still unclear how long the vaccine protection will last or whether a booster vaccination will be necessary in the future, present data do not show a significant drop of the antibody titers over time.

For Cervarix®, it has been demonstrated that after 8.4 years and 9.4 years, respectively (Roteli-Martins et al. 2012; Naud et al. 2011), all vaccinated women are still seropositive and that the vaccine titers for HPV 16 and 18 continue to be many times higher than the natural antibody titer. Cervarix® vaccination led to a significantly higher antibody titer than Gardasil® (Einstein et al. 2009).

15.3 Indications for HPV Vaccination

This chapter will refer to Gardasil 9® as the HPV vaccine of choice and the indications approved by the American Food and Drug Administration (FDA) as of August 2020 (prescribing information).

Gardasil 9® is approved for both genders aged 9–45. The prescribing information specifically points out that only lesions caused by the nine specific HPV types may be prevented and that vaccination does not obviate the need for screening.

15.3.1 HPV Vaccination for Children and Adolescents

HPV vaccination is approved from the age of 9. Due to the purely prophylactic nature of the HPV vaccines, vaccination is most effective if done before the time of first sexual intercourse. Also, the likelihood of HPV infection increases with an increasing number of sexual partners (Paavonen et al. 2007). In addition, antibody titers triggered by the vaccine are higher in younger individuals. Therefore, girls and boys should be vaccinated as early as possible.

- The FDA lists the following conditions for women, which may be prevented by HPV vaccination:
  - Cervical, vulvar, vaginal, anal, oropharyngeal, and other head and neck cancers.
  - Genital warts (condyloma acuminata).
  - Cervical intraepithelial neoplasia (CIN) grade 2/3 and cervical adenocarcinoma in situ (AIS).
  - Cervical intraepithelial neoplasia (CIN) grade 1.
  - Vulvar intraepithelial neoplasia (VIN) grades 2 and 3.
  - Vaginal intraepithelial neoplasia (VAIN) grades 2 and 3.
  - Anal intraepithelial neoplasia (AIN) grades 1, 2, and 3.
- The respective conditions for men are:
  - Anal, oropharyngeal, and other head and neck cancers.
  - Genital warts (condylomata acuminata).
  - Anal intraepithelial neoplasia (AIN) grades 1, 2, and 3.

Although sexual intercourse is the most likely mode of HPV infection, other routes of transmission play a significant role and may influence HPV vaccine effectiveness even when given at an early age.

Doerfler et al. (2009) found that HPV high risk DNA is present in the anogenital area of approximately 14% of girls prior to coitarche after sexual abuse had been ruled out. Shew et al. (2013) identified HPV DNA in 10 out of 22 adolescents (age 14–17 years), who denied previous penetrative sex. However, seven of the ten HPV positive girls reported noncoital behavior that may have contributed to HPV infection.

In a review of the literature on non-sexual modes of HPV transmission, Sabeena et al. (2017) found numerous evidence that both horizontal (through autoinoculation, heteroinoculation, and fomites) and vertical (e.g. during delivery) transmission of HPV infection are possible. However, some modes of transmission can be ruled out such as the use of swimming pools or toilets.

15.3.2 HPV Vaccination for Men

HPV vaccination has primarily been developed for the prevention of cervical cancer. However, as Stanley already pointed out in 2012 (Stanley 2012), about 5% of all cancers are HPV-related including cancer of the larynx, head and neck, and penis. Furthermore, genital warts caused by HPV types 6 and 11 are a significant health risk which is also not gender-specific. Vaccination also protects homosexual men and thus eliminates discrimination.

Furthermore, by vaccinating the male population, herd immunity can be achieved more quickly, thus lowering the overall HPV disease burden.

Another important aspect that advocates HPV vaccination of men is the lack of screening strategies for practically all HPV-related diseases that affect men.

Overall, the nonavalent HPV vaccine protects from infection with low-risk HPV types that are responsible for more than 90% of all genital warts and from infection with high-risk HPV types that are responsible for 90% of anal cancers and significant proportions of oropharyngeal and penile cancers (Lieblong et al. 2019).

About one-third of the HPV vaccination programs of the 107 WHO member states, who have introduced the vaccination, are gender neutral, i.e. HPV vaccination is also available to men (Bruni et al. 2021).

15.3.3 Catch-Up HPV Vaccination

The American Cancer Society (ACS) guideline of 2020 recommends vaccination at the ages of 9 and 12 and at the same time encourages health care providers to offer vaccination at the age of 9 or 10. HPV vaccination up to the age of 26 is then called "catch-up vaccination" and recommended to all individuals who have not been adequately vaccinated so far (Saslow et al. 2020). In contrast to European regulations, who do not set an upper age limit for HPV vaccination, HPV vaccines in the USA are only licensed for use in adults up to 45 years.

The ACS does not recommend catch-up vaccination for individuals 27–45 years old because of low effectiveness and an insufficient cancer prevention potential.

Based on the available literature, the ACS argues that, compared to vaccination up to the age of 26, vaccination of 27–45-year-old adults will prevent only 0.5% of cancers, 0.4% of cervical precancers, and 0.3% of genital warts over the next 100 years.

HPV testing prior to catch-up HPV vaccination is not recommended (Gross et al. 2020), as no testing systems exist that reliably predict vaccination benefits. The detection of HPV proteins or HPV-specific antibodies is not suitable and not sufficiently validated for routine diagnostics. Detection methods used in the vaccination studies were developed by the respective pharmaceutical companies and are not commercially available.

With Gardasil 9® covering nine HPV types including cross-protection of closely related genotypes, a certain degree of HPV protection is likely, regardless of age or sexual activity.

Despite the fact that the ACS does not endorse shared decision-making due to a lack of sufficient guidance on the selection of patients who might benefit (Saslow et al. 2020), many patients will still require individual counseling.

15.3.4 HPV Vaccination Following Treatment for Cervical Dysplasia

Subgroup analysis of the original Gardasil® vaccine studies suggested that patients still benefit from HPV vaccination if they develop cervical dysplasia despite previous vaccination, as patients within the vaccinated cohort have a significantly lower likelihood of recurrence following dysplasia treatment (Joura et al. 2012).

At the time, it was assumed that the sequence "HPV vaccination – diagnosis of CIN – reduced probability of recurrence" also applies to the sequence "diagnosis of CIN – HPV vaccination – reduced probability of recurrence." Therefore, Kang et al. (2013) vaccinated 351 patients 1 week after CIN treatment and compared the respective recurrence rates with a group of patients who had not been vaccinated. Indeed the recurrence rate in the vaccinated group was significantly lower (9 versus 27 patients).

In the meantime, two randomized trials, both from Italy (Ghelardi et al. 2018; Pieralli et al. 2018) have shown the efficacy of prophylactic vaccination with Gardasil® around the time of CIN treatment for a reduced likelihood of subsequent disease recurrence. Ghelardi et al. found that the risk of subsequent high grade cervical disease was reduced by 81.2% (95% CI 34.3–95.7%) when vaccination was started 30 days after surgery.

In the study by Pieralli et al. the first injection of the quadrivalent vaccine was given 3 months after treatment for CIN. Significantly less patients in the vaccine group had a recurrence compared to untreated patients (3.4% versus 13.5%, respectively).

In both studies, women until the age of 45 years were included.

There is evidence that HPV vaccination is able to significantly reduce the recurrence rate of cervical intraepithelial neoplasia. Previously unvaccinated women up to the age of 45 years should be counseled regarding the potential benefits of post-treatment vaccination.

15.4 Efficacy of HPV Vaccination

Previous studies on HPV vaccination did not allow the conclusion that the incidence of cancer, in particular cervical cancer, can actually be reduced by the vaccine. Instead, cervical intraepithelial neoplasia and other precancerous lesions served as surrogate markers, as it is reasonable to assume that a reduction of the incidence of high-grade dysplasia will lead to a long-term decline of cancer incidence.

A Cochrane review (Arbyn et al. 2018) concluded that HPV vaccines are highly efficient, although, so far, the duration of the studies is too short to draw definitive conclusions on the outcome of cervical cancer. No vaccine related deaths were identified.

However, Arbyn et al. (2018) have been strongly criticized by Jørgensen et al. (2018), who claimed that the selection of trials for the review had been biased, and nearly half of relevant trials were not included, triggering a discussion on trial eligibility criteria (Heneghan and Onakpoya 2019).

Finally, after more than 15 years of HPV vaccination worldwide, there is growing evidence that HPV vaccination is highly effective within a real-life setting in countries that have achieved a high level of coverage. Thus, the results from the initial licensing studies on HPV vaccination for both Gardasil® and Cervarix® (Castellsague et al. 2011; FUTURE II Study Group 2007; Garland et al. 2007; Lehtinen et al. 2012) have been confirmed.

15.4.1 Real-Life Effectiveness of HPV Vaccines

In 2011 and 2013, Australia, which from early on achieved a vaccination coverage of more than 70%, could observe a dramatic decline of genital warts (condylomata acuminata), the majority of which is caused by HPV 6 and 11. Furthermore, in 2011, the first Australian data on real-life effectiveness on high grade cervical abnormalities in women up to the age of 18 years were published by Brotherton et al. (2011).

More recently, Markowitz et al. (2019) determined type-specific HPV DNA (HPV 6/11/16/18 of the quadrivalent vaccine, Gardasil®) in cytology specimens from 20–29-year-old women in two time periods: 2012–2013 and 2015–2016, respectively, and found a decline of type-specific HPV prevalence by 78% among 20–24-year-old women and by 38% among 25–29-year-old women. Furthermore, a decline was also observed in non-vaccinated women as evidence of herd immunity.

Through data obtained from the Finnish cancer registry, Luostarinen et al. (2018) presented the first real-life evidence that HPV vaccination indeed protects against invasive cancer associated with HPV: Two age-aligned cohorts of vaccinated and non-vaccinated women were compared. Whereas ten cases of invasive cancer were identified in non-vaccinated women (8 cervical cancers, one vulvar cancer, one oropha-

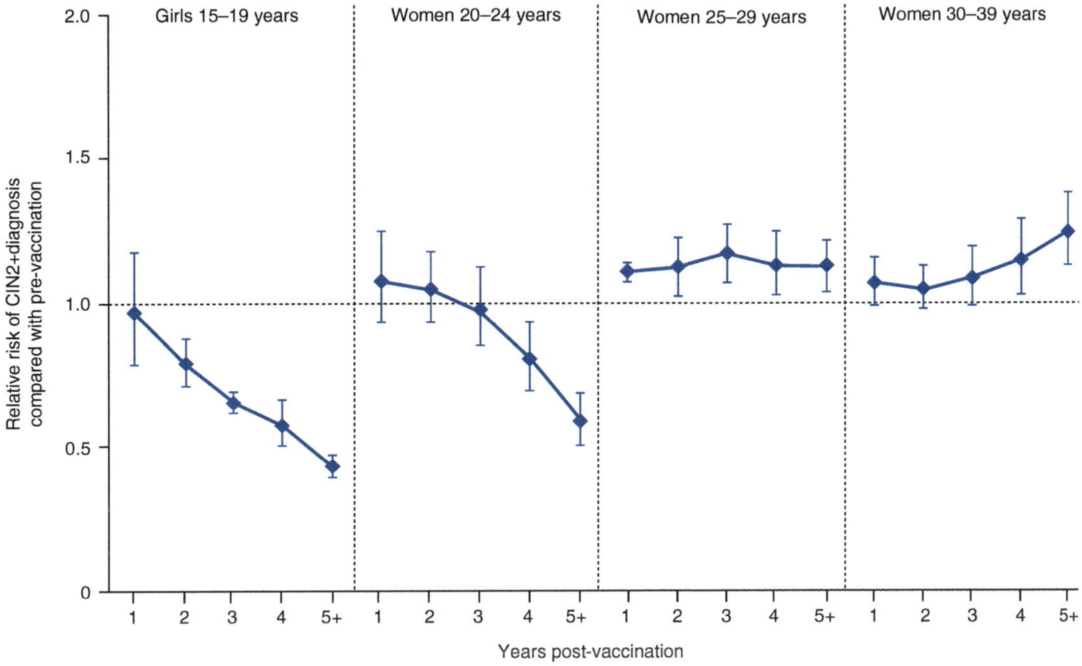

Fig. 15.2 Changes in CIN2+ diagnosis among girls and women during the first 7 years after HPV vaccination (bivalent vaccines, girls only, countries with high vaccination coverage). The most dramatic reduction can be observed in the 15- to 19-year-old group (51%) followed by the 20- to 24-year-old women (31%), whereas no change is seen in older women, who usually did not receive HPV vaccination (Drolet et al. 2019)

ryngeal cancer), no cancer cases occurred in the vaccinated group.

Drolet et al. (2019) performed a systemic review and meta-analysis to determine the population level impact. HPV 16 and 18 prevalence had decreased by 83% among 13- to 19-year-old girls 5–8 years after vaccination. Among 20- to 24-year-old girls, prevalence was also reduced by 66%. Anogenital wart diagnoses decreased significantly depending on the age of the population studied: 67% (15–19 years), 54% (20–24 years), and 31% (25–29 years), respectively. Most importantly, CIN2+ diagnosis was reduced dramatically. Five to nine years after vaccination, CIN2+ decreased by 51% in the 15–19 year age group, and by 31% in women aged 20–24 years (Fig. 15.2).

As can be expected, vaccination programs covering boys and programs with a high vaccination coverage had a greater population impact and led to a more pronounced herd effect.

15.4.2 HPV Vaccination Efficacy in Glandular Lesions

Apparently, all three HPV vaccines are effective in glandular lesion. This is a significant advantage of HPV vaccination, as diagnosis of glandular lesions by cytopathology and colposcopy is unsatisfactory.

Lehtinen et al. (2012) demonstrated that Cervarix® is able to lower the occurrence of cervical adenocarcinoma in situ. A study by de Sanjose et al. (2010) suggests that the efficacy in prevention of glandular lesions may be even higher compared to prevention of squamous cell lesions (Table 15.2), as a high percentage of cervical adenocarcinomas and also adenocarcinoma in situ are associated with HPV genotypes 18 and 45.

Whereas cross-protection against HPV 45 could be assumed for Gardasil® and Cervarix® due to the structural similarities between HPV

Table 15.2 Frequency of HPV types in adenocarcinomas versus squamous cell carcinomas (de Sanjose et al. 2010)

	Incidence (%)	
HPV type	Adenocarcinoma	Squamous cell carcinoma
16	50	62
18	32	8
45	12	5
Total	**94**	**75**

18 and 45, HPV 45 is part of the Gardasil 9® vaccination. Overall, up to 94% of all glandular lesions may be prevented by vaccination.

In the meantime, real-life data for AIS are available: AIS incidence rates are also declining due to HPV vaccination (Cleveland et al. 2019). In the younger age group (21 to 24 years), a decrease of 22.1% has been observed.

15.4.3 Prophylaxis of Condylomata Acuminata through Gardasil®

Both the original Gardasil® vaccine and the newer Gardasil 9® are directed against the two low-risk HPV genotypes HPV 6 and 11, which are not cancer-related. However, HPV 6 and 11 are responsible for the vast majority of genital warts (condylomata acuminata), which to date are the most common sexually transmitted disease. Also, the high recurrence rate after medical or surgical treatment makes condylomata a major health-care problem.

In Australia, where the quadrivalent HPV vaccine Gardasil® was introduced in 2007 for both schoolchildren and as catch-up vaccination for women up to 27 years, there is increasing evidence that prevention of condylomata acuminata is very efficient. Already in 2011, Read et al. (2011) observed that the number of patients with genital warts treated in a large STD clinic in Melbourne had dropped dramatically since the introduction of Gardasil® vaccination. This decline was most pronounced in young women under the age of 21 and less drastic for women aged 21–29. In addition, young men were significantly less frequently affected by condylomata, which can be interpreted as herd immunity. No effect was seen in women and men older than 29 years, i.e., cohorts that had not had access yet to HPV vaccination.

At the time this observational study had been conducted in Australia, Gardasil® vaccination had been available to the female population only. Therefore, no effect on the frequency of genital warts in homosexual men was observed.

A summary of data from eight Australian centers treating patients with sexually transmitted diseases showed among other things, that in 2011, not a single woman under the age of 21 was diagnosed with condylomata acuminata after having been vaccinated with Gardasil® (Ali et al. 2013).

In the presence of recurrent condylomata acuminata including non-gynecologic locations, Yang et al. (2019) surprisingly observed a therapeutic-like vaccination effect of Gardasil®. Fourteen out of thirty patients (47%) had a complete clinical response, and five patients (17%) had a partial response. The authors suggest that vaccination may be an alternative treatment option for selected patients (multiple warts, problematic lesion locations, and uncooperative patients).

15.4.4 Statistic Modeling of HPV Vaccination Impact

Early on, modeling studies have been done in order to predict the HPV vaccination impact (Schneider et al. 2007), as no registry data had yet been available. Now that real-life data have been generated, recent modeling studies are able to make predictions about the future of cervical cancer and its precursors.

A study from Australia (Hall et al. 2019) concluded that if high vaccination coverage and concomitant screening can be maintained and defining an elimination threshold of four new cases per 100,000 women annually, cervical cancer can be eliminated as a public health problem in Australia within the next 20 years.

Brisson et al. (2020) published another modeling study on the effectiveness of HPV vaccination on the elimination of cancer, i.e. a reduction by 97%, specifically in low income and lower middle income countries, and concluded that cervical cancer can ultimately (100 years) be eradicated by vaccination in combination with twice-lifetime screenings.

Saslow et al. (2020) from the American Cancer Society (ACS) state:

"Vaccination of all children between ages 9 and 12 years will prevent >90% of the cervical, oropharyngeal, anal, vaginal, vulvar, and penile cancers that are caused by HPV and, combined with screening and the treatment of cervical precancers, can lead to the first elimination of a cancer in history."

15.5 Adverse Reactions of HPV Vaccination and the Risk of Serotype Replacement

The adverse reaction profiles of Gardasil® and Cervarix® were similar to those of other vaccines and were not significantly different when compared directly (Einstein et al. 2009). Most frequently, skin reactions at the injection site are seen within 5 days of vaccination (77.1%) as well as mild or moderate headaches (16.6%).

Early on, the two HPV vaccines have been suspected to be the cause of serious illness. For example, the onset of multiple sclerosis had been diagnosed around the time of HPV vaccination. Sutton et al. (2009) observed five such cases that occurred within 21 days of Gardasil® vaccination. Ultimately, no causal relationship between multiple sclerosis and HPV vaccination was found.

Moreira et al. (2016) performed a combined analysis of seven clinical trials using the quadrivalent Gardasil® and came to the conclusion that the vaccine is well tolerated in the targeted age group of 9- to 26-year-old subjects. Injection site adverse effects were more common for the nonavalent compared to the quadrivalent vaccine. Otherwise, the safety profile was similar for both vaccines.

As early as 2000, Garnett and Waddell (2000) voiced concern about the possibility of the so-called serotype replacement, i.e., the elimination of HPV 16 and 18 through vaccination and the subsequent increased prevalence of other high-risk HPV serotypes. Similarly, vaccination against low-risk types HPV 6 and 11 and their elimination may also lead to replacement by high-risk serotypes.

Man et al. (2020) constructed a transmission model in which a vaccine virus and a non-vaccine type compete. They concluded that, although so far post-vaccination surveillance data appear to be reassuring, it is still too early to rule out serotype replacement. Therefore, it is important to monitor non-vaccine HPV serotypes in order to be able to recognize a shift toward serotype replacement.

15.6 Impact of HPV Vaccination on Secondary Screening

Present screening strategies need to be modified constantly due to the HPV vaccination related decrease of CIN prevalence.

Lei et al. (2020) could demonstrate from Swedish registry data that HPV vaccination lowers the positive predictive value of cytology. This effect is more pronounced when vaccination is done at an earlier age. The authors therefore discuss either to decrease the intensity of screening in these women or to adopt primary HPV screening with partial HPV genotyping as HPV16/18 positivity in vaccinated women is more likely to represent persistent infection than in non-vaccinated women.

Due to the decrease in the positive predictive value of cytology in vaccinated women and thus the increasing inefficiency of cytology, Sundström et al. (2021) predict that HPV based screening in combination with appropriate biomarkers will become the preferred method of screening including very young women.

References

Ali H, Donovan B, Wand H, Read TR, Regan DG, Grulich AE et al (2013) Genital warts in young Australians five years into national human papillomavirus vaccination programme: national surveillance data. BMJ 346:f2032. https://doi.org/10.1136/bmj.f2032

Arbyn M, Xu L, Simoens C, Martin-Hirsch PP (2018) Prophylactic vaccination against human papillomaviruses to prevent cervical cancer and its precursors. Cochrane Database Syst Rev 207(11):1753–1241. https://doi.org/10.1002/14651858.CD009069.pub3

Brisson M, Kim JJ, Canfell K, Drolet M, Gingras G, Burger EA et al (2020) Impact of HPV vaccination and cervical screening on cervical cancer elimination: a comparative modelling analysis in 78 low-income and lower-middle-income countries. Lancet 395(10224):575–590. https://doi.org/10.1016/S0140-6736(20)30068-4

Brotherton JM, Fridman M, May CL, Chappell G, Saville AM, Gertig DM (2011) Early effect of the HPV vaccination programme on cervical abnormalities in Victoria, Australia: an ecological study. Lancet 377(9783):2085–2092. https://doi.org/10.1016/S0140-6736(11)60551-5

Bruni L, Saura-Lázaro A, Montoliu A, Brotons M, Alemany L, Diallo MS et al (2021) HPV vaccination introduction worldwide and WHO and UNICEF estimates of national HPV immunization coverage 2010-2019. Prev Med 144:106399. https://doi.org/10.1016/j.ypmed.2020.106399

Castellsague X, Munoz N, Pitisuttithum P, Ferris D, Monsonego J, Ault K et al (2011) End-of-study safety, immunogenicity, and efficacy of quadrivalent HPV (types 6, 11, 16, 18) recombinant vaccine in adult women 24-45 years of age. Br J Cancer 105(1):28–37. https://doi.org/10.1038/bjc.2011.185

Cleveland AA, Gargano JW, Park IU, Griffin MR, Niccolai LM, Powell M et al (2019) Cervical adenocarcinoma in situ: human papillomavirus types and incidence trends in five states, 2008–2015. Int J Cancer 10:645. https://doi.org/10.1002/ijc.32340

de Sanjose S, Quint WG, Alemany L, Geraets DT, Klaustermeier JE, Lloveras B et al (2010) Human papillomavirus genotype attribution in invasive cervical cancer: a retrospective cross-sectional worldwide study. Lancet Oncol 11(11):1048–1056. https://doi.org/10.1016/S1470-2045(10)70230-8

Doerfler D, Bernhaus A, Kottmel A, Sam C, Koelle D, Joura EA (2009) Human papilloma virus infection prior to coitarche. Am J Obstet Gynecol 200(5):487–485. https://doi.org/10.1016/j.ajog.2008.12.028

Drolet M, Bénard É, Pérez N, Brisson M, HPV Vaccination Impact Study Group (2019) Population-level impact and herd effects following the introduction of human papillomavirus vaccination programmes: updated systematic review and meta-analysis. Lancet. https://doi.org/10.1016/S0140-6736(19)30298-3

Einstein MH, Baron M, Levin MJ, Chatterjee A, Edwards RP, Zepp F et al (2009) Comparison of the immunogenicity and safety of Cervarix and Gardasil human papillomavirus (HPV) cervical cancer vaccines in healthy women aged 18-45 years. Hum Vaccin 5(10):705–719

Garland SM, Hernandez-Avila M, Wheeler CM, Perez G, Harper DM, Leodolter S et al (2007) Quadrivalent vaccine against human papillomavirus to prevent anogenital diseases. N Engl J Med 356(19):1928–1943

Garnett GP, Waddell HC (2000) Public health paradoxes and the epidemiological impact of an HPV vaccine. J Clin Virol 19(1–2):101–111. http://doi.org/S1386-6532(00)00129-3

Ghelardi A, Parazzini F, Martella F, Pieralli A, Bay P, Tonetti A et al (2018) SPERANZA project: HPV vaccination after treatment for CIN2. Gynecol Oncol 151(2):1–6. https://doi.org/10.1016/j.ygyno.2018.08.033

Gross G, Wieland U, Wemer RN (2020) Evidenz- und konsensbasierte Leitlinie: Impfprävention HPV-assoziierter Neoplasien. AWMF-Register Nr.: 082–002

Hall MT, Simms KT, Lew J-B, Smith MA, Brotherton JM, Saville M et al (2019) The projected timeframe until cervical cancer elimination in Australia: a modelling study. Lancet Public Health 4(1):e19–e27. https://doi.org/10.1016/S2468-2667(18)30183-X

Hausen zur H (2009) Papillomaviruses in the causation of human cancers - a brief historical account. Virology 384(2):260–265. https://doi.org/10.1016/j.virol.2008.11.046

Heneghan C, Onakpoya I (2019) Editors' response to concerns over the publication of the Cochrane HPV vaccine review was incomplete and ignored important evidence of bias. BMJ Evid Based Med 24(1):1–4. https://doi.org/10.1136/bmjebm-2018-111108

Hildesheim A, Herrero R, Wacholder S, Rodriguez AC, Solomon D, Bratti MC et al (2007) Effect of human papillomavirus 16/18 L1 virus like particle vaccine among young women with preexisting infection: a randomized trial. JAMA 298(7):743–753

Jørgensen L, Gøtzsche PC, Jefferson T (2018) The Cochrane HPV vaccine review was incomplete and ignored important evidence of bias. BMJ Evid Based Med 23(5):165–168. https://doi.org/10.1136/bmjebm-2018-111012

Joura EA, Garland SM, Paavonen J, Ferris DG, Perez G, Ault KA et al (2012) Effect of the human papillomavirus (HPV) quadrivalent vaccine in a subgroup of women with cervical and vulvar disease: retrospective pooled analysis of trial data. BMJ 344:e1401. https://doi.org/10.1136/bmj.e1401

Joura EA, Giuliano AR, Iversen OE, Bouchard C, Mao C, Mehlsen J et al (2015) A 9-valent HPV vaccine against infection and intraepithelial neoplasia in women. N Engl J Med 372(8):711–723. https://doi.org/10.1056/NEJMoa1405044

Kang WD, Choi HS, Kim SM (2013) Is vaccination with quadrivalent HPV vaccine after loop electrosurgical excision procedure effective in preventing recurrence in patients with high-grade cervical intraepithelial neoplasia (CIN2-3)? Gynecol Oncol. https://doi.org/10.1016/j.ygyno.2013.04.050

Kaufmann AM, Nieland JD, Jochmus I, Baur S, Friese K, Gabelsberger J et al (2007) Vaccination trial with HPV16 L1E7 chimeric virus-like particles in women suffering from high grade cervical intraepithelial neoplasia (CIN 2/3). Int J Cancer 121(12):2794–2800. https://doi.org/10.1002/ijc.23022

Lehtinen M, Paavonen J, Wheeler CM, Jaisamrarn U, Garland SM, Castellsague X et al (2012) Overall efficacy of HPV-16/18 AS04-adjuvanted vaccine against grade

3 or greater cervical intraepithelial neoplasia: 4-year end-of-study analysis of the randomised, double-blind PATRICIA trial. Lancet Oncol 13(1):89–99. https://doi.org/10.1016/S1470-2045(11)70286-8

Lei J, Ploner A, Lehtinen M, Sparén P, Dillner J, Elfström KM (2020) Impact of HPV vaccination on cervical screening performance: a population-based cohort study. Br J Cancer 123(1):155–160. https://doi.org/10.1038/s41416-020-0850-6

Lieblong BJ, Montgomery BEE, Su LJ, Nakagawa M (2019) Natural history of human papillomavirus and vaccinations in men: a literature review. Health Sci Rep 2(5):e118. https://doi.org/10.1002/hsr2.118

Luostarinen T, Apter D, Dillner J, Eriksson T, Harjula K, Natunen K et al (2018) Vaccination protects against invasive HPV-associated cancers. Int J Cancer 142(10):2186–2187. https://doi.org/10.1002/ijc.31231

Man I, Vänskä S, Lehtinen M, Bogaards JA (2020) Human papillomavirus genotype replacement: still too early to tell? J Infect Dis 445:2. https://doi.org/10.1093/infdis/jiaa032

Markowitz LE, Naleway AL, Lewis RM, Crane B, Querec TD, Weinmann S et al (2019) Declines in HPV vaccine type prevalence in women screened for cervical cancer in the United States: evidence of direct and herd effects of vaccination. Vaccine 37(29):3918–3924. https://doi.org/10.1016/j.vaccine.2019.04.099

Moreira ED, Block SL, Ferris D, Giuliano AR, Iversen O-E, Joura EA et al (2016) Safety profile of the 9-valent HPV vaccine: a combined analysis of 7 phase III clinical trials. Pediatrics 138(2):e20154387. https://doi.org/10.1542/peds.2015-4387

Naud P, Roteli-Martins CM, De Carvalho N, et al (2011) HPV-16/18 vaccine: sustained immunogenicity and efficacy to 9.4 years. Abstract no. O-18.04]. 27th International Papillomavirus Conference; 2011 Sep 17–22; Berlin

Paavonen J, Jenkins D, Bosch FX, Naud P, Salmerón J, Wheeler CM et al (2007) Efficacy of a prophylactic adjuvanted bivalent L1 virus-like-particle vaccine against infection with human papillomavirus types 16 and 18 in young women: an interim analysis of a phase III double-blind, randomised controlled trial. Lancet 369(9580):2161–2170. https://doi.org/10.1016/S0140-6736(07)60946-5

Pieralli A, Bianchi C, Auzzi N, Fallani MG, Bussani C, Fambrini M et al (2018) Indication of prophylactic vaccines as a tool for secondary prevention in HPV-linked disease. Arch Gynecol Obstet 189(2):1–6. https://doi.org/10.1007/s00404-018-4926-y

Read TR, Hocking JS, Chen MY, Donovan B, Bradshaw CS, Fairley CK (2011) The near disappearance of genital warts in young women 4 years after commencing a national human papillomavirus (HPV) vaccination programme. Sex Transm Infect 87(7):544–547. https://doi.org/10.1136/sextrans-2011-050234

Roteli-Martins CM, Naud P, De Borba P, Teixeira JC, De Carvalho NS, Zahaf T et al (2012) Sustained immunogenicity and efficacy of the HPV-16/18 AS04-adjuvanted vaccine: up to 8.4 years of follow-up. Hum Vaccin Immunother 8(3):390–397. https://doi.org/10.4161/hv.18865

Sabeena S, Bhat P, Kamath V, Arunkumar G (2017) Possible non-sexual modes of transmission of human papilloma virus. J Obstet Gynaecol Res 43(3):429–435. https://doi.org/10.1111/jog.13248

Saslow D, Andrews KS, Manassaram-Baptiste D, Smith RA, Fontham ETH, American Cancer Society Guideline Development Group (2020) Human papillomavirus vaccination 2020 guideline update: American Cancer Society guideline adaptation. CA: A Cancer J Clin Am Cancer Soc. https://doi.org/10.3322/caac.21616

Schneider A, Hammerschmidt T, Schwarz TF, Rogoza RM, Ferko N, Siebert U (2007) Langfristige Public-Health-Effekte einer Impfung gegen Zervixkarzinom in Deutschland. Geburtsh Frauenheilk 67: 850–858

Shew ML, Weaver B, Tu W, Tong Y, Fortenberry JD, Brown DR (2013) High frequency of human papillomavirus detection in the vagina before first vaginal intercourse among females enrolled in a longitudinal cohort study. J Infect Dis 207(6):1012–1015. https://doi.org/10.1093/infdis/jis775

Stanley M (2012) Perspective: vaccinate boys too. Nature 488(7413):S10. https://doi.org/10.1038/488S10a

Stanley M, Dull P (2018) HPV single-dose vaccination: impact potential, evidence base and further evaluation. Vaccine 36(32 Pt A):4759–4760. https://doi.org/10.1016/j.vaccine.2018.02.076

Strasser T (1978) Reflections on cardiovascular diseases. Interdiscip Sci Rev 3:225–230

Sundström K, Herweijer E, Wang J (2021) Cervical screening in high-income countries: the need for quality assurance, adjunct biomarkers and rational adaptation to HPV vaccination. Prev Med 144:106382. https://doi.org/10.1016/j.ypmed.2020.106382

Sutton I, Lahoria R, Tan I, Clouston P, Barnett M (2009) CNS demyelination and quadrivalent HPV vaccination. Mult Scler 15(1):116–119. https://doi.org/10.1177/1352458508096868

Yang M-Y, Son J-H, Kim G-W, Kim H-S, Ko H-C, Kim M-B et al (2019) Quadrivalent human papilloma virus vaccine for the treatment of multiple warts: a retrospective analysis of 30 patients. J Dermatolog Treat 30(4):405–409. https://doi.org/10.1080/09546634.2018.1527006

Psychological Considerations of Screening and Triage

16

Contents

The psychological burden of Pap smear and HPV screening as well as colposcopic triage is quite significant and frequently underestimated. In this chapter, the psychological effects and possible strategies to alleviate stressful situations are discussed.

16.1 Psychological Effects of Screening for Cervical Cancer

In Pap test-based screening, it is unlikely that an abnormal Pap smear is associated with cancer diagnosis. Rather, the majority of abnormal smears are due to preneoplasia including low-grade dysplasia (LSIL), which does not require treatment. In addition, a significant number of patients are confronted with inconclusive Pap smears such as ASC-US. However, from a patient's perspective, this is perceived differently. The necessity of colposcopic triage or even a minor abnormality that requires a follow-up exam after a shortened interval can become a major psychological burden.

Lauver et al. (1999) interviewed women with an abnormal Pap smear result. Above all, women were concerned that they would not properly understand the meaning of the Pap smear diagnosis. Also, the fear of cancer, infertility, and sexual transmission of HPV infection in general was expressed.

Frederiksen et al. (2015) performed a meta-analysis of quantitative studies measuring psychological outcomes in women with histologically confirmed CIN diagnosis. Only 16 studies were identified meeting the selection criteria. A negative psychological impact of diagnosis and treatment of CIN was evident. Pap smear results had similar psychological consequences as a CIN diagnosis. Furthermore, psychological outcomes several years after diagnosis were not different between patients with CIN compared to patients with an actual diagnosis of cervical cancer, i.e., many women considered the diagnosis of intraepithelial lesions as grave as the diagnosis of actual cancer.

R. J. Lellé, V. Küppers, *Colposcopy*, https://doi.org/10.1007/978-3-030-85388-4_16

To a young symptom-free and healthy woman, the cytopathologic ASC-US diagnosis may signal that she is now considered "a patient." Many young women may experience that they are confronted for the first time with a potentially life-threatening disease such as cancer.

The fact that a colposcopy clinic is not a "cancer clinic" but rather a specialized diagnostic unit to identify patients who may need minor surgery to avoid a possible future cancer risk is not easily understood by the patients.

As there is a widespread anxiety of cancer within our society, a variety of expressions used by both patients and health-care professionals may further trigger this anxiety, as illustrated by the following examples.

"Carcinoma In Situ"

This is an alternative histological expression for certain high-grade squamous intraepithelial lesions. Unfortunately, the WHO in its latest revision of histopathologic nomenclature (WHO Classification of Tumours Editorial Board 2020) still considers the expression "squamous cell carcinoma in situ" to be acceptable. Patients are prone to misinterpret "carcinoma in situ" as invasive carcinoma.

"High-Risk Virus," "Cancer Virus," "Cancer Vaccine"

As human papilloma viruses are traditionally subdivided into low- and high-risk types, the expression "HPV high risk" might be misinterpreted to imply a "high risk for cancer." Sometimes HPV are outright called "cancer viruses," or the HPV vaccine is mislabeled "cancer vaccine," which it is not. All of this is in stark contrast to the frequent occurrence of these so-called "high-risk" virus types, mostly in healthy individuals.

Unfortunately, the scientific fact that the majority of precancers of the lower genital tract is HPV related has led to the labeling of these diseases as "sexually transmitted."

Women, regardless of the severity of their diagnosis, which may range from a minor Pap smear abnormality to the diagnosis of cervical cancer, are confronted with the concept of personal responsibility and guilt regarding sexuality. Disease may be regarded as "punishment" for unsanctioned sexual practice.

A positive HPV test result may trigger a critical analysis of sexual behavior of oneself as well as of present or past sexual partners. In a monogamous relationship, HPV positivity may be erroneously considered a sign of infidelity.

The HPV diagnosis may also cause a feeling of uncleanliness and the fear to infect the partner. Overall, potential relationship problems may be exacerbated.

Lerman et al. (1991) found that about a quarter of the women surveyed felt impaired in their day-to-day activities by the diagnosis of an abnormal screening result. Half of women reported a negative impact on their sex life, and 40% suffered from sleep disorders.

Using the Impact of Event Scale, Sharp et al. (2011) demonstrated a significant mental distress in women with low-grade abnormal cervical cytology who underwent colposcopy. Psychological distress was not even alleviated, if colposcopy was normal.

Obviously, colposcopic examination has both distressing and calming effects. According to Jones et al. (1996), patients preferred immediate colposcopy to a repeat Pap smear, when low-grade dysplasia was suspected. However, 47% of women who underwent immediate colposcopy still stated that they were afraid of cancer versus 33% of patients monitored by cervical cytology.

The patients' psychological distress level is particularly high during pregnancy, as the diagnosis of any type of cervical abnormality may be perceived as a direct threat to one's own life and that of the unborn child.

16.2 Strategies to Reduce Psychological Distress

O'Connor et al. (2016) analyzed the entire sensory experience of women during colposcopy, i.e., beyond fear and pain. Obviously, a lack of preparatory information on what kind of sensations to expect during colposcopy, contributed to having a negative sensory experience of this procedure.

Health-care professionals are not able to intuitively register the level of psychological distress the patient is experiencing. An outwardly calm patient does not necessarily cope better with her feelings of anxiety. Therefore, several questionnaires have proven useful to provide objective evaluation of anxiety:

- PEAPS-Q (Psychosocial Effects of Abnormal Pap Smear Questionnaire) by Bennetts et al. (1995) and Stinnett (2000).
- CDDQ (Cervical Dysplasia Distress Questionnaire) by Shinn et al. (2004), which has been developed from the PEAPS-Q.

A study conducted by Handelzalts et al. (2015) on pain and anxiety in relation to colposcopy shows that young patients (pain management) and patients who are examined for the first time (anxiety management) require particular attention.

Patients can be reassured most effectively through education. The involvement of another health-care professional such as a certified nurse may be helpful to partly overcome anxiety (Lauver et al. 1999; Gath et al. 1995).

Ideally, the education process starts prior to the actual colposcopy consultation. Patients need to be made aware that a cancer diagnosis is rare and that colposcopy is carried out to clarify the diagnosis and to carry out preventive measures.

If biopsies are taken during colposcopy examination, results should be obtained expeditiously and communicated to the patient to further reduce anxiety levels (Gath et al. 1995).

Video colposcopy is a valuable tool to improve both education and communication with the patient, as the patient is actively involved in the diagnostic workup. Also, this leads to a better understanding of the anatomic structures involved. According to Nugent and Tamlyn-Leaman (1992), about 40% of women surveyed did not know the location of the cervix. According to a randomized study by Walsh et al. (2004), video colposcopy can significantly reduce anxiety. However, this could not be confirmed by a more recent prospective randomized trial (Hilal et al. 2017). As there were no indications that video colposcopy increases anxiety during or after colposcopy, the authors consider it useful for educational purposes only.

Also, Hilal et al. (2018) could not confirm the anxiety-reducing effect of classical music (Mozart) during colposcopy clinic, again using a strict prospective randomized trial format.

References

Bennetts A, Irwig L, Oldenburg B, Simpson JM, Mock P, Boyes A et al (1995) PEAPS-Q: a questionnaire to measure the psychosocial effects of having an abnormal pap smear. Psychosocial Effects of Abnormal Pap Smears Questionnaire. J Clin Epidemiol 48(10):1235–1243. 089543569500015V [pii]

Frederiksen ME, Njor S, Lynge E, Rebolj M (2015) Psychological effects of diagnosis and treatment of cervical intraepithelial neoplasia: a systematic review. Sex Transm Infect 91(4):248–256. https://doi.org/10.1136/sextrans-2014-051754

Gath DH, Hallam N, Mynors-Wallis L, Day A, Bond SA (1995) Emotional reactions in women attending a UK colposcopy clinic. J Epidemiol Community Health 49(1):79–83

Handelzalts JE, Krissi H, Levy S, Broitman M, Binyamin L, Peled Y (2015) Multidimensional associations of pain and anxiety before and after colposcopy. Int J Gynaecol Obstet 131(3):297–300. https://doi.org/10.1016/j.ijgo.2015.05.038

Hilal Z, Alici F, Tempfer CB, Seebacher V, Rezniczek GA (2017) Video colposcopy for reducing patient anxiety during colposcopy: a randomized controlled trial. Obstet Gynecol 130(2):411–419. https://doi.org/10.1097/AOG.0000000000002127

Hilal Z, Alici F, Tempfer CB, Rath K, Nar K, Rezniczek GA (2018) Mozart for reducing patient anxiety during colposcopy: a randomized controlled trial. Obstet Gynecol 132(4):1047–1055. https://doi.org/10.1097/AOG.0000000000002876

Jones MH, Singer A, Jenkins D (1996) The mildly abnormal cervical smear: patient anxiety and choice of management. J R Soc Med 89(5):257–260

Lauver DR, Baggot A, Kruse K (1999) Women's experiences in coping with abnormal Papanicolaou results and follow-up colposcopy. J Obstet Gynecol Neonatal Nurs 28(3):283–290

Lerman C, Miller SM, Scarborough R, Hanjani P, Nolte S, Smith D (1991) Adverse psychologic consequences of positive cytologic cervical screening. Am J Obstet Gynecol 165(3):658–662. 0002-9378(91)90304-A [pii]

Nugent LS, Tamlyn-Leaman K (1992) The colposcopy experience: what do women know? J Adv Nurs 17(4):514–520

O'Connor M, Waller J, Gallagher P, Martin CM, O'Leary J, D'Arcy T et al (2016) Exploring women's sensory experiences of undergoing colposcopy and related procedures: implications for preparatory sensory information provision. J Psychosom Obstet Gynecol 37(4):137–146. https://doi.org/10.1080/0167482X.2016.1197905

Sharp L, Cotton S, Carsin AE, Gray N, Thornton A, Cruickshank M, Little J (2011) Factors associated with psychological distress following colposcopy among women with low-grade abnormal cervical cytology: a prospective study within the Trial Of Management of Borderline and Other Low-grade Abnormal smears (TOMBOLA). Psycho-Oncology 22:368. https://doi.org/10.1002/pon.2097

Shinn E, Basen-Engquist K, Le T, Hansis-Diarte A, Bostic D, Martinez-Cross J et al (2004) Distress after an abnormal Pap smear result: scale development and psychometric validation. Prev Med 39(2):404–412. https://doi.org/10.1016/j.ypmed.2004.02.004. S0091743504000763 [pii]

Stinnett BA (2000) Use of psychosocial effects of Abnormal Pap Smears Questionnaire (PEAPS-Q) in a community hospital colposcopy clinic. J Low Genit Tract Dis 4(1):34–39

Walsh JC, Curtis R, Mylotte M (2004) Anxiety levels in women attending a colposcopy clinic: a randomised trial of an educational intervention using video colposcopy. Patient Educ Couns 55(2):247–251. https://doi.org/10.1016/j.pec.2003.09.012. S0738399103003008 [pii]

WHO Classification of Tumours Editorial Board (2020) Female genital tumours. IARC Press, Lyon

Cervical Cancer Prevention, Diagnosis, and Management Within a Low-Resource Environment

17

Contents

Cancer screening strategies that have been developed for industrialized resource-rich countries are not feasible within a low-resource environment. For example, morphology-based techniques such as cytopathology require a large number of trained personnel and a sophisticated infrastructure. However, alternative methods such as visual inspection (VIA and VILI) have proven to be effective and will be described in detail.

17.1 Introduction

Many aspects of cervical cancer screening presented in previous chapters reflect the situation in Western industrialized regions such as Europe and the USA. However, it does not represent the global situation. The majority of the world's population does not have access to cervical cancer screening. Whereas the vast majority of cervical cancer cases—about 85%—occur in developing countries, strategies developed for resource-rich developed countries cannot be transferred directly to other countries. For example, morphology-based methods such as cytopathology would not be successful in sub-Saharan African nations due to an extreme shortage of pathologists as well as a total lack of trained technicians (Adesina et al. 2013). Under the best of circumstances, these countries have one tenth of the number of pathologists compared to Western countries. Therefore, alternative screening strategies are needed that take into account local conditions such as the geographical situation, the specific epidemiologic data, and especially the availability of trained personnel.

In this chapter, an introduction will be given to cervical cancer screening and treatment within a low-resource environment. Frequent reference is

R. J. Lellé, V. Küppers, *Colposcopy*, https://doi.org/10.1007/978-3-030-85388-4_17

made toward Tanzania as one of the sub-Saharan African nations as well as Indonesia, a vast archipelago located in the Far East, both countries with a very high cervical cancer incidence thriving to establish effective cervical cancer screening methods.

17.2 Worldwide Cervical Cancer Statistics

From a global perspective, the world cancer burden has been growing considerably within the last several years, and cancer incidence will continue to rise. Unfortunately, the strongest impact will be felt in low- and middle-income countries. Most of these countries are ill-equipped to cope with early detection and prevention strategies. Therefore, cancer diagnosis is delayed until the patient suffers from advanced stage disease, which in most cases is not amenable to effective and curative treatment, even under the best of circumstances.

The extent of this problem becomes clear through the World Cancer Report published in 2014 by the World Health Organization (Stewart and Wild 2014). The worldwide cancer burden is expected to increase by 70% within the next two decades.

For cervical cancer, an annual increase of the global cancer burden of 0.6% between 1980 and 2010 has been calculated (Forouzanfar et al. 2011).

Even high-income countries will not be able to effectively treat and cure a large number of cancer patients as the cost of personalized cancer medicine is increasing exponentially. Therefore, the primary focus should be on cancer prevention and—if not feasible—on early detection of disease.

There are only two types of cancer which can be prevented effectively, i.e., lung cancer, by cessation of smoking, and cervical cancer, by HPV vaccination and/or screening for cervical precancer.

Arbyn et al. (2011) determined the worldwide burden of cervical cancer for the year 2008. They estimated 530,000 cases and 275,000 deaths from the disease. A map of the global age-standardized incidence rate clearly reflects the close relationship between poverty and cervical cancer occurrence (Fig. 17.1) and mortality (Fig. 17.2), respectively.

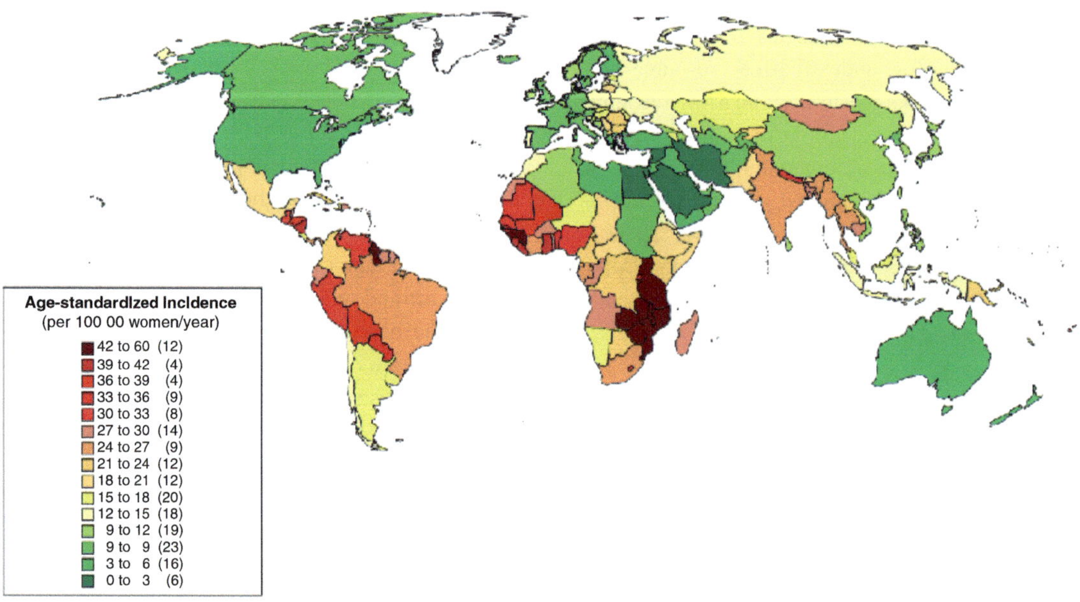

Fig. 17.1. Global age-standardized cervical cancer incidence per 100,000 women/year for 2008. The number in brackets corresponds to the number of countries within the respective cervical cancer incidence range (Arbyn et al. 2011)

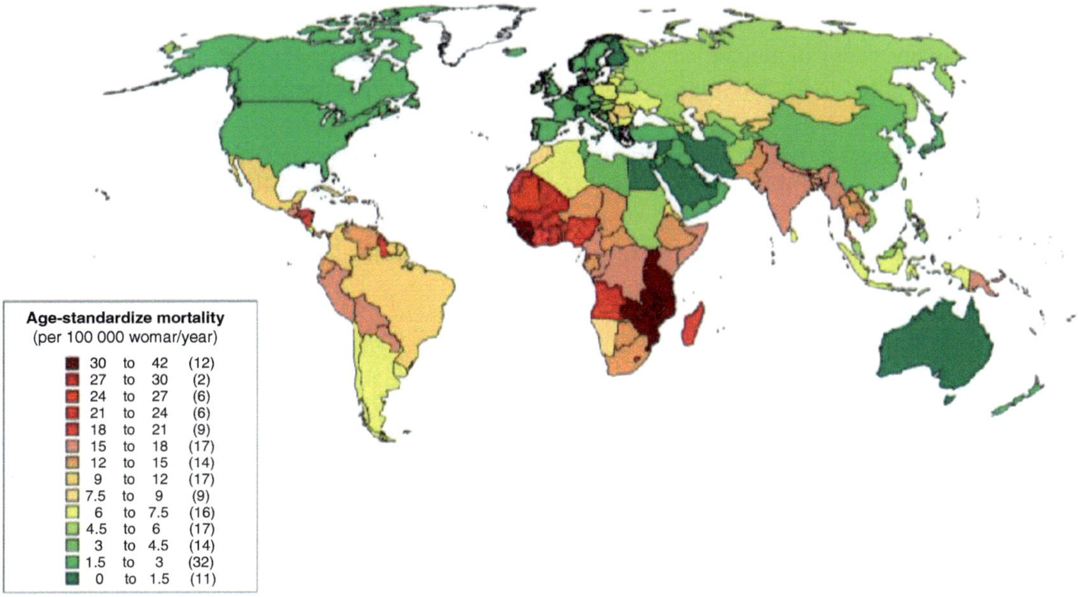

Fig. 17.2 Global age-standardized cervical cancer mortality per 100,000 women/year for 2008. The number in brackets corresponds to the number of countries within the respective cervical cancer mortality range (Arbyn et al. 2011)

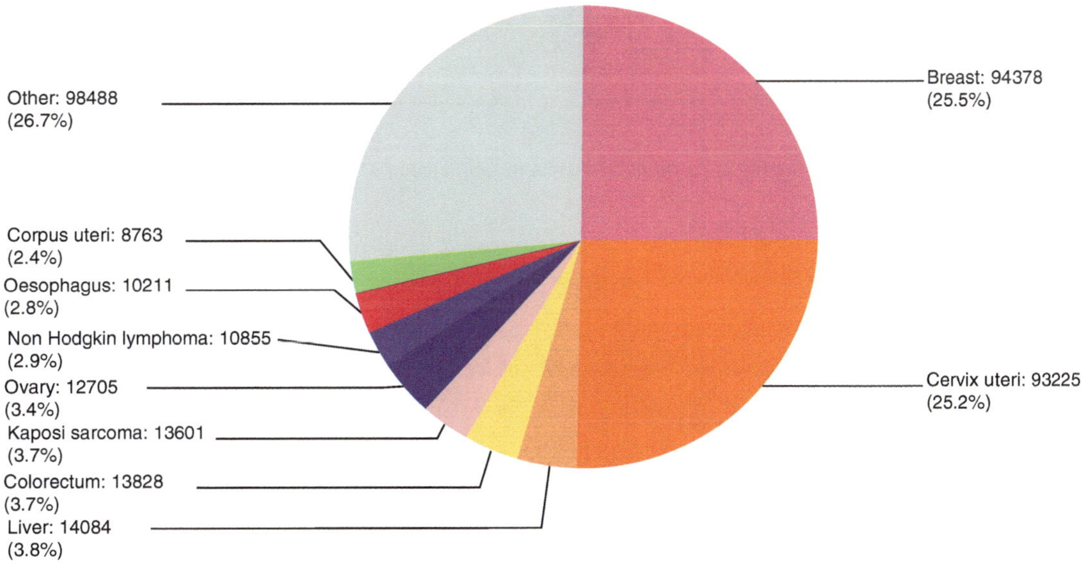

Fig. 17.3 Estimated cancer incidence proportions in women in sub-Saharan Africa, 2012 (Stewart and Wild 2014)

The above mentioned WHO report clearly demonstrates that the heaviest burden for carcinoma of the cervix lies within the poorest regions of the world such as the countries of sub-Saharan Africa. According to this report, cervical cancer is the second most common cancer in women in sub-Saharan Africa accounting for about one quarter of all female cancers (Fig. 17.3).

This proportion is almost equal to the proportion of breast cancer which is considered by far the most frequent female cancer worldwide.

Looking at cancer mortality, cervical cancer is the most frequent cause of female cancer death with 23.2% compared to 19.3% in breast cancer (Fig. 17.4).

Due to the high incidence and prevalence of both breast cancer and cervical cancer in the countries of sub-Saharan Africa, women are considerably more likely to die from cancer than men. When looking at the estimated 5-year mortality proportions of the adult population encompassing both genders, breast cancer (22.6%) and cervical cancer (18.1%) are constituting a considerable heavier cancer mortality burden than, for example, carcinoma of the prostate, the most frequent male cancer (10.3%) (Fig. 17.5).

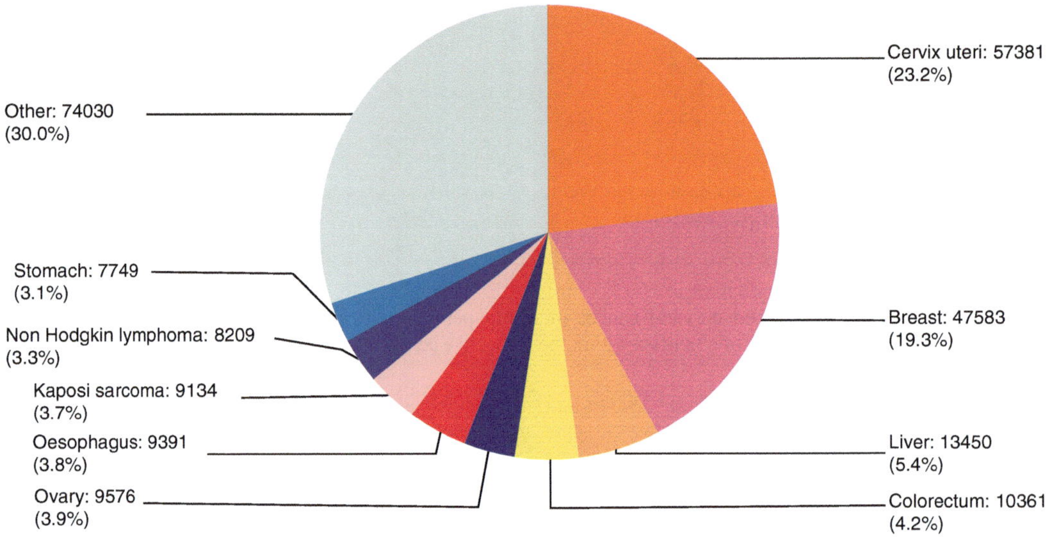

Fig. 17.4 Estimated cancer mortality proportions in women in sub-Saharan Africa, 2012 (Stewart and Wild 2014)

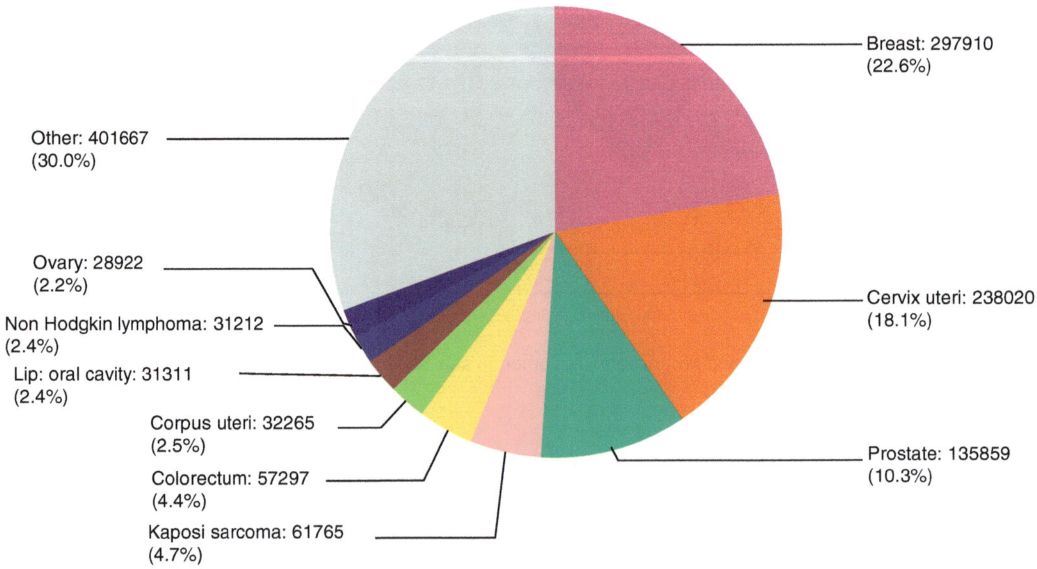

Fig. 17.5 Estimated cancer 5-year mortality proportions (adult population, both sexes combined) in sub-Saharan Africa, 2012 (Stewart and Wild 2014)

Silkensen et al. (2018) state that we are presently *"at a crossover point with cervical cancer mortality exceeding maternal deaths during childbirth"* (Fig. 17.6).

Besides sub-Saharan Africa with the highest cervical cancer incidence worldwide, special consideration should be given to East and Central Asia as it is the most populous region with 57% of the world population living in these countries. Although cancer distribution is different from sub-Saharan Africa, another preventable type of cancer, lung cancer, plays a significant role (10.1%) and is leading cancer mortality statistics; carcinoma of the cervix remains a major problem with 9.6% of all female cancer cases (Fig. 17.7) and 8.2% of female cancer deaths.

As this chapter will particularly focus on experiences from Tanzania and Indonesia, some specific data on these two countries are given below.

Tanzania is part of sub-Saharan Africa having one of the highest cancer incidence and mortality rates worldwide. According to Arbyn et al. (2011), the age-standardized incidence rate is 51/100,000 (Fig. 17.8).

Similarly, Indonesia's cervical cancer incidence and mortality are high, ranking as number

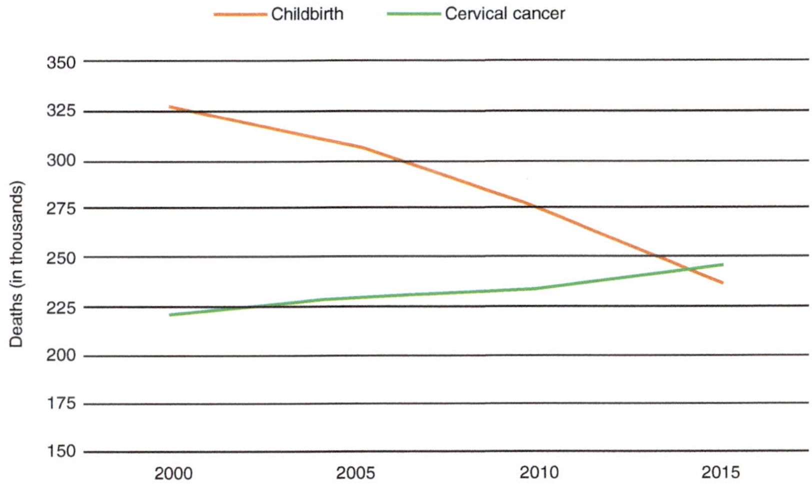

Fig. 17.6 Global burden of death from childbirth and cervical cancer (2000–2015) (Silkensen et al. 2018)

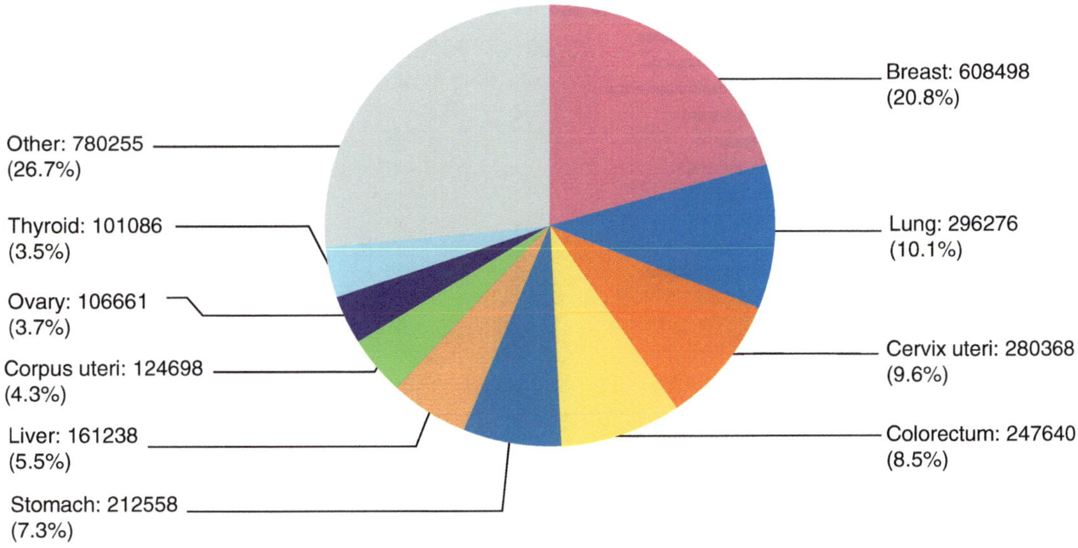

Fig. 17.7 Estimated cancer incidence proportions in women in East and Central Asia, 2012 (Stewart and Wild 2014)

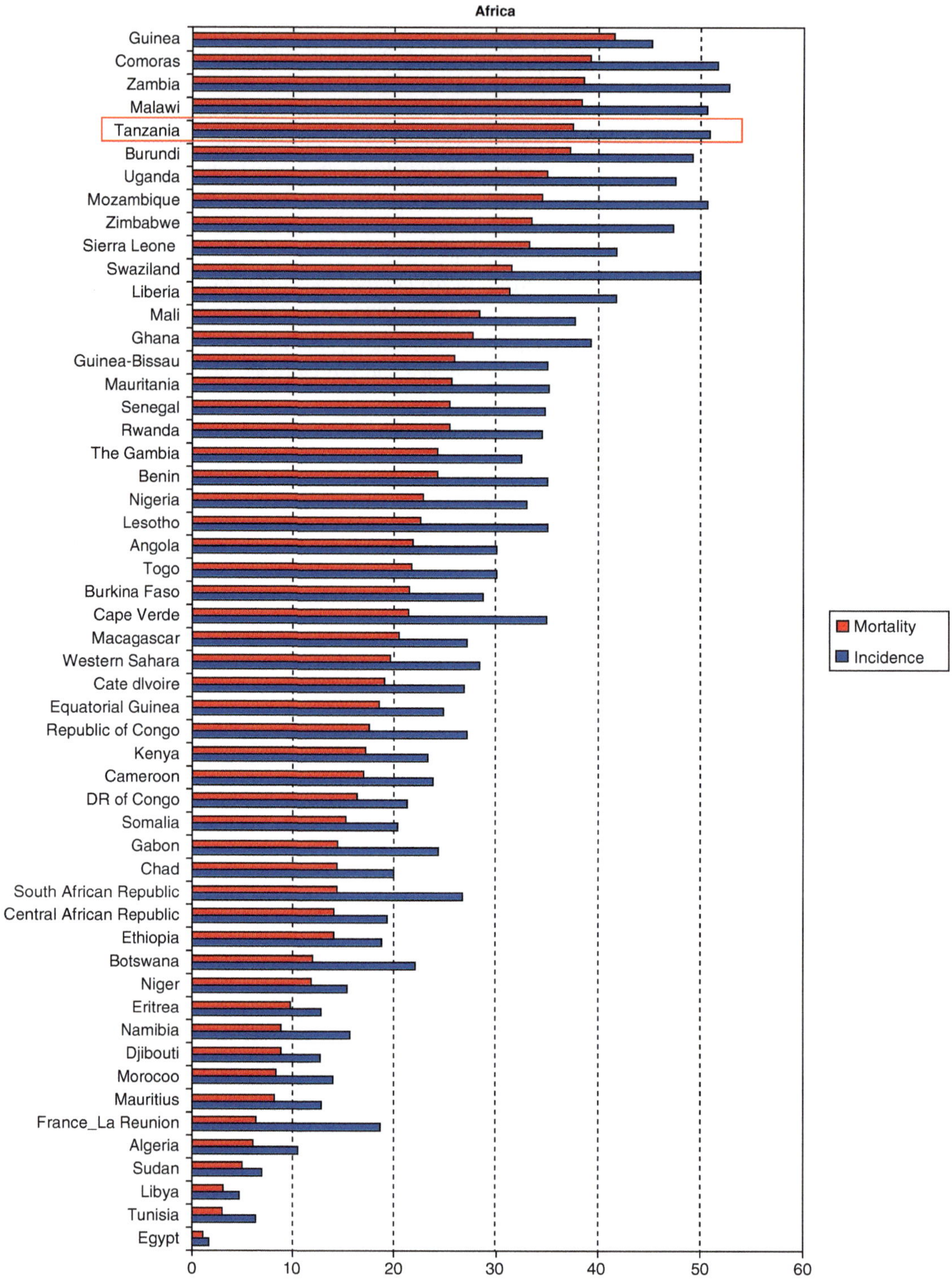

Fig. 17.8 Age-standardized cervical cancer incidence and mortality per 100,000 women/year in Africa (Arbyn et al. 2011)

14 out of 46 Asian countries. Looking at histopathological diagnosis as collected from 13 different laboratories between 1988 and 1991 (Tjindarbumi and Mangunkusumo 2002), cervical carcinoma was by far the most frequent primary cancer diagnosed (28.66–29.63%) followed by breast cancer (17.77–19.52%). In fact, due to the high incidence of these two leading cancers in women, cancer was diagnosed almost twice as frequently in women than in men (65% versus 35%).

A more detailed analysis of the Indonesian data by Oemati et al. (2011) highlights the fact that due to the high overall incidence of female organ cancer, women in Indonesia are about twice as likely to suffer from cancer as are men.

As in many countries, there is not yet a national cancer registry in Indonesia. However, indirectly, through statistics of pathology reports, it can be concluded that female cancers are by far the most common entity overall. According to Aziz (2009), cervical cancer was the most frequent pathological cancer diagnosis in 2002 (30.8%) when the numbers from male and female patients were combined, whereas the breast was the second most common cancer site (21.0%).

This again illustrates the fact that women carry the heaviest cancer burden compared to men if there is no effective cancer prevention program.

According to the above-quoted analysis of cervical cancer incidence and mortality by Arbyn et al. (2011), Indonesia ranks 14th within 46 Asian countries (Fig. 17.9).

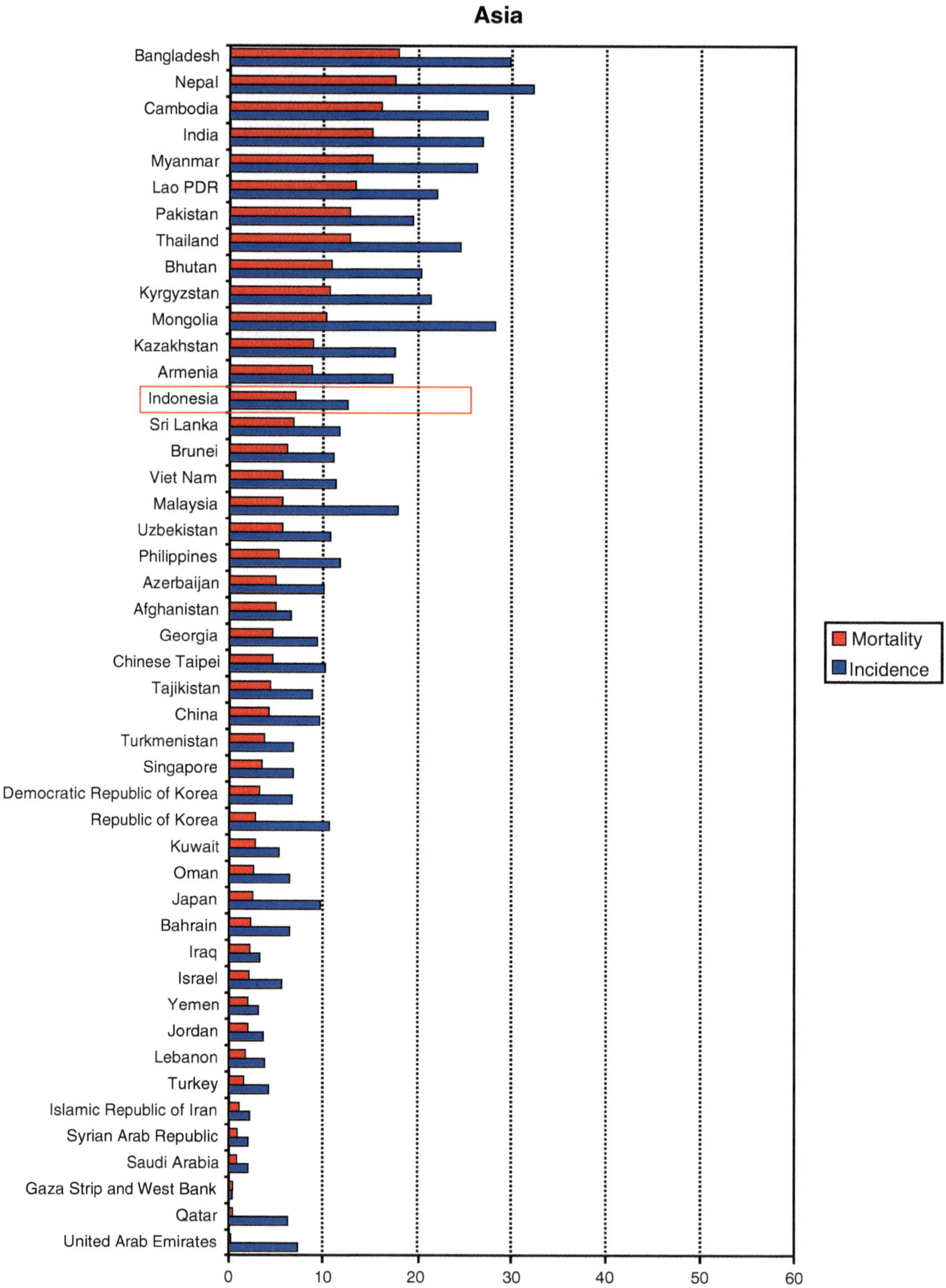

Fig. 17.9 Age-standardized cervical cancer incidence and mortality per 100,000 women/year in Asia (Arbyn et al. 2011)

17.3 Cervical Cancer Prevention

17.3.1 Barriers to Cervical Cancer Prevention

In order to establish a functioning cancer prevention program, barriers preventing the target population to participate in the intended program need to be identified.

Islam et al. (2017) studied the key barriers of cervical and breast cancer screening in low- and middle-income countries through a systematic literature review and came to the conclusion that health policy makers need to implement educational interventions as an integral part of screening programs.

Lim and Ojo (2017) analyzed the available literature on barriers to utilizing cervical cancer screening in one of the more problematic low-resource environments, i.e., sub-Saharan Africa. Among those barriers are accessibility such as the proximity to a screening facility and the amount of time needed to have the screening test performed. Furthermore, knowledge and attitude of patients are most important. Lim and Ojo point out that in two of the studies analyzed (Gharoro and Ikeanyi 2006; Mutyaba et al. 2007), only 14% and 19% of female health-care workers, respectively, participated in cervical screening programs themselves and might therefore not be a sufficient source of knowledge and cannot serve as role models to their female patients.

Specific studies on the acceptability of vaccination and screening have been done both in Tanzania and Indonesia.

Deborah Watson-Jones from the London School of Hygiene and Tropical Medicine and her colleagues have studied the feasibility of HPV vaccination in the north of Tanzania (Remes et al. 2012; Watson-Jones et al. 2012a, b).

The HPV vaccine is typically administered to adolescent or pre-adolescent girls. This is an age group that is not typically targeted by vaccination programs in these countries. As the vaccine is designed to prevent a sexually transmitted disease, promotion of the vaccine within the community is crucial.

In order to assess HPV vaccine acceptability, semi-structured interviews and group discussions were conducted with parents, schoolgirls, teachers, health workers, and religious leaders of both Muslim and Christian faith (Remes et al. 2012). The most important aspect was found to be adequate information for parents, especially regarding side effects and the potential impact on fertility.

Watson-Jones et al. (2012a, b) compared two different delivery strategies for the vaccine (quadrivalent Gardasil®). Using coverage by dose as the primary outcome parameter, class-based vaccination was superior to age-based vaccination.

Similar studies on vaccine and screening acceptability were done in Indonesia.

A questionnaire study performed in the Yogyakarta Province of Indonesia (Endarti et al. 2018) showed insufficient knowledge regarding cervical cancer, HPV, screening, and HPV vaccination of approximately two-thirds of the female participants (192 young women, 100 mothers of girls aged 12–15, and 100 adult women). However, 90% or more tended to accept HPV vaccination.

Another study on cancer screening awareness in Indonesia (Anwar et al. 2018) confirmed a strong association between awareness of Pap smear/mammography/breast self-examination and higher education as well as family income. Overall, only 20% of women surveyed were aware of the Pap test, and only 28% of these women had been screened by it.

According to a descriptive cross-sectional study conducted in West-Java, Indonesia (Hassan et al. 2018), the willingness and acceptance of cervical cancer screening by married women of reproductive age is high. Although 83% never had any education on cervical cancer, 91% expressed willingness to participate in such education and 83% already said that they would participate in cervical cancer screening using VIA.

Jaspers et al. (2011) interviewed 746 parents with at least one daughter and found parental acceptance to be high. On the other hand, the overall knowledge on cervix cancer or HPV was low. Several barriers to vaccine acceptance were identified. Interestingly, religion (56% Muslim, 21% Hindu, 23% Christian) did not play a significant role with only 11.3% of interviewees considering it an influence on their decision.

This is confirmed by Widiasih and Nelson (2018) who interviewed 20 Muslim women, ten from urban areas and ten from rural areas of West Java Province, Indonesia, in order to determine the role of Muslim husbands who traditionally play a major role in family life and may influence women's health and cancer resources. Widiasih et al. found that Muslim husbands both from urban and rural areas actively supported to promote women's health. However, there was a lack of support regarding cancer screening, emphasizing a need to improve the Muslim husbands' awareness of the importance of screening.

Self-testing may be another strategy to overcome barriers of screening. A pilot study in Makassar, Indonesia, showed that HPV self-testing is feasible and may be an alternative way of screening within this environment (Chandra et al. 2017).

17.3.2 Primary Prevention: HPV Vaccination

Considering the complex infrastructure required for a secondary screening program for cervical cancer and its precursors, it would be logical to give priority to the establishment of a HPV vaccination program that would be capable to prevent the majority of cervical cancers. Especially with the advent of the nonavalent vaccine Gardasil 9®, there is hope that cervical cancer might be altogether eradicated at some point in the future.

Although high-risk HPV type distribution may differ between countries, HPV 16/18 vaccines such as Gardasil® and Cervarix® and especially Gardasil 9® should all be able to significantly reduce the HPV-related disease burden.

Still, HPV type distribution in different countries differs significantly. According to the following data, HPV 52 occurs frequently in addition to HPV 16 and 18.

For example, in rural Ethiopia, 13.2% of women were HPV high-risk positive when tested with the Hybrid capture test (Ruland et al. 2006). In another study from the same area (Leyh-Bannurah et al. 2014), 15.8% of women were positive. HPV typing identified HPV 16 as the most common phenotype (24.4%) followed by HPV 52 (11.6%), HPV 56 (10.5%), and HPV 31 (10.5%).

In Indonesia, HPV 18 appears to play a prominent role in cervical cancer. When 74 consecutive Indonesian cervical cancer samples were tested, 71 of which were HPV positive, 39.4% contained HPV 18 DNA (Schellekens et al. 2004). HPV 16 was still the most frequently occurring high-risk HPV type with 43.7% of samples. In a group of cervical samples from 209 Indonesian patients without neoplastic disease, 13.4% contained some type of high-risk HPV (De Boer et al. 2006). Four samples (1.9%) were positive for HPV 16 and 5 (2.4%) were positive for HPV 18, which points to a high prevalence of HPV 18 within the population.

A third Indonesian study (Vet et al. 2008) gave a slightly different picture of HPV distribution. The most prevalent types were HPV 52 (23.2%), 16 (18.0%), 18 (16.1%), and 39 (11.8%). In 20.7% of patients, multiple types were identified. HPV 52 is one of six HPV high-risk types covered by the nonavalent vaccine (Joura et al. 2015).

In Tanzania, HPV type distribution within the rural and urban population has also been studied extensively, both in HIV-positive and HIV-negative women (Dartell et al. 2012). Using the HC2 test for screening of HPV high-risk positivity, 20.1% of women tested positive. HIV-positive women had a significantly higher prevalence of high-risk HPV, i.e., 46.7% compared to 17.2% for HIV-negative women. Among HC2-positive samples, HPV 52 was the most frequent HPV type both in HIV-negative (20.5%) and HIV-positive women (25.6%). No particular high-risk HPV type was significantly more common in HIV-positive women.

The most extensive analysis of HPV type distribution in invasive cancer was done by de Sanjose et al. (2010). They concluded that HPV types 16, 18, 31, 33, 35, 45, 52, and 58 should

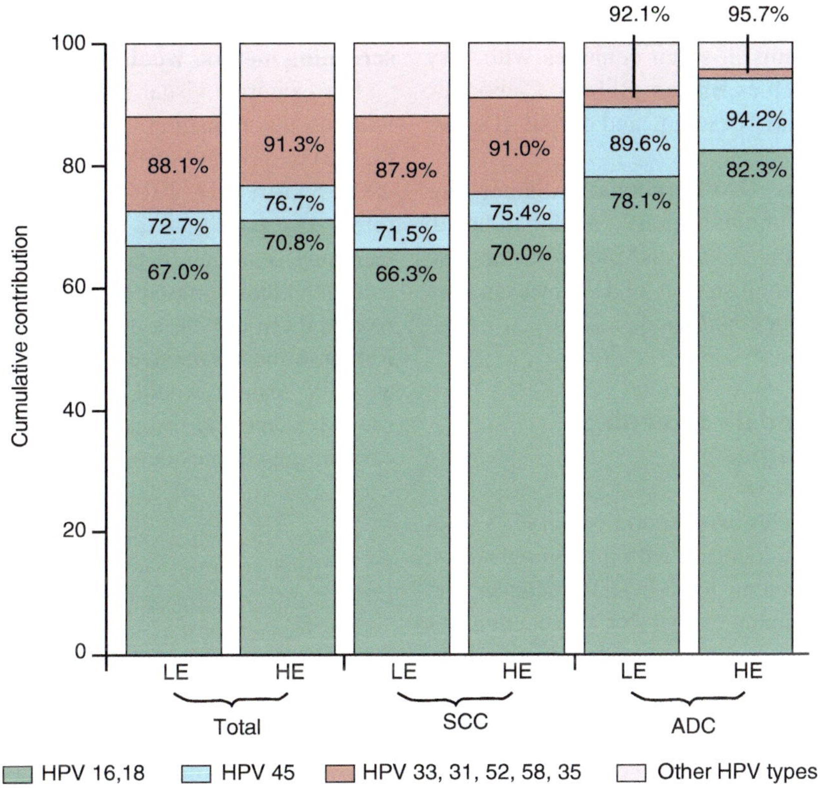

Fig. 17.10 Worldwide HPV type distribution in cervical cancer specimens. LE = lower estimate of type-specific contribution. HE = higher estimate of type-specific contribution. SCC = squamous cell carcinoma. ADC = adenocarcinoma (de Sanjose et al. 2010)

be given priority when developing vaccines (Fig. 17.10).

Looking at worldwide HPV type distribution in women with normal cytology (Clifford et al. 2005), significant heterogeneity was found. For example, European women were significantly more likely to be infected with HPV 16 than women living in sub-Saharan Africa. Particularly within Asia, there was significant heterogeneity. This needs to be taken into account regarding the design of HPV screening tests as well as the development of effective HPV vaccines.

Goldie et al. (2008) performed a financial analysis by estimating averted cervical cancer cases and deaths and calculated cost-effectiveness of HPV 16/18 vaccination of young adolescent girls. Seventy-two countries with low resources were included. Indeed, vaccination was found to be very cost-effective. For example, for Tanzania a 50.7% reduction in lifetime risk of cervical cancer was calculated. Disability-adjusted life years (DALY) averted were calculated as 50,119. The respective calculations for Indonesia were 56.7% risk reduction and 79,675 DALYs averted.

In Indonesia, where presently visual inspection with acetic acid is considered the screening method of choice, a cost-utility analysis clearly demonstrates that the addition of HPV vaccination of children and adolescents is indeed cost-effective (Setiawan et al. 2016). Statistical modeling for the Indonesian population also shows that HPV vaccination, with quadrivalent Gardasil®, will be very cost-effective, especially when catch-up vaccination is implemented (Kosen et al. 2017).

Of course, there are numerous obstacles for primary prevention through HPV vaccination in a low-resource environment, the high costs for the vaccine being just one of them. However, the Gardasil® vaccines, donated by the manufacturer, has been used successfully to launch HPV vaccination programs in seven countries with very low income such as Bhutan, Bolivia, Cambodia, Cameroon, Haiti, Lesotho, and Nepal (Ladner et al. 2012).

In addition, GAVI (Global Alliance for Vaccines and Immunization)[1], a global health partnership of the private and public sector, also sponsors the establishment of HPV vaccination programs in poor countries.

17.3.3 Secondary Screening Strategies

As many obstacles exist to implement HPV vaccination in poor countries with limited resources, secondary screening for cervical precancer and cancer will remain crucial for these countries in the foreseeable future. In addition, immediate action is mandated to act on the already high prevalence of disease.

Gakidou et al. (2008), who analyzed the coverage of cervical cancer screenings in 57 countries, stated that cytological screening coverage in developing countries is on average 19% compared to 63% in more developed countries. The lowest coverage was found for Bangladesh (1%) and the highest for Brazil (73%) (Fig. 17.11).

Furthermore, women who are at highest risk for cervical cancer, i.e., older and poorer women, are even less likely to be screened.

As can be expected, there is a direct relationship between wealth and the likelihood of cervical cancer screening (Fig. 17.12).

Screening strategies successfully used in high-income countries will not be feasible and less effective within a low-resource environment and vice versa. As a rule of thumb, the more cases of the condition or disease are to be expected, the more acceptable a less sensitive screening method would be.

For example, visual inspection of the cervix without magnification has been shown to be highly effective in India (Sankaranarayanan et al. 2009; Shastri et al. 2014), whereas it would perform very poorly in a European country like Germany with a 50-year history of cervical cancer screening based on the Pap test. In other words, there are "less needles in the haystack." Rather, a more sensitive screening method such as HPV testing would be required to further improve screening results in areas with very low cervical cancer prevalence.

- The following screening methods are listed according to increasing sensitivity:
  - Speculum exam
  - VIA or VILI
  - Colposcopy
  - Pap test
  - HPV test
  - (Future) molecular markers
- An increase in sensitivity will result in a decrease in specificity, whereas future molecular markers might have the potential to be both more sensitive and more specific than the presently available screening strategies.

Using less sensitive and less specific methods in a low-resource environment can only be a temporary solution. However, as Sankaranarayanan et al. (2015) point out, *"Despite all its limitations, implementation of VIA in low- and middle-income countries will facilitate the building up of infrastructure and human resources that may facilitate the introduction of affordable HPV tests in the future."*

In 2013, the World Health Organization has published guidelines on the selection of

[1] www.gavi.org.

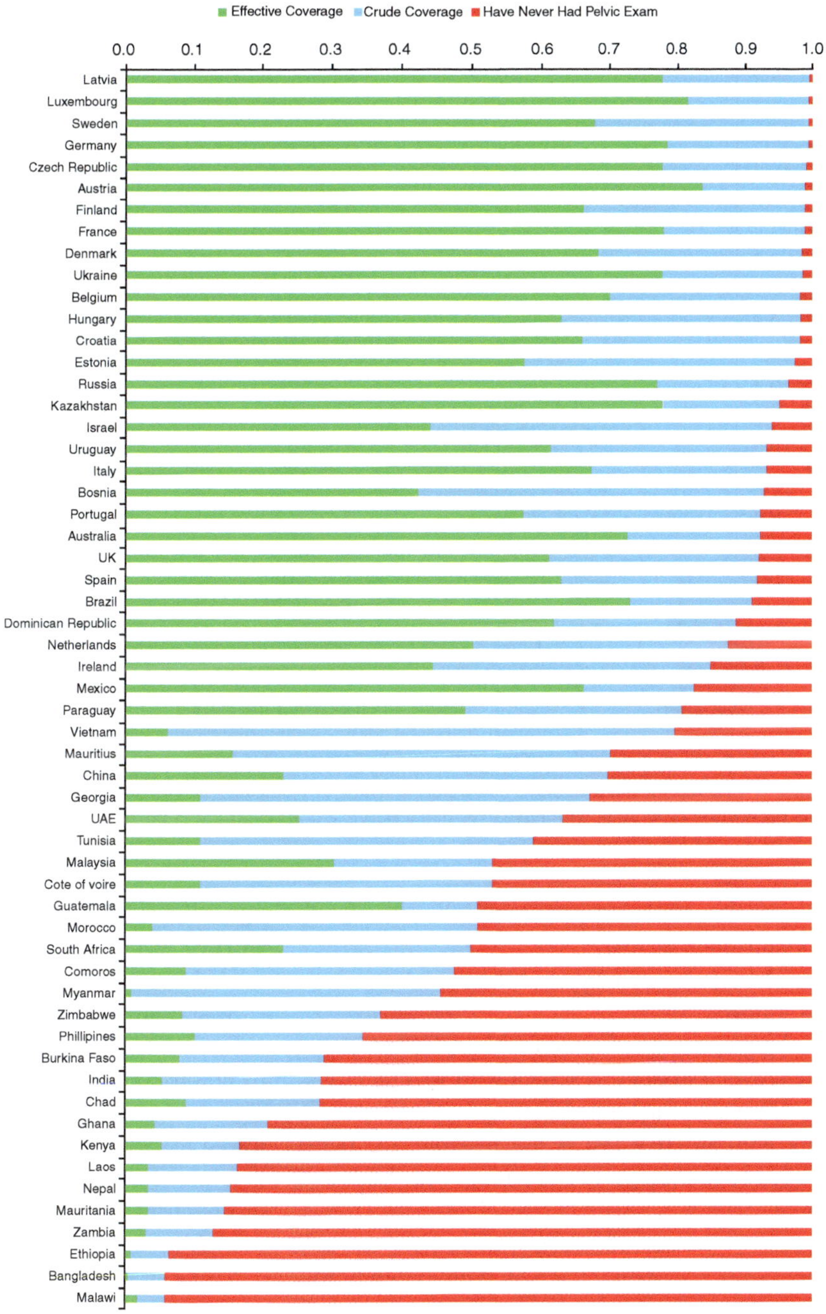

Fig. 17.11 Screening coverage for women ages 25–64. Crude coverage is defined as the proportion of women who have ever had a pelvic exam. Effective coverage is the proportion of women who report that they have had a pelvic exam as well as a Pap smear within the last 3 years (Gakidou et al. 2008)

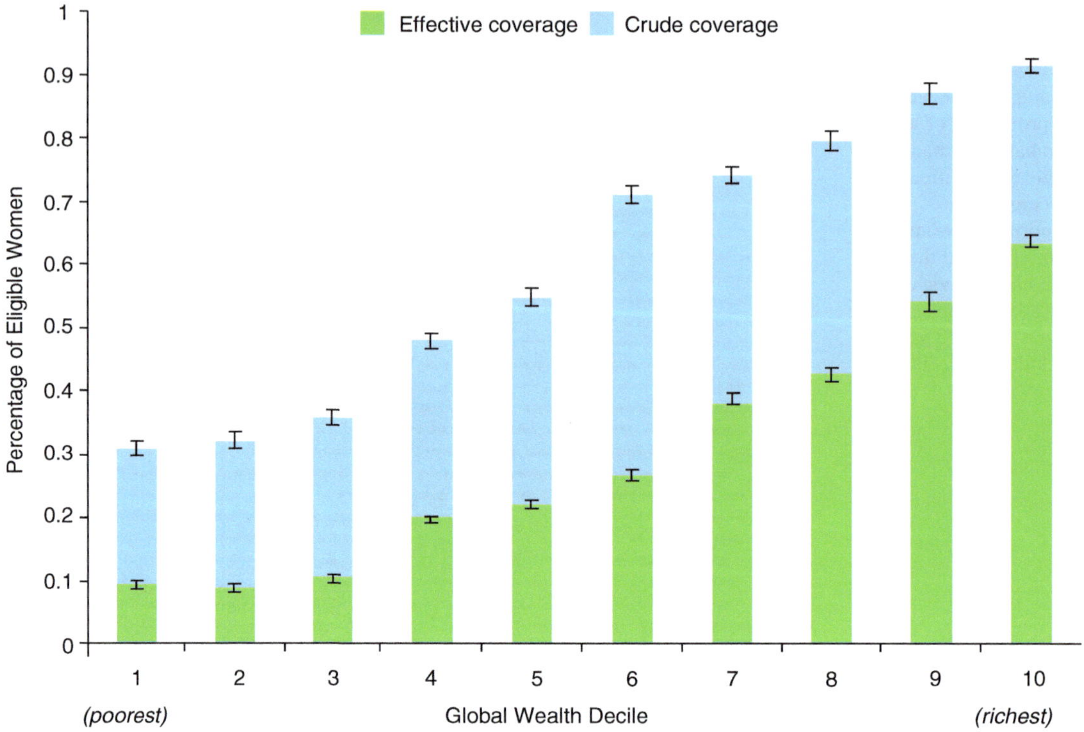

Fig. 17.12 Screening coverage by global wealth decile across 57 countries. Effective coverage is the proportion of women who report that they have had a pelvic exam as well as a Pap smear within the last 3 years. Crude coverage is the proportion of women who have ever had a pelvic exam (Gakidou et al. 2008)

secondary screening strategies (World Health Organization 2013).

The recommendations of the expert panel are as follows:

Use a strategy of screen with an HPV test and treat over a strategy of screen with VIA and treat. In resource-constrained settings, where screening with an HPV test is not feasible, the panel suggests a strategy of screening with VIA and treat.

Use a strategy of screen with an HPV test and treat over a strategy of screen with cytology followed by colposcopy (with or without biopsy) and treat. However, in countries where an appropriate/high-quality screening strategy with cytology followed by colposcopy already exists, either an HPV test or cytology followed by colposcopy could be used.

Use a strategy of screen with VIA and treat over a strategy of screen with cytology followed by colposcopy (with or without biopsy) and treat. The recommendation for VIA over cytology followed by colposcopy can be applied in countries that are currently considering either program or countries that currently have both programs available.

Use a strategy of screen with an HPV test and treat over a strategy of screen with an HPV test followed by colposcopy (with or without biopsy) and treat.

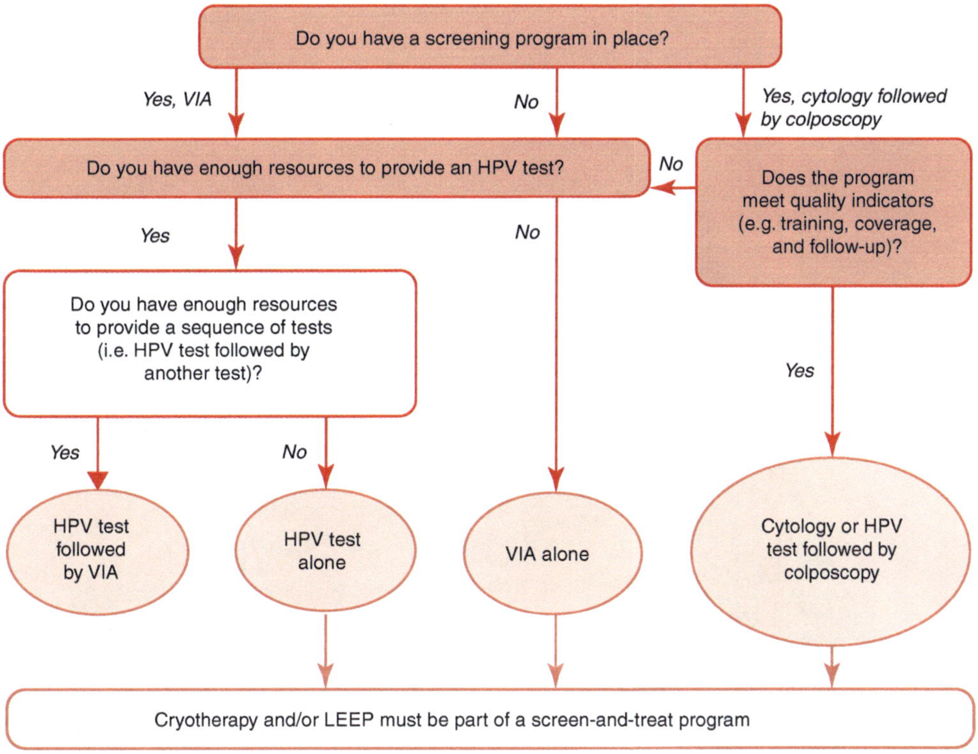

Fig. 17.13 Decision-making algorithm for program managers regarding the selection of an appropriate secondary cervical cancer screening program (World Health Organization 2013)

Use either a strategy of screen with an HPV test followed by VIA and treat or a strategy of screen with an HPV test and treat.

Use a strategy of screen with an HPV test followed by VIA and treat over a strategy of screen with VIA and treat.

Use a strategy of screen with an HPV test followed by VIA and treat over a strategy of screen with cytology followed by colposcopy (with or without biopsy) and treat.

Use a strategy of screen with an HPV test followed by VIA and treat over a strategy of screen with an HPV test followed by colposcopy (with or without biopsy) and treat.

In addition, a detailed algorithm for program managers is provided (Fig. 17.13).

In countries where cervical cancer is an endemic disease, all health personnel should be familiar with cervical cancer screening techniques. In medical schools, both theoretical and practical training have to be part of the curriculum, so that upon graduation, doctors will be capable to provide screening services (Fig. 17.14).

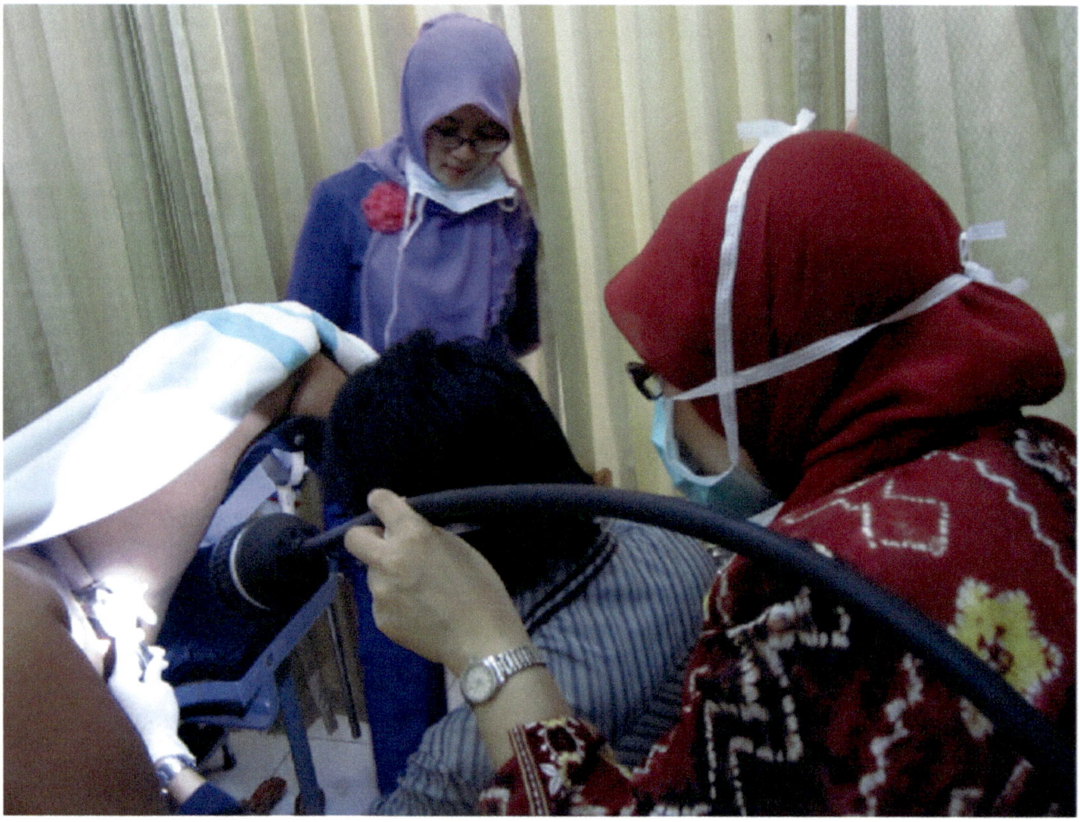

Fig. 17.14 Medical students from Muhammadiyah University, Yogyakarta, Indonesia, receiving practical teaching on visual screening for cervical neoplasia

17.3.3.1 Pap Test

The Pap test has been at the core of cervical screening efforts within the last 60 years.

At present, the Pap test can be considered the gold standard of cervical cancer screening. In fact, Pap test screening is the most effective screening strategy ever conceived for any cancer.

In comparison, to mammography screening for early detection of breast cancer, cytological screening does not only aim toward early detection of the disease in order to decrease mortality. Rather, most cervical cancer cases can be prevented through detection and treatment of precancers.

The reduction of cervical cancer incidence and mortality in many regions of the world is largely due to effective screening based on Pap smear testing.

However, there are a number of reasons why cytological screening cannot be implemented as the primary screening tool in a low-resource environment.

Cytology screening requires a large number of qualified Pap smear readers. These individuals need constant training and retraining as well as a comprehensive system of quality control. There does not exist a sufficient number of doctors trained as pathologists to provide these services. In sub-Saharan Africa, the lack of pathologists is most striking as documented by Adesina et al. (2013). These countries have at best one tenth of the pathology coverage compared to high-resource countries (Fig. 17.15). At the time of this survey, Tanzania had only 23 pathologists which corresponds to 1 pathologist per 1,877,739 people. Somalia did not have a single pathologist, and Benin, Burundi, Eritrea, Lesotho, Swaziland, and Gambia had only one pathologist each. Therefore, not even basic standards of cancer care can be upheld, let alone additional services provided such as cytological screening or the supervision of trained Pap smear readers.

As Pap smear screening is not feasible as a point of care procedure, slides need to be labeled, col-

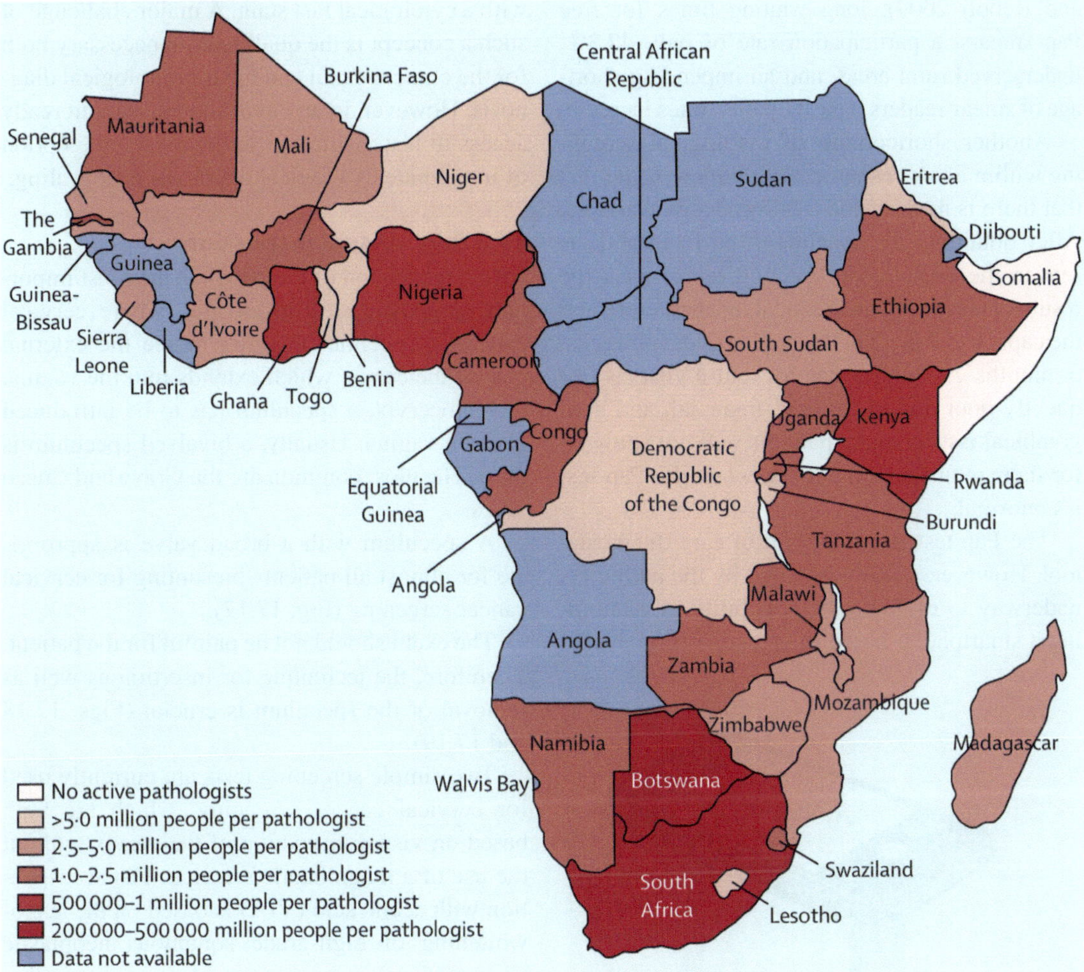

Fig. 17.15 Population per pathologist in sub-Saharan Africa (Adesina et al. 2013)

lected, and sent to a specialized facility. Therefore, a recall system is mandatory. Patients with abnormal test results need to be retested or further evaluated through colposcopy and biopsy. And all of these measures should be done in a timely manner. Thus, a sophisticated infrastructure is required with multiple visits of patients.

In a highly screened population such as Germany, the percentage of abnormal Pap smears will be very low. Marquardt et al. (2014) found a 1.58% positive rate including ASC-US. In contrast, Bayer (2011), who established a cytological screening program at the Ifisi Mission Hospital in the Southern Highlands of Tanzania, found a positive rate of 20–22% in the initial screening rounds. Overall, only 300 patients were screened. This means that every fifth patient screened cytologically would have to be recalled to undergo at least one further diagnostic step.

If HIV prevalence is high, the number of abnormal smears will also increase due to the higher prevalence of precancer and cancer and also because inflammatory changes and ASC-US diagnoses will become more frequent. In the study of Bayer (2011), up to 44% of HIV-positive women had abnormal Pap test results.

Despite these obstacles mentioned above, Malaysia succeeded in establishing a Pap smear-based cancer screening program. However, Malaysia still faces major challenges, making its cytological screening program less effective compared to high-resource countries (Othman and Rebolj 2009): long waiting times for free Pap smears, a participation rate of only 47.3%, underserved rural areas, and an impending shortage of smear-readers if participation rates increase.

Another shortcoming of cytological screening within a low-resource environment is the fact that there is no "see and treat" concept available. After obtaining the specimen, the fixed slide is sent to the pathologist who will report back the results. Depending on the local infrastructure and the capacity of the lab, this will take days, weeks, or months. As compliance for return visits is frequently poor due to cultural, financial, and geographical issues, many patients will not show up for their return appointments, when the Pap test is abnormal.

The Pap test is not a point of care diagnostic tool. However, a study initiated by the authors is underway to evaluate the feasibility of combining a smartphone-based microscope (Fig. 17.16) with a cytological fast stain. A major challenge of such a concept is the qualification necessary both for the clinical exam and the morphological diagnosis. However, in an environment without ready access to histopathological diagnosis, the option of immediate cytological diagnosis is appealing.

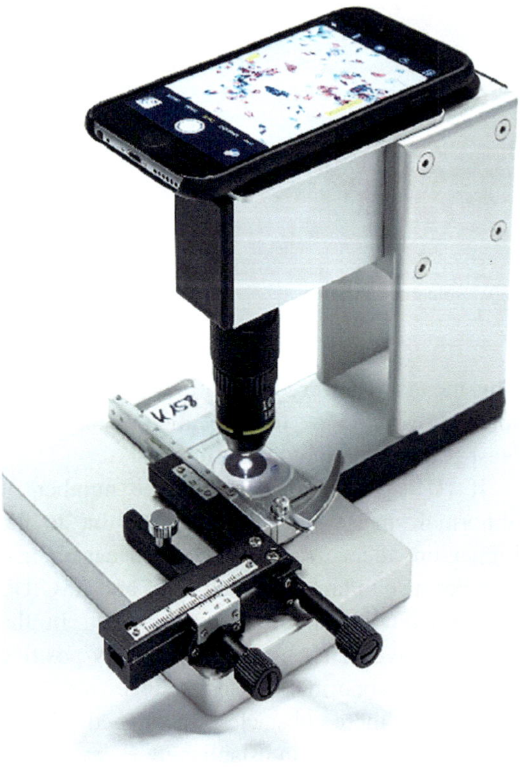

Fig. 17.16 A commercially available smartphone-based microscope (www.smartskope.com) has been modified to provide the stability and accuracy needed for cytopathological evaluation. The device is battery operated

17.3.3.2 Visual Inspection

Visual inspection of the cervix is the most important diagnostic step in an area where cervical cancer is endemic. In order to see the external part of the cervix which extends into the vagina, the ectocervix, a speculum has to be introduced into the vagina. Usually, a bivalved speculum is used. The most common are the Grave and Cusco types.

A speculum with a broad valve is appropriate for almost all patients presenting for cervical cancer screening (Fig. 17.17).

The exam should not be painful for the patient. Therefore, the technique for insertion as well as removal of the speculum is crucial (Figs. 17.18 and 17.19).

Two simple screening tests are currently used for cervical cancer screening, which are both based on visual inspection of the cervix without the use of a magnification device. Visual inspection with acetic acid (VIA) is based on the acetowhitening of high-grade squamous neoplastic tissue. Visual inspection with Lugol's iodine (VILI) identifies the yellow non-iodine uptake areas of the cervix and their relation to the transformation zone in order to define the subgroup of screening patients who might have high-grade precancer.

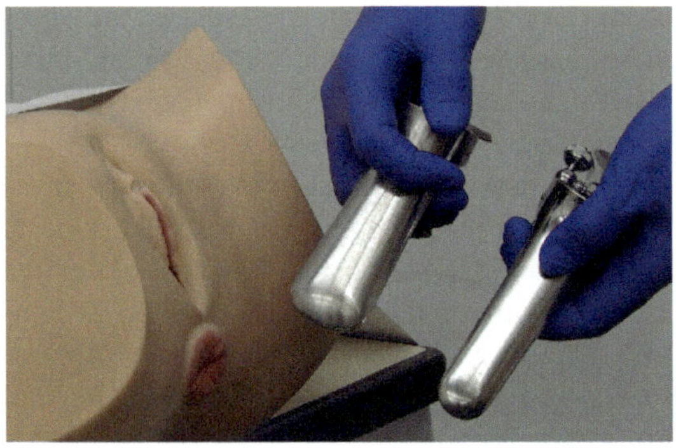

Fig. 17.17 A speculum with a broad valve (left) is preferable for optimal visualization of the external cervix

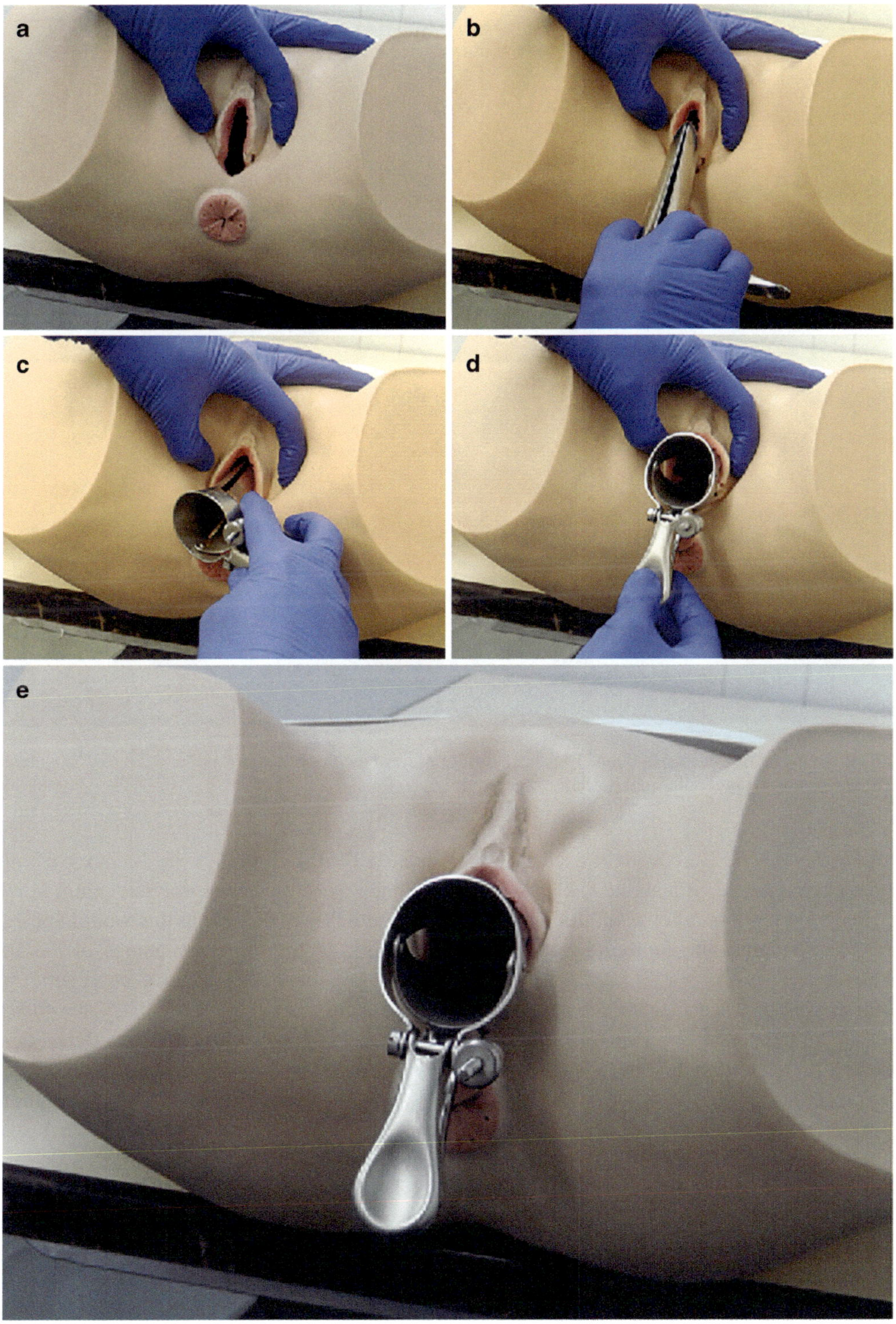

Fig. 17.18 Insertion of the Cusco speculum. The labia are spread sideways (**a**). As the vulvar opening has a vertical axis, the speculum is inserted accordingly, and pressure is applied posteriorly (**b**, **c**) as this area is less tender than the clitoral region of the vulva. The closed speculum is then rotated clockwise by 90° (**d**), opened and fixed by turning the screw (**e**). Then a visual inspection is performed without further need to adjust the speculum during the exam

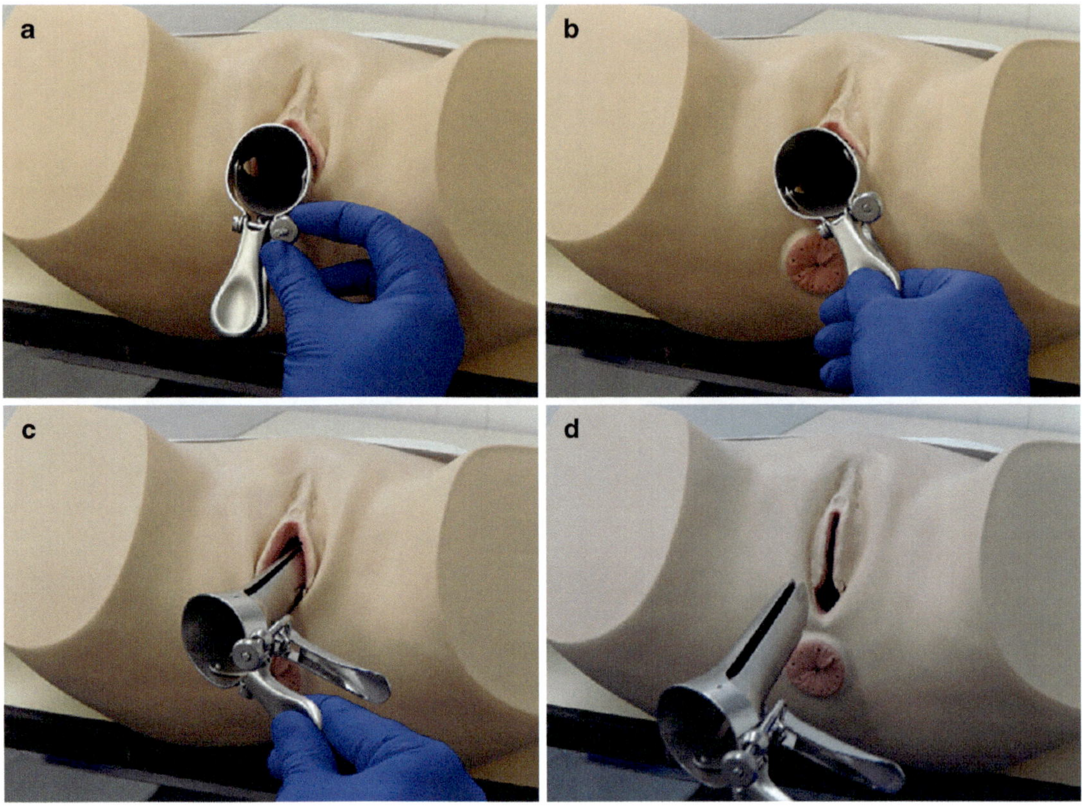

Fig. 17.19 Removal of Cusco speculum. The speculum is unscrewed completely (**a**) and turned by 90° counterclockwise (**b**) before removing it with light posterior pressure (**c**, **d**)

Both VIA and VILI are widely used in low-resource environments, as a single visit approach is feasible with treatment consisting of cryotherapy for those patients who are found to be VIA or VILI positive.

Both in rural Indonesia (Domingo et al. 2008) as well as in Tanzania (The United Republic of Tanzania 2011), VIA/VILI is the official cervical cancer prevention strategy.

17.3.3.2.1 Visual Inspection with Acetic Acid (VIA)

Rationale and Effectiveness of VIA

For a long time, researchers from India have been active in the search for effective cervical cancer prevention strategies. According to Shastri et al. (2014), 23% of all cervical cancer patients worldwide are from India with 123,000 new cases diagnosed every year and 67,000 cervical cancer-related deaths. Initially, the Indian government planned to adopt Pap smear screening; however, India quickly realized that this would not be feasible due to the huge percentage of the Indian population that needs to be screened with limited health-care resources. Also, a single, once in a lifetime Pap smear does not lead to a reduction of cervical cancer mortality (Sankaranarayanan et al. 2009). Therefore, visual inspection of the cervix using acetic acid has been studied extensively.

The pivotal study on VIA screening in India was published by Surendra Shastri from the Tata Memorial Hospital in Mumbai in 2014 (Shastri et al. 2014). In this prospective randomized study, 75,360 women were screened by VIA and compared to 76,178 women who served as controls. Patients were between 34 and 64 years of age. In accordance with limited personnel resources, all VIA exams were performed by primary health-care workers who underwent 4 weeks of training. VIA screening was performed every 2 years, as a previous study by Sankaranarayanan et al. (2009) had already demonstrated that a single VIA examination does not reduce cancer mortality. Therefore, four rounds of screening were done every 2 years followed by monitoring for disease every 2 years thereafter with a total follow-up of 12 years. At the completion of follow-up, cervical cancer mortality was down 31% in the screening group compared to the control group. Shastri et al. concluded that biannual VIA screening could prevent 22,000 cancer deaths annually in India and 72,600 cancer deaths worldwide in resource-poor environments.

This study by Shastri et al. has raised considerable ethical concerns because of its prospective randomized design (Suba 2016; Bagcchi 2014; Labani & Astana 2014). "No screening" was considered the standard of care, thus accepting a considerable number of women dying from cervical cancer: 254 women in unscreened control groups from several Indian cervical cancer prevention trials have died of the disease. Suba (2016) concludes his critique by saying: *"You can't let people die to show something you already know."*

In their response, Sankaranarayanan et al. (2014) state: *"We reiterate that our studies conducted in India by Indian scientists and clinicians are of the highest order of scientific and ethical merit and we completely refute the said allegations."* The authors argue that in the year 2000, when these trials were initiated, it was unknown whether these screening strategies would lead to a significant reduction of cancer mortality. Definitely, future trial designs will need to take into account that the standard of care has changed by now (Sankaranarayanan et al. 2014).

In 2012, the World Health Organization published the results of a VIA/cryotherapy demonstration project conducted in six sub-Saharan countries (World Health Organization 2012). Overall, 19,579 patients were screened. VIA positivity was 10.1% ranging from 5.7% to 28.0% (Table 17.1).

Two hundred forty-three patients (12.3%) did not fulfill the eligibility criteria for cryotherapy as the lesion extended into the cervical canal or was located at the vaginal wall. Of 1737 women (87.7%) fulfilling eligibility criteria, cryotherapy was performed in 1058 patients (60.9%).

Table 17.1 VIA test results in six sub-Saharan countries (World Health Organization 2012)

	Total number of women screened	Number of VIA-positive women
Tanzania	5390	524 (9.7%)
Malawi	1221	151 (12.4%)
Zambia	1381	386 (28.0%)
Nigeria	5529	317 (5.7%)
Uganda	2312	180 (7.8%)
Madagascar	3746	422 (11.3%)
Total	19,579	1980 (10.1%)

In Tanzania, Ngoma et al. (2010) evaluated cervical cancer screening by visual inspection (n = 10,378). All patients in this study underwent colposcopy. Biopsies were obtained if colposcopy was abnormal. Compared to this standard, VIA sensitivity for CIN2+ diagnosis was 60.6% (95% CI 42.1–77.1%), and specificity was 98.2% (95% CI 97.9–98.4%). The respective results for sensitivity of VILI were higher than for VIA (see below). The Tanzanian screening study clearly illustrates the scope of the problem: out of 10,378 women screened, the diagnosis of invasive cervical cancer was several times higher than the diagnosis of CIN2+: 200 (1.9%) versus 33 (0.32%).

For Indonesia, Vet et al. (2012) documented screening results of 22,040 women (33.9% from Jakarta, 36.3% from Tasikmalaya in West Java, and 29% from the Island of Bali). Screening was performed by trained medical doctors using VIA. If VIA was positive, biopsies were obtained, and the patient was treated immediately with cryotherapy. VIA was positive in 4.4% of women. The positive predictive value of VIA for CIN2+ was 29.7% with a specificity of 98.1%. The prevalence of CIN2+ lesions was 1.15% and of invasive cancer 0.18%.

The effectiveness of VIA is not undisputed. However, even colposcopy screening is inferior to Pap test screening. VIA screening uses the same principle as colposcopy, i.e., the effect of a 5% solution of acetic acid on preneoplastic tissue, however without magnification and without histological diagnosis. Ajenifuja et al. (2013) did

Table 17.2 Strengths and limitations of VIA and HPV testing (Silkensen et al. 2018)

VIA strengths	VIA limitations
Affordable; low per-capita screening costs	High inter-operator variability
Point-of-care results; treatment or referral decisions can be taken in the some visit	Problematic sensitivity, especially for older women with endocervical lesions
Useful for downstaging of cancers in previously unscreened women	Need for investments in high-intensity quality assurance efforts
HPV testing strengths	**HPV testing limitations**
Point-of-care testing or centralized testing, dependent on testing platform and local needs	Majority of HPV infections (especially in young women) are transient and clinically non-significant
Simplicity and potential scalability of self-collection of samples	Lack of specificity for precancer
Reproducible results; not rater-dependent	Higher per-capita tests costs than VIA
Economical due to longer screening intervals possible for HPV-negative women	

a study on VIA for cervical screening in rural Nigeria, calling into question the reproducibility of VIA. Seven health-care workers with a 2-year experience were retrained for 2 weeks using the IARC manual (Sankaranarayanan and Wesley 2003). Subsequently, VIA screening results were monitored for these seven individuals and showed a wide range of VIA diagnoses, thus questioning the reliability and reproducibility of VIA within this setting.

Rodriguez et al. (2004) found that VIA, or rather VIA using twofold magnification (VIAM), is not effective when cytological and/or HPV screening is already established. When patients were screened 5 years after they had had negative cytological results and a negative HPV test, VIAM was not sensitive enough to detect incident high-grade dysplasia.

In Indonesia, where presently visual inspection with acetic acid is considered the screening method of choice, a statistical modeling study (Setiawan et al. 2016) showed that the combination of VIA and HPV screening reduces the incidence of cervical cancer by 58.5% compared to a reduction of only 7.9% through VIA. In absolute numbers, this corresponds to 25 cancer deaths per 100,000 prevented by VIA and 98 deaths prevented by the combined strategy.

Silkensen et al. (2018) come to the conclusion that in the near future cervical cancer screening in a low-resource environment will shift from visual inspection with acetic acid to screening through a molecular marker, presently HPV analysis. These tests will be based on the platform of an already established VIA program.

A unique advantage of HPV screening is self-sampling offering an alternative option to women who might otherwise not participate in cervical cancer screening.

A major problem of VIA screening is the so-called scale-up challenge. On one hand, efforts of scaling up an already established screening program remains a major goal. On the other hand, this requires significant resources for quality assurance including the recruitment and training and continuous retraining of providers (Silkensen et al. 2018).

Table 17.2 summarizes the strengths and limitations of VIA and HPV screening according to Silkensen et al. (2018).

According to WHO guidelines, VIA screening should be replaced by HPV screening as soon as the necessary infrastructure and funding are available (World Health Organization 2014a, b). Nevertheless, VIA screening is the first step toward cervical cancer screening for developing countries with a high prevalence of cervical cancer.

As Sankaranarayanan et al. (2015) state: *"Despite all its limitations, implementation of VIA screening in LMICs[2] will facilitate the building up of infrastructure and human resources that may facilitate the introduction of affordable HPV tests in future."*

[2]LMICs = low- and middle-income countries.

Practice of VIA

One of the major advantages of visual screening is the fact that it does not necessarily have to be performed by physicians but can be done by healthcare professionals such as nurses and midwives or specifically trained personnel. For effective visual screening, continuous training is crucial.

For the Tanzanian study performed by Ngoma et al. (2010), the IARC manual (Sankaranarayanan and Wesley 2003) was used as the basis for a 5-day training program including lectures and discussion of photographs of VIA/VILI-positive and VIA/VILI-negative cases as well as practical training on volunteers. The test positive rate for VIA (3.8%) and VILI (4.8%) fluctuated throughout the study period. Peaks of test positivity were seen immedi-

- For VIA screening, the following items are required/recommended:
  - Examination table with stirrups.
  - Any table that can be used as an improvised examination table.
  - Light source.
  - Ideally a battery-operated LED light source is used which has a very low energy consumption. A headlamp is preferable to a flashlight (Figs. 17.20 and 17.21).
  - Sterile specula (Cusco or Grave).
  - Examination gloves.
  - Cotton swabs.
  - Acetic acid 5%.

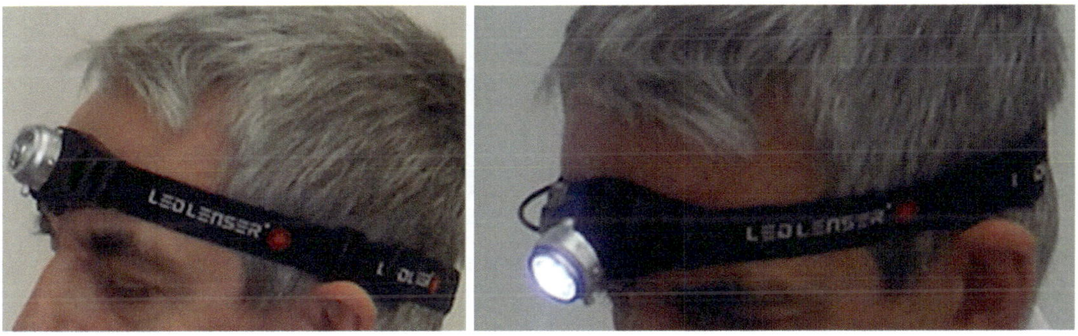

Fig. 17.20 A headlamp with battery-saving LED bulbs that can be tilted is preferable to a flashlight, as it leaves both hands free for examination

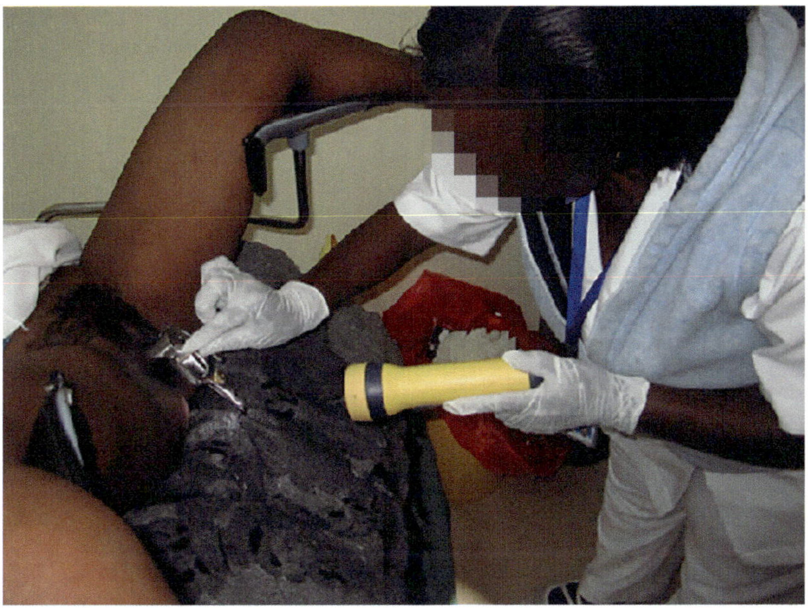

Fig. 17.21 VIA using a flashlight. After insertion of the speculum, 5% acetic acid is applied to the cervix and visual inspection performed using a flashlight

Acetic acid can be freshly prepared by adding 5 mL of glacial acetic acid into 95 mL of distilled water. However, careless handling of the concentrated acid may lead to injury of the skin. Furthermore, application of the undiluted solution to the cervix and vagina has severe consequences. The National Alert Network (NAN) operated by the American Institute for Safe Medication Practices issued a warning[3] on the use of glacial acetic acid as it had been mistakenly applied topically in four instances without dilution, resulting in severe burns and permanent scarring (Network 2013). Consequently, NAN recommends to remove glacial acetic acid from stock and clearly states: *"Glacial acetic acid has no use in its current form in clinical medicine."*

Alternatively, vinegar available from grocery stores can be used (Fig. 17.22).

However, not all brands of clear vinegar are suitable. A concentration of 5% must be ensured without any other ingredients such as salt. The brands available in Tanzania (Fig. 17.23) are summarized in Table 17.3.

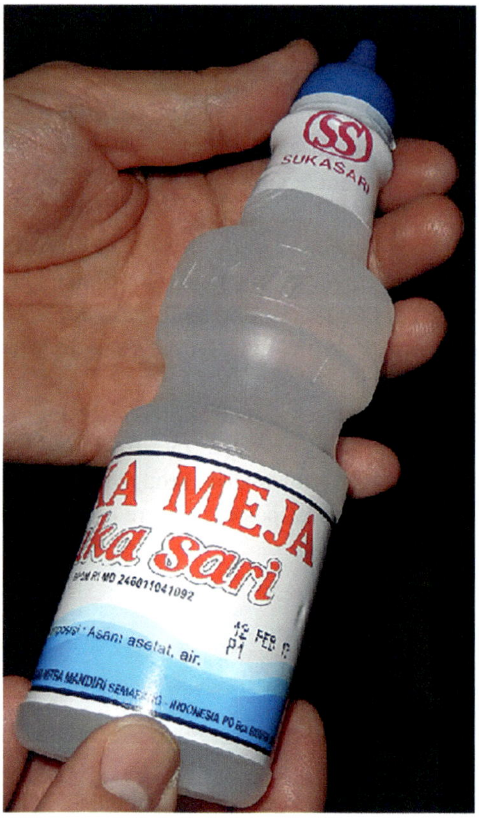

Fig. 17.22 "Cuka meja" or table vinegar as used for cooking in Indonesia for visual screening (VIA)

- VIA screening is done as follows:
  1. (Written) informed consent is obtained from the patient.
  2. The patient's history including the gynecologic and obstetric history is obtained.
  3. The HIV status is documented or the appropriate tests are performed.
  4. The patient is placed in a lithotomy position.
  5. The vulva and the perineal and anal areas are inspected for ulcerations, warts, or any other abnormalities.
  6. The speculum is moistened using clean water or normal saline and carefully introduced into the vagina.
  7. Possible bleeding and the characteristics of the vaginal discharge are noted.
  8. 5% acetic acid is liberally applied to the cervix and upper vagina, and the vaginal mucus is gently wiped off as much as possible.
  9. The cervical os is identified as well as the transformation zone and squamocolumnar junction if visible.
  10. VIA positivity is evaluated 1 min after the application of the acetic acid.

[3]https://www.ismp.org/NAN/files/20130121.pdf.

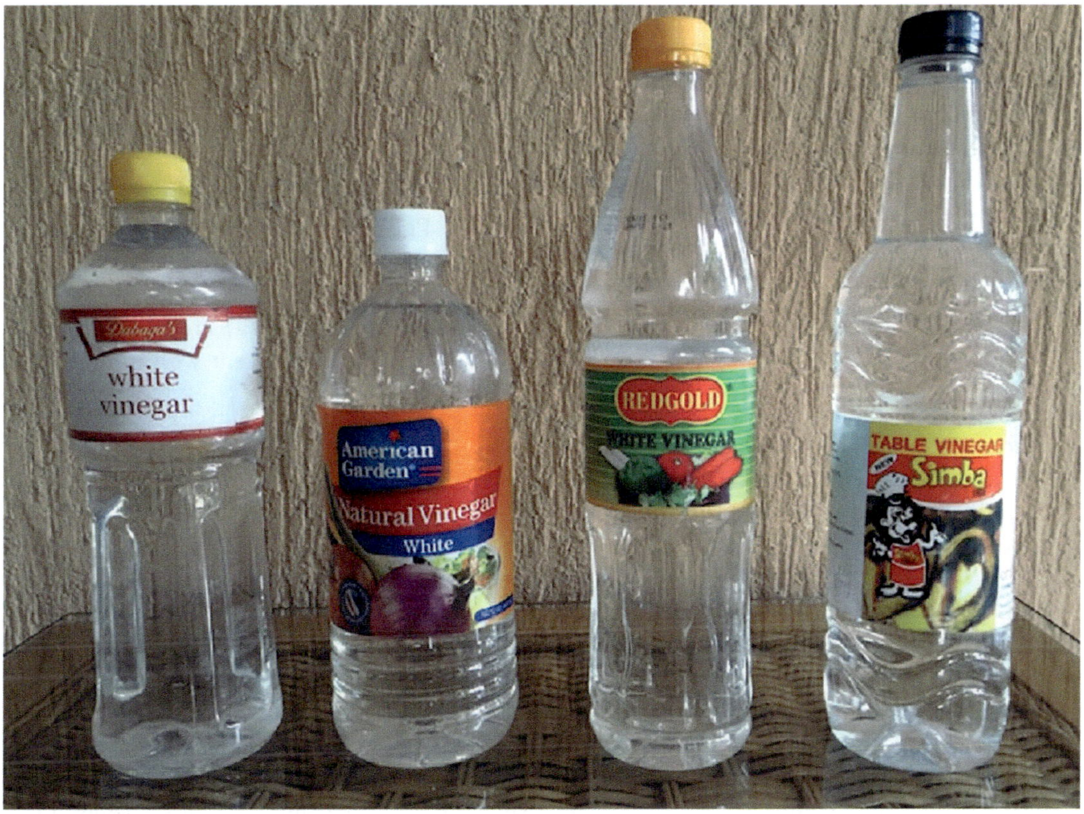

Fig. 17.23 Different brands of table vinegar available in Tanzania

Table 17.3 Properties of different brands of table vinegar in Tanzania. The American Garden brand ("Simba") is the most appropriate for use in visual screening

	Manufacturer	Contents	Size	Price
				Tanzanian shillings
Dabaga	Tanzania	4%	930 mL	1600
		+ salt		
American Garden	USA	5%	946 mL	6800
Redgold	Tanzania	No concentration given	965 mL	1500
Simba	Tanzania	No concentration given	1000 mL	1500

It is best to decide after the application of acetic acid whether the squamocolumnar junction is visible or not, as this cannot be reliably done, when the surface of the cervix is partially or completely obscured by cervical mucus or vaginal secretions.

When teaching visual inspection of the cervix, particular emphasis should be placed on the technique of speculum insertion and removal in order to optimally visualize the cervix and vagina as well as to minimize the discomfort to the patient.

Cervical screening programs performing VIA (or any other method) frequently integrate breast examination, as breast cancer is one of the most common cancers in women. However, in contrast to cervical cancer screening, there is no evidence that clinical breast examination (inspection and palpation) and breast self-examination significantly reduce breast cancer mortality, neither in countries with routine mammography screening nor within a low-resource environment (Nelson et al. 2009).

In 2011, the Tanzanian Ministry of Health and Social Welfare has established service delivery guidelines for cervical cancer prevention (The United Republic of Tanzania 2011). In this chapter, these guidelines will be used to illustrate how VIA can be integrated into a screening program with a very high frequency of cervical cancer. The Tanzanian guidelines state: *"VIA, combined with immediate treatment of precancerous lesions with cryotherapy in a single visit approach, will be the secondary prevention strategy used in Tanzania."*

Target Population

The target age group is 30–50 years of age. For Tanzania, this translates into an absolute number of 3.9 million women to be screened or 3.19 million women, if a coverage of 80% is attained (numbers projected for the year 2010). On request, younger or older women are screened also after counseling. Tanzania plans to eventually expand its target population to 25–59 years.

Women who previously underwent total hysterectomy due to benign conditions such as fibroids do not require screening.

For HIV-infected women, there is no age limit. Women who test HIV positive should be screened regardless of age once they have been sexually active with a yearly interval regardless of test results.

In women with negative screening results and no significant risk factors, screening may be stopped at the age of 59. Postmenopausal women may be screened using the Pap test.

VIA-Negative Patients

- VIA negativity is defined as any of the following findings (Sankaranarayanan and Wesley 2003):
  - No acetowhite lesions on the cervix
  - Polyps that protrude from the cervical canal
  - Nabothian cysts
  - Smooth acetowhite areas, which are partially transparent with ill-defined margins
  - Smooth acetowhite areas with well-defined or indefinite margins detached from the squamocolumnar junction (satellite lesions)

Cervical ectopy, atrophy, or inflammation may complicate cervical assessment.

Cervical ectopy is a physiological condition in which the columnar epithelium protrudes from the cervical canal and may cover large portions (Fig. 17.24) or the entire ectocervix (Figs. 17.25 and 17.26). The columnar epithelium does not always undergo metaplasia and will therefore not be acetowhite. Exposed columnar epithelium may bleed on touch and further complicate differential diagnosis to invasive disease.

VIA-negative patients are followed-up every 3 years. HIV-positive women are followed yearly. If patients are VIA negative on three con-

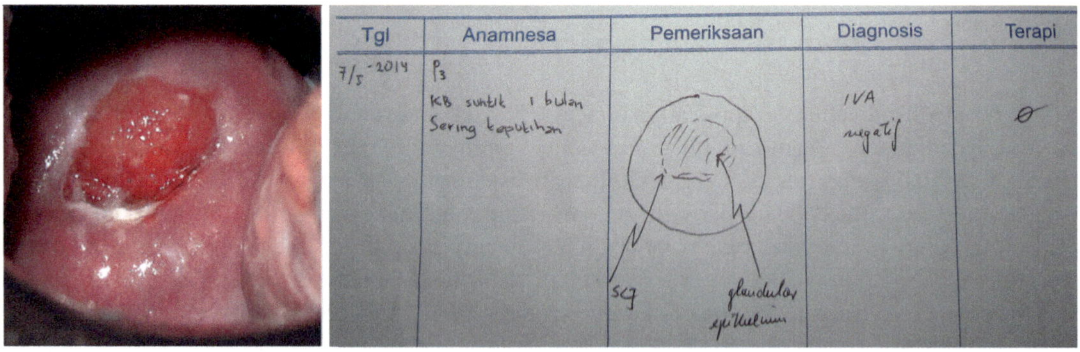

Fig. 17.24 Cervical ectopy covering the anterior (ventral) aspect of the cervix. A 48-year-old woman presented for screening at PKU Muhammadiyah Pakem hospital in Central Java, Indonesia, complaining of white discharge starting 1 month ago. This constitutes a normal finding (VIA negative)

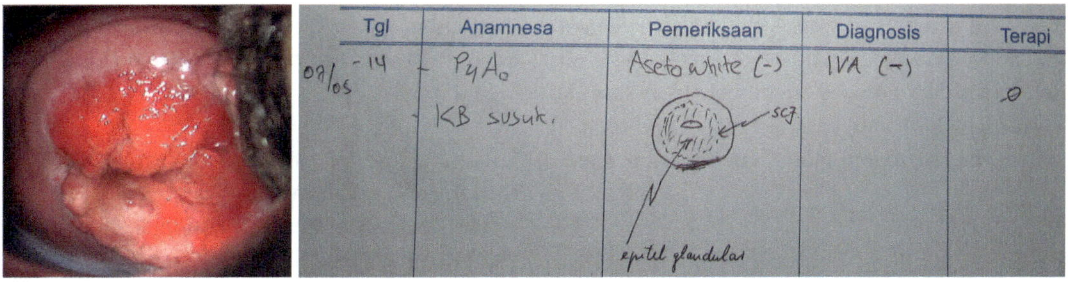

Fig. 17.25 Cervical ectopy of the entire ectocervix. A 40-year-old woman presented for screening at PKU Muhammadiyah Pakem hospital in Central Java, Indonesia. There is discrete acetowhitening of the right dorsal quadrant from immature metaplasia. According to colposcopy nomenclature, this would be a "minor change" and regarded as VIA negative

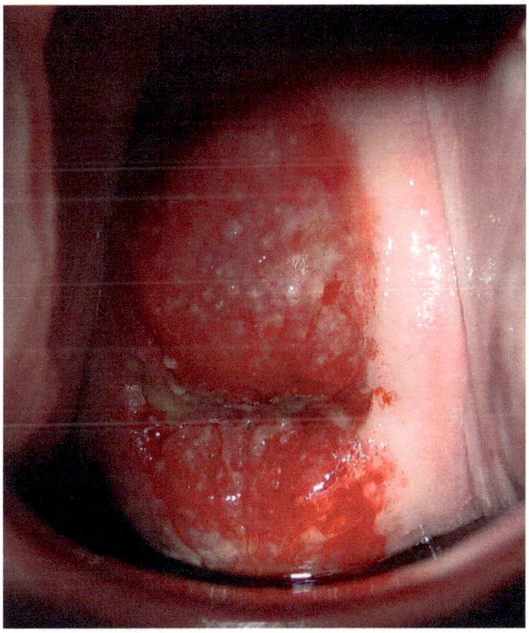

Fig. 17.26 Cervical ectopy with partial transformation and pronounced vessels which are bleeding on touch (VIA negative). A 38-year-old woman presented for screening at Kulon Progo in Central Java, Indonesia. On VIA, invasive cancer cannot be ruled out

secutive visits, the screening interval may also be extended to 3 years.

However, the Tanzanian guidelines correctly state that high coverage rates of more than 80% are more important to the success of the cervical cancer prevention program than a high screening frequency of individual patients.

VIA-Positive Patients

- VIA positivity is defined as any of the following findings (modified; Sankaranarayanan and Wesley 2003):
  - Any intensely white areas which are opaque with well-defined margins close to the squamocolumnar junction and/or close to the cervical os
  - Condyloma and leukoplakia close to the squamocolumnar junction

Patients with VIA-positive findings are counseled and preferably treated on the same day with cryosurgery ("screen and treat") or LEEP.

According to the Johns Hopkins Program for International Education in Gynecology and Obstetrics (JHPIEGO),[4] 7405 women were entered into screening programs performed in Tanzania between April 2010 and September 2012. A total

[4]www.jhpiego.com.

of 532 women (7.2%) were found to be VIA positive, and 414 women who were cryotherapy eligible received same-day treatment. In Indonesia, JHPIEGO claims to have screened and treated (single-visit approach) more than 50,000 women.

Suspicious for Cancer

- On visual inspection, overt cervical cancer usually presents with one of three characteristics or a combination thereof:
  - Tissue defect (ulceration), both small (a few millimeters in diameter) and large (destroying the entire cervix as well as part of the vagina)
  - Abnormal growth of tissue (exophytic, papillary, or cauliflower-like), which may also encompass the entire cervix and upper vagina
  - A pronounced asymmetry, e.g., between the anterior and the posterior part of the cervix

Microinvasive cervical carcinoma cannot be reliably diagnosed by visual inspection but will most likely be diagnosed as HSIL/VIA positive. Even if not diagnosed correctly, microinvasive disease might still be treated successfully with cryosurgery or LEEP.

If there is any suspicion of cancer on VIA, invasion should be confirmed or ruled out by cervical biopsies.

Squamocolumnar Junction Not Visible/ Atrophy and Inflammation

If the squamocolumnar junction is not visible, the Tanzanian guidelines recommend Pap smear screening instead of VIA. However, it should be noted that this poses several problems. Apart from the costs and lack of high-capacity Pap smear screening facilities and the low number of pathologists in Tanzania, visualization of the squamocolumnar junction will be difficult to perform without the aid of a colposcope, especially if no acetic acid is applied prior to the inspection of the cervix.

Furthermore, in many instances a major change (type 2) lesion may be seen on VIA exam that partially extends beyond the cervical os. Without evidence of invasive disease, these patients would benefit from local treatment such as LEEP.

Atrophy of the cervix may also complicate VIA (Figs. 17.27, 17.28, and 17.29). The identification of CIN2+ disease is more difficult in older patients, especially in postmenopause, as the squamocolumnar junction is usually not visible. Although atrophy will not be confused with cancer, intracervical manifestations of cancer can not be diagnosed at an early stage.

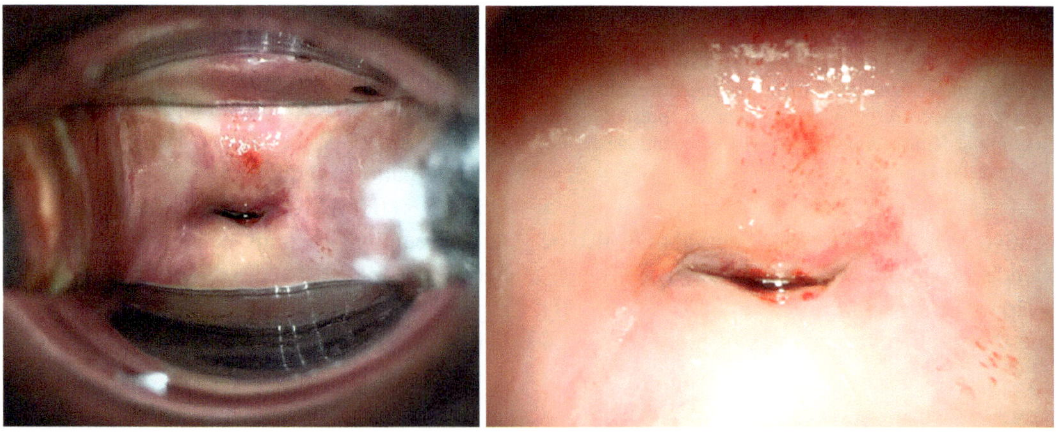

Fig. 17.27 Atrophy. The squamocolumnar junction is not visible. The patient is 70 years old and HIV negative. She presented for cervical cancer screening at META Referral Hospital, Mbeya, Tanzania. Although she is not part of the target population, visual screening is done on all patients who present to any of the Tanzanian screening centers

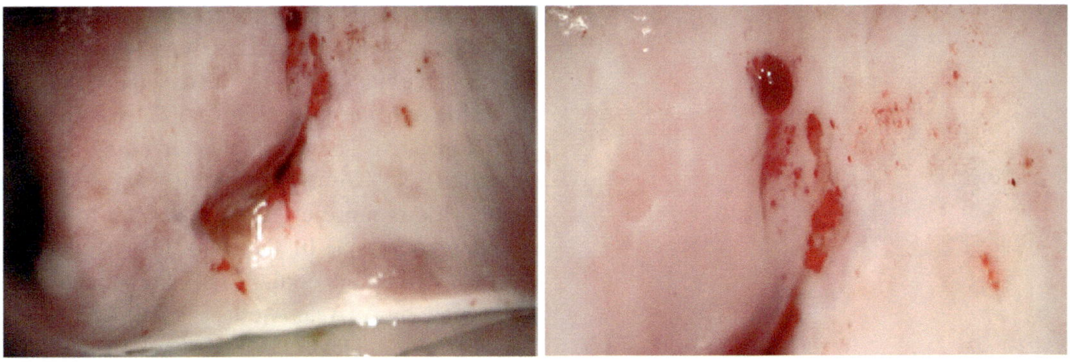

Fig. 17.28 Atrophy with petechial bleeding after application of acetic acid. The squamocolumnar junction is not visible. The 53-year-old patient is HIV positive and complained of lower back pain. She presented for screening at META Referral Hospital, Mbeya, Tanzania. Visual inspection is unsatisfactory in this patient. A Pap smear was obtained and found to be normal (Fig. 17.29)

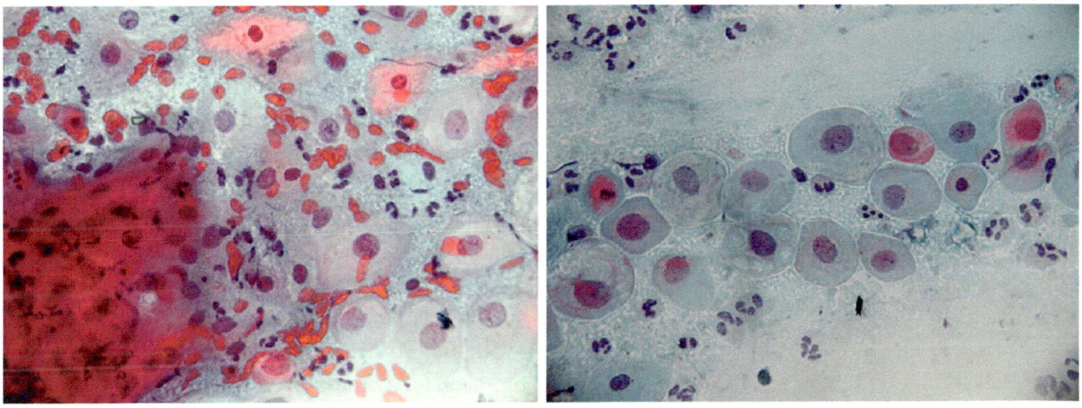

Fig. 17.29 Normal Pap smear with atrophy with parabasal cells (see Fig. 17.28)

Patients with inflammatory changes (cervicitis) may present with copious yellowish/greenish discharge, a swollen diffusely red cervix, or a strawberry-like pattern of the squamous epithelium due to tiny abrasions (Figs. 17.30, 17.31, and 17.32). Inflammation frequently occurs, if a high percentage of patients is HIV positive. With the exception of HPV-based screening programs, this will interfere with the accuracy of both VIA and Pap test. The respective screening tests should be repeated 2–4 weeks following antibiotic treatment. Unfortunately, in Tanzania no local antibiotics that can be applied directly to the vagina and cervix are available. This frequently leads to overtreatment with widespread use of broad spectrum antibiotics in the absence of pelvic inflammatory disease.

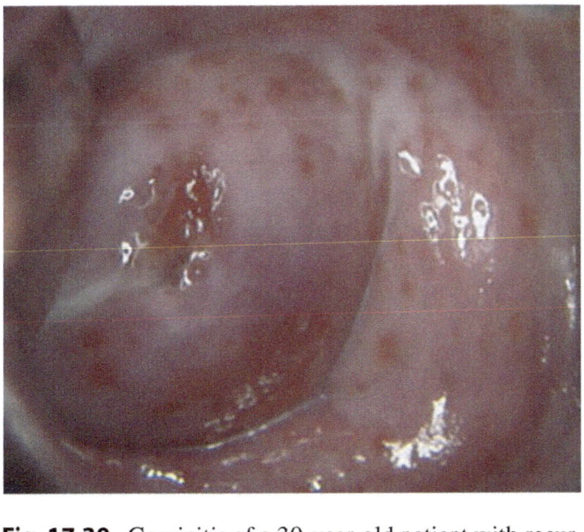

Fig. 17.30 Cervicitis of a 30-year-old patient with recurrent fungal infections

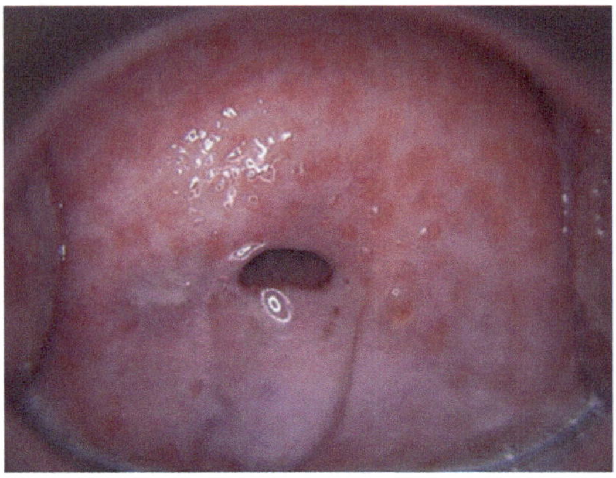

Fig. 17.31 Cervicitis

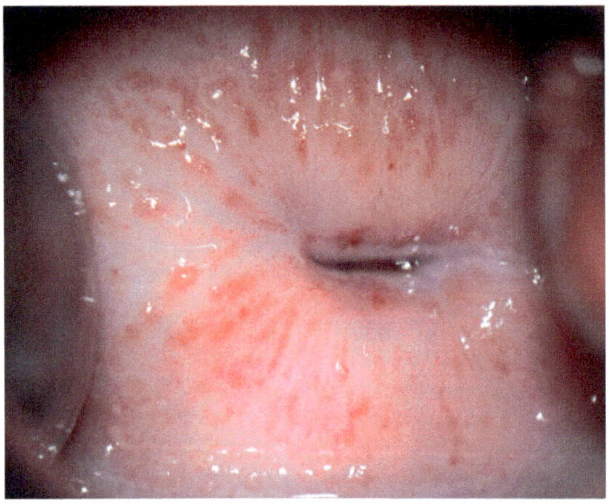

Fig. 17.32 Cervicitis as well as atrophy. A 34-year-old HIV-positive patient complaining of irregular menstrual bleeding presented to the cervical cancer screening unit at META Referral Hospital, Mbeya, Tanzania

17.3.3.2.2 Visual Inspection with Lugol's Iodine (VILI)

VILI is another visual test that involves staining of the cervix with Lugol's iodine. Normal cells take up the iodine stain and appear a mahogany brown, whereas precancerous cervical lesions appear yellow.

Rationale and Effectiveness of VILI

In colposcopy, the application of Lugol's solution (Schiller's test) is mostly used as an add-on after inspection of the cervix and vagina subsequent to acetic acid. Prior to surgery, Lugol's solution is most useful to outline the area that needs to be treated and to identify healthy non-dysplastic tissue that needs to be spared. However, Lugol's solution may also be used as the basis of a stand-alone screening test using the naked eye only.

Although interpretation of VILI-positive and VILI-negative lesions might not be as straightforward as VIA evaluation, there is evidence that VILI is more effective than VIA in detecting preneoplasia. In the Tanzanian study conducted by Ngoma et al. (2010), all patients were screened by VIA as well as VILI, and results were blinded. Of 33 HSIL cases, VIA and VILI detected 20 CIN2+ cases (61%) and missed 2 cases (6%). VILI detected 11 cases (33%) that were missed by VIA, whereas none of the CIN2/CIN3 lesions diagnosed by VIA were missed by VILI. Sensitivity of VILI was superior to VIA: 93.9% versus 60.6%, respectively.

In a comprehensive meta-analysis by Fokom-Domgue et al. (2015) comparing the two methods, VILI was significantly more sensitive than VIA for the diagnosis of preneoplastic diseases of the cervix (95.1% versus 87.2%). However, the meta-analysis had been limited to studies conducted in sub-Saharan countries.

Large studies comparing the impact of VILI screening on cervical cancer mortality are not yet available, so at present, no definite conclusions on the effectiveness of VILI can be drawn.

Practice of VILI

- Sankaranarayanan and Wesley (2003) give the following instructions for the preparation of a 5% solution:
  - Dissolve 10 g of potassium iodide in 100 mL distilled water.
  - Add 5 g of iodine after the potassium iodide is fully dissolved.
  - Stir well until all the iodine flakes have fully dissolved.

Lugol's iodine is kept in a tightly closed brown glass bottle and can be stored for up to 1 month.

In Sankaranarayanan and Wesley's (2003) manual on visual screening, VIA and VILI are treated equally. The material and procedure required for examination and preparation of the patient including informed consent, positioning of the patient, external examination, speculum exam, etc., are identical to the VIA exam. Lugol's iodine is then applied to the cervix using a cotton swab. The solution should be handled carefully as its stains will be difficult to remove. As with acetic acid, it is applied liberally onto the cervix as well as the upper vagina. Excess fluid is removed with a dry cotton swab.

As a rule, dark brown areas which are called Lugol positive are not dysplastic or neoplastic. All other areas that are Lugol negative are carefully noted. These areas will either be pale, whitish, or yellow. For interpretation of VILI, the position of these areas in relation to the transformation zone and the squamocolumnar junction is important.

As with VIA, the result of the exam may be:

- VILI negative
- VILI positive
- Suspicious for cancer
- Squamocolumnar junction not visible/inflammatory changes.

The definition of VILI-positive and VILI-negative is more complex compared to VIA. VILI is considered positive, if thick yellow iodine-negative areas are seen with well-defined borders. These must be located within the transformation adjacent to the squamocolumnar junction. If the squamocolumnar junction is not visible, the iodine non-uptake area should be close to the cervical os. If the entire cervix is iodine negative and densely yellow, this may also considered VILI positive.

The following findings are to be interpreted as VILI negative:

- The squamous epithelium turns black or dark brown, whereas the columnar epithelium does not take up the iodine solution.
- Patches of unstained or light brown areas are seen with poorly defined borders.
- A leopard skin pattern, which may be a sign of inflammation.
- Several small iodine-negative areas which are further away from the squamocolumnar junction or one or several larger lesions forming more complex patterns having clearly defined margins. Again these lesions are far away from the squamocolumnar junction.

17.3.3.2.3 Alternative Colposcopy Devices

Although colposcopy is not recommended for screening, several investigators have been trying to enhance VIA through portable devices that provide a low magnification of around 4×. One of these instruments, the Muenster Colposcopic Magnification Device (Lellé 2007), has already been discussed (Chap. 7). Below, some of these devices are presented that may be useful in future screening settings.

The Gynocular® is a portable monocular colposcope, which provides 5×, 8×, and 12× resolutions (Nessa et al. 2014; Ngonzi et al. 2013) (Fig. 17.33).

Through the widespread use of affordable high-performance smartphones, which are constantly improved, new options are available to document colposcopic images. Using standard hardware and software, good-quality colposcopic images can be obtained (Fig. 17.34).

Yeates et al. (2016) studied VIA enhanced by smartphone cervicography (SEVIA = smartphone enhanced VIA) on 1072 Tanzanian women. Examination was done by five nonphysician providers who received feedback by expert viewers within minutes, so that within 1 month,

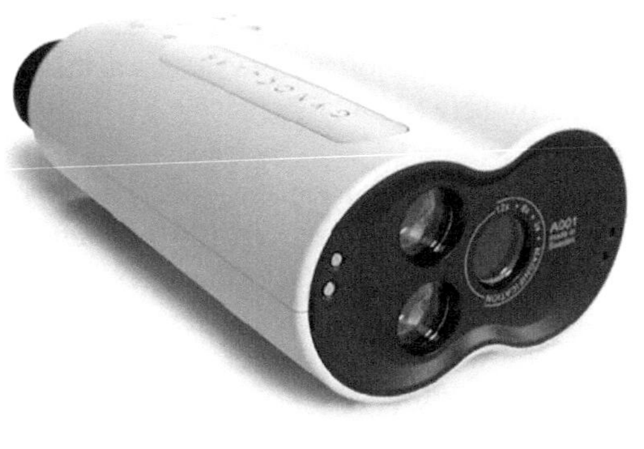

Fig. 17.33 Gynocular®, a portable monocular colposcopic device with resolutions of up to 12×

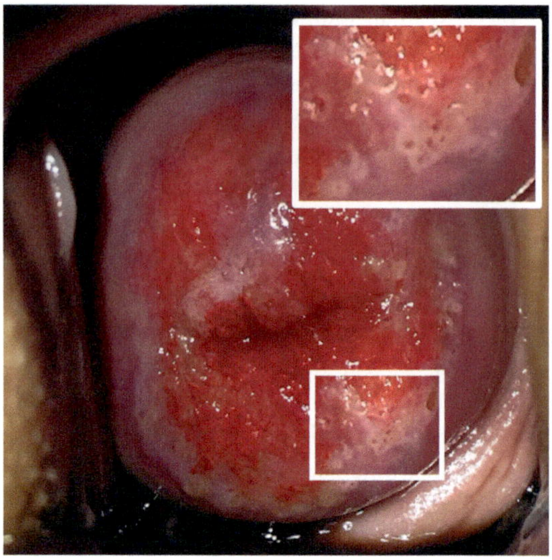

Fig. 17.34 Smartphone image of the cervix (major change within a large atypical transformation zone). The original image has been recorded in the Tagged Image File Format (TIFF) which is a lossless graphics format (file size: 6.3 MB). An iPhone 6 plus has been used with the "Camera+" app (www.cameraplus.com), as the settings can be optimized for colposcopic photography

the agreement rate between providers and experts was 97%. Several smartphones had been tested prior to initiation of the study, and the iPhone 5S was selected for clarity and resolution of images as well as ease of use.

According to Ricard-Gauthier et al. (2015), 96% of smartphone images were classified as very good or acceptable for evaluation, when 88 HPV-positive women from Madagascar were screened and 7 (8%) women with CIN2+ disease were identified. The on-site physician achieved a diagnostic sensitivity of 28.6% (95% CI 3.7–71%), whereas the offsite physicians achieved a sensitivity between 42.9% (95% CI 9.9–81.6%) and 85.7% (95% CI 42.1–99.6%).

In order to further enhance smartphone performance, Mink and Peterson (2016) founded a startup company manufacturing a colposcopic smartphone adapter and created a special colposcopy software. It was called the "enhanced visual assessment" (EVA) system (Fig. 17.35).

Lam et al. (2015) created an optical vaginal probe that is attached to a smartphone. The device is called "point of care tampon" (POCkeT) and is introduced directly into the vagina without the need of a speculum (Fig. 17.36).

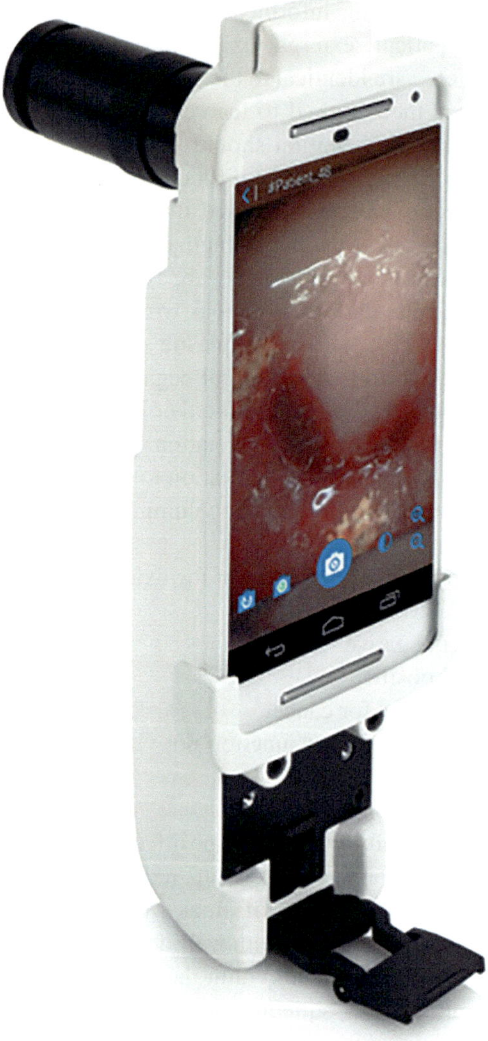

Fig. 17.35 The "enhanced visual assessment" (EVA) system that is attached to a smartphone and can be used as a colposcope

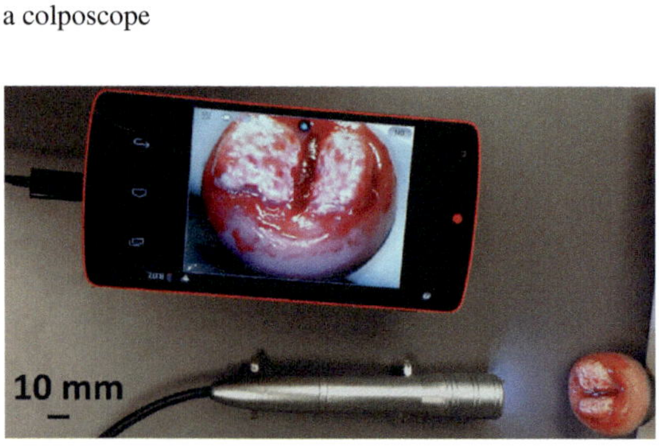

Fig. 17.36 The "point of care tampon" (POCkeT), a vaginal probe that can be introduced directly into the vagina without a speculum (Lam et al. 2015)

17.3.3.3 HPV Test

HPV screening has several advantages for low-income countries. Compared to both cytopathological and visual screening (VIA, VILI), HPV testing is less subjective and well standardized. Thus, reproducibility is higher. Furthermore, HPV test results are less dependent on the quality of the specimen, which is a major problem of the Pap test.

Although sensitivity of the HPV test is high with up to 96% (Cuzick et al. 2006; Koliopoulos et al. 2007), its specificity is too low to allow treatment of all HPV-positive patients without prior triage.

Whereas a single round of cytological screening will not significantly reduce the number of women with advanced cervical cancer and its associated mortality, a single HPV test (HC2) has been shown to lead to a significant decline in the rate of advanced cancers (Sankaranarayanan et al. 2009). Furthermore, the fact that the age-standardized rate of invasive cancer among women with negative Pap smear results or negative VIA is more than four times the rate among HPV-negative women demonstrates the high negative predictive value that is associated with a negative HC2 test result.

The strengths and limitations of VIA and HPV testing have already been summarized in Table 17.2.

A Chinese study (Wu et al. 2005) compared four different screening methods: VIA, colposcopy, ThinPrep® cytopathology, and HPV testing using HC2. The authors concluded that the HPV test is the best choice for primary screening, as it had the highest sensitivity (88.89%) and the highest negative predictive value (97.10%) compared to the other screening modalities studied.

The major obstacles for the introduction of HPV testing in low-resource countries are the lack of infrastructure and of course the higher costs compared to visual inspection. Qiagen, the company producing the Hybrid Capture HPV test (HC2), has developed the so-called careHPV® test which is a less expensive alternative to the HC2 test. The careHPV® test is able to detect 14 different HPV high-risk subtypes: 16, 18, 31, 33, 35, 39, 45, 51, 52, 56, 58, 59, 66, and 68. The test principle and the laboratory procedure are similar to the HC2 test. However, the time to perform the assay is much shorter: 2.5 h compared to 5 h for the HC2. Also, instead of hybridization on microplates, monoclonal antibody-coated magnetic beads are used. The careHPV® test is a low-throughput test with 24–90 samples processed simultaneously. No running water or electricity is required. The testing equipment can run on a battery. The test can also withstand temperature fluctuations.

The careHPV® test has been widely tested in various countries such as China (Ying et al. 2014; Qiao et al. 2008; Lin et al. 2014), Brazil (Lorenzi et al. 2013), Nigeria (Gage et al. 2012), India (Labani et al. 2014), and Thailand (Trope et al. 2013). A high agreement between HC2 and the careHPV® test has been demonstrated. careHPV® testing has also been shown to work well with self-sampled material.

Although Tanzanian guidelines clearly specify VIA in combination with cryotherapy as a single-visit approach as the method of choice for cervical cancer screening, the Tanzanian ministry recommends to introduce HPV testing as soon as a suitable test becomes available and affordable. Once HPV testing is used as the primary screening strategy, VIA can be used as triage of HPV-positive patients.

This is consistent with WHO guidelines that also recommend VIA triage after HPV testing (World Health Organization 2014a, b). Patients are treated only if both VIA and HPV test are positive (Fig. 17.37).

An important aspect of HPV screening is its potential for self-testing. Belinson et al. (2001) studied several screening methods in Shanxi Province, a rural area of China. For detection of CIN2+, the sensitivity and specificity of self-testing were 83% and 86%, respectively. Using the careHPV® methodology, a Brazilian study by Lorenzi et al. (2013) also came to a favorable conclusion: HPV high-risk detection rates did not differ between self-sampled specimens and those obtained by health-care professionals.

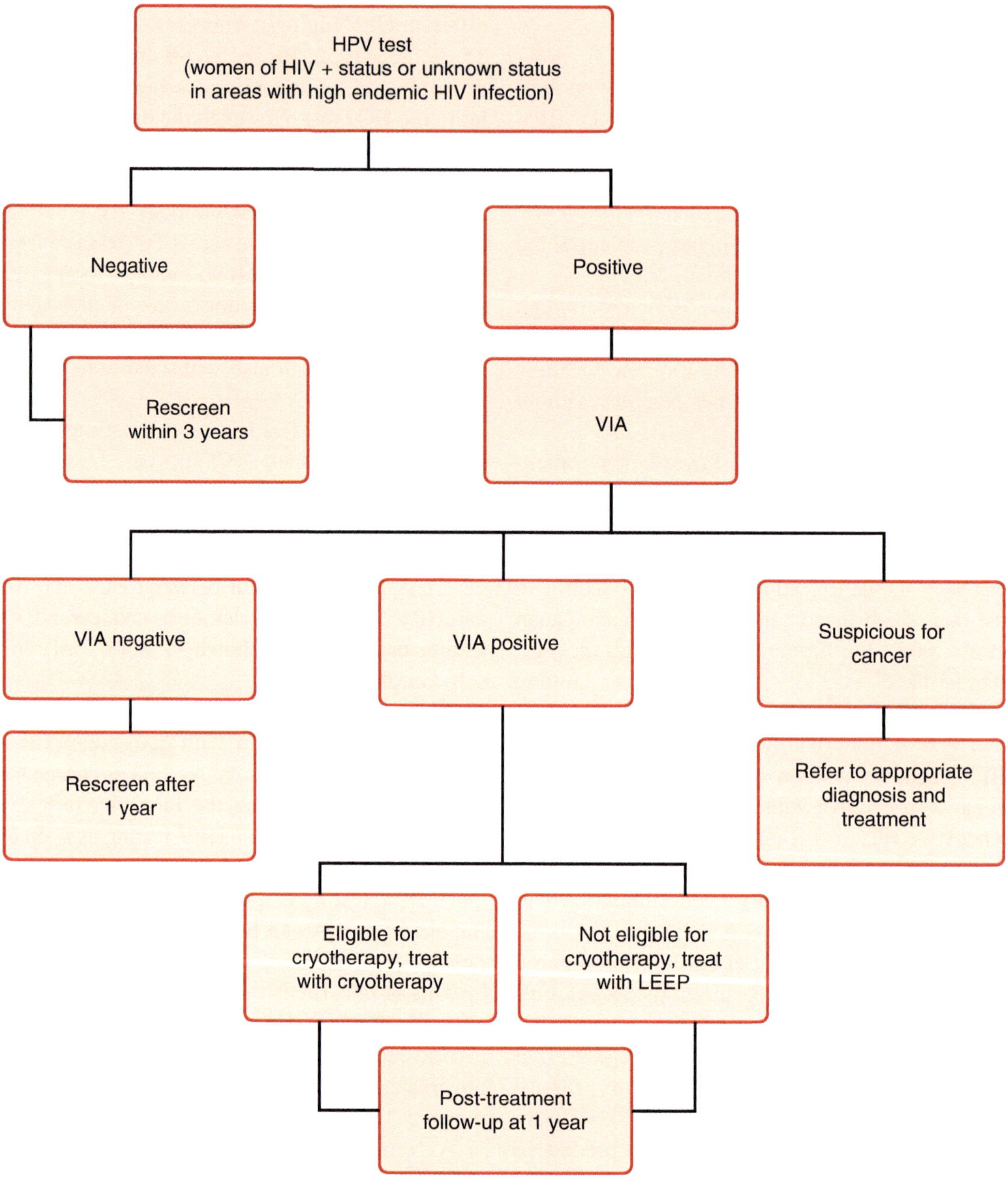

Fig. 17.37 Treatment algorithm if HPV testing is used as the primary screening tool for preinvasive and invasive cervical disease according to WHO guidelines (World Health Organization 2014a, b)

17.3.3.4 HPV and HIV Infection

On numerous occasions in this chapter, the close relationship between HPV-related disease and HIV infection has been pointed out. In HIV-positive patients, CIN and other precancers will develop more frequently and progress more rapidly toward invasive disease. Therefore, based on data by Petry et al. (1994, 1996) as well as others, CIN has been recognized as an AIDS-defining disease.

Furthermore, the immunological interactions between the human immunodeficiency virus and the papilloma virus are presently the subject of an ongoing study (2H study) by the Department of Infectious Diseases and Tropical Medicine of the Ludwig Maximilian University of Munich in collaboration with the Mbeya Medical Research Center (MMRC), Mbeya, Tanzania.

As a consequence of HIV being a strong risk factor for cervical disease, Mwanahamuntu et al. (2009) suggest to link screening strategies such as VIA and cryosurgery to already established HIV care centers as has been done, for instance, in Zambia.

17.3.3.5 Reporting of Screening Results

Systematic documentation is crucial for follow-up as well as quality assurance of a screening program. The WHO (2014a, b) has proposed a form for the screening visit (Fig. 17.38) which may be adapted to the requirements of a specific program.

Fig. 17.38 Sample form for documentation of a screening visit (World Health Organization 2014a, b)

Client information

Individual ID [ ][ ] [ ][ ] [ ][ ] [ ][ ] [ ][ ][ ][ ]
Region District Facility Year Individual

Name: ____________________

Date of birth: [ ][ ] / [ ][ ] / [ ][ ][ ][ ] or **estimaged age at last birthday:** [ ][ ]

Contact Information (Address, phone, etc.)

____
____
____
____

Center name and code ____________________ [ ][ ]

Date of the visit [ ][ ]/[ ][ ]/[ ][ ][ ][ ]

Clinical file reference ____________________

Previously screened (1: Yes, 2: No, 3: Do not know) [ ]

HPV DNA/cytology sample taken (1: Yes, 2: No) [Complete the laboratory form] [ ]

Laboratory specimen identification ____________________

Date of the test result appointment for
HPC DNA/cytology [keep the form until this date] [ ][ ]/[ ][ ]/[ ][ ][ ][ ]

Screening test result (use only the row corresponding to the test used)

VIA/VILI result (0: Not done, 1: Negative, 2: Positive, 3: Suspect cancer) [ ]

HPV DNA result (0: Not done, 1: Negative, 2: Positive) [ ]

Cytology result [ ]
(0: Inadequate, 1: Normal, 2: Inflammation, 3: ASCUS, 4: LSIL, 5: HSIL,
6: Invasive carcinoma, 7: Inconclusive, 8: Other, describe____________________)

Action taken [ ]
(1: Reassured and advised to retest after time period designated by national or program policy, 2: Treatment by cryotherapy, 3: Referred for diagnosis/treatment at the secondary health center, 4: Referred for invasive cancer management, 5: other, describe________
____________________)

If referred, referral center name and code ____________________ [ ] [ ]

17.3.4 Treatment of Preinvasive Disease

Treatment methods for preinvasive disease have already been described in previous chapters. The following chapter presents a more detailed description emphasizing the respective role within a low-resource environment.

Cold-knife conization is not included. Although it may be used in select circumstances as for patients with adenocarcinoma in situ, the World Health Organization guidelines of 2013 (World Health Organization 2013) expressively state that it should not be used as part of a screen and treat strategy.

In addition, the World Health Organization has published guidelines on the treatment of high-grade squamous intraepithelial neoplasia as well as adenocarcinoma in situ (World Health Organization 2014a, b).

- The following recommendations for women with histologically confirmed high-grade cervical disease (HSIL)—regardless of HIV status—are given by the WHO expert panel. In brackets the quality of statistical evidence is given:
  - Use cryotherapy over no treatment (very low).
  - Use LEEP over no treatment (low).
  - Use cold-knife conization over no treatment (low).
  - Use either cryotherapy or LEEP in women for whom either cryotherapy or LEEP is appropriate to use and available (very low).
  - Use cryotherapy over cold-knife conization in women for whom either cryotherapy or cold-knife conization is appropriate to use (very low evidence).
  - Use LEEP over cold-knife conization in women for whom either LEEP or cold-knife conization is appropriate to use (very low evidence).
  - For women with histologically confirmed AIS disease—regardless of HIV status—cold-knife conization is recommended over LEEP (very low evidence).

If VIA is considered the primary screening tool as is the case in most low-resource environments, then the WHO recommends the use of cryotherapy, preferably within a single visit (World Health Organization 2014a, b). If patients are not eligible for cryotherapy (see below), removal of the VIA positive area by LEEP is recommended (Fig. 17.39).

Although same-day treatment is recommended, it is not feasible in the majority of cases because of a variety of reasons, ranging from permission from the patients' spouses to equipment failure. According to the WHO screening demonstration project conducted in six sub-Saharan countries including Tanzania (Peramiho/Moshi region) (World Health Organization 2012), same-day cryotherapy could only be achieved in 39.1% of patients who were eligible. In 8.4% of patients, cryotherapy had been delayed for more than 90 days.

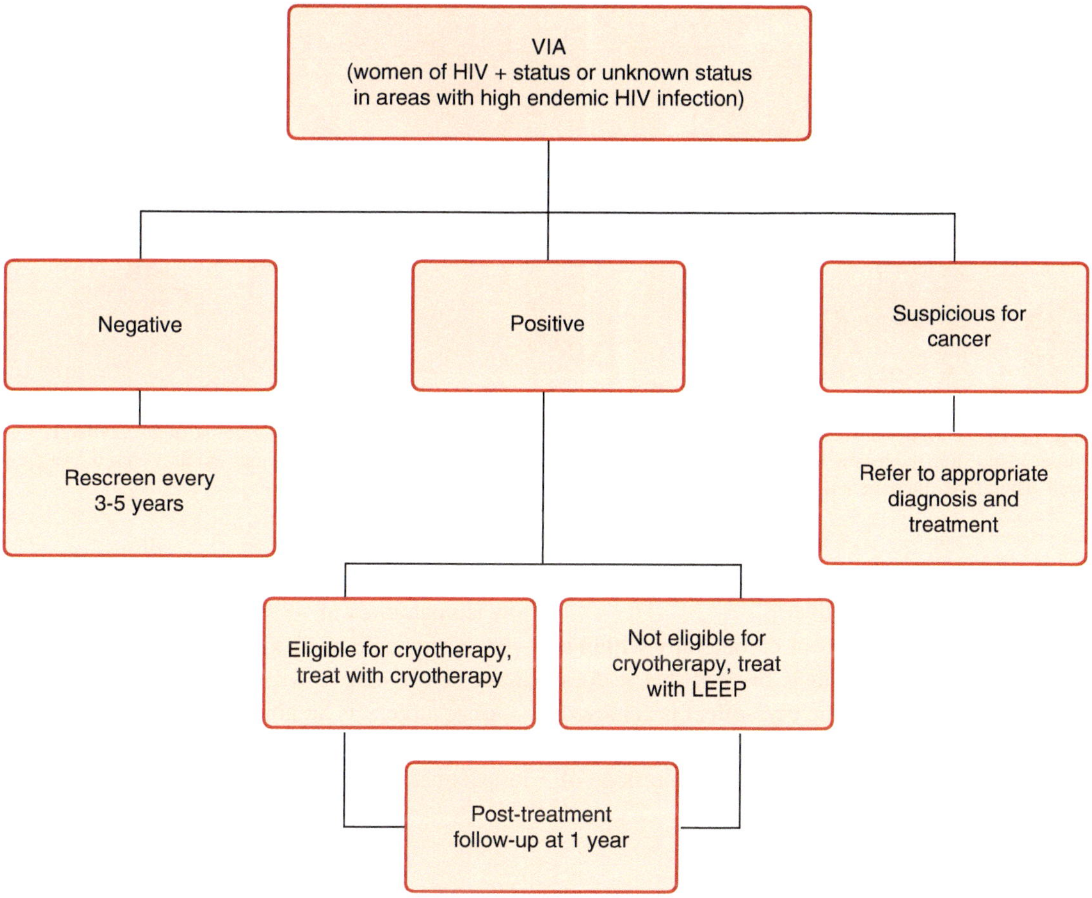

Fig. 17.39 Treatment algorithm if VIA is used as the primary screening tool for preinvasive and invasive cervical disease according to WHO guidelines (World Health Organization 2014a, b)

17.3.4.1 Cryotherapy

Cryotherapy is the treatment of choice for the removal of high-grade disease (CIN2 or CIN3) as suspected by visual inspection (VIA).

Cryotherapy can thus be performed within a single-visit approach. As it does not necessarily require biopsy confirmation of dysplasia, it is ideal for areas without a sufficient number of pathologists. Furthermore, treatment by cryotherapy can be performed by a nurse or midwife without the need for general or local anesthesia.

If the VIA exam yields a positive result, patients are considered for cryotherapy, if the following criteria are met:

1. The patient gives her consent.
2. The lesion can be fully visualized.
3. The lesion involves less than 75% of the cervix.
4. The lesion does not extend onto the vagina (Fig. 17.40).
5. The tip of the cryogun covers the entire lesion (less than 2 mm of the lesion beyond the cryo-tip).
6. The cervix is not deformed anatomically and allows effective application of the cryo-tip.

If the patient declines cryotherapy, VIA is repeated after 1 year. If the lesion cannot be fully visualized, covers more than 75% of the cervix, and/or is too large for the cryo-tip, LEEP should be considered.

Preferably, cryotherapy (or LEEP) is performed on the same day. In pregnant women,

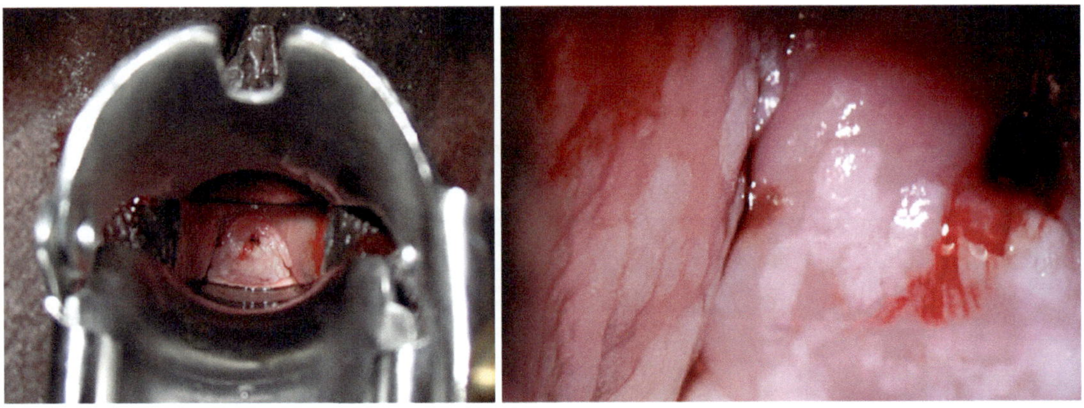

Fig. 17.40 A VIA-positive lesion in a 29-year-old patient who is HIV positive with a T4 count of 225 cells/μL. On closer inspection, the lesion does not only cover more than 75% of the cervical surface but also extends onto the vaginal wall. Therefore, the patient does not qualify for cryosurgery

treatment should be deferred and performed about 12 weeks after delivery.

One of the advantages of cryotherapy within a low-resource environment is the fact that it does not require electricity. The cryo-effect is achieved through refrigerant gases, either carbon dioxide or nitrous oxide ("laughing gas"). Decompression of these gases within the cryo-tip will achieve very low temperatures of −89 °C for nitrous oxide and −68 °C for carbon dioxide. Freezing of cervical tissue below −20 °C will result in necrosis.

Cryosurgery is an ablative technique that will destroy the tissue rather than remove it as does loop excision (LEEP).

- The steps for cryotherapy are as follows (The United Republic of Tanzania 2011; Sellors and Sankaranarayanan 2003) (Figs. 17.41, 17.42, 17.43, 17.44, and 17.45):
  - Check for exclusion criteria (see above).
  - Check for informed consent.
  - Insert speculum (Cusco or Grave).
  - Apply 5% acetic acid and/or Lugol's solution and repeat visual inspection.
  - Local anesthesia is not required.
  - Select the adequate cryo-tip.
  - Firmly apply the cryo-probe onto the cervix.
  - Make sure that the vaginal wall does not touch the tip. This may require a wooden spatula to distance the vaginal wall from the tip (Fig. 17.44).
  - Set timer and trigger the cryogun.
  - Perform cryotherapy either as "single-freeze" procedure (5 min of continuous freezing) or "double-freeze" procedure (3 min of freezing, 5 min of thawing, 3 min of freezing). Watch for the formation of a 3–5 mm ice ball around and beyond the tip.
  - Allow for thawing before removing the cryo-gun.
  - Check for bleeding. Supply sanitary pads. Do not use vaginal packs.
  - Provide instructions to the patient. The patient must be advised not to douche, not to use tampons, and not to have sexual intercourse.
  - Have patient return for follow-up visit after 3 months.

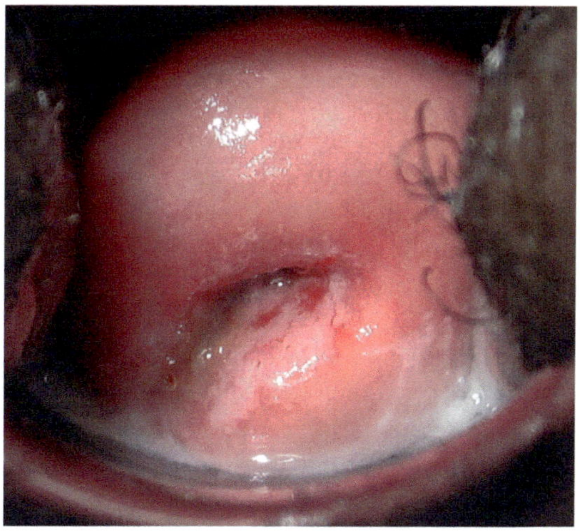

Fig. 17.41 Cryosurgery. A 31-year-old patient with unknown HIV status presented for screening at Mbeya Referral Hospital, Tanzania, and was found to be VIA positive. The acetowhite lesion is mainly located on the posterior (dorsal) two quadrants of the cervix. It extends close to the cervical canal. However, it can be completely covered with the cryo-tip, and the patient is eligible for cryotherapy according to the "screen and treat" approach

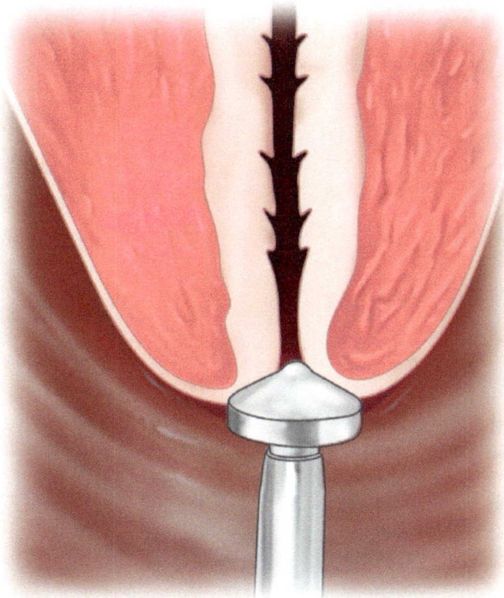

Fig. 17.43 For cryotherapy of cervical dysplasia, the cryo-tip is placed onto the outer cervix. Lesions within or extending too far into the cervical canal cannot be treated effectively by cryotherapy

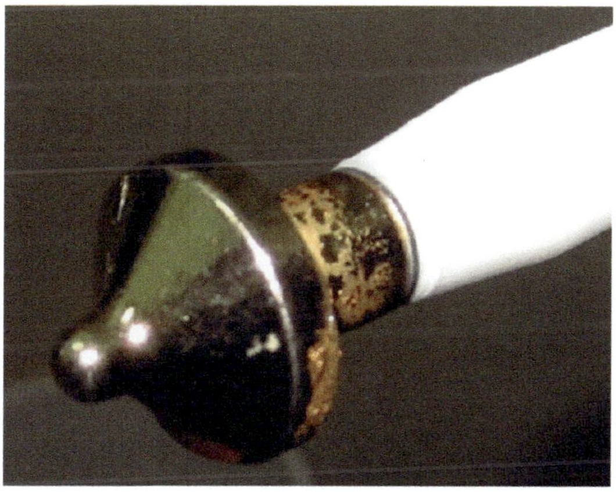

Fig. 17.42 Cryosurgery. The cryo-tip has a "cowboy head" configuration which partially reaches inside the cervical canal

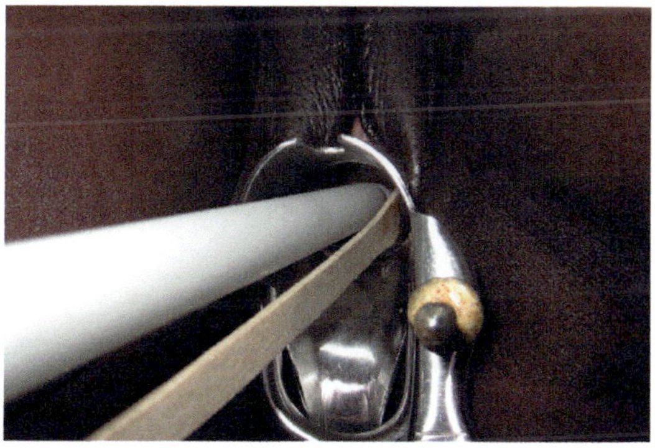

Fig. 17.44 Cryosurgery. A wooden spatula is used to distance the vaginal wall from the cryo-tip

Usually, wound healing of the cervix occurs fast. Following cryotherapy, complete healing of the cervix is to be expected after 4–6 weeks (Fig. 17.46). For up to 4 weeks, there will be a significant watery discharge. Postoperative bleeding is rare.

There is evidence that wound healing is considerably delayed in HIV-positive patients. Pfaendler et al. (2015) studied 101 cryotherapy

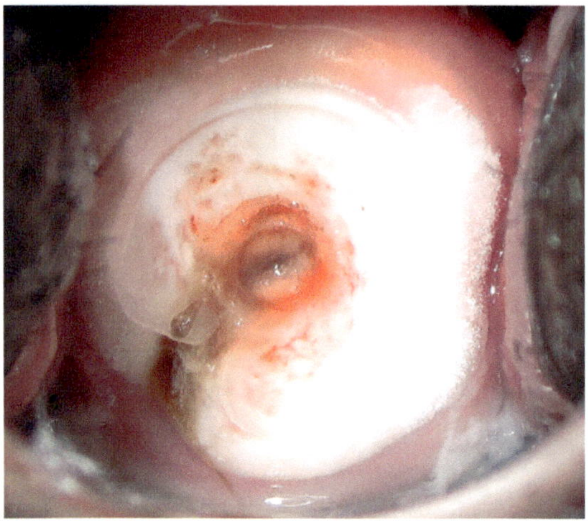

Fig. 17.45 Cryosurgery. Cervix immediately after freezing with the cryo-tip

eligible HIV-positive women in Zambia and found that even 12 weeks postoperatively only 65% of patients experienced complete healing of the cervix. Healing was especially delayed in women over the age of 30.

It is important to tell the patient that no adverse effects are to be expected on fertility or on future pregnancies.

Vet et al. (2012), who evaluated VIA screening within a single-visit approach in Indonesia, saw 53.9% of women treated by cryotherapy for follow-up 6 months after the procedure. VIA was repeated and a Pap test performed. The overall cure rate was 92.0%.

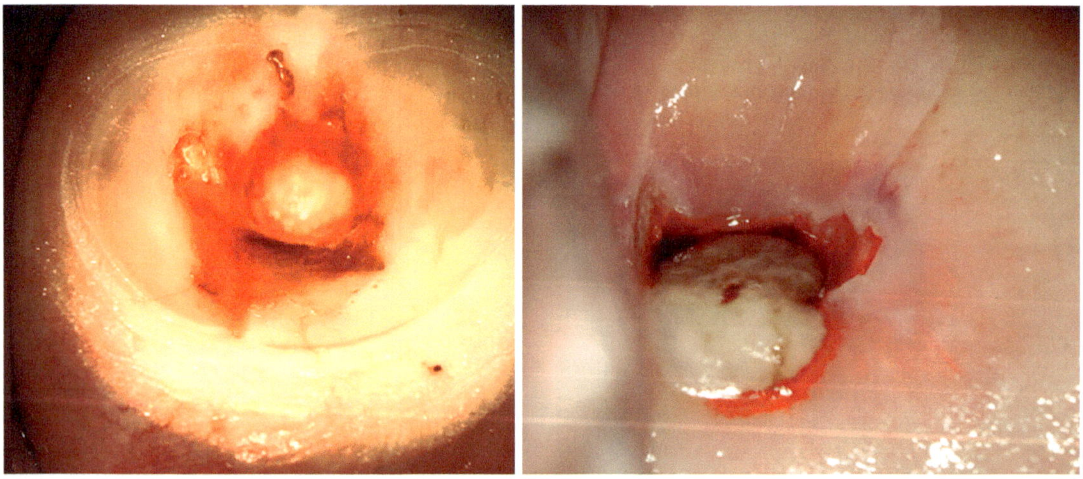

Fig. 17.46 Cryosurgery. A 39-year-old HIV-negative patient underwent cryotherapy for a VIA-positive lesion. On the left the cervix immediately following surgery is shown, and on the right 4 weeks later: the cervical wound has healed completely. No significant scarring has occurred, and the squamocolumnar junction is partially visible

17.3.4.2 Loop Electrosurgical Excision Procedure (LEEP)

Loop excision should be performed when there are contraindications to cryosurgery. In comparison to cryosurgery, LEEP requires considerably more expertise and training and should be done by a doctor. The equipment has to have a reliable source of electricity and is more expensive, and bleeding during or after the procedure is an important issue. Nevertheless, it is not a very difficult procedure to master. Before performing loop excision on a patient, the surgeon can practice excision and coagulation on animal meat or liver in order to get a feeling for the properties of the electrosurgical instruments and different settings of the generator.

Targeted cervical surgery such as loop resection should be performed under colposcopic guidance. Therefore, the surgeon should practice handling of the equipment using the colposcope.

LEEP is an ablative procedure. Thus, histopathological examination is possible so that microinvasive cancer would be diagnosed.

Whereas cryosurgery is performed without anesthesia, it might be advisable to use spinal anesthesia depending on the overall experience of the surgeon and his staff. Also, LEEP performed on patients within a low-resource environment is likely to require a larger resection volume especially in HIV-positive patients. Local anesthesia by injection of the anesthetic directly into the cervix is described below.

The main goal of LEEP is the complete excision of the precancerous cervical lesion. Although it can be advantageous to be able to document the complete histopathologic removal with margins that are not overly compromised by thermal artifact, several pieces of material obtained by using a small or intermediate loop (multiple-pass technique, Fig. 17.47) are also acceptable instead of the so-called one-pass technique (Fig. 17.48).

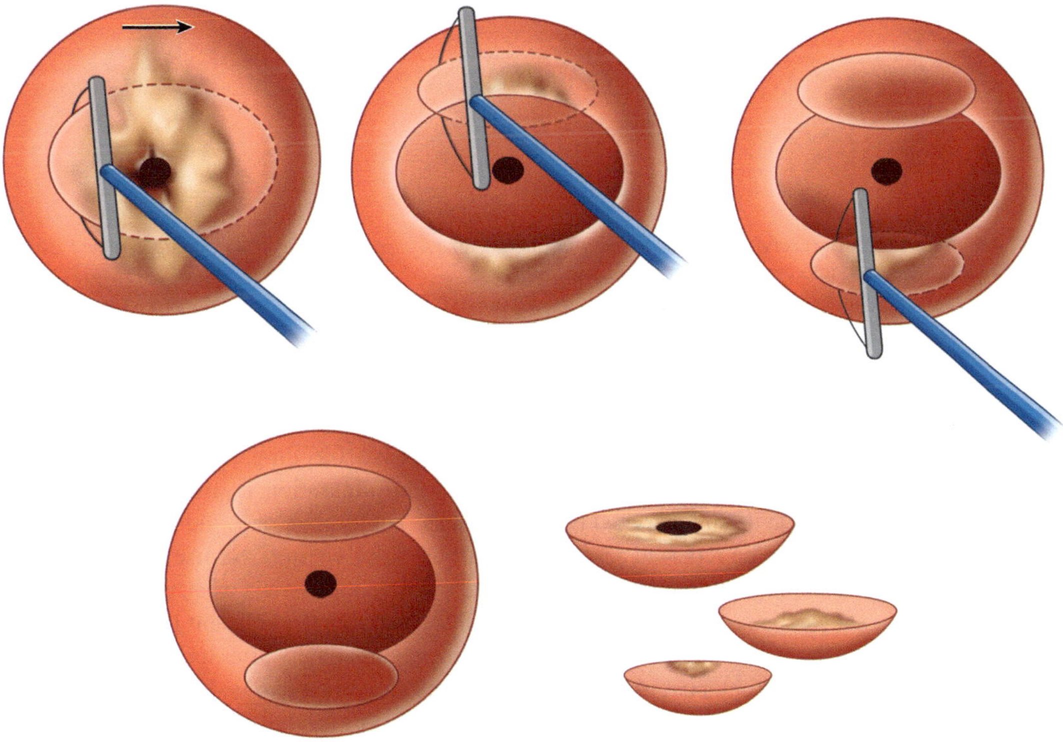

Fig. 17.47 Loop electrosurgical excision procedure (LEEP) of the cervix using the multiple-pass technique. This is acceptable as the main goal of the procedure is the complete removal of the lesion as visualized through colposcopy. Histopathologic demonstration of free margins is secondary

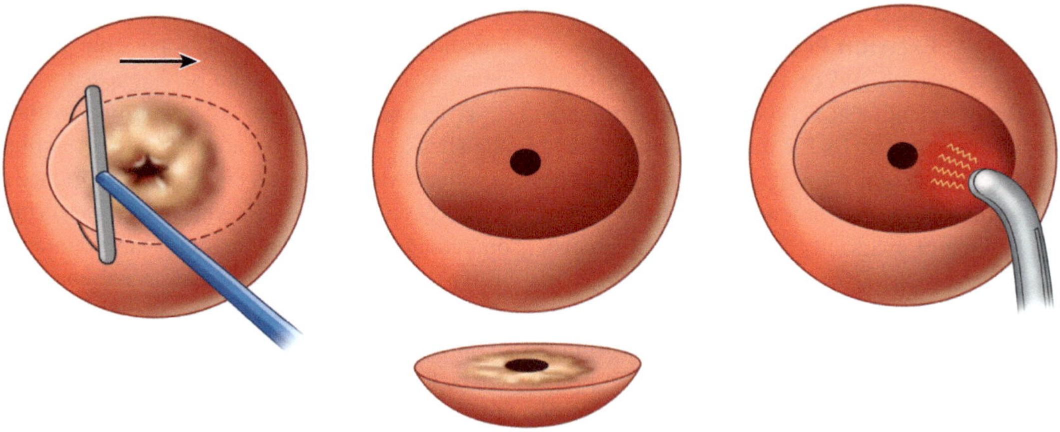

Fig. 17.48 Loop electrosurgical excision procedure (LEEP) of the cervix using one-pass technique to remove a cone-like specimen

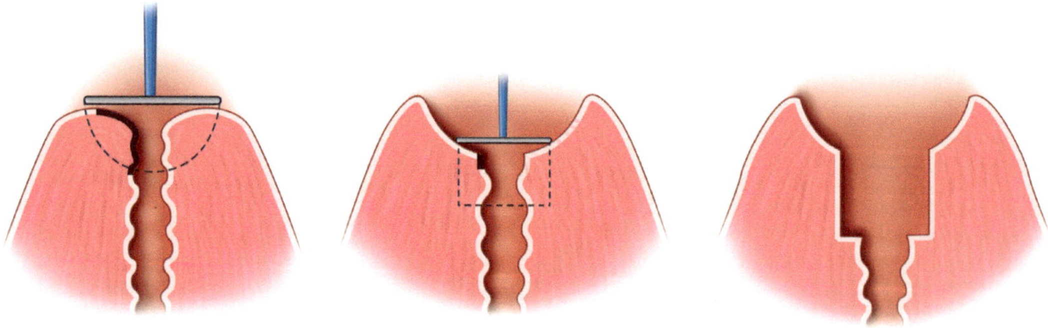

Fig. 17.49 With LEEP, intracervical lesions that cannot be adequately treated by cryosurgery are resected using a small loop that is inserted into the cervical canal

Lesions which extend into the endocervical canal and cannot be adequately treated by cryosurgery are resected using a small loop that is inserted into the cervical canal (Fig. 17.49). Thus, a cylinder-shaped piece of tissue is removed. If further resection of endocervical tissue is required, this step may be repeated several times. Ultimately, the entire tissue surrounding the endocervical canal can be removed.

Adequate hemostasis is essential to LEEP and is almost always achieved by coagulation or rather fulguration. If the generator is set to fulguration mode, it will generate sparks between the electrode and the tissue without direct tissue contact. Only rarely sutures are needed to stop excessive bleeding. When electrosurgical coagulation/fulguration is available, the use of Monsel's solution is not indicated. However, Monsel's solution may be useful, if a patient comes back to the clinic a week or two following the procedure due to persistent light to moderate bleeding. Immediately after loop resection, vaginal packs should be avoided in order to be able to diagnose postoperative bleeding.

- The steps for LEEP are as follows (The United Republic of Tanzania 2011; Sellors and Sankaranarayanan 2003) (Figs. 17.50, 17.51, 17.52, 17.53, and 17.54):
  - Check for informed consent.
  - Consider spinal or local anesthesia.
  - Introduce speculum (e.g., Cusco or Grave), preferably with an insulating cover (Fig. 17.50).
  - Attach smoke evacuator to speculum or use suction tube.
  - Apply 5% acetic acid and/or Lugol's solution and repeat visual inspection.
  - Perform local anesthesia: inject the local anesthetic a few millimeters into the periphery of the cervix either at 12, 3, 6, and 9 o'clock position or at 12, 4, and 8 o'clock as well as into the cervical canal. Use xylocaine, preferably without adrenaline. Addition of a vasoconstricting agent (vasopressin) is optional.
  - The appropriate type of loop is selected.
  - The generator is activated (handle switch or food pedal) just prior to touching the surface of the tissue.
  - The loop is gently guided through the tissue without pressure.
  - Use forceps to remove resected tissue.
  - These steps may be repeated multiple times.
  - Measure resection volume (Chap. 8) and document.
  - Obtain adequate hemostasis with a ball electrode set to fulguration mode.
  - Before discharging the patient, check for bleeding. Supply sanitary pads. Avoid the use of vaginal packs.
  - Provide instructions to the patient. The patient needs to be advised not to douche, not to use tampons, and not to have sexual intercourse.
  - Have patient return for follow-up visit after 3 months.

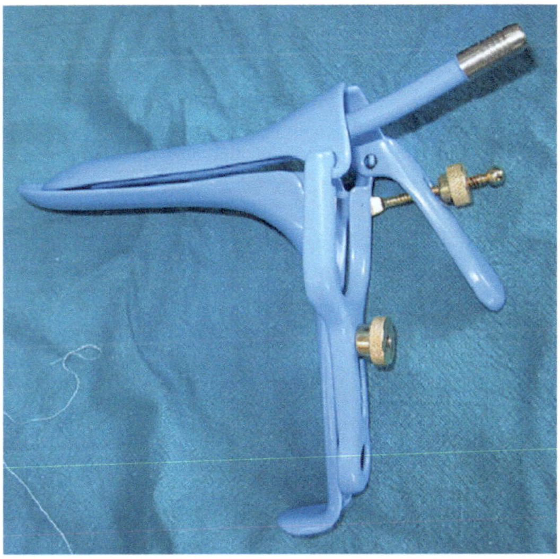

Fig. 17.50 LEEP. Grave's speculum with insulating cover and attachment for smoke evacuation

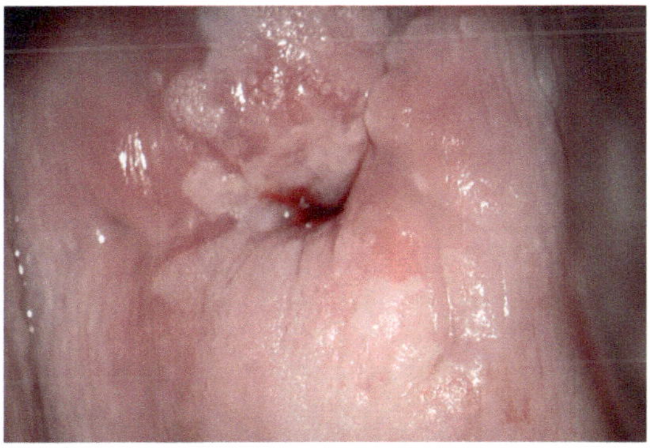

Fig. 17.51 LEEP. A 39-year-old HIV-positive patient who suffers from tuberculosis. At the time of cervical cancer screening at Mbeya Referral Hospital, Tanzania, she was found to be VIA positive. The acetowhite lesion covers more than 75% of the cervix and extends into the cervical canal. Therefore, she does not fulfill the eligibility criteria for cryotherapy and is referred for loop resection

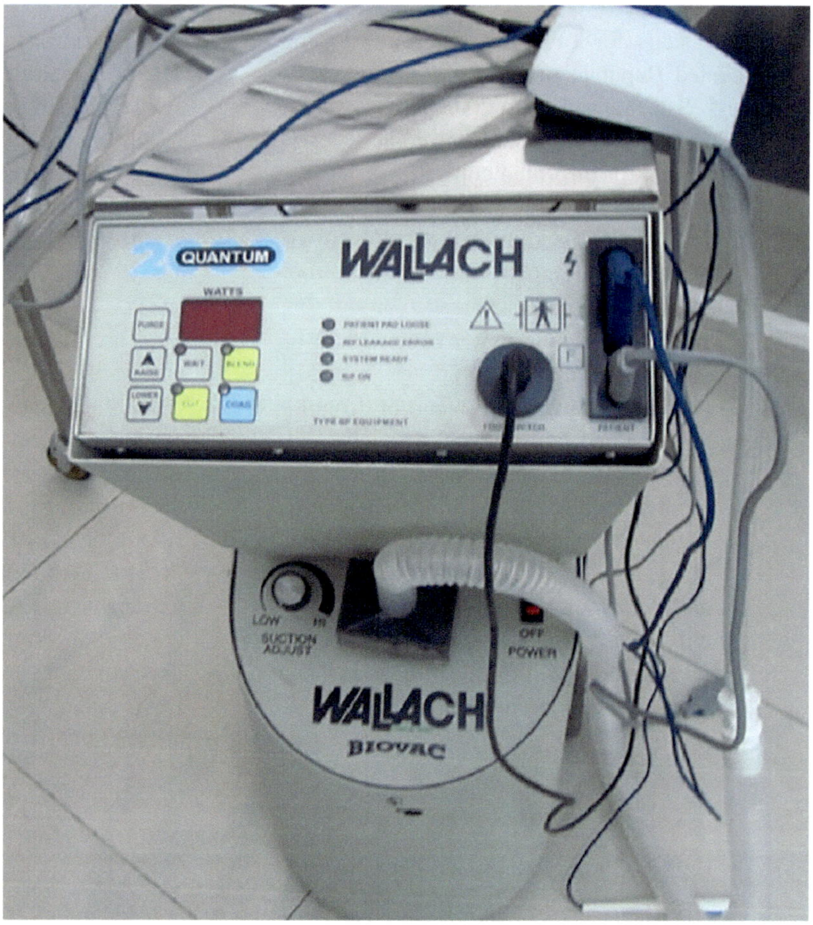

Fig. 17.52 LEEP. Electric generator with integrated suction device

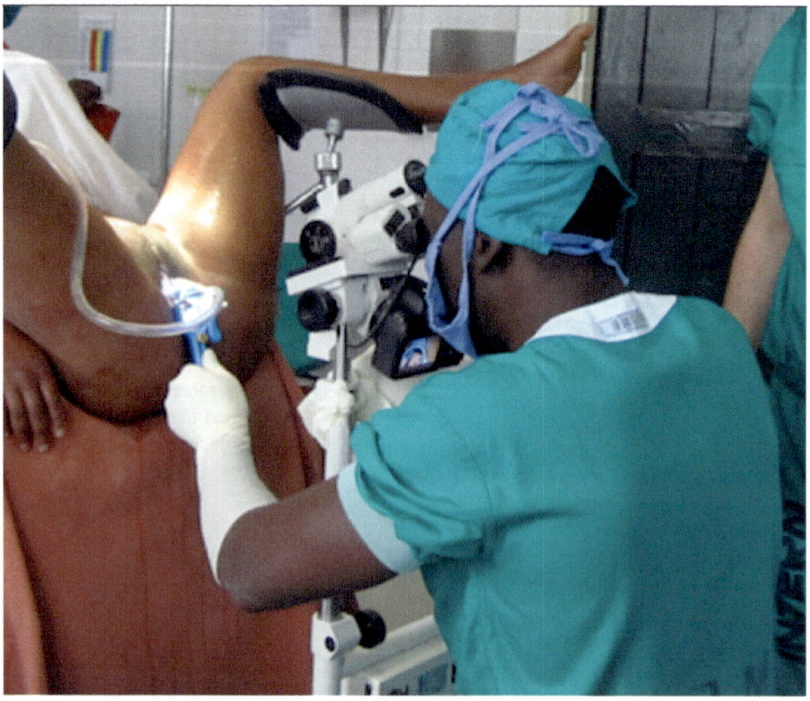

Fig. 17.53 LEEP. The loop resection is done under colposcopic guidance (7.5×)

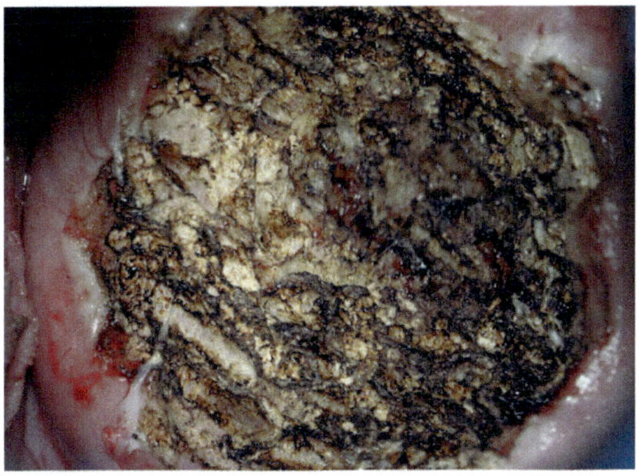

Fig. 17.54 LEEP. Treatment result immediately after loop resection and coagulation/fulguration

17.3.4.3 Hysterectomy

Hysterectomy is not a suitable option for treatment of preinvasive cervical disease. Compared to cryotherapy and LEEP, hysterectomy is a major surgical procedure with a significant complication rate. This is especially true for a low-resource environment which involves higher infection rates, the lack of blood units if unexpected bleeding arises, and the reduced ability to deal with anesthesia complications.

Furthermore, there is a significant risk for VAIN following hysterectomy for CIN (Schockaert et al. 2008). The incidence of VAIN will be even higher in HIV-positive patients.

However, occasionally hysterectomy may be a viable treatment option for high-grade cervical intraepithelial dysplasia, even when there are no concomitant hysterectomy indications such as e.g. symptomatic fibroids or prolapse. Here are some circumstances when hysterectomy might be considered:

- On visual inspection and/or colposcopy, microinvasive disease cannot be ruled out.
- Histopathologic examination is not available or only after a considerable time interval (more than 6 weeks).
- Patient compliance is low; hence, it is unlikely that the patient will return to the hospital. Also, the traveling distance to the hospital might be long and the infrastructure limited.

17.3.4.4 Vaginal and Vulvar Dysplasia

Treatment of both vaginal and vulvar dysplasia in a low-resource environment is an unsolved problem. Although there are no data on its prevalence, it will occur more frequently in patients with a compromised immune system such as HIV infection.

Local resection of both vaginal and vulvar diseases is feasible only if there are only a few localized lesions. However, in HIV-infected patients, VIN and VAIN tend to be multifocal and may cover large areas.

17.4 Cervical Carcinoma

17.4.1 Visual Cervical Cancer Diagnosis

Symptoms of cervical cancer such as irregular/intermenstrual, postmenopausal and/or postcoital bleeding, foul-smelling or watery discharge, and abdominal or back pain are not specific and highly unreliable when trying to establish the clinical diagnosis of cervical cancer.

However, in most instances, a visual diagnosis of cervical cancer will be possible, especially as most patients will be diagnosed with advanced-stage disease within a low-resource environment.

Two characteristic signs of cancer are exophytic tissue growth (Figs. 17.55b, c and 17.57a, f, g) and necrosis (Fig. 17.55a) which will leave a defect of the entire cervix or a part of it. Sometimes exophytic growth and necrosis occur concomitantly (Figs. 17.55f and 17.56b, c). Sometimes, visual signs are less typical (Figs. 17.56d and 17.57c, e). However, in combination with palpation and the presence of a nodular mass extending onto the vagina and/or toward the parametria, the clinical diagnosis can be established. Occasionally, the cervix cannot be visualized due to extensive bleeding (Fig. 17.56e).

In FIGO stage IVA disease, i.e., invasion of the bladder, part of the bladder mucosa may be visible (Figs. 17.56f and 17.57h).

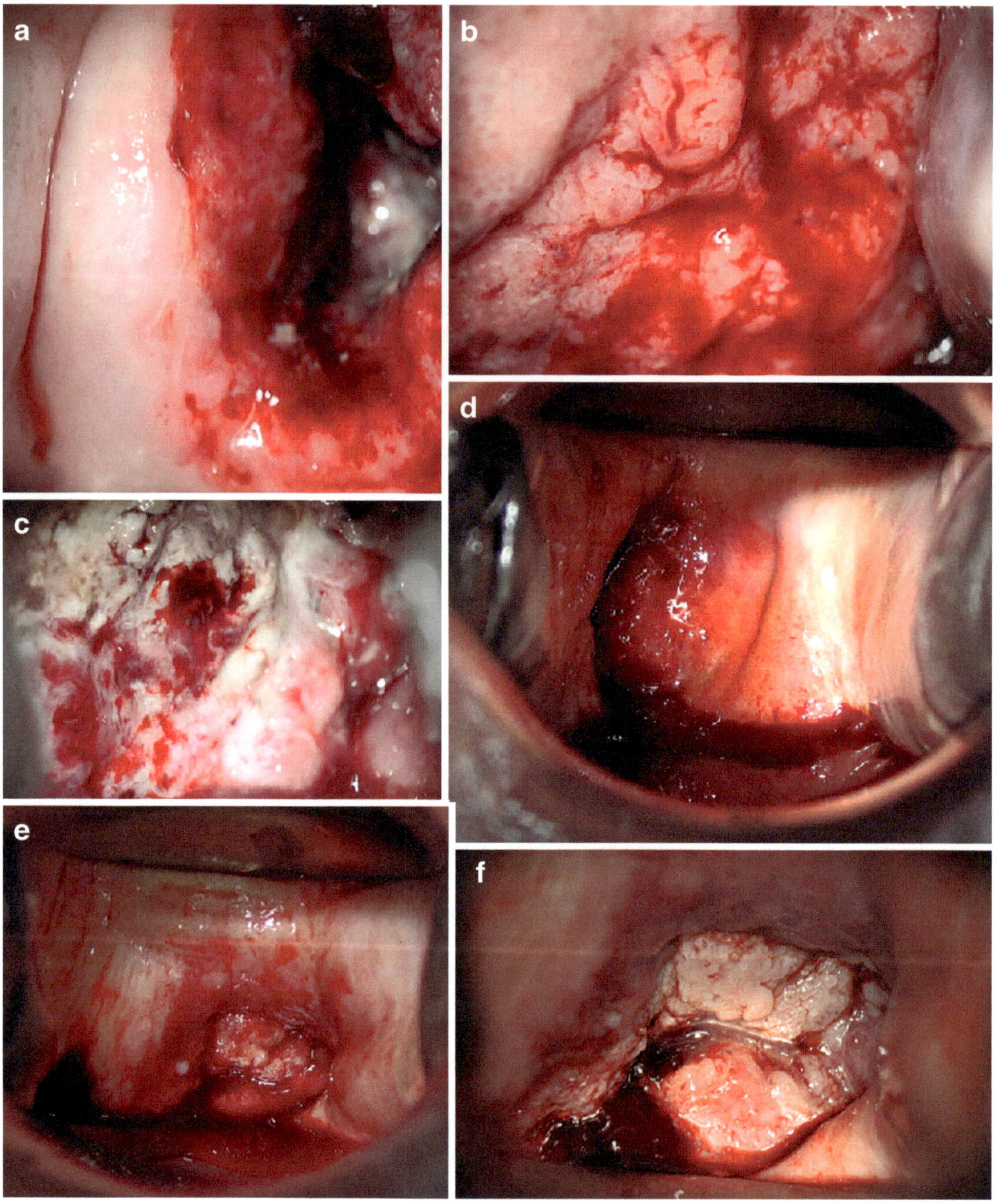

Fig. 17.55 (**a**–**f**) Visual inspection: cervical cancer compilation

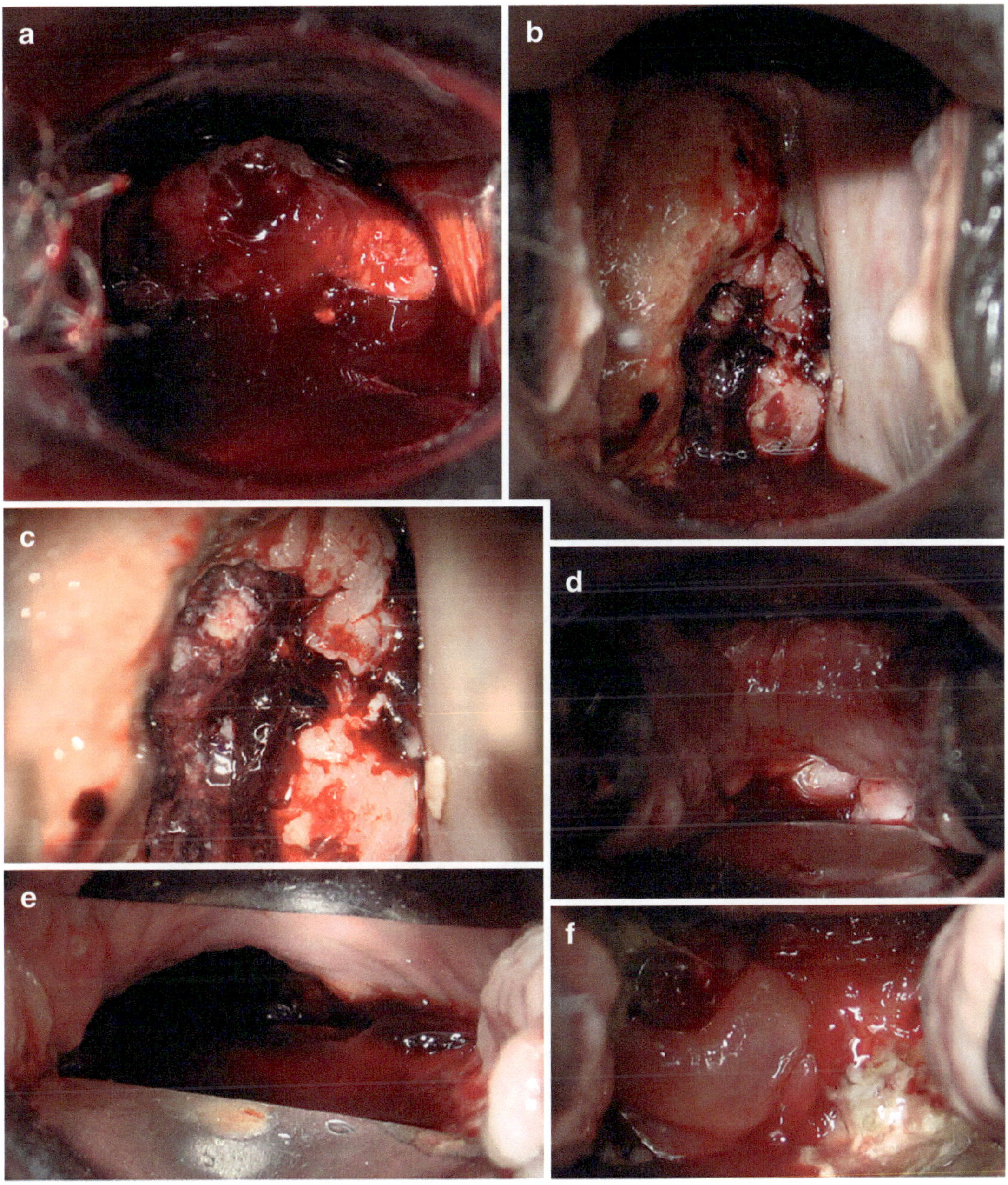

Fig. 17.56 (**a**–**f**) Visual inspection: cervical cancer compilation

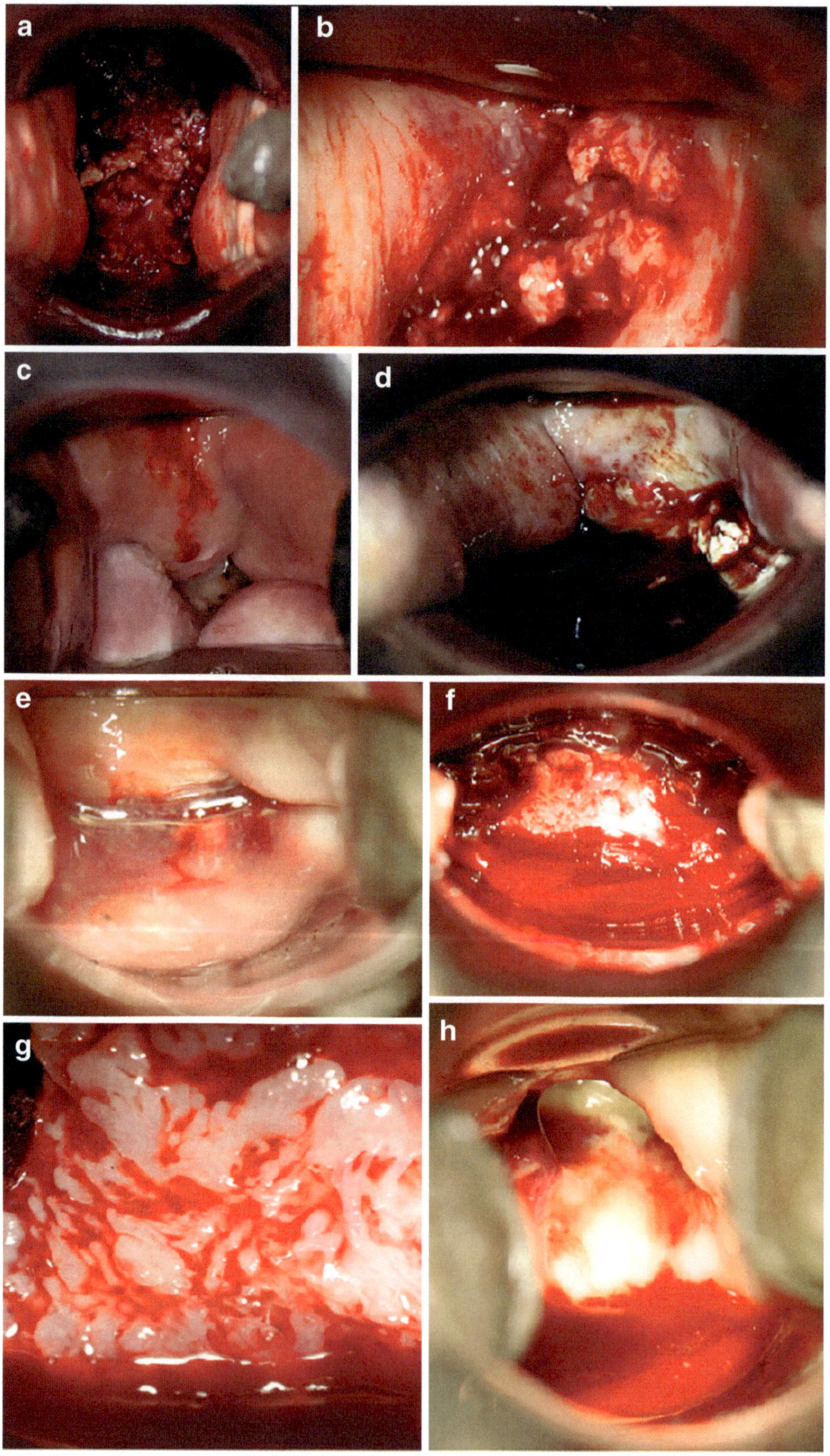

Fig. 17.57 (**a**–**h**) Visual inspection: cervical cancer compilation

17.4.2 Pitfalls of Cervical Cancer Diagnosis

In most cases of advanced cervical cancer, visual diagnosis without the benefit of histopathological confirmation is feasible. However, treatment of cervical cancer based on a clinical diagnosis is a major compromise made necessary and justified by a lack of resources. One should always realize that occasionally even the most experienced clinicians may be misled. Here are a few examples of potential pitfalls of visual cervical cancer diagnosis.

Myoma or fibroids of the uterus are the most frequently occurring tumors of the uterus which are almost always benign (Fig. 17.58).

Occasionally, a fibroid will extend into the uterine cavity and become pedunculated. Eventually it will be "born" through the cervical canal due to the contractions of the uterus ("myoma in statu nascendi") (Figs. 17.59 and 17.60). Such a myoma may be confused with an exophytic mass as seen in advanced cervical carcinoma: When there is no sufficient blood supply of the pedunculated fibroid, it may become necrotic and lead to the wrong diagnosis if no histopathologic examination is performed.

Advanced gestational trophoblastic neoplasia (GTN), in particular choriocarcinoma protruding from the cervix or involving the cervix (Fig. 17.61), may be misdiagnosed as carcinoma of the cervix, especially in an environment where a histopathological diagnosis is not readily available.

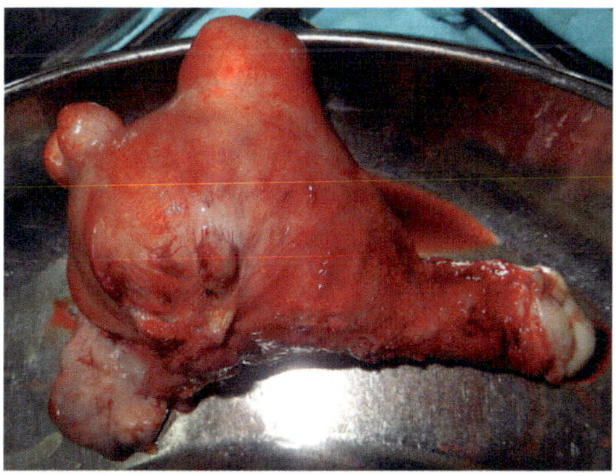

Fig. 17.58 Uterus with multiple fibroids (META Referral Hospital, Mbeya, Tanzania)

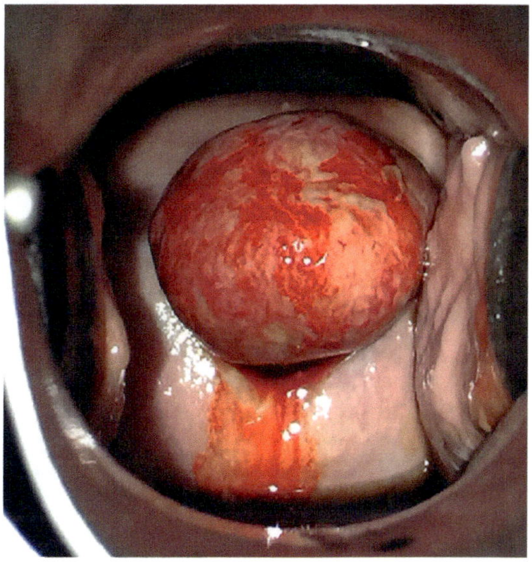

Fig. 17.59 Fibroid protruding from the cervical canal, so-called "myoma in statu nascendi." Occasionally this finding may be confused with an exophytic mass in cervical cancer

Even on microscopic exam, GTN may mimic cervical carcinoma (Jordan and Randall 2011). The patient's history, probably revealing a previous pregnancy as well as β-HCG measurements in urine and/or blood will lead to the correct diagnosis, which is critical for the appropriate treatment. However, no history of a recent delivery or abortion does not rule out GTN. Narita et al. (2003) observed a 53-year-old patient with an epithelioid trophoblastic tumor initially interpreted as cervical cancer which originated after a spontaneous delivery 25 years ago. Furthermore, extrauterine choriocarcinoma located in the cervix must also be taken into account, although this is a very rare entity (Kairi-Vassilatou et al. 2018).

Occasionally, vaginal metastases from GTN can be observed.

Whereas cervical carcinoma will be treated by surgery and/or radiation therapy, the treatment of choice for any type and stage of GTN is primary chemotherapy, in particular methotrexate. When using the appropriate chemotherapy treatment,

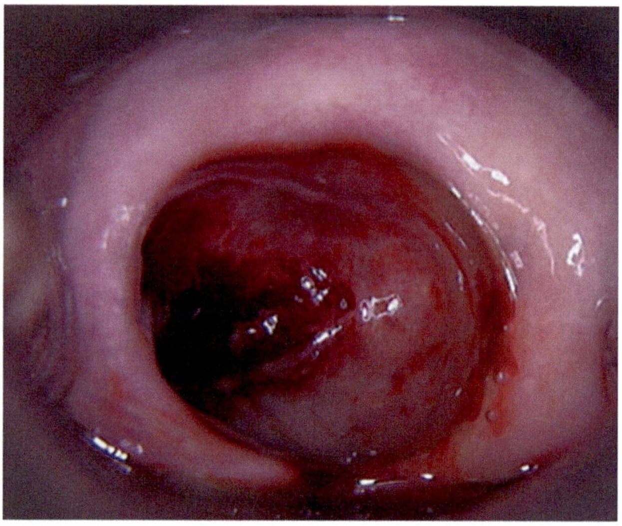

Fig. 17.60 "Myoma in statu nascendi"

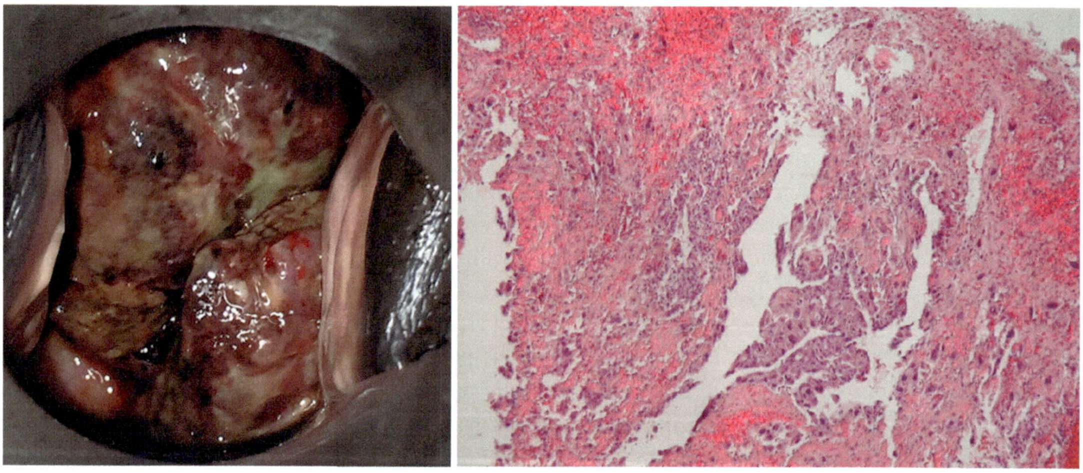

Fig. 17.61 A 47-year-old patient with an 8 cm mass protruding from the cervix referred to Mbeya Referral Hospital, Tanzania, after a clinical diagnosis of advanced cervical carcinoma. Biopsy revealed gestational choriocarcinoma

the vast majority of patients will be cured, even those with metastatic disease.

In some patients with GTN, hysterectomy may be advisable to stop uterine bleeding. However, surgical intervention may prove dangerous or even fatal when the cancer has already spread beyond the uterus and involves adjacent pelvic organs resulting in massive intraoperative bleeding.

Schistosomiasis or bilharzia, a parasitic disease caused by the *Schistosoma*-type flatworm, is endemic in many parts of the world, particularly in Africa, and frequently involves the female genital tract. It has long been suspected that schistosomiasis facilitates HIV as well as HPV infection (Poggensee and Feldmeier 2001; Feldmeier et al. 1995; Petry et al. 2003). A study on cervical biopsies in northern Tanzania revealed a 37% prevalence of female genital tract schistosomiasis (Poggensee et al. 2000). In Malawi, 65% of biopsies were found to be positive (Kjetland et al. 1996).

Cervical manifestations of *Schistosoma haematobium* are described as "sandy patches" which are acetonegative and may be situated inside or outside the transformation zone and

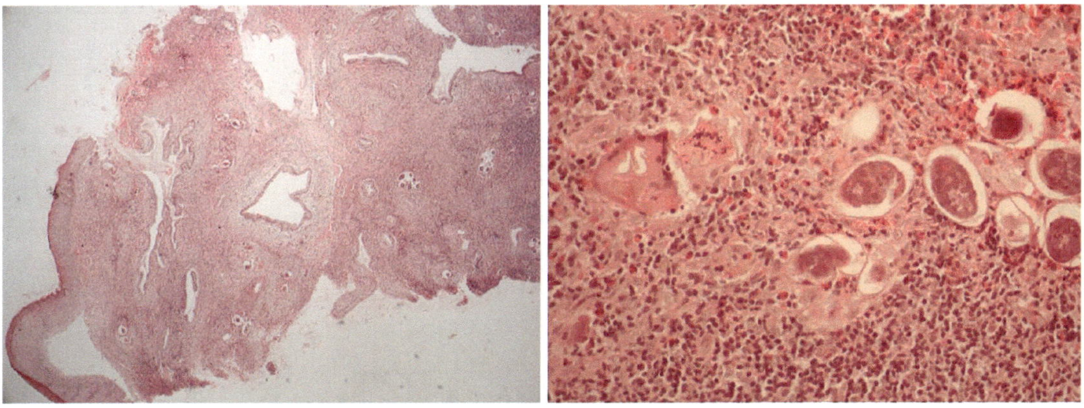

Fig. 17.62 Cervical schistosomiasis diagnosed as VIA positive in a 28-year-old woman. In this particular case, cervical biopsy had been performed prior to treatment of the presumed cervical dysplasia. Histological exam did not show squamous dysplasia. Instead, multiple schistosome eggs can be seen within the transformation zone (Contributed by Dr. Josefo Ferro, Department of Pathology, Catholic University of Mozambique and Beira Central Hospital)

are not enhanced by green light. Furthermore, atypical vessels may be seen (Kjetland et al. 2012). As cervical schistosomiasis has also been described as cauliflower-like growth, nodular hypertrophy, as well as ulcerative and polypoid lesions (Poggensee and Feldmeier 2001), it may be misinterpreted as cervical carcinoma. Also, misinterpretation of VIA positivity may occur (Fig. 17.62).

17.4.3 Management of Patients with Invasive Cervical Carcinoma

In the WHO screening project (World Health Organization 2012) conducted in six sub-Saharan countries including Tanzania, 326 women out of 19,579 women screened (1.7%) had lesions suspicious of cancer at the time of screening. Further investigation of these lesions proved to be unsatisfactory in the vast majority of patients (Fig. 17.63). Only 96 women (29.4%) were further evaluated. Out of the 77 patients with cancer, 64 women (83.1%) had advanced stage disease and were offered chemoradiation. It is unclear how many patients actually underwent the recommended treatment.

In the WHO data, no surgical treatment by radical hysterectomy is documented. Thirteen patients were offered abdominal hysterectomy. However, no details are given if these 13 patients actually suffered from invasive disease or precancer only.

Without screening, the majority of patients diagnosed with cervical cancer will present with advanced stage disease as shown in Fig. 17.64. Twenty-one out of 29 patients (72%) were inoperable with FIGO stage IIIA disease or higher.

In a statistical analysis of 137 patients presenting to Universitas Diponegoro, Semarang, located in Central Java, Indonesia, in 2010 (Suryapratama 2012), 81% of patients presented with stage III or IV disease (Fig. 17.65).

A retrospective analysis of 1709 patients with cervical cancer treated at Dr. Cipto Mangunkusumo Hospital in Jakarta, Indonesia, between 2012 and 2016 showed that 80.34% of patients presented at an advanced stage (Winarto et al. 2018). The most common histological type was moderately differentiated squamous cell carcinoma without lymphovascular space involvement.

In addition, in many low-income countries, availability of radiation treatment is limited. Both Tanzania and Ethiopia have a single treatment facility for the entire country. Furthermore, in Ethiopia only external beam radiation is available but no brachytherapy. Patients who are able to secure treatment for themselves have signifi-

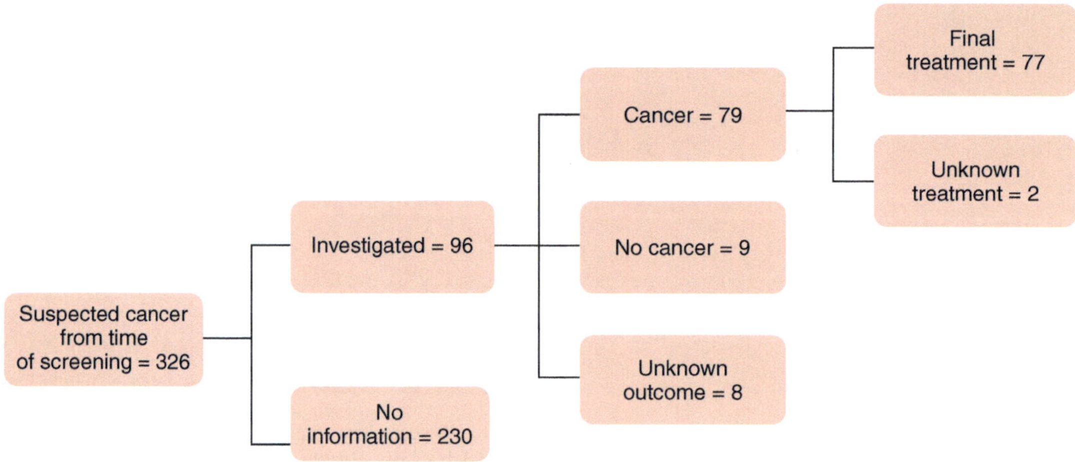

Fig. 17.63 Further investigation of 326 out of 19,579 patients (1.7%) suspected of cervical cancer at the time of visual screening in six sub-Saharan countries (World Health Organization 2012)

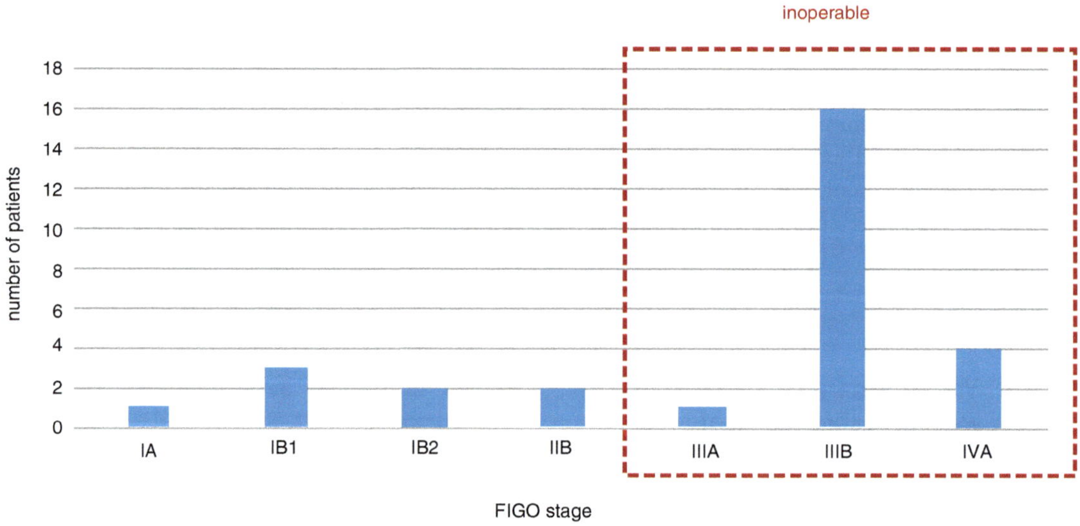

Fig. 17.64 FIGO stage of patients with a clinical diagnosis of cervical cancer in Mbeya, Tanzania (personal experience of one of the authors, R.L., on three consecutive visits in 2015 and 2016). Whereas early-stage IIB disease may still be amenable to radical surgery, when radiotherapy is not available, patients with FIGO stages III and IV are definitely inoperable

cant waiting periods until the beginning of the radiation therapy and undergo progression of disease as demonstrated by Kantelhardt et al. (2014) for Ethiopia. After a median waiting time of 3.8 months, the proportion of patients with stage IIIB/IVA disease almost doubled (33.5% increasing to 63.9%).

When systematic screening is instituted in a previously unscreened population, a large number of patients with invasive cancer will be diagnosed initially as has been shown, for example, by a Tanzanian screening study (Ngoma et al. 2010). The initial cervical cancer detection rate was 1.9%. However, 20% of patients were found to still have stage I disease, and 41% had stage II disease. Consequently, patients whose cervical cancer is detected within a screening program are diagnosed earlier and may have a more favorable prognosis.

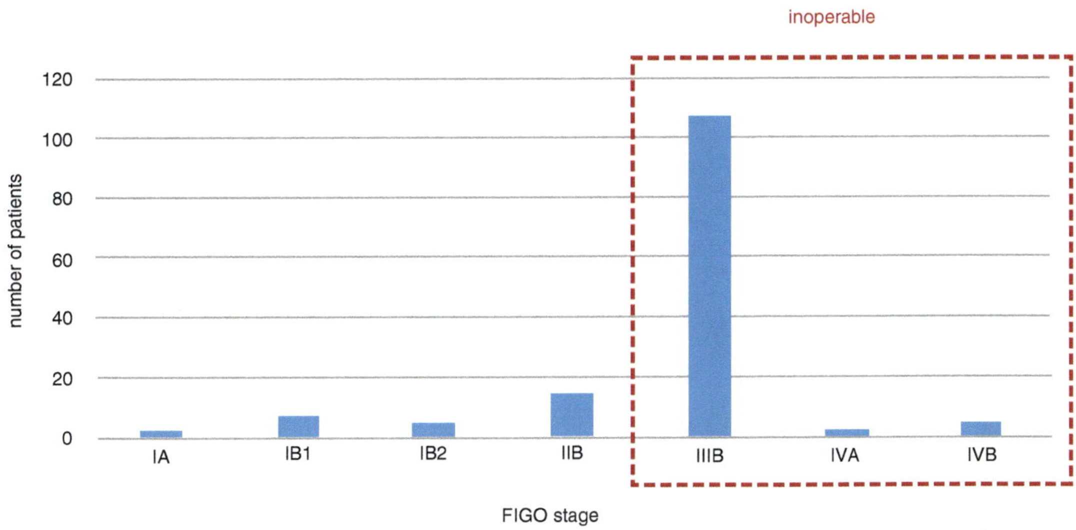

Fig. 17.65 FIGO stage distribution of cervical cancer patients at Universitas Diponegoro, Semarang, Indonesia. Only 11% of women were potentially operable. The vast majority of patients (78%) presented with FIGO stage IIIB disease (Suryapratama 2012)

17.4.3.1 Special Treatment Considerations (META Hospital, Mbeya, Tanzania)

17.4.3.1.1 Radiation Therapy

Unfortunately, primary combined radiation therapy (teletherapy and brachytherapy) as well as cisplatin chemotherapy as radiosensitizer is not an option for most patients at META hospital in Tanzania as there is only one treatment facility located in Dar es Salaam (Fig. 17.66).

Therefore, all patients who present with early stage disease (< FIGO IIIB) and will tolerate a 3–4-h surgical intervention should be considered as candidates for surgery.

Surgical treatment for cervical cancer consists of a Piver class III resection (Piver et al. 1974). For this type of surgery, the uterine artery is transected at its origin from the internal iliac artery. The parametria are cut as close to the pelvic sidewall as possible.

The surgical strategies summarized below are making several compromises and have to take into account the specific situation at the META Hospital at Mbeya, Tanzania, as well as the high number of patients with advanced-stage cervical cancer.

Particularly, the lack of a radiation therapy facility at Mbeya and the poor accessibility of the treatment center at Dar es Salaam influence treatment decisions and will make it necessary to deviate from established international guidelines of cancer treatment.

Of course, it should be one of the primary aims of Tanzanian health-care politics to establish adequate access to radiation therapy facilities, especially in the Southern Highlands of Tanzania.

17.4.3.1.2 Pelvic Lymph Node Dissection

According to the medical literature, pelvic lymph node involvement is an indication for adjuvant radiation therapy in combination with cisplatin chemotherapy (Peters et al. 2000). This type of treatment is indicated even for patients with only one lymph node metastasis. Unfortunately, adjuvant therapy cannot improve overall survival. However, it will lower the likelihood of pelvic recurrence which in turn may lead to poor quality of life due to fistula formation and other symptoms of local disease progression.

At the present time, access to adjuvant chemoradiation is limited for patients of the Mbeya region. Therefore, systematic pelvic lymph node dissection should not be performed routinely, as the surgical procedure in itself is not of any proven therapeutic value and, in the absence of adjuvant radiation therapy, of no immediate therapeutic consequence.

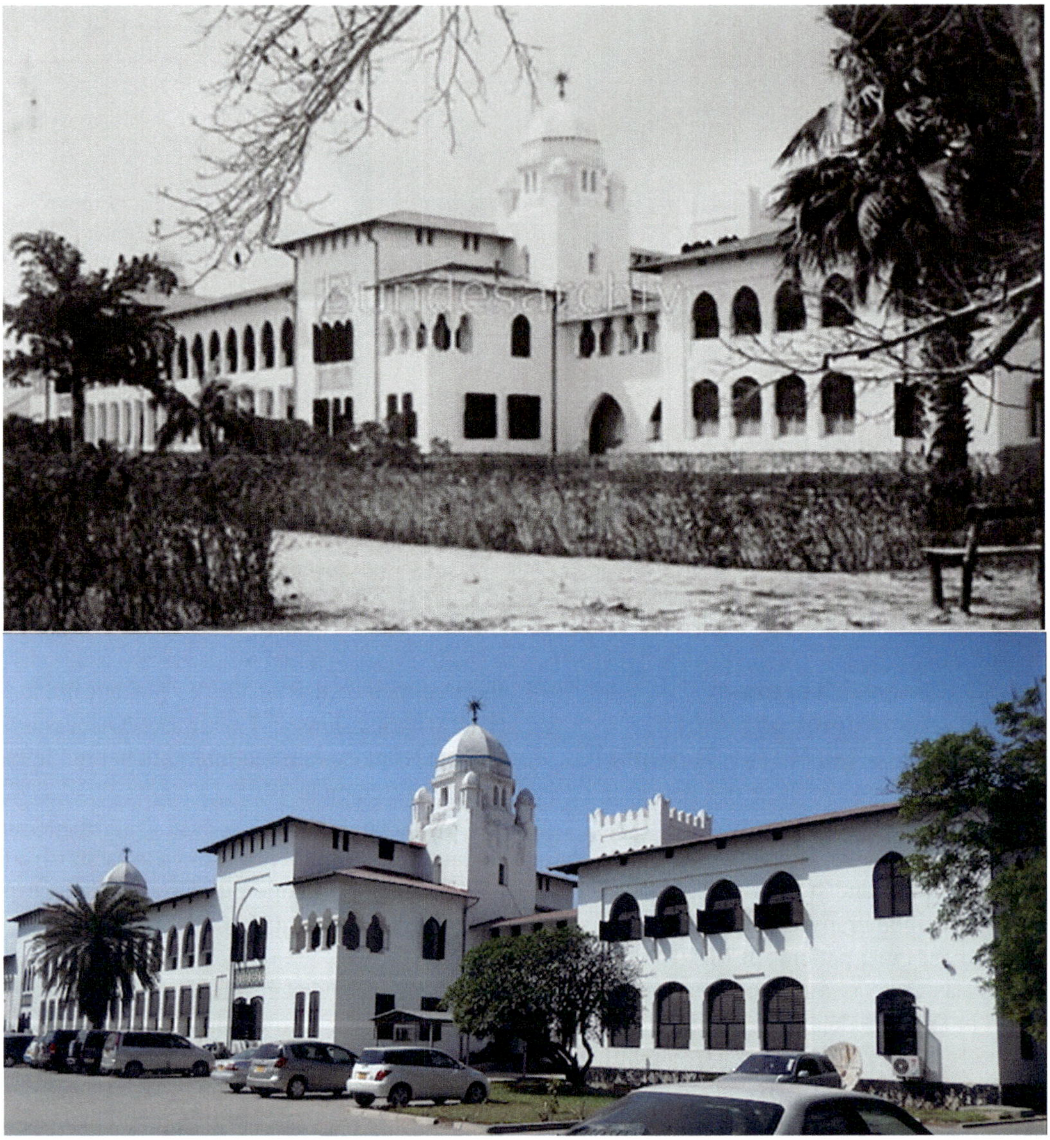

Fig. 17.66 Ocean Road Cancer Institute (ORCI) in Dar es Salaam, Tanzania. The former building founded by the German colonial government in 1895 is still in use [upper image: Bundesarchiv Bild 105-D 0 A6176, Foto: Dobbertin, Walter 1906/1914]. ORCI houses the only radiation therapy treatment facility in the entire country

Instead, a thorough evaluation of both the pelvic and the paraaortic regions should precede radical hysterectomy. Suspicious lymph nodes should be removed, although there is no evidence that debulking surgery is of any real benefit to patients with lymph node involvement. Rather it should be noted that these patients do not benefit from radical surgery, if they receive radiation therapy (Richard et al. 2008).

17.4.3.1.3 Neoadjuvant Chemotherapy

Neoadjuvant or induction chemotherapy would be an option to downstage advanced cervical cancer in order to avoid primary radiation therapy and to eventually perform radical surgery. It has long been established that cervical cancer is highly chemosensitive with a response rate of up to 90% (Dottino et al. 1991). However, highly toxic regimens have to be used such as cisplatin and bleomycin, in order to achieve these response rates. In an environment where chemotherapy with any of these drugs is not routinely applied, neoadjuvant chemotherapy should not be used. Furthermore, there are no reliable data available, that neoadjuvant chemotherapy improves overall survival.

17.4.3.1.4 FIGO Staging

In cervical cancer, treatment decision regarding surgery versus radiation therapy is made through bimanual examination using the FIGO staging system. Patients with hydronephrosis or a nonfunctioning kidney are classified as having stage IIIB disease, even in the absence of pelvic sidewall involvement. Therefore, proper FIGO staging always includes evaluation of the kidneys—either by ultrasound or by intravenous pyelogram.

Patients up to stage IIB may undergo surgery. However, if radiation therapy is available, stages IB2/IB3, IIA, and IIB should be treated by primary radiation therapy in order to avoid adjuvant irradiation, which would be administered postoperatively. For this may lead to increased morbidity as the highly traumatized surgical field has to be treated.

Interestingly, a highly experienced group of gynecologic surgeons from Japan has reported data on patients with FIGO IIB disease, who were surgically treated (Kasamatsu et al. 2009). Forty-eight percent of these patients were found to have a negative pelvic lymph node status. Furthermore, 50% of patients who were thought to have parametrial involvement on clinical exam were found to have disease limited to the cervix. Of those patients who had pathologically proven parametrial involvement, radical hysterectomy was technically feasible in 99% of cases. Nevertheless, adjuvant radiation therapy was indicated in 47% due to pelvic lymph node metastases or histologically proven parametrial involvement.

17.4.3.1.5 Preservation of the Ovaries and Bilateral Salpingectomy

According to data published by Shimada et al. (2006), ovaries can safely be preserved in younger patients diagnosed with squamous cell carcinoma of the cervix, whereas in patients with adenocarcinoma, bilateral salpingo-oophorectomy should be considered. According to Shimada et al., ovarian metastasis occurred in only 0.79% of patients with squamous cell carcinoma of the cervix with FIGO stage IB or IIB disease compared to 5.31% in patients with adenocarcinoma.

Recent studies have provided evidence that what have been traditionally thought to be primary ovarian tumors originate in the fallopian tubes and subsequently involve the ovary (Kurman and Shih 2010). Therefore, whenever the ovaries are preserved, bilateral salpingectomy should be performed.

17.4.3.2 Postoperative Bladder Dysfunction

The rate of urodynamic bladder dysfunction after radical hysterectomy for cervical carcinoma is as high as 72% on long-term follow-up (Plotti et al. 2011). The most traumatic surgical steps are vaginal, anterior, and posterior parametrial resection, when part of the parasympathetic fibers which arise from the S3 and S4 nerve roots are damaged in a Piver class III radical hysterectomy. Therefore, Chamberlain et al. (1991) suggest removal of the indwelling urinary catheter on day 6 with documentation of subsequent voiding volumes as well as urinary volumes remaining in the bladder. Repeated overextension of the bladder may lead to permanent damage of bladder function.

17.4.3.3 Preservation of Fertility

In many cultures, preservation of fertility is considered tantamount. Whereas in the vast majority of patients with invasive cervical cancer fertility preservation is not possible, conization or resection by LEEP may be acceptable in FIGO stage IA1 disease. However, this requires a thorough histopathological workup. The potential lack of follow-up exams, including colposcopy, needs to be taken into account. In many instances, total hysterectomy will be the safer option.

This is also true for fertility preservation when treating FIGO stage IB disease by radical trachelectomy (Abu-Rustum et al. 2006; Schneider et al. 2012). Overall experience with this procedure is limited and follow-up of patients as well as special monitoring of subsequent pregnancies are mandatory.

17.4.3.4 Summary: Radical Surgery for Cervical Cancer

- Systematic pelvic lymph node dissection should not be performed if adjuvant radiation therapy for patients with positive lymph node status is not available.
- Suspicious pelvic lymph nodes should be removed and send to histopathologic evaluation.
- Patients with FIGO stage IB1, IB2, IB3, and IIA disease should undergo a Piver class III radical hysterectomy.
- Patients with FIGO stage IIB disease might also benefit from primary surgery and should be explored surgically.
- In young patients, ovarian preservation should be considered. However, the relatively high percentage of ovarian metastases in patients with cervical adenocarcinoma should be kept in mind.
- When ovaries are preserved, bilateral salpingectomy should be performed.
- A strict postoperative voiding schedule should be established for patients undergoing radical hysterectomy in order to prevent overextension of the urinary bladder with subsequent permanent damage of bladder function.

17.5 Conclusions and Outlook

Awareness of the problem of cervical cancer burden on a political and governmental level is urgently needed to overcome the lack of prioritization in many low-resource countries. Tsu and Levin (2008) point to the *"unfair burden older women are carrying and the broad benefits that could be achieved by implementing HPV vaccination for young adolescent girls and appropriate screening and treatment programmes for women in their 30s and 40."*

In this chapter, alternative screening and treatment strategies have been discussed which are suitable for low- and middle-income countries. Some of these strategies are identical to established or future strategies in high-income countries, such as HPV screening, whereas some strategies are quite different and only suitable for regions with a high prevalence of disease such as visual screening in combination with a "see and treat" or "screen and treat" approach.

The most useful concept for cervical cancer prevention is HPV vaccination of girls and possibly boys at an early age. This is true for all countries regardless of their resources.

As pointed out earlier, HPV vaccination has been surprisingly underused in the USA as well as in most European countries despite its availability.

Once effective HPV vaccination coverage has been achieved, the requirements for secondary screening methods will change significantly on a global scale. As Sankaranarayanan et al. (2015) point out, existing screening programs in high-income countries will need to be adjusted to the effects of these vaccination programs as cytopathology-based screening programs will no longer be sensitive enough. Also, short screening intervals (3 years) or very short intervals (1 year) will no longer be appropriate in the postvaccination era.

In the long term, cervical cancer screening strategies will be similar in all countries. Sankaranarayanan et al. (2015) conclude: *"In the postvaccination scenario, HPV testing-based, low-intensity screening with raised age at initiating screening and few screening rounds at wide intervals such as 7 or 10 years seems to be the most suitable option for screening in all countries."*

17.6 Further Reading and Online Resources

Numerous teaching resources are available online free of charge from the WHO[5] and the IARC as well as others. Several of these resources have been quoted in this chapter.

The World Health Organization has published a manual called "Comprehensive Cervical Cancer Control. A guide to essential practice." The second edition of this free 408-page manual was published in 2014 (World Health Organization 2014a, b). Indeed, the main focus of this WHO publication is the practice of cervical cancer prevention, diagnosis, and treatment. Detailed suggestions are made to future program directors, including suggestions for consent forms and other documentation.

Another publication by the International Agency for Research on Cancer (IARC) from Sankaranarayanan and Wesley on visual screening for cervical neoplasia published in 2003 (Sankaranarayanan and Wesley 2003) is a practice-oriented manual both on VIA and VILI and is ideal as a primer for health service personnel and can be used as course material. Similarly, Sellors and Sankaranarayanan have published a manual on colposcopy and treatment of CIN (Sellors and Sankaranarayanan 2003).

In addition, the WHO/IARC have published a handbook on "Cervix Cancer Screening" in 2005 (World Health Organization 2005).

In addition, a trainee's handbook on VIA, HPV testing, and cryotherapy has been published by the WHO in 2017 (World Health Organization. Regional Office for South-East Asia 2017).

The Johns Hopkins Program for International Education in Gynecology and Obstetrics (JHPIEGO) provides online VIA teaching material as a high-resolution poster that can be downloaded and printed (Blumenthal et al. 2007).[6] This poster shows typical images of the cervix: VIA negative, VIA positive, cancer, and post-cryotherapy.

[5]https://screening.iarc.fr/manuals.php.

[6]http://reprolineplus.org/resources/cervical-cancer-prevention-learning-resource-package-atlas-visual-inspection-cervix-acetic.

References

Abu-Rustum NR, Sonoda Y, Black D, Levine DA, Chi DS, Barakat RR (2006) Fertility-sparing radical abdominal trachelectomy for cervical carcinoma: technique and review of the literature. Gynecol Oncol 103(3):807–813. https://doi.org/10.1016/j.ygyno.2006.05.044. S0090-8258(06)00420-3 [pii]

Adesina A, Chumba D, Nelson AM, Orem J, Roberts DJ, Wabinga H et al (2013) Improvement of pathology in sub-Saharan Africa. Lancet Oncol 14(4):e152–e157. https://doi.org/10.1016/S1470-2045(12)70598-3

Ajenifuja KO, Gage JC, Adepiti AC, Wentzensen N, Eklund C, Reilly M et al (2013) A population-based study of visual inspection with acetic acid (VIA) for cervical screening in rural Nigeria. Int J Gynecol Cancer 23(3):507–512. https://doi.org/10.1097/IGC.0b013e318280f395

Anwar SL, Tampubolon G, Van Hemelrijck M, Hutajulu SH, Watkins J, Wulaningsih W, PILAR Research Network (2018) Determinants of cancer screening awareness and participation among Indonesian women. BMC Cancer 18(1):208. https://doi.org/10.1186/s12885-018-4125-z

Arbyn M, Castellsague X, de Sanjose S, Bruni L, Saraiya M, Bray F, Ferlay J (2011) Worldwide burden of cervical cancer in 2008. Ann Oncol 22(12):2675–2686. https://doi.org/10.1093/annonc/mdr015

Aziz MF (2009) Gynecological cancer in Indonesia. J Gynecol Oncol 20(1):8–10. https://doi.org/10.3802/jgo.2009.20.1.8

Bagcchi S (2014) Cervical cancer screening trials in India spark controversy. BMJ 348(April):g3038–g3038. https://doi.org/10.1136/bmj.g3038

Baldur-Felskov B, Mwaiselage J, Faber MT, Kjaerem M, Cour CD de la, Munk C, et al (2019) Factors associated with a cervical high-grade lesion on cytology or a positive visual inspection with acetic acid among more than 3300 Tanzanian women. Trop Med Int Health 24:229–37.

Bayer E (2011) Zervixzytologie am Ifisi Missionshospital in Mbalizi/Mbeya/Tanzania (Cervical cytology in Ifisi Mission Hospital in Mbalizi/Mbeya/Tanzania). Verh Dtsch Ges Zyt 27:68–69

Belinson J, Qiao YL, Pretorius R, Zhang WH, Elson P, Li L et al (2001) Shanxi Province Cervical Cancer Screening Study: a cross-sectional comparative trial of multiple techniques to detect cervical neoplasia. Gynecol Oncol 83(2):439–444. https://doi.org/10.1006/gyno.2001.6370. S0090-8258(01)96370-X [pii]

Blumenthal PD, McIntosh N, Crump S, Elabd S, Lewison D (2007) Cervical cancer prevention learning resource package: atlas of visual inspection of the cervix with acetic acid

Chamberlain DH, Hopkins MP, Roberts JA, McGuire EJ, Morley GW, Wang CC (1991) The effects of early removal of indwelling urinary catheter after radical hysterectomy. Gynecol Oncol 43(2):98–102

Chandra R, Rauf S, Malinta U (2017) Human papilloma virus self testing as an alternative method for cervical cancer screening. J Nurs Sci Health 5:114–119. https://doi.org/10.32771/inajog.v5i2.531

Clifford GM, Gallus S, Herrero R, Munoz N, Snijders PJ, Vaccarella S et al (2005) Worldwide distribution of human papillomavirus types in cytologically normal women in the International Agency for Research on Cancer HPV prevalence surveys: a pooled analysis. Lancet 366(9490):991–998

Cuzick J, Clavel C, Petry KU, Meijer CJ, Hoyer H, Ratnam S et al (2006) Overview of the European and North American studies on HPV testing in primary cervical cancer screening. Int J Cancer 119(5):1095–1101. https://doi.org/10.1002/ijc.21955

Dartell M, Rasch V, Kahesa C, Mwaiselage J, Ngoma T, Junge J et al (2012) Human papillomavirus prevalence and type distribution in 3603 HIV-positive and HIV-negative women in the general population of Tanzania. Sex Transm Dis 39(3):201–208. https://doi.org/10.1097/OLQ.0b013e31823b50ad

De Boer R, Burris H, Monnier A, Mouridsen H, O'Shaughnessy J, McIntyre K et al (2006) The head to head trial: letrozole vs anastrozole as adjuvant treatment of postmenopausal patients with node positive breast cancer. J Clin Oncol 24:10672

Domingo EJ, Noviani R, Noor MR, Ngelangel CA, Limpaphayom KK, Thuan TV et al (2008) Epidemiology and prevention of cervical cancer in Indonesia, Malaysia, the Philippines, Thailand and Vietnam. Vaccine 26(Suppl 1):M71–M79. https://doi.org/10.1016/j.vaccine.2008.05.039

Dottino PR, Plaxe SC, Beddoe AM, Johnston C, Cohen CJ (1991) Induction chemotherapy followed by radical surgery in cervical cancer. Gynecol Oncol 40(1):7–11

Endarti D, Satibi S, Kristina SA, Farida MA, Rahmawanti Y, Andriani T (2018) Knowledge, perception, and acceptance of HPV vaccination and screening for cervical cancer among women in Yogyakarta Province, Indonesia. Asian Pac J Cancer Prev 19(4):1105–1111. https://doi.org/10.22034/APJCP.2018.19.4.1105

Feldmeier H, Krantzi I, Poggensee G (1995) Female genital schistosomiasis: a neglected risk factor for the transmission of HIV? Trans R Soc Trop Med Hyg 89(2):237. https://doi.org/10.1016/0035-9203(95)90512-X

Fokom-Domgue J, Combescure C, Fokom-Defo V, Tebeu PM, Vassilakos P, Kengne AP, Petignat P (2015) Performance of alternative strategies for primary cervical cancer screening in sub-Saharan Africa: systematic review and meta-analysis of diagnostic test accuracy studies. BMJ 351:h3084. https://doi.org/10.1136/bmj.h3084

Forouzanfar MH, Foreman KJ, Delossantos AM, Lozano R, Lopez AD, Murray CJ, Naghavi M (2011) Breast and cervical cancer in 187 countries between 1980 and 2010: a systematic analysis. Lancet 378(9801):1461–1484. https://doi.org/10.1016/S0140-6736(11)61351-2

Gage JC, Ajenifuja KO, Wentzensen N, Adepiti AC, Stoler M, Eder PS et al (2012) Effectiveness of a simple rapid human papillomavirus DNA test in rural Nigeria. Int J Cancer 131(12):2903–2909. https://doi.org/10.1002/ijc.27563

Gakidou E, Nordhagen S, Obermeyer Z (2008) Coverage of cervical cancer screening in 57 countries: low average levels and large inequalities. PLoS Med 5(6):e132. https://doi.org/10.1371/journal.pmed.0050132

Gharoro EP, Ikeanyi EN (2006) An appraisal of the level of awareness and utilization of the Pap smear as a cervical cancer screening test among female health workers in a tertiary health institution. Int J Gynecol Cancer 16(3):1063–1068. https://doi.org/10.1111/j.1525--1438.2006.00579.x

Goldie SJ, O'Shea M, Campos NG, Diaz M, Sweet S, Kim S-Y (2008) Health and economic outcomes of HPV 16,18 vaccination in 72 GAVI-eligible countries. Vaccine 26(32):4080–4093. https://doi.org/10.1016/j.vaccine.2008.04.053

Hassan RB, Armawan E, Arya IFD (2018) Visual inspection test with acetic acid for cervical cancer screening: willingness and acceptability among reproductive age and married women. Althea Med J 5(2):98–104. https://doi.org/10.15850/amj.v5n2.1419

Islam RM, Billah B, Hossain MN, Oldroyd J (2017) Barriers to cervical cancer and breast cancer screening uptake in low-income and middle-income countries: a systematic review. Asian Pac J Cancer Prev 18(7):1751–1763. https://doi.org/10.22034/APJCP.2017.18.7.1751

Jaspers L, Budiningsih S, Wolterbeek R, Henderson FC, Peters AAW (2011) Parental acceptance of human papillomavirus (HPV) vaccination in Indonesia: a cross-sectional study. Vaccine 29(44):7785–7793. https://doi.org/10.1016/j.vaccine.2011.07.107

Jordan S, Randall LM (2011) Differentiating squamous cell carcinoma of the cervix and epithelioid trophoblastic tumor. Int J Gynecol Cancer 21:918

Joura EA, Giuliano AR, Iversen OE, Bouchard C, Mao C, Mehlsen J et al (2015) A 9-valent HPV vaccine against infection and intraepithelial neoplasia in women. N Engl J Med 372(8):711–723. https://doi.org/10.1056/NEJMoa1405044

Kairi-Vassilatou E, Papakonstantinou K, Grapsa D, Kondi-Paphiti A, Hasiakos D (2018) Primary gestational choriocarcinoma of the uterine cervix. Report of a case and review of the literature. Int J Gynecol Cancer 17(4):921–925. https://doi.org/10.1111/j.1525--1438.2006.00852.x

Kantelhardt EJ, Moelle U, Begoihn M, Addissie A, Trocchi P, Yonas B et al (2014) Cervical cancer in Ethiopia: survival of 1,059 patients who received oncologic therapy. Oncologist 19(7):727–734. https://doi.org/10.1634/theoncologist.2013-0326

Kasamatsu T, Onda T, Sawada M, Kato T, Ikeda S (2009) Radical hysterectomy for FIGO stage IIB cervical cancer: clinicopathological characteristics and prognostic evaluation. Gynecol Oncol 114(1):69–74. https://doi.org/10.1016/j.ygyno.2009.03.026. S0090-8258(09)00197-8 [pii]

Kjetland EF, Poggensee G, Helling-Giese G, Richter J, Sjaastad A, Chitsulo L et al (1996) Female genital schistosomiasis due to Schistosoma haematobium Clinical and parasitological findings in women in rural Malawi. Acta Trop 62(4):239–255. https://doi.org/10.1016/S0001-706X(96)00026-5

Kjetland EF, Leutscher PDC, Ndhlovu PD (2012) A review of female genital schistosomiasis. Trends Parasitol 28(2):58–65. https://doi.org/10.1016/j.pt.2011.10.008

Koliopoulos G, Arbyn M, Martin-Hirsch P, Kyrgiou M, Prendiville W, Paraskevaidis E (2007) Diagnostic accuracy of human papillomavirus testing in primary cervical screening: a systematic review and meta-analysis of non-randomized studies. Gynecol Oncol 104(1):232–246. https://doi.org/10.1016/j.ygyno.2006.08.053

Kosen S, Andrijono A, Ocviyanti D, Indriatmi W (2017) The cost-effectiveness of quadrivalent human papillomavirus vaccination in Indonesia. Asian Pac J Cancer Prev 18(7):2011–2017. https://doi.org/10.22034/APJCP.2017.18.7.2011

Kurman RJ, Shih IM (2010) The origin and pathogenesis of epithelial ovarian cancer: a proposed unifying theory. Am J Surg Pathol 34(3):433–443. https://doi.org/10.1097/PAS.0b013e3181cf3d79

Labani S, Asthana S (2014) Cervical cancer screening trials in India and ethical issues. J Nurs Sci Health 26(3):211–212

Labani S, Asthana S, Sodhani P, Gupta S, Bhambhani S, Pooja B et al (2014) CareHPV cervical cancer screening demonstration in a rural population of north India. Eur J Obstet Gynecol Reprod Biol 176:75–79. https://doi.org/10.1016/j.ejogrb.2014.03.006

Ladner J, Besson M-H, Hampshire R, Tapert L, Chirenje M, Saba J et al (2012) Assessment of eight HPV vaccination programs implemented in lowest income countries. BMC Public Health 12(1):370. https://doi.org/10.1186/1471-2458-12-370

Lam CT, Krieger MS, Gallagher JE, Asma B, Muasher LC, Schmitt JW et al (2015) Design of a Novel Low Cost Point of Care Tampon (POCkeT) colposcope for use in resource limited settings. PLoS One 10(9):e0135869. https://doi.org/10.1371/journal.pone.0135869

Lellé RJ (2007) Die Münster-Kolposkopielupe - eine Alternative zum konventionellen Kolposkop. Geburtshilfe Frauenheilkd 67:154–155

Leyh-Bannurah S-R, Prugger C, de Koning MN, Goette H, Lellé RJ, Ferlay J et al (2014) Cervical human papillomavirus prevalence and genotype distribution among hybrid capture 2 positive women 15 to 64 years of age in the Gurage zone, rural Ethiopia. Infect Agents Cancer 9(1):33. https://doi.org/10.1186/1750-9378-9-33

Lim JNW, Ojo AA (2017) Barriers to utilisation of cervical cancer screening in Sub Sahara Africa: a systematic review. Eur J Cancer Care 26(1):e12444. https://doi.org/10.1111/ecc.12444

Lin C-Q, Chen F, Liu B, Zhang Y-Z, Cui X-L, Li A-M et al (2014) A parallel study of careHPV and Hybrid Capture 2 human papillomavirus DNA testing for cervical cancer screening in rural China. J Virol Methods 202:73–78. https://doi.org/10.1016/j.jviromet.2014.03.002

Lorenzi AT, Fregnani JHTG, Possati-Resende JC, Neto CS, Villa LL, Longatto-Filho A (2013) Self-collection for high-risk HPV detection in Brazilian women using the careHPV™ test. Gynecol Oncol 131(1):131–134. https://doi.org/10.1016/j.ygyno.2013.07.092

Marquardt K, Kolankowska I, Pfandzelter R (2014) Jahresstatistik Zervixzytologie. Der Frauenarzt 55(8):732–733

Mink J, Peterson C (2016) MobileODT: a case study of a novel approach to an mHealth-based model of sustainable impact. mHealth 2(4):12

Mutyaba T, Faxelid E, Mirembe F, Weiderpass E (2007) Influences on uptake of reproductive health services in Nsangi community of Uganda and their implications for cervical cancer screening. Reprod Health 4(1):4. https://doi.org/10.1186/1742-4755-4-4

Mwanahamuntu MH, Sahasrabuddhe VV, Pfaendler KS, Mudenda V, Hicks ML, Vermund SH et al (2009) Implementation of "see-and-treat" cervical cancer prevention services linked to HIV care in Zambia. AIDS 23(6):1–5. https://doi.org/10.1097/QAD.0b013e3283236e11.00002030-200903270-00001 [pii]

Narita F, Takeuchi K, Hamana S, Ohbayashi C, Ayata M, Maruo T (2003) Epithelioid trophoblastic tumor (ETT) initially interpreted as cervical cancer. Int J Gynecol Cancer 13(4):551–554. https://doi.org/10.1046/j.1525-1438.2003.13311.x. https://doi.org/10.1093/annonc/mdy375.013. academic.oup.com

Nelson HD, Tyne K, Naik A, Bougatsos C, Chan BK, Humphrey L (2009) Screening for breast cancer: an update for the U.S. Preventive Services Task Force. Ann Intern Med 151(10):727–737. https://doi.org/10.7326/0003-4819-151-10-200911170-00009

Nessa A, Roy JS, Chowdhury MA, Khanam Q, Afroz R, Wistrand C, et al (2014) Evaluation of the accuracy in detecting cervical lesions by nurses versus doctors using a stationary colposcope and Gynocular in a low-resource setting. BMJ Open 4:e005313.

Network NA (2013) Warning! Severe burns and permanent scarring after glacial acetic acid (= 99.5%) mistakenly applied topically

Ngoma T, Muwonge R, Mwaiselage J, Kawegere J, Bukori P, Sankaranarayanan R (2010) Evaluation of cervical visual inspection screening in Dar es Salaam, Tanzania. Int J Gynaecol Obstet 109(2):100–104. https://doi.org/10.1016/j.ijgo.2009.11.025

Ngonzi J, Bajunirwe F, Wistrand C, Mayanja R, Altman D, Thorsell M, et al (2013) Agreement of colposcope and gynocular in assessment of cervical lesions by swede score: a randomized, crossover pilot trial. J Low Genit Tract Dis 17:372–7.

Oemati R, Rahajeng E, Kristanto AY (2011) Tumor's Prevalence and Influence's Factors in Indonesia. Bul Penelit Kesehat 39(4):190–204

Othman NH, Rebolj M (2009) Challenges to cervical screening in a developing country: the case of Malaysia. Asian Pac J Cancer Prev 10(5):747–752

Peters WA III, Liu PY, Barrett RJ, Stock RJ, Monk BJ, Berek JS et al (2000) Concurrent chemotherapy and pelvic radiation therapy compared with pelvic radiation therapy alone as adjuvant therapy after radical surgery in high-risk early-stage cancer of the cervix. J Clin Oncol 18(8):1606–1613

Petry KU, Scheffel D, Bode U, Gabrysiak T, Kochel H, Kupsch E et al (1994) Cellular immunodeficiency enhances the progression of human papillomavirus-associated cervical lesions. Int J Cancer 57(6):836–840

Petry KU, Kochel H, Bode U, Schedel I, Niesert S, Glaubitz M et al (1996) Human papillomavirus is associated with the frequent detection of warty and basaloid high-grade neoplasia of the vulva and cervical neoplasia among immunocompromised women. Gynecol Oncol 60(1):30–34

Petry KU, Scholz U, Hollwitz B, von Wasielewski R, Meijer CJLM (2003) Human papillomavirus, coinfection with Schistosoma hematobium, and cervical neoplasia in rural Tanzania. Int J Gynecol Cancer 13(4):505–509. https://doi.org/10.1046/j.1525-1438.2003.13301.x

Piver MS, Rutledge F, Smith JP (1974) Five classes of extended hysterectomy for women with cervical cancer 44:265–72.

Pfaendler KS, Sahasrabuddhe VV, Katundu K, Mwanahamuntu MH, Kapambwe S, Vermund SH, Parham GP (2015) Factors associated with post-cryotherapy wound healing among HIV-infected women in a low-resource Sub-Saharan African setting. Gynecol Oncol 137:69. https://doi.org/10.1016/j.ygyno.2015.01.165

Plotti F, Angioli R, Zullo MA, Sansone M, Altavilla T, Antonelli E et al (2011) Update on urodynamic bladder dysfunctions after radical hysterectomy for cervical cancer. Crit Rev Oncol Hematol 80(2):323–329. https://doi.org/10.1016/j.critrevonc.2010.12.004

Poggensee G, Feldmeier H (2001) Female genital schistosomiasis: facts and hypotheses. Acta Trop 79(3):193–210. https://doi.org/10.1016/S0001-706X(01)00086-9

Poggensee G, Kiwelu I, Weger V, Göppner D, Diedrich T, Krantz I, Feldmeier H (2000) Female genital schistosomiasis of the lower genital tract: prevalence and disease-associated morbidity in northern Tanzania. J Infect Dis 181(3):1210–1213. https://doi.org/10.1086/315345

Qiao Y-L, Sellors JW, Eder PS, Bao Y-P, Lim JM, Zhao F-H et al (2008) A new HPV-DNA test for cervical-cancer screening in developing regions: a cross-sectional study of clinical accuracy in rural China. Lancet Oncol 9(10):929–936. https://doi.org/10.1016/S1470-2045(08)70210-9

Remes P, Selestine V, Changalucha J, Ross DA, Wight D, de Sanjosé S et al (2012) A qualitative study of HPV vaccine acceptability among health workers, teachers, parents, female pupils, and religious leaders in northwest Tanzania. Vaccine 30(36):5363–5367. https://doi.org/10.1016/j.vaccine.2012.06.025

Ricard-Gauthier D, Wisniak A, Catarino R, van Rossum AF, Meyer-Hamme U, Negulescu R et al (2015) Use of smartphones as adjuvant tools for cervical cancer screening in low-resource settings. J Low Genit Tract Dis 19(4):295–300. https://doi.org/10.1097/LGT.0000000000000136

Richard SD, Krivak TC, Castleberry A, Beriwal S, Kelley JL III, Edwards RP, Sukumvanich P (2008) Survival for stage IB cervical cancer with positive lymph node involvement: a comparison of completed vs. abandoned radical hysterectomy. Gynecol Oncol 109(1):43–48. https://doi.org/10.1016/j.ygyno.2007.12.002. S0090-8258(07)00978-X [pii]

Rodriguez AC, Morera LA, Bratti C, Herrero R, Cox JT, Morales J et al (2004) Performance of direct visual inspection of the cervix with acetic acid and magnification in a previously screened population. J Low Genit Tract Dis 8(2):132–138

Ruland R, Prugger C, Schiffer R, Regidor M, Lellé RJ (2006) Prevalence of human papilloma virus infection in women in rural Ethiopia. Eur J Epidemiol 21(9):727–729

de Sanjose S, Quint WG, Alemany L, Geraets DT, Klaustermeier JE, Lloveras B et al (2010) Human papillomavirus genotype attribution in invasive cervical cancer: a retrospective cross-sectional worldwide study. Lancet Oncol 11(11):1048–1056. https://doi.org/10.1016/S1470-2045(10)70230-8

Sankaranarayanan R, Wesley RS (2003) A practical manual on visual screening for cervical neoplasia. IARC Press, p Lyon

Sankaranarayanan R, Nene BM, Shastri SS, Jayant K, Muwonge R, Budukh AM et al (2009) HPV screening for cervical cancer in rural India. N Engl J Med 360(14):1385–1394. https://doi.org/10.1056/NEJMoa0808516. 360/14/1385 [pii]

Sankaranarayanan R, Nene BM, Shastri S, Esmy PE, Rajkumar R, Muwonge R et al (2014) Response to article titled "US-funded measurements of cervical cancer death rates in India: scientific and ethical concerns" by Eric J Suba. Indian J Med Ethics 11(3):175–178

Sankaranarayanan R, Qiao YL, Keita N (2015) The next steps in cervical screening. Women Health 11(2):201–212. https://doi.org/10.2217/whe.14.70

Schellekens MC, Dijkman A, Aziz MF, Siregar B, Cornain S, Kolkman-Uljee S et al (2004) Prevalence of single and multiple HPV types in cervical carcinomas in Jakarta, Indonesia. Gynecol Oncol 93(1):49–53. https://doi.org/10.1016/j.ygyno.2003.12.015

Schneider A, Erdemoglu E, Chiantera V, Reed N, Morice P, Rodolakis A et al (2012) Clinical recommendation radical trachelectomy for fertility preservation in patients with early-stage cervical cancer. Int J Gynecol Cancer 22(4):659–666. https://doi.org/10.1097/IGC.0b013e3182466a0e

Schockaert S, Poppe W, Arbyn M, Verguts T, Verguts J (2008) Incidence of vaginal intraepithelial neoplasia after hysterectomy for cervical intraepithelial neoplasia: a retrospective study. Am J Obstet Gynecol 199(2):113.e1–113.e5. https://doi.org/10.1016/j.ajog.2008.02.026. S0002-9378(08)00172-5 [pii]

Sellors JW, Sankaranarayanan R (2003) Colposcopy and treatment of cervical intraepithelial neoplasia. A beginner's manual. IARC Press, Lyon

Setiawan D, Dolk FC, Suwantika AA, Westra TA, Wilschut JC, Postma MJ (2016) Cost-utility analysis of human papillomavirus vaccination and cervical screening on cervical cancer patient in Indonesia. Val Health Reg Iss 9:84–92. https://doi.org/10.1016/j.vhri.2015.10.010

Shastri SS, Mittra I, Mishra GA, Gupta S, Dikshit R, Singh S, Badwe RA (2014) Effect of VIA screening by primary health workers: randomized controlled study in Mumbai, India. J Natl Cancer Inst 106:dju009. https://doi.org/10.1093/jnci/dju009

Shimada M, Kigawa J, Nishimura R, Yamaguchi S, Kuzuya K, Nakanishi T et al (2006) Ovarian metastasis in carcinoma of the uterine cervix. Gynecol Oncol 101(2):234–237. https://doi.org/10.1016/j.ygyno.2005.10.004. S0090-8258(05)00879-6 [pii]

Silkensen SL, Schiffman M, Sahasrabuddhe V, Flanigan JS (2018) Is It Time to move beyond visual inspection with acetic acid for cervical cancer screening? Glob Health Sci Pract 6(2):242–246. https://doi.org/10.9745/GHSP-D-18-00206

Stewart BW, Wild CP (2014) World cancer report 2014. International Agency for Research on Cancer, WHO, Geneva

Suba EJ (2016) US-funded measurements of cervical cancer death rates in India: scientific and ethical concerns. Indian J Med Ethics 11(3):167–175

Suryapratama SA. (2012) Karakteristik penderita kanker serviks di RSUP Dr. Kariadi Semarang tahun 2010. Fakultas Kedokteran Universitas Diponegoro

The United Republic of Tanzania Ministry of Health and Welfare S (2011) Tanzania service delivery guidelines for cervical cancer prevention and control

Tjindarbumi D, Mangunkusumo R (2002) Cancer in Indonesia, present and future. Jpn J Clin Oncol 32(Suppl):S17–S21

Trope LA, Chumworathayi B, Blumenthal PD (2013) Feasibility of community-based careHPV for cervical cancer prevention in rural Thailand. J Low Genit Tract Dis 17(3):315–319. https://doi.org/10.1097/LGT.0b013e31826b7b70

Tsu VD, Levin CE (2008) Making the case for cervical cancer prevention: what about equity? Reprod Health Matt 16(32):104–112. https://doi.org/10.1016/S0968-8080(08)32411-2

Vet JN, de Boer MA, van den Akker BE, Siregar B, Lisnawati, Budiningsih S et al (2008) Prevalence of human papillomavirus in Indonesia: a population-based study in three regions. Br J Cancer 99(1):214–218

Vet JN, Kooijman JL, Henderson FC, Aziz FM, Purwoto G, Susanto H et al (2012) Single-visit approach of cervical cancer screening: see and treat in Indonesia. Br J Cancer 107(5):772–777. https://doi.org/10.1038/bjc.2012.334

Watson-Jones D, Baisley K, Ponsiano R, Lemme F, Remes P, Ross D et al (2012a) Human papillomavirus vaccination in Tanzanian schoolgirls: cluster-randomized trial comparing 2 vaccine-delivery strategies. J Infect Dis 206(5):678–686. https://doi.org/10.1093/infdis/jis407

Watson-Jones D, Tomlin K, Remes P, Baisley K, Ponsiano R, Soteli S et al (2012b) Reasons for receiving or not receiving HPV vaccination in primary schoolgirls in Tanzania: a case control study. PLoS One 7(10):e45231. https://doi.org/10.1371/journal.pone.0045231

Widiasih R, Nelson K (2018) Muslim husbands' roles in women's health and cancer: the perspectives of Muslim women in Indonesia. Asian Pac J Cancer Prev 19(6):1703–1709. https://doi.org/10.22034/APJCP.2018.19.6.1703

Winarto H, Kusuma D, Anggraeni TD, Andrijono, Purwoto G, Purbadi S et al (2018) Clinicopathologic characteristics of cervical cancer patients at Dr. Cipto Mangunkusumo Hospital, Jakarta, Indonesia, January 2012–December 2016. Adv Sci Lett 24(9):6433–6436. https://doi.org/10.1166/asl.2018.12738

World Health Organization (2005) IARC handbooks of cancer prevention. Cervix cancer screening. IARC Press, Lyon

World Health Organization (2012) Prevention of cervical cancer through screening using visual inspection with acetic acid (VIA) and treatment with cryotherapy. In: A demonstration project in six African countries: Malawi, Madagascar, Nigeria, Uganda, the United Republic of Tanzania, and Zambia. WHO Document Production Services, Geneva

World Health Organization (2013) WHO guidelines for screening and treatment of precancerous lesions for cervical cancer prevention. WHO, Geneva

World Health Organization (2014a) Comprehensive cervical cancer control. A guide to essential practice, 2nd edn. WHO, Geneva

World Health Organization (2014b) WHO guidelines for treatment of cervical intraepithelial neoplasia 2–3 and adenocarcinoma in situ: cryotherapy, large loop excision of the transformation zone, and cold knife conization. WHO, Geneva

World Health Organization. Regional Office for South-East Asia (2017) Training of health staff in VIA, HPV detection test and cryotherapy - trainees' handbook. World Health Organization. Regional Office for South-East Asia, New Delhi. https://apps.who.int/iris/handle/10665/259001

Wu S, Meng L, Wang S, Ma D (2005) A comparison of four screening methods for cervical neoplasia. Int J Gynecol Obstet 91(2):189–193. https://doi.org/10.1016/j.ijgo.2005.08.013

Yeates KE, Sleeth J, Hopman W, Ginsburg O, Heus K, Andrews L et al (2016) Evaluation of a smartphone-based training strategy among health care workers screening for cervical cancer in Northern Tanzania: the Kilimanjaro method. J Glob Oncol 2:356. https://doi.org/10.1200/JGO.2015.001768

Ying H, Jing F, Fanghui Z, Youlin Q, Yali H (2014) High-risk HPV nucleic acid detection kit–the *care*HPV test –a new detection method for screening. Sci Rep 4(1):4704. https://doi.org/10.1038/srep04704

18 Clinical Scenarios for Colposcopy Training

Contents

This is an important part of this textbook.
In this chapter, common and less common scenarios from a colposcopy clinic are discussed to provide a practical approach to colposcopy training.

Please note:
The 2011 Rio nomenclature of colposcopy (Bornstein et al. 2012a, b) is applied whenever appropriate (gray box).
All colposcopy images are called "adequate" using the definition by Bornstein et al. (2012a, b): "The examination may be obscured by *inflammation*, *bleeding*, or *scarring*."
National and international guidelines have been changing over time. Some patients have not been optimally managed at the time. However, ideal or exemplary scenarios are rarely encountered in real life. Therefore, none of the individual facts including discrepant findings have been altered in order to reflect the routine of colposcopy clinics in different environments. Each of these scenarios is followed by a critical commentary.

R. J. Lellé, V. Küppers, *Colposcopy*, https://doi.org/10.1007/978-3-030-85388-4_18

18.1 Cervical Dysplasia

18.1.1 Overtreatment of LSIL/CIN1

A 21-year-old patient has had an abnormal Pap test suspecting LSIL, possibly also HSIL/CIN2. On colposcopy, a large ectopy is seen with a small band of thin acetowhite epithelium located adjacent to the squamocolumnar junction with a discrete mosaic formation.

- Adequate colposcopy
- Squamocolumnar junction visible
- T1
- Abnormal colposcopic findings: thin acetowhite epithelium close to the squamocolumnar junction (minor change) Fig. 18.1

A biopsy from 12 o'clock is taken and does not show cervical intraepithelial neoplasia. The repeat Pap smear (ThinPrep®) suggests LSIL. The Hybrid capture II test is positive for both low- and high-risk virus DNA.

Fourteen months later, colposcopy is repeated and the results are unchanged. Another biopsy from 12 o'clock is obtained and shows LSIL (CIN1). Subsequently, CO_2 laser vaporization of the transformation zone is performed.

One year later, the patient, now 23 years old, is seen for follow-up colposcopy. Now, the ectocervix is covered completely by mature Lugol-positive squamous epithelium. However, the squamocolumnar junction is no longer visible (T3). Peripherally at 5 o'clock, a small acetowhite area with sharp borders is present which stains Lugol-negative (minor change) (Fig. 18.2).

Now, the ThinPrep® Pap smear is normal, and the Hybrid capture II test has become negative.

Commentary

Low-grade dysplasia (LSIL/CIN1) in such a young patient should not be treated as CIN1 is not considered a condition that requires treatment any more. The probability of spontaneous regression is high, and surgery may lead to complications in future pregnancies.

When Pap smear screening is initiated at an early age and at a short interval, the diagnosis of ASC-US or LSIL is increasingly likely and may lead to overtreatment, as patients will be under increasing psychological stress due to several repeat exams and request surgical removal of the cellular changes.

CO_2 laser treatment is a somewhat more gentle alternative to LEEP and appears to have been "successful" as the Pap smear result returned to normal, and the HPV test was negative, which will not always be the case. However, the squamocolumnar junction is no longer visible.

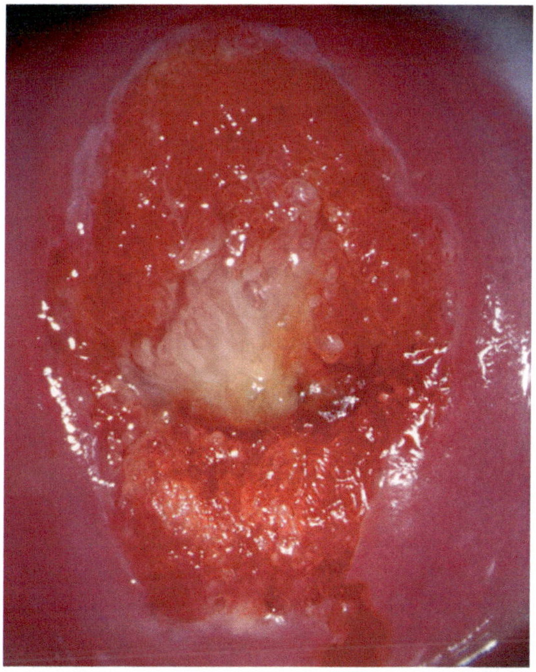

Fig. 18.1 Minor change. At the periphery of a large ectopy, a small band of transparent acetowhite epithelium is seen

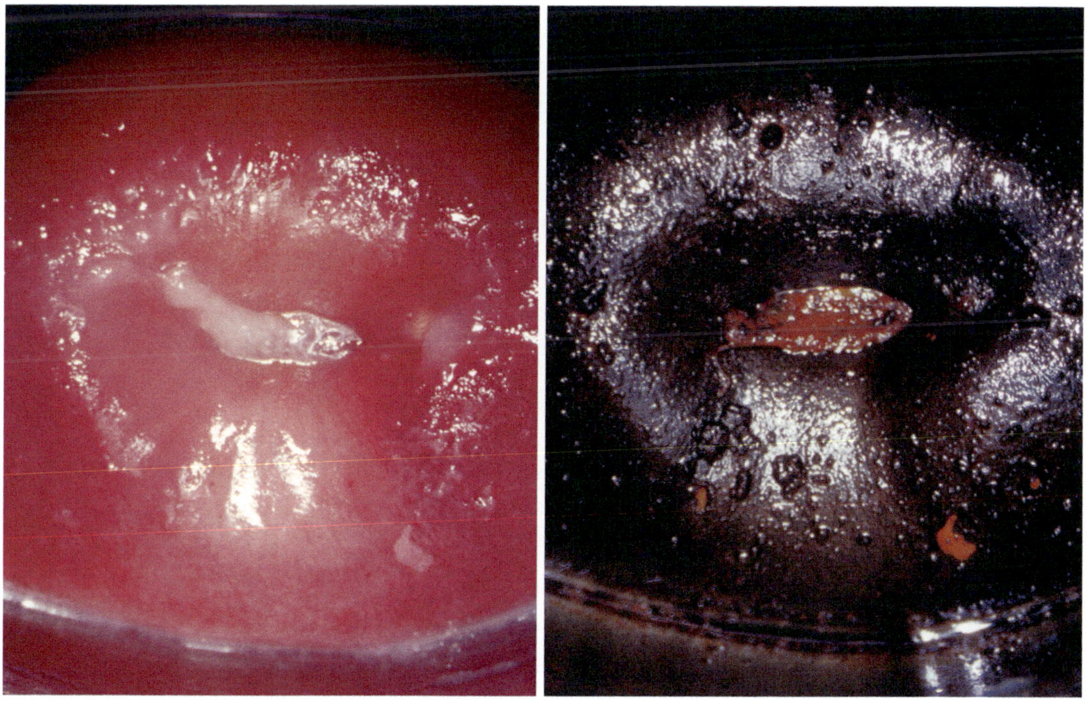

Fig. 18.2 Although only LSIL had been verified in this 21-year-old patient, CO_2 laser vaporization has been performed. The ectocervix is normal. However, the squamocolumnar junction cannot be visualized any more (T3)

18.1.2 Cervix Before and After CO_2 Laser Treatment for CIN2

A 38-year-old nulligravid patient is suspected of having LSIL/HSIL (CIN2) on her routine Pap smear. On colposcopy, a large ectopy is seen which is partially covered by mature metaplastic epithelium. Within the dorsal quadrants, abnormal opaque acetowhite epithelium is seen with sharp borders and irregular mosaic.

- Adequate colposcopy
- Squamocolumnar junction visible
- T1
- Abnormal colposcopic findings: opaque acetowhite epithelium within the dorsal quadrants (major change)
  Fig. 18.3

A biopsy is obtained from 7 o'clock using a small electrosurgical loop and shows moderate dysplasia (CIN2). The repeat Pap smear at the time of colposcopy suggest HSIL/CIN2. The Hybrid capture II test is HPV high-risk positive. The patient is subsequently treated by CO_2 laser vaporization.

Five months later, the squamocolumnar junction is still visible with a circular area of thin acetowhite epithelium with regular punctation (Fig. 18.4). The Pap test (ThinPrep®) is normal, and the HPV test has become negative.

Commentary

Postoperatively, there is a significant tissue loss of the ectocervix despite the fact that the CO_2 laser had been used for vaporization instead of loop or laser resection. A less radical procedure might have been advisable as the patient is nulligravid.

The acetowhite staining seen on follow-up colposcopy is due to metaplastic tissue that has developed postoperatively (also see Chap. 9).

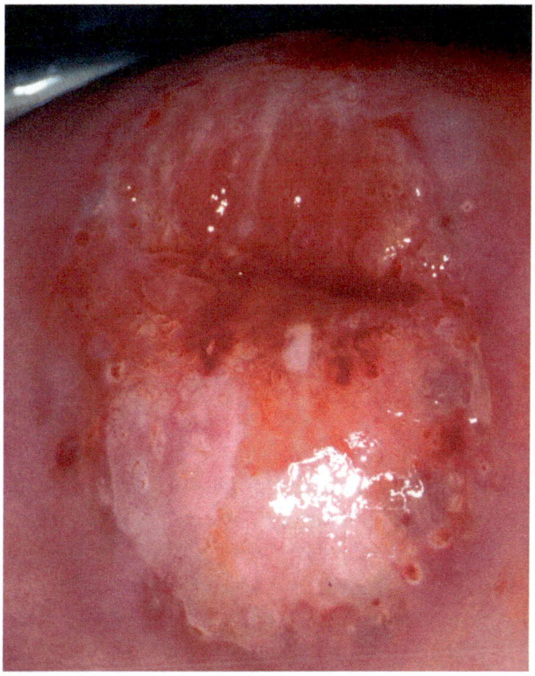

Fig. 18.3 A 38-year-old patient with major change located in the dorsal quadrants

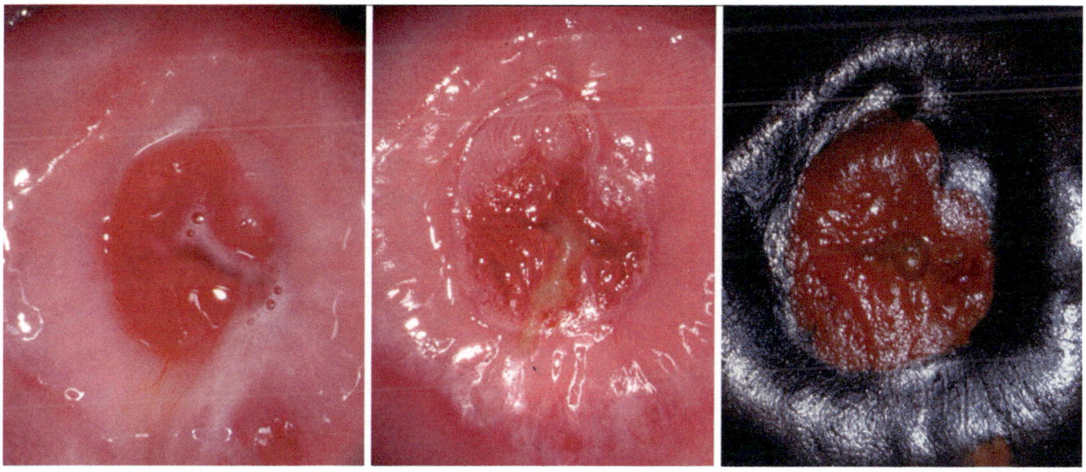

Fig. 18.4 Cervix 5 months after LEEP for HSIL/CIN2

18.1.3 Cervix Before and After LEEP for CIN2

Four years earlier, a 29-year-old patient has given birth by cesarean section due to pre-eclampsia. Two months before the current examination, a routine Pap smear shows HSIL/CIN2. The HPV test (HC2) is positive at the time. A tissue sample is obtained and moderate dysplasia (CIN2) is diagnosed.

On colposcopy, the squamocolumnar junction is partially located within the cervical canal but can be visualized. Ventrally and adjacent to the cervical canal, a thick and opaque acetowhite area can be seen.

- Adequate colposcopy
- Squamocolumnar junction visible
- T2
- Abnormal colposcopic findings: ventral two quadrants with opaque acetowhite epithelium (major change) Fig. 18.5

The ThinPrep® Pap test is indicative of HSIL/CIN3, whereas the Hybrid capture II is negative for HPV DNA.

The patient is greatly disturbed by the diagnosis and urges a speedy operation. A LEEP resection is carried out under local anesthesia at the express request of the patient. The LEEP specimen shows low-grade dysplasia only.

Six months later, a well-preserved ectocervix is seen with normal colposcopic findings. The squamocolumnar junction can still be visualized (Fig. 18.6). On cytologic exam (ThinPrep®), persistence of HSIL/CIN2 is suspected. However, the HPV test (HC2) is negative.

The patient wishes to become pregnant. A repeat colposcopy is recommended after 6 months.

Commentary

The clinical scenario highlights several problems, which are not uncommon in a colposcopy clinic.

Obviously, the HPV test is false negative as HSIL of the cervix had already been confirmed by biopsy. In the clinical context described above, HPV testing is not indicated (Lellé 2007).

On posttreatment follow-up, the Pap test still indicates HSIL. Although the HPV test is negative, this result has to be seen in the context of a prior negative test result and does not rule out persistent disease.

The desire of the young patient to become pregnant in the near future is understandable and does not need to be delayed any further, as in the event of persistent cervical dysplasia, pregnancy does not worsen the clinical course of precancerous disease, which can be monitored throughout pregnancy.

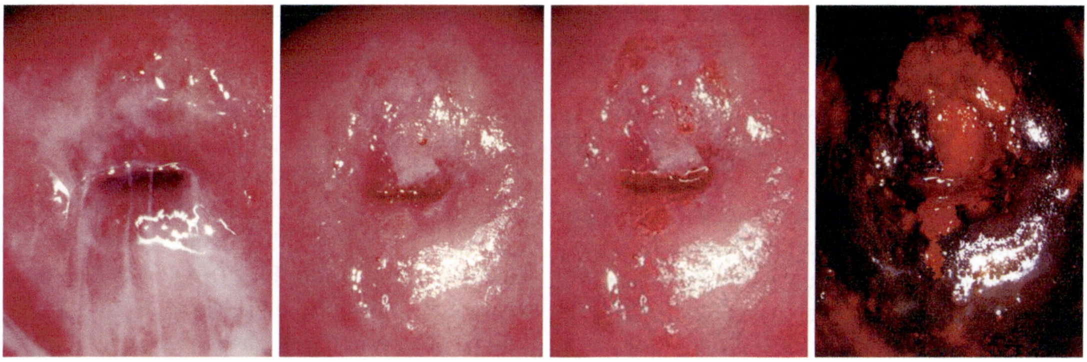

Fig. 18.5 A 29-year-old patient with HSIL/CIN2 on biopsy at 12 o'clock (major change)

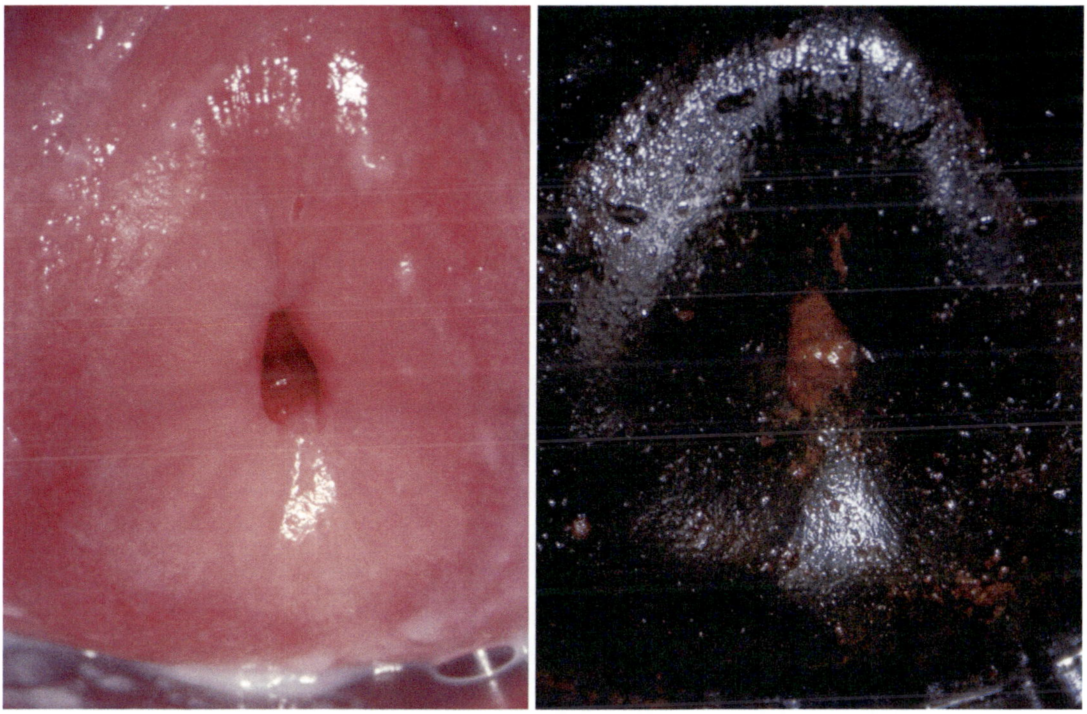

Fig. 18.6 Cervix 6 months after LEEP. The squamocolumnar junction can be visualized (T2). The entire ectocervix is iodine positive

18.1.4 Cervix Before and After LEEP for CIN2

A 36-year-old patient was found to have an abnormal Pap smear (LSIL, possibly HSIL/CIN2) the previous year. At the time, the patient was pregnant. After delivery, a repeat Pap smear is still indicative of cervical dysplasia.

On colposcopy, the squamocolumnar junction is visible. At 1 o'clock there is a thick acetowhite area next to a delicate mosaic.

- Adequate colposcopy
- Squamocolumnar junction visible
- T1
- Abnormal colposcopic findings: left ventral quadrant with dense acetowhite epithelium (major change)
  Fig. 18.7

Targeted biopsy reveals HSIL/CIN2. The Hybrid capture II test is positive for high-risk HPV DNA. The patient undergoes loop resection.

Seven months later, the patient presents with a good postoperative result: there is no stenosis of the cervical canal, and the squamocolumnar junction is visible. At 3 o'clock there is a Nabothian cyst which is covered by mature Lugol-positive squamous epithelium (Fig. 18.8). The Pap smear is normal. However, the Hybrid capture test is still positive for HPV high-risk DNA.

Commentary
After successful dysplasia treatment, the HPV test will be negative in most patients. However, 20–30% of patients remain HPV positive. HPV positivity is not synonymous with persistence of dysplasia. The American Gynecological Society (ACOG) accepts the HPV test as a "test of cure" based on a low level of evidence (ACOG 2016). If the HPV test is positive, another colposcopic examination 6–12 months after treatment of HSIL is recommended.

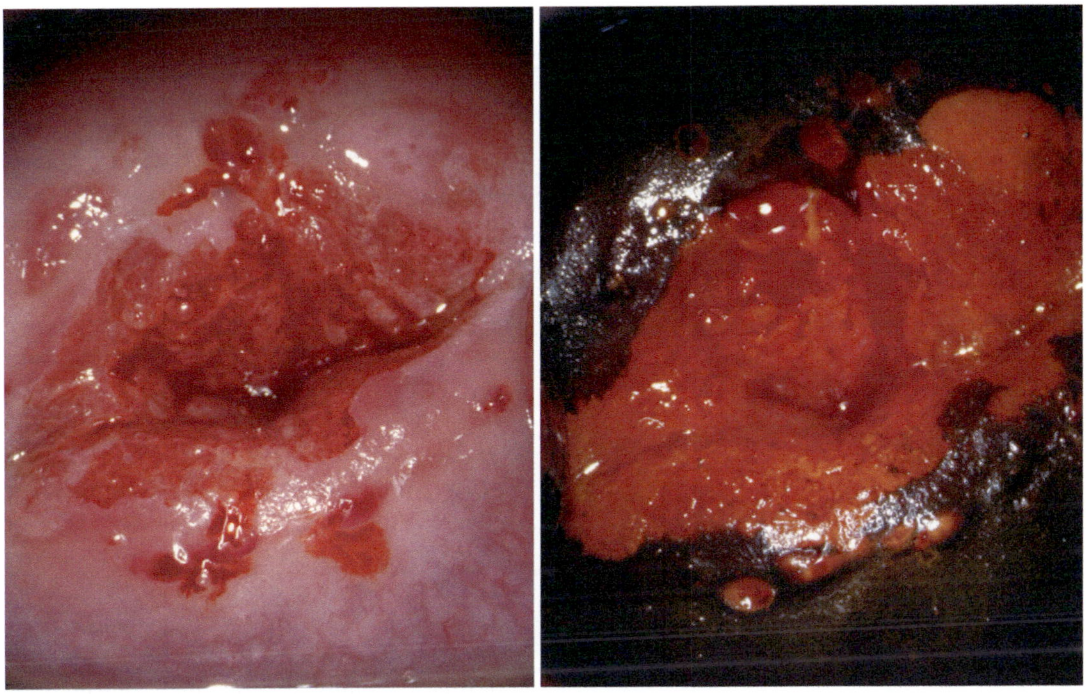

Fig. 18.7 A 36-year-old patient with major change on colposcopy (T1)

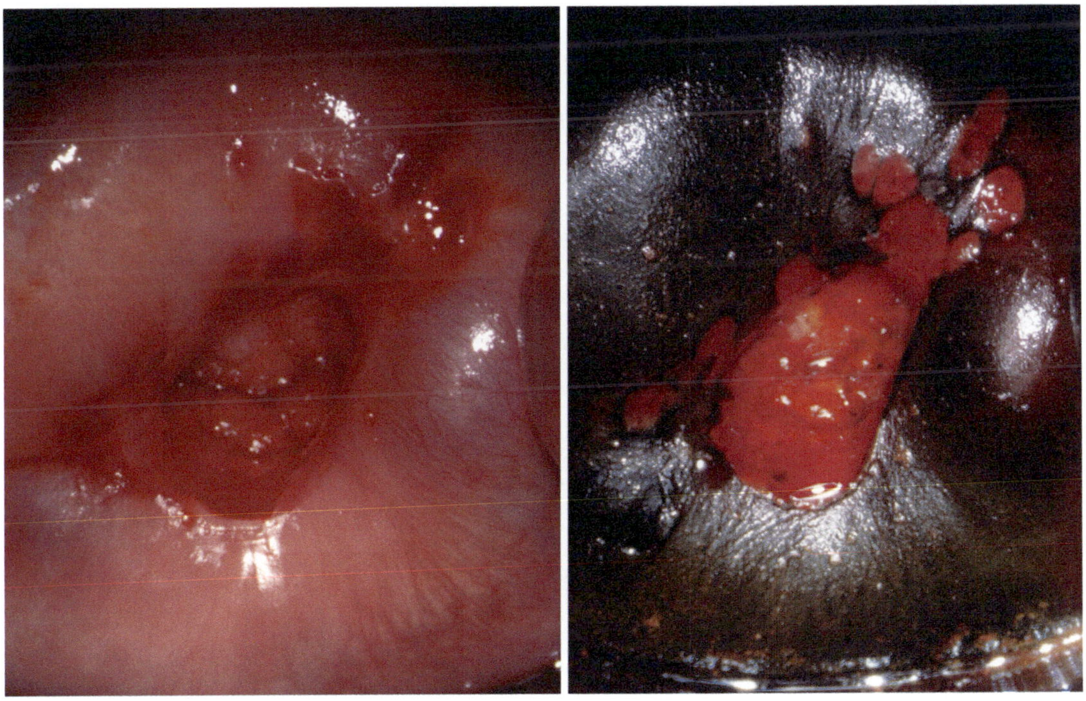

Fig. 18.8 Cervix 7 months after LEEP

18.1.5 Cervix Before and After LEEP for CIN3

The patient is 40 years old. Six months earlier, HSIL/CIN2 was suspected on a routine Pap test. Colposcopic exam reveals a large ectopic area, partially covered by squamous metaplasia. A thick opaque acetowhite area with slightly raised borders covers part of the dorsal quadrants. The abnormal epithelium stains Lugol-negative.

- Adequate colposcopy
- Squamocolumnar junction visible
- T1
- Abnormal colposcopic findings: left and right dorsal quadrant with thick and opaque acetowhite epithelium (major change)
  Fig. 18.9

A biopsy is obtained from 6 o'clock and reveals HSIL/CIN3. A repeat Pap smear is positive for HSIL/CIN2 only. As can be expected, the Hybrid capture II test is HPV positive.

Under colposcopic guidance, the atypical transformation zone is removed using a small loop which is passed through the tissue several times.

The result 6 months later is satisfactory. The ectocervix is Lugol-positive. The squamocolumnar junction can be visualized using Kogan speculum (Fig. 18.10). The Pap smear is normal, and the HPV test (HC2) has become negative.

Commentary
A large transformation zone can only be removed in the shape of a cone or a cylinder by removing a considerable amount of tissue, if a one-pass technique is used with a large electrosurgical loop. Alternatively, a small loop may be used which is passed through the tissue several times. Complete resection is ensured by operating under colposcopic magnification and not by the demonstration of histologically free margins.

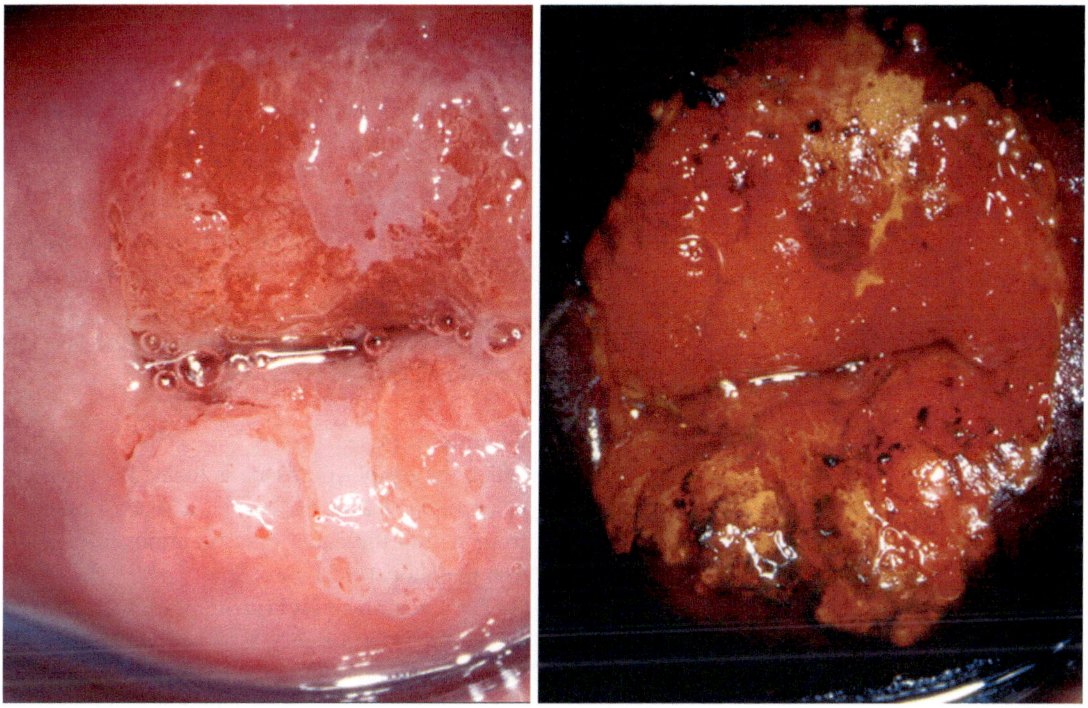

Fig. 18.9 A 40-year-old patient with opaque acetowhite epithelium dorsally (major change)

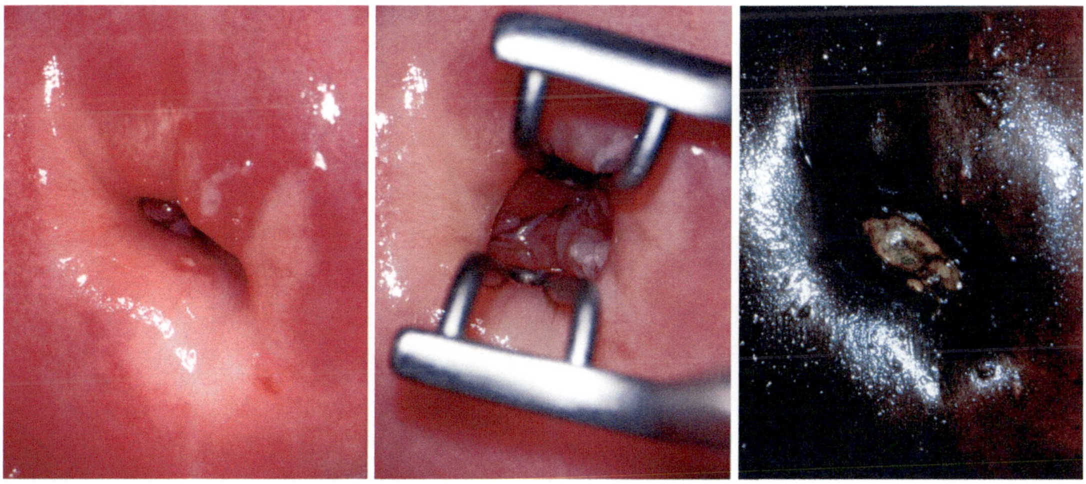

Fig. 18.10 Seven months following loop resection, the entire ectocervix is Lugol-positive, whereas the squamocolumnar junction can still be visualized (T2)

18.1.6 Cervix Before and After LEEP for CIN3

A 39-year-old woman has had abnormal smears for more than a year. On colposcopic examination, a small but dense acetowhite area is visible ventrally close to the cervical canal. The entire squamocolumnar junction can be visualized by opening the cervix with a cotton swab.

- Adequate colposcopy
- Squamocolumnar junction visible through manipulation with a cotton swab
- T2
- Abnormal colposcopic findings: dense acetowhite area at 12 to 1 o'clock close to and partially within the cervical canal (major change)
  Fig. 18.11

Biopsy of the acetowhite area reveals HSIL/CIN3. The Pap smear (ThinPrep®) rather suggests moderate dysplasia (HSIL/CIN2), and the Hybrid capture II test is positive for HPV high-risk DNA.

Using the electrosurgical loop, both an external and an internal cylinder is resected, which are both positive for CIN3. However, the endocervical curettage is free of dysplasia.

Eight months later, the patient presents to the colposcopy clinic for follow-up. The ectocervix is normal and stains Lugol-positive (Fig. 18.12). The Pap test is negative, and the HC2 test has turned negative.

Commentary

When the dysplastic tissue is located completely or partially within the cervix, a second cylinder from within the canal may be removed in addition to endocervical curettage.

The negative Hybrid capture test result 8 months after surgery is a very reliable indicator of complete removal of the dysplastic tissue, certainly more reliable than a free resection margin.

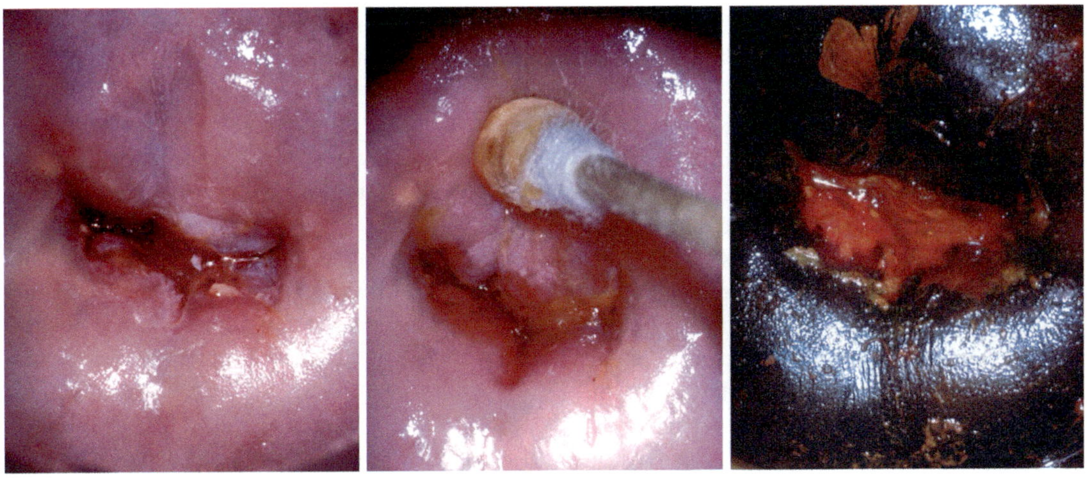

Fig. 18.11 Major change at the 12 to 1 o'clock position extending into the cervical canal (T2)

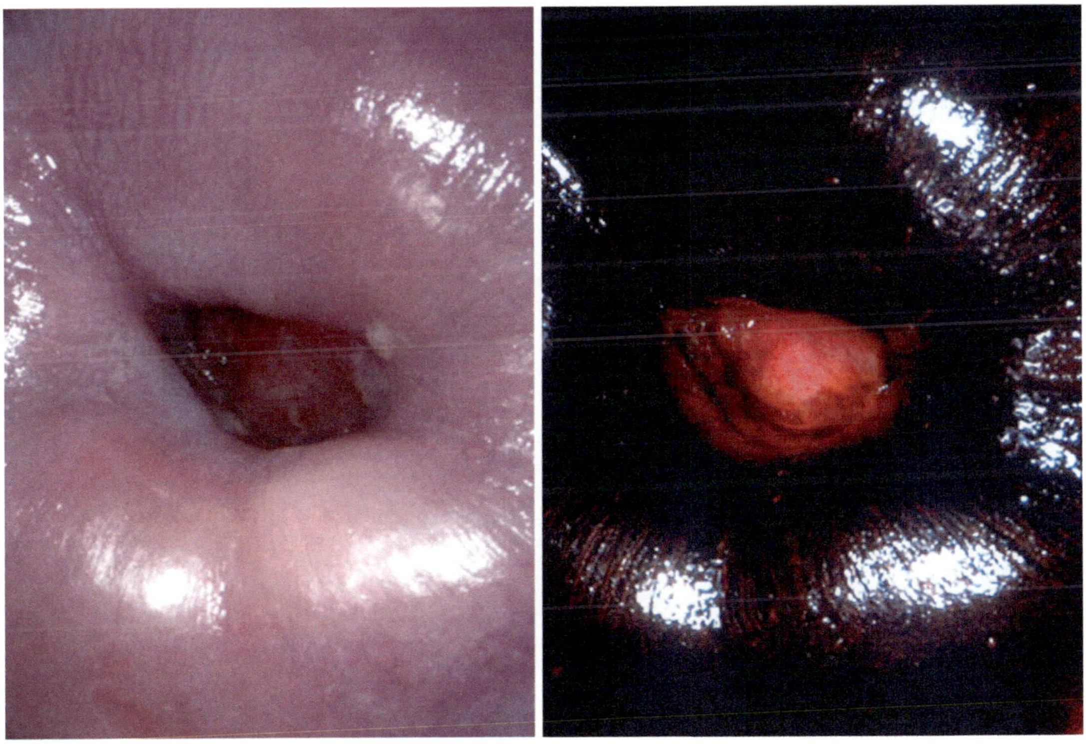

Fig. 18.12 Eight months after LEEP resection, the cervical epithelium is normal, and the squamocolumnar junction is still visible

18.1.7 Cervix Before and After LEEP for CIN3

A 34-year-old patient is suspected to have low-grade cervical dysplasia based on the Pap smear. Since she wants to get pregnant in the near future, she is referred to the colposcopy clinic.

The squamocolumnar junction is visible with the aid of the Kogan speculum. The epithelium of the dorsal cervical quadrants shows a marked acetowhite reaction. Whereas close to the cervical canal, the acetowhite epithelium is Lugol-negative, there is a Lugol-positive stain toward the periphery.

- Adequate colposcopy
- Squamocolumnar junction visible with Kogan speculum
- T2
- Abnormal colposcopic findings: right and left dorsal quadrants with dense acetowhite area (major change)
  Fig. 18.13

A tissue sample is obtained from 6 o'clock close to the cervical canal, which shows cervical intraepithelial neoplasia grades 1, 2, and 3. Subsequently, the tissue is removed using a medium-sized loop. The specimen is marked with a suture at 12 o'clock. Final histopathologic evaluation reveals HSIL. The resection margins are free, and the endocervical curettage is negative.

Eleven months later, the squamocolumnar junction is still visible. The squamous epithelium of the ectocervix is completely Lugol-positive (Fig. 18.14), and the ThinPrep® Pap smear is normal with a negative HPV test (HC2).

Shortly afterward, the patient has an uneventful pregnancy with spontaneous delivery.

Commentary

A one-time LSIL Pap test result is not necessarily an indication for colposcopic triage. However, in a patient who wishes to get pregnant immediately, further evaluation may be justified. In this particular clinical scenario, a high-grade SIL was indeed identified and treated.

On histopathological exam, specimen margins were free of disease. Nevertheless, as pointed out earlier, a negative HPV test result is a more reliable indicator of complete removal.

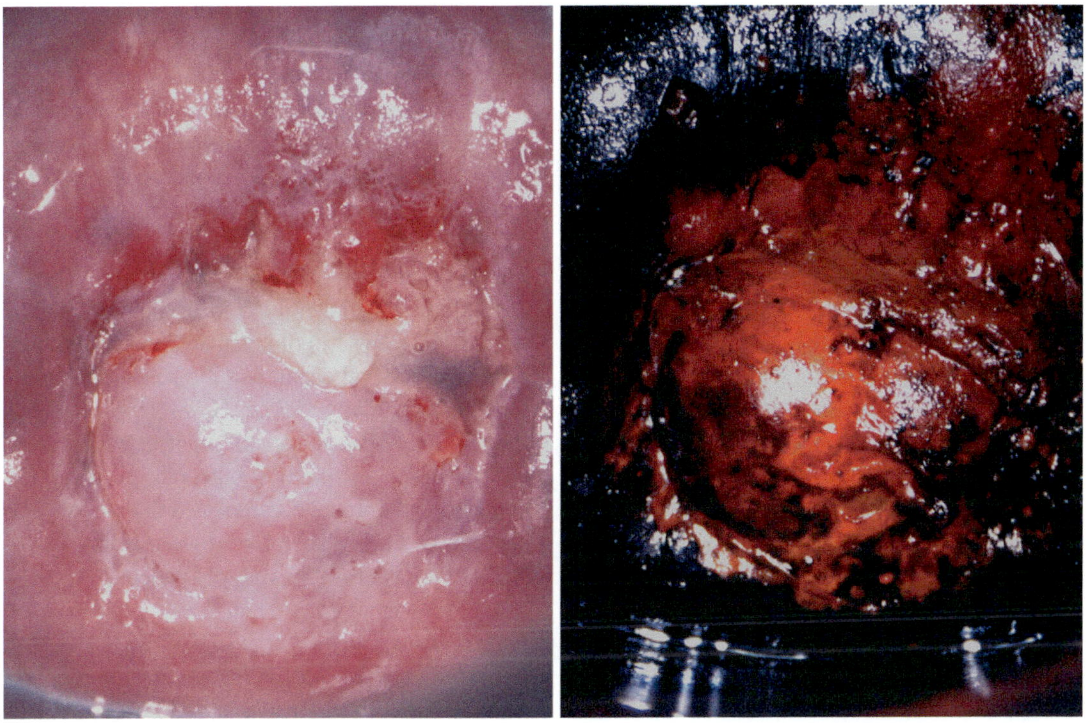

Fig. 18.13 Cervix of a 34-year-old patient with a dense acetowhite area dorsally (major change)

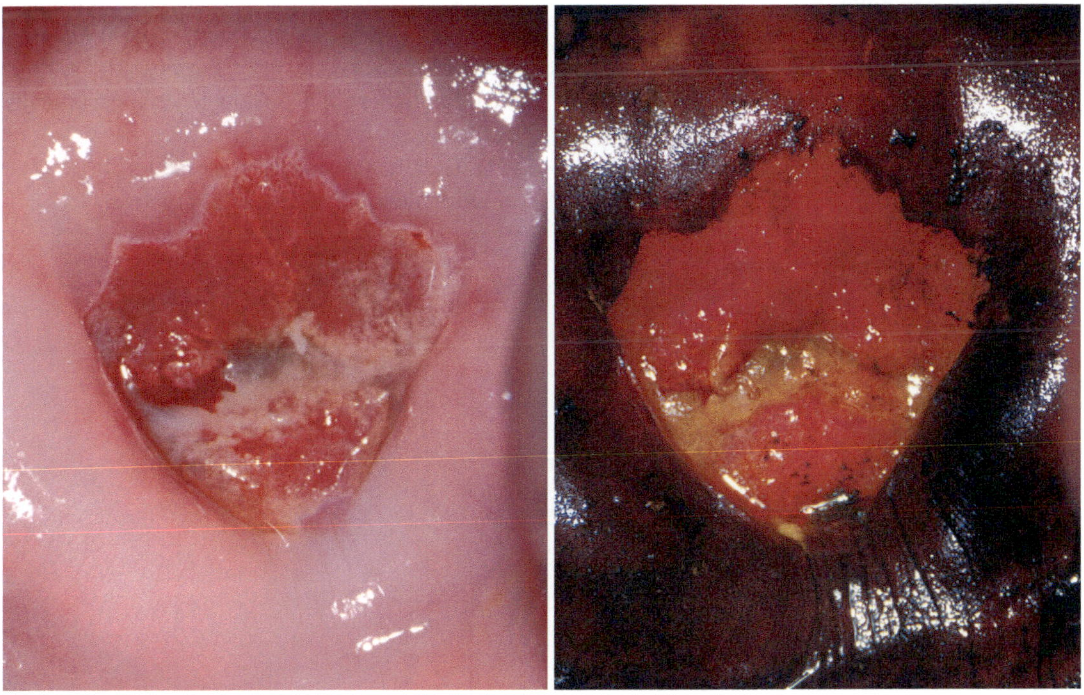

Fig. 18.14 Eleven months after loop resection, the ectocervix is Lugol-positive. The squamocolumnar junction is clearly visible (T1)

18.1.8 Cervix Before and After LEEP for CIN3

A 45-year-old patient has been treated for genital warts (condylomata acuminata). A ThinPrep® Pap smear taken during the gynecologic consultation indicates HSIL/CIN3. Before application of the acetic acid solution, a small plaque of hyperkeratosis is visible at a 5 o'clock position. After application of acetic acid, this area is less conspicuous, and it stains Lugol-negative.

The acetowhite reaction is most pronounced within the ventral quadrants. The tissue is densely acetowhite and opaque. After the acetic acid reaction has partially subsided, the vascular structures, which cause the phenomenon of punctation and mosaic, can be observed more clearly.

- Adequate colposcopy
- Squamocolumnar junction visible with Kogan speculum
- T2
- Abnormal colposcopic findings: right and left dorsal quadrants with dense acetowhite area (major change) Fig. 18.15

A CIN3 diagnosis is established by targeted biopsy from the ventral part of the cervix close to the cervical canal.

The patient undergoes surgery with electrosurgical resection of the atypical transformation zone using a large loop, and a second specimen from inside the cervical canal is obtained using a smaller loop. Both specimens are positive for CIN3, including the tissue from endocervical curettage.

Eight months later, the ectocervix appears to be normal and stains Lugol-positive. There is no stenosis of the cervical canal, and the squamocolumnar junction is partially visible (Fig. 18.16). However, the ThinPrep® Pap smear still suggests HSIL/CIN3, and the HC2 test is HPV high risk positive. The endocervical curettage is repeated and shows persistence of CIN3. Therefore, hysterectomy is discussed with the now 46-year-old patient.

Commentary

Despite extensive LEEP resection of the cervix with two different-sized loops, high-grade dysplasia had not been eliminated within the cervical canal. Therefore, hysterectomy is an acceptable treatment option, if the patient has been made aware of the risk of subsequent vaginal intraepithelial neoplasia. Before surgery, the vagina needs to be thoroughly evaluated colposcopically to rule out pre-existent VAIN.

If the patient wants to preserve fertility, cervical amputation would be an alternative.

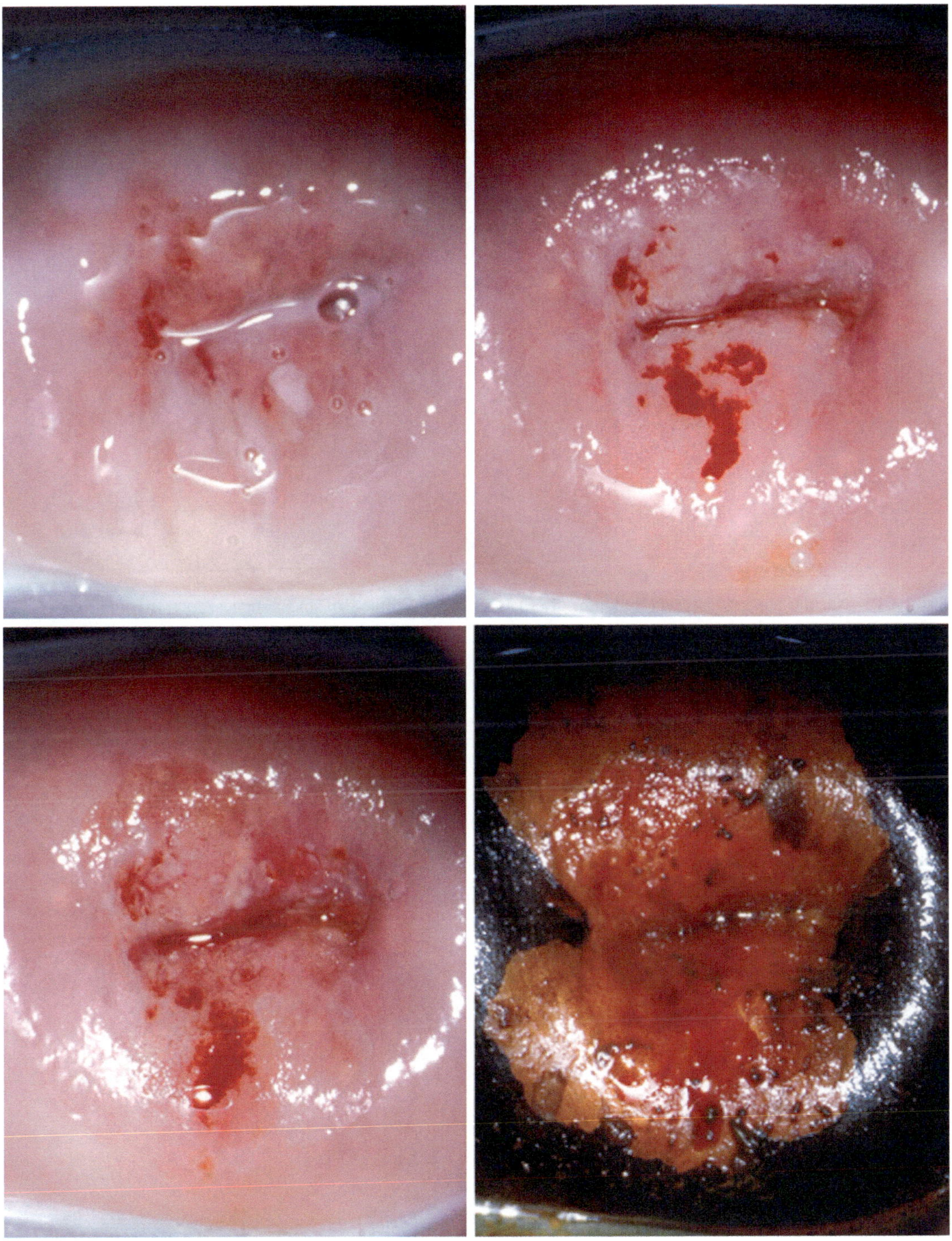

Fig. 18.15 Major change of the dorsal cervical quadrants

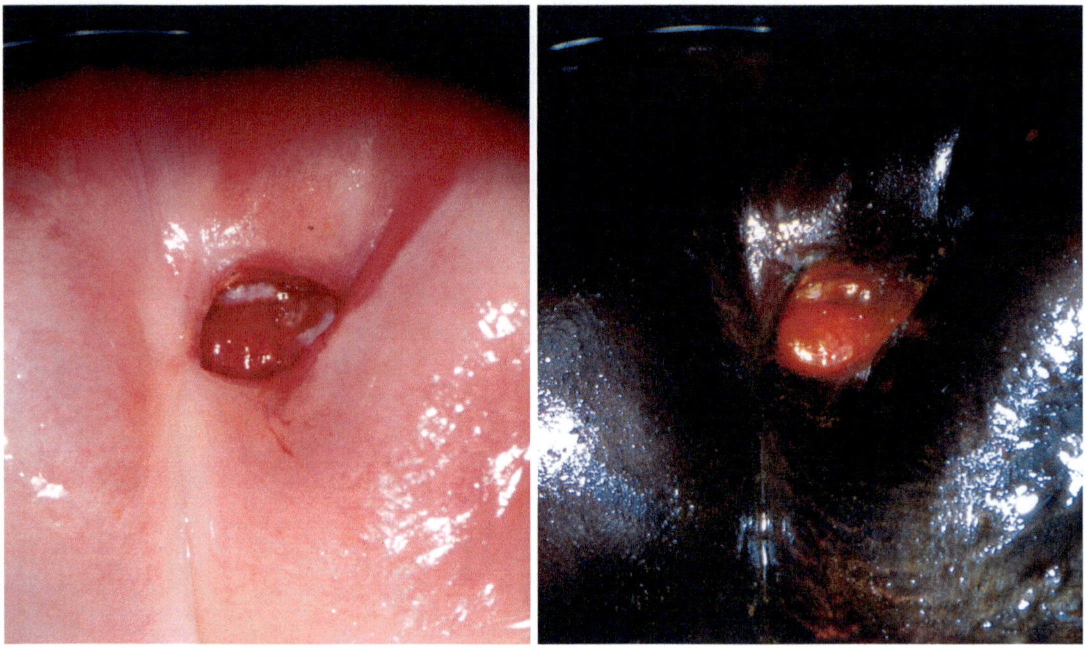

Fig. 18.16 Normal-appearing cervix 8 months after LEEP. However, the Pap smear suggests persistent HSIL

18.1.9 Cervix Before and After LEEP and CO_2 Laser Treatment for CIN3

The patient is 34 years old, G1 P0. Presently, she is scheduled for ICSI (intracytoplasmic sperm injection) due to infertility of her partner. According to the patient, a Pap smear taken 6 months ago had been abnormal and she is referred to the colposcopy clinic.

On colposcopy, the squamocolumnar junction can be visualized using the Kogan speculum. A large opaque acetowhite and Lugol-negative area with sharp borders is identified. All four quadrants are involved. Close to the cervical canal and at the 3 o'clock position, the tissue is particularly dense and slightly raised (inner border lesion).

- Adequate colposcopy
- Squamocolumnar junction visible with Kogan speculum
- T2
- Abnormal colposcopic findings: all four quadrants with dense acetowhite area, inner border lesion at 3 o'clock (major change)
  Fig. 18.17

ThinPrep® Pap smear shows HSIL/CIN3, which is confirmed by targeted biopsy. As expected, the Hybrid capture II test is positive for HPV high-risk DNA.

The tissue around the cervical canal is resected with a small electrosurgical loop, and the peripheral tissue is vaporized with the CO_2 laser.

Four months later, the squamocolumnar junction can still be visualized with the Kogan speculum. Ventrally, the cervix shows both punctation and mosaic (Fig. 18.18). The Pap test is normal.

Commentary

Prior to fertility treatment, cervical screening should be performed.

Targeted biopsy should be obtained from the site of the inner border lesion as this is a pathognomonic sign of HSIL.

In the right ventral quadrant, the lesion extends far into the periphery of the ectocervix. There may be only low-grade dysplasia present in this area. In order to limit the tissue loss, a combination of loop electrosurgical resection and CO_2 laser vaporization has been used for treatment.

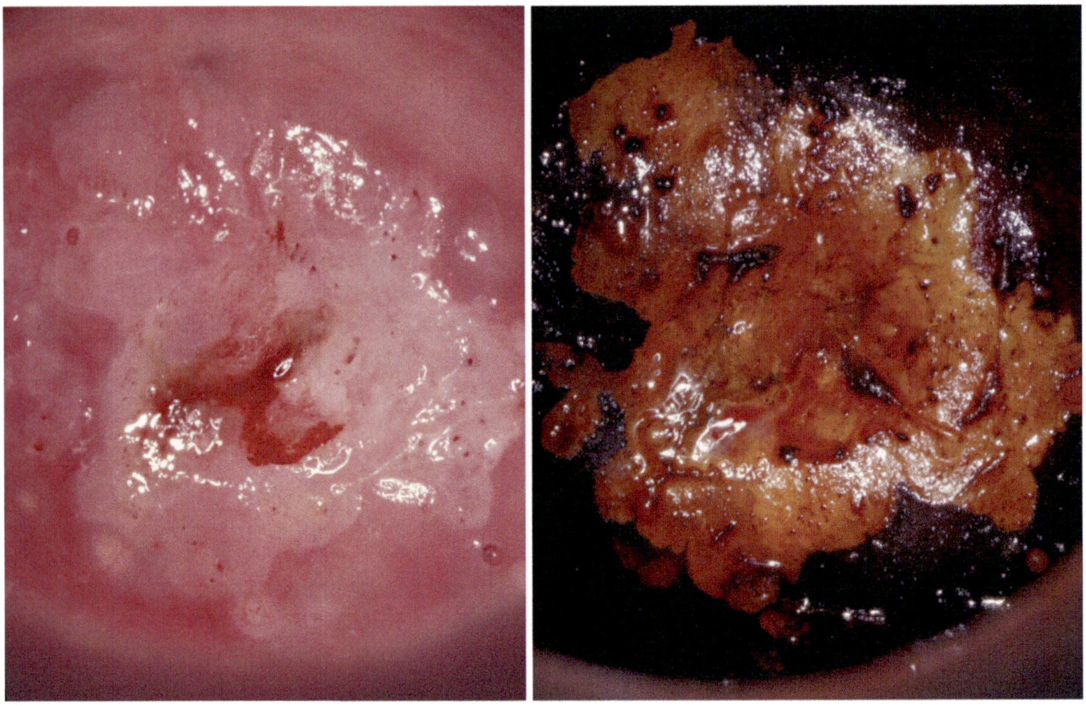

Fig. 18.17 A 34-year-old patient with HSIL/CIN3. There is dense acetowhite epithelium (major change) located within all four quadrants of the cervix. There is a so-called inner border lesion at 3 o'clock

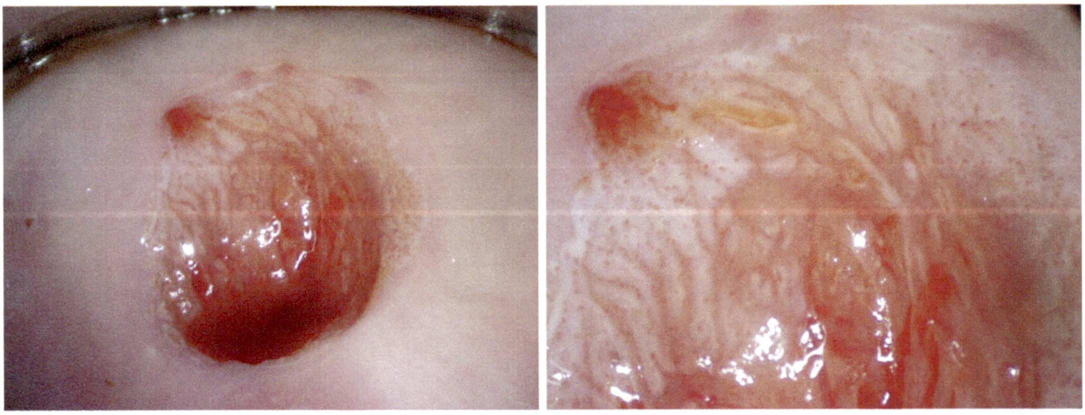

Fig. 18.18 Four months after LEEP and CO_2 laser vaporization. Although a pattern of punctation and mosaic is present, there is no evidence of persistent disease

18.1.10 Cervix Before and After LEEP and CO_2 Laser Treatment for CIN3

A 23-year-old nulligravid patient has an abnormal Pap smear result suspecting HSIL/CIN3 and is referred to colposcopic triage. A large ectopy is seen with partial metaplastic transformation. The squamocolumnar junction can be identified clearly. The major change lesion is located within the ventral quadrants as well as the right dorsal quadrant, showing a coarse and irregular mosaic.

- Adequate colposcopy
- Squamocolumnar junction visible
- T1
- Abnormal colposcopic findings: ventral and right dorsal quadrants with dense acetowhite area and irregular mosaic (major change)
  Fig. 18.19

The ThinPrep® test also indicates HSIL/CIN3, and the Hybrid capture II test is positive for HPV high-risk DNA. A biopsy at 12 o'clock confirms the diagnosis of CIN3. In the subsequent operation, the main lesion is resected with a small electrosurgical loop. The remaining area of the transformation zone is vaporized with the CO_2 laser.

At the follow-up in the colposcopy clinic 6 months later, a small ectopy has formed again (Fig. 18.20), so the squamocolumnar junction is still visible (T1). The cytological smear is normal, and the Hybrid capture II test is now HPV negative.

Commentary

With a large atypical transformation zone of the type shown here, a "classic" cold-knife conization or even a one-pass resection with a large electrosurgical loop would lead to an unacceptable tissue defect in this young nulligravid patient. CO_2 laser vaporization alone or in combination with targeted loop resection under colposcopic guidance is more appropriate.

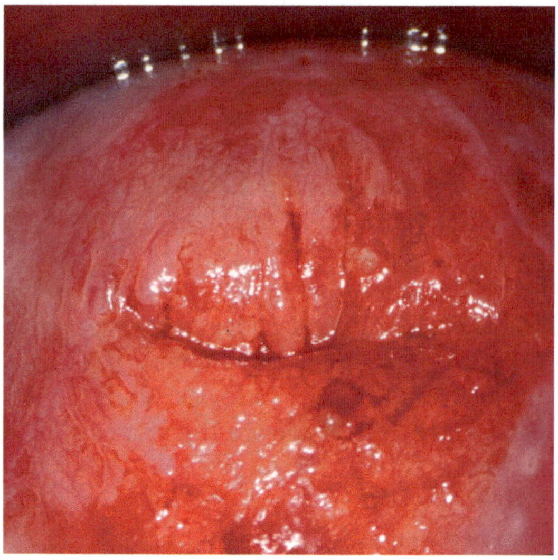

Fig. 18.19 A 23-year-old patient with HSIL/CIN3. A large partially atypical ectopy/transformation zone is seen

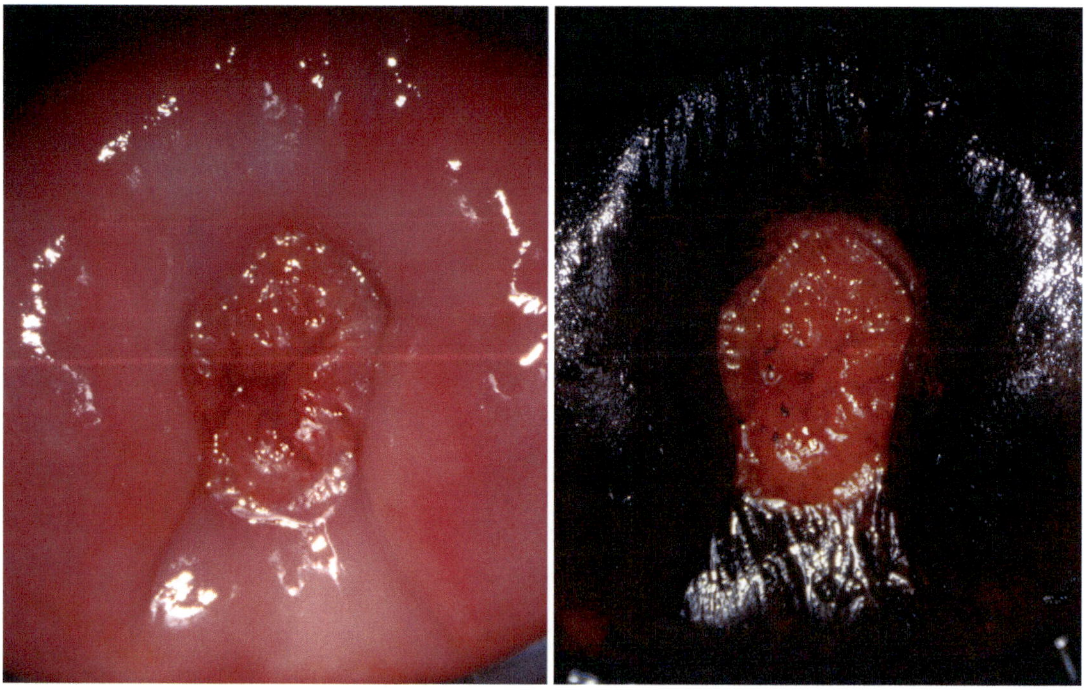

Fig. 18.20 Six months after loop resection, there is an obvious tissue defect. A small ectopy has developed again (T1)

18.1.11 Cervix Before and After LEEP and CO_2 Laser Treatment for CIN3

The patient is 25 years old and has not been pregnant yet. One year earlier, CIN1/CIN2 had been suspected on the routine Pap test. HPV typing had been done revealing HPV 16 DNA.

On colposcopy, the squamocolumnar junction can be visualized with the Kogan speculum. The cervical canal is surrounded by opaque acetowhite epithelium with a typical inner border lesion at 11 o'clock.

- Adequate colposcopy
- Squamocolumnar junction visible with the aid of the Kogan speculum
- T2
- Abnormal colposcopic findings: all four quadrants with dense acetowhite area close to the cervical canal and inner border lesion at 11 o'clock (major change). Fig. 18.21

The biopsy taken from the inner border lesion confirms the diagnosis of CIN3, whereas the Pap smear suggests HSIL/CIN2. The HC2 test is positive for HPV high-risk DNA.

During the subsequent operation, only part of the ectocervix is resected (LEEP), and the transformation zone is otherwise vaporized by CO_2 laser to a depth of approximately 7 mm.

Ten months later, colposcopy shows a good treatment result with the clearly visible squamocolumnar junction and no cervical stenosis (Fig. 18.22). The ThinPrep® Pap smear is normal, and the HPV test (HC2) has become negative.

Commentary

If the diagnosis of cervical dysplasia has been confirmed preoperatively by targeted biopsy, if the squamocolumnar junction can be seen, and if there are no discrepancies to the cytological diagnosis, all requirements for CO_2 laser vaporization without the need of further tissue resection are met. With laser vaporization only, the risk of premature birth appears to be the lowest (Kyrgiou et al. 2006).

A favorable result has been achieved by surgical treatment as seen on follow-up colposcopy: the amount of tissue loss is acceptable. There is no stenosis of the cervical canal, and the squamocolumnar junction is clearly visible. However, such optimal results are not reliably achieved as individual wound healing does not solely depend on surgical technique (Martin-Hirsch et al. 2000).

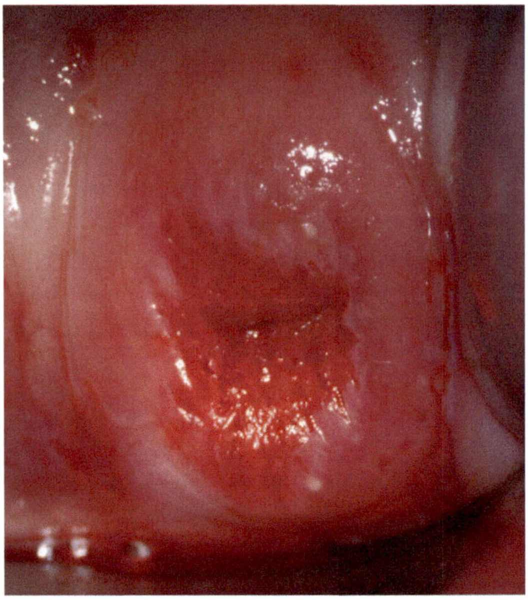

Fig. 18.22 Ten months after treatment by LEEP in combination with CO_2 laser vaporization, there is no significant tissue defect, and the entire transformation zone is visible (T1)

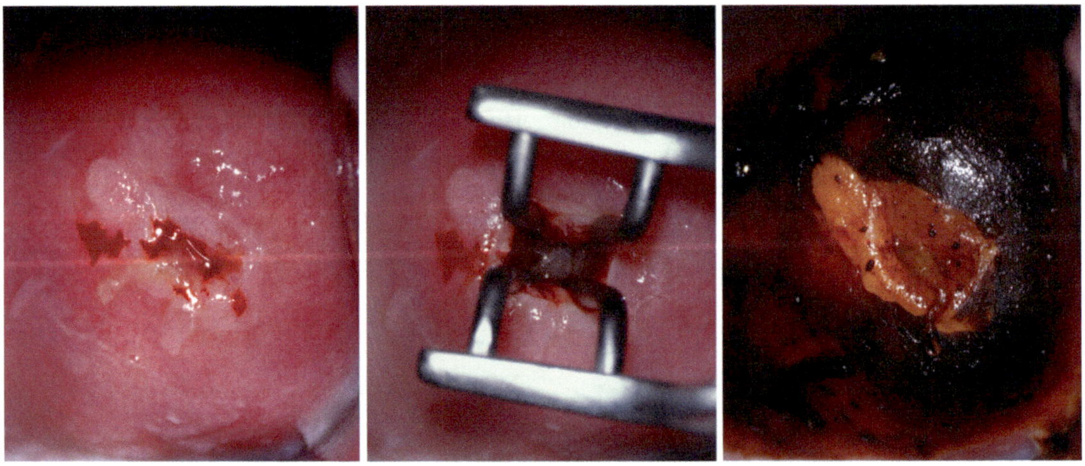

Fig. 18.21 A 25-year-old patient with HSIL/CIN3 on targeted biopsy (major change within all four quadrants). The squamocolumnar junction can be fully visualized with a Kogan speculum (T2)

18.1.12 Cervix Before and After LEEP and CO_2 Laser Treatment for CIN3

The patient is 32 years old. She has no children but plans to become pregnant in the coming year. Five and a half years ago, she underwent conization for HSIL/CIN3. One year ago, the Pap smear started to be abnormal again indicating HSIL/CIN2 disease.

Colposcopy shows a fairly well-preserved cervix without stenosis, although the squamocolumnar junction is no longer visible. Almost the entire surface of the ectocervix is covered by coarse mosaic which extends to the upper vagina. The abnormal epithelium is Lugol-negative.

- Adequate colposcopy
- Squamocolumnar junction not visible
- T3
- Abnormal colposcopic findings: all four quadrants with course mosaic that extends onto the upper vagina (major change) Fig. 18.23

The ThinPrep® Pap smear indicates HSIL/CIN2, and the Hybrid capture test is positive for HPV high-risk DNA. DNA cytophotometry shows aneuploidy with DNA values of up to 30 c.

The patient undergoes surgery. The tissue close to the cervical canal and partly from inside the cervical canal is removed with a small electrosurgical loop. The peripheral areas and the upper vagina are treated with the CO_2 laser.

After 3 months, the cervix has healed completely (Fig. 18.24). The squamocolumnar junction is partially visible. At 6 o'clock, there is a small thin acetowhite area (minor change). ThinPrep® Pap smear is now normal, and the HC2 test has become negative. A biopsy at 6 o'clock is negative for dysplasia.

Commentary

In the past, some authors (Grote et al. 2004) have advocated the use of DNA cytometry as a marker of disease progression. Aneuploidy may suggest a higher probability that low-grade dysplasia will develop into high-grade disease. Nowadays, the relatively complex and expensive procedure is rarely done anymore. In the scenario described above, the DNA cytometry result did not directly affect management decisions.

Despite two prior surgeries, the cervix of this nulligravid patient is still well preserved. The combination of limited loop resection and CO_2 laser vaporization may help to limit tissue loss.

The acetowhite reaction of the epithelium at 6 o'clock 3 months after surgery is most likely due to immature metaplasia. However, biopsy should be done to rule out persistent or recurrent disease.

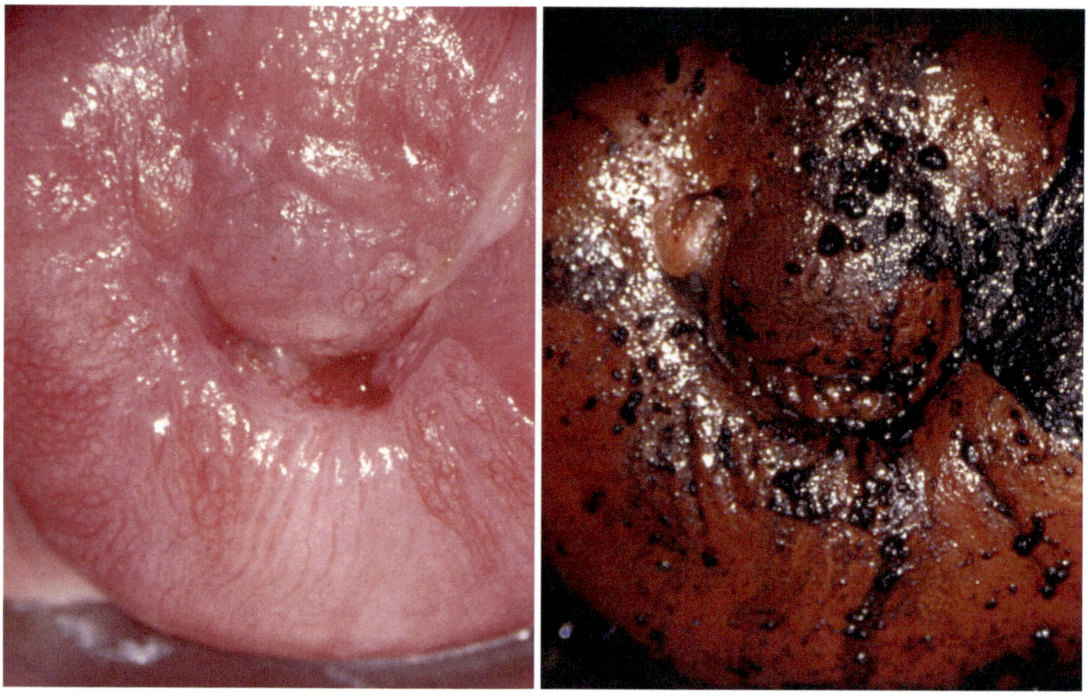

Fig. 18.23 Recurrent HSIL/CIN2. A 32-year-old patient underwent conization for HSIL/CIN3 five and a half years prior

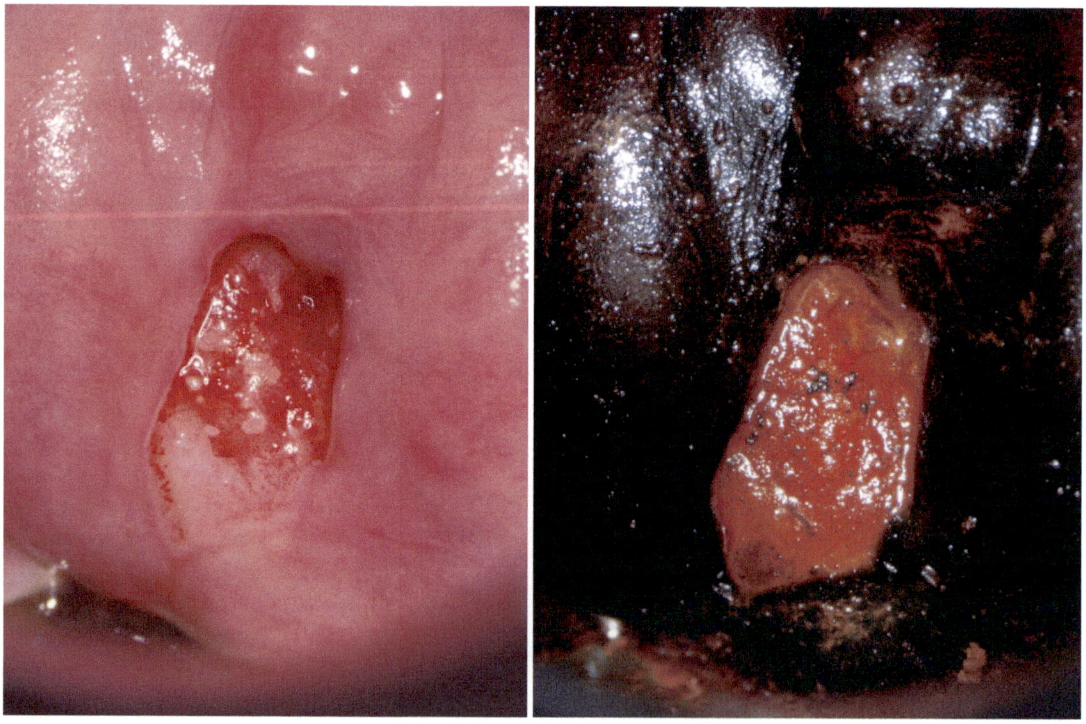

Fig. 18.24 Cervix 3 months after repeat LEEP and CO_2 laser surgery for HSIL/CIN2. At six o'clock, there is a small area of acetowhite epithelium (minor change)

18.1.13 Cervix Before and After LEEP and CO_2 Laser Treatment for CIN3

In a 25-year-old nulligravid patient, an abnormal cervical smear was noted for the first time 5 months earlier (HSIL/CIN2). The patient wants to become pregnant in the near future.

Colposcopy is done, and the squamocolumnar junction can clearly be identified. At 11 o'clock, an area of coarse hyperkeratosis is noted. Prominent vessels can be seen both on the dorsal quadrants of the cervix and the right ventral quadrant. After application of the acetic acid solution, a raised and irregular mosaic is visible.

- Adequate colposcopy
- Squamocolumnar junction visible
- T1
- Abnormal colposcopic findings: dorsal quadrants and right ventral quadrant with hyperkeratosis and dense acetowhite area and irregular mosaic (major change)
  Fig. 18.25

Biopsy at 12 o'clock shows HSIL, whereas the repeat Pap smear is only indicative of low-grade dysplasia. The HPV test (HC2) is high-risk HPV DNA positive.

The central part of the lesion is resected using an electrosurgical loop, whereas the periphery is treated with CO_2 laser.

Seven months later, the patient returns to the colposcopy clinic. Visibility of the squamocolumnar junction has been preserved. The entire ectocervix is Lugol-positive (Fig. 18.26), and the cytological smear is normal with a negative HC2 test result.

Commentary

Leukoplakia can typically be seen before the application of acetic acid. Hyperkeratosis of the non-keratinizing squamous epithelium of the cervix is a rather unspecific condition, which may be associated with condylomata, local inflammation, squamous cell dysplasia (CIN1 to 3), and keratinizing squamous cell carcinomas.

In contrast to the phenomenon of "inner border lesion," leukoplakia is not necessarily the area with the highest degree of dysplasia. The choice of the biopsy site should therefore be based on the usual criteria and be chosen close to the cervical canal.

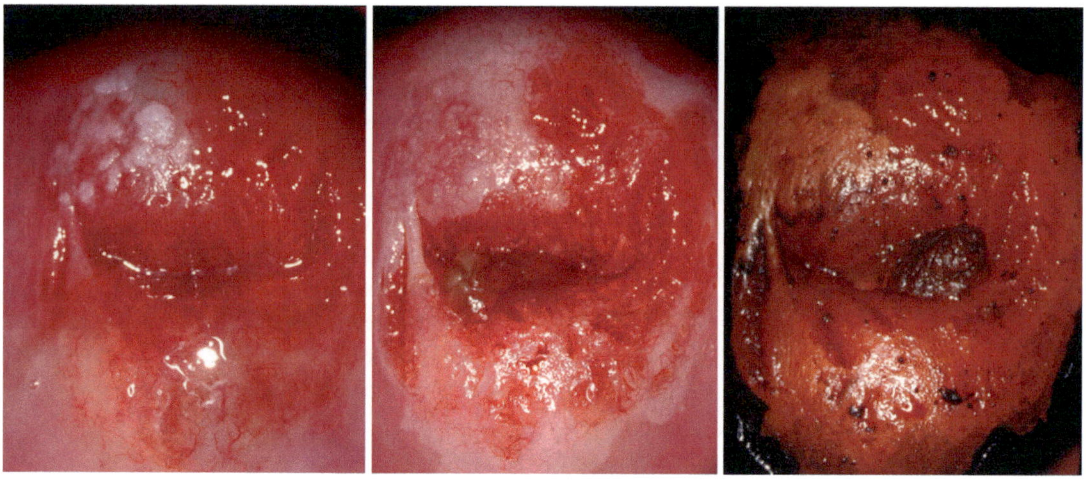

Fig. 18.25 A 25-year-old nulligravid patient with HSIL of the cervix (major change). At 11 o'clock, there is a prominent area of hyperkeratosis

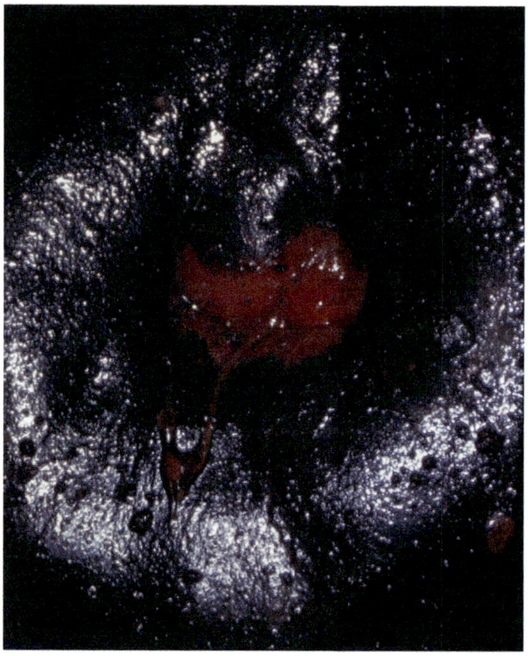

Fig. 18.26 Satisfactory result with a type T1 transformation zone 7 months after LEEP and CO_2 laser surgery

18.1.14 CIN3 Presenting with Prominent Vessels

A 37-year-old patient, P3, had an abnormal Pap smear for the first time 9 months prior suspecting only low-grade SIL. A repeat Pap smear indicated high-grade neoplasia, possibly CIN2, and the patient is referred to colposcopy.

The squamocolumnar junction is visible when applying the Kogan speculum. There is a mature transformation zone with numerous conspicuous blood vessels covering most of the ectocervix. These resemble the large dilated blood vessels overlying Nabothian cysts with regular branching and no evidence of atypia. After application of acetic acid, these vessels recede to a large extent behind a delicate and diffuse staining of the squamous epithelium. At 3 o'clock, the acetowhite reaction is slightly more pronounced. On Schiller's test, a large part of the transformation remains iodine-negative.

- Adequate colposcopy
- Squamocolumnar junction visible with the Kogan speculum
- T2
- Abnormal colposcopic findings: all four quadrants with large regular vessels that recede behind a delicate and diffuse acetowhite staining (minor change) Fig. 18.27

Although the colposcopic appearance is not typical for high-grade dysplasia, the Pap smear now suspects HSIL/CIN3 disease, and the HPV test (HC2) is positive. Biopsy at 3 o'clock confirms the diagnosis of CIN3.

The Lugol-negative area is resected/vaporized with a combined LEEP/CO_2 laser approach. Endocervical curettage is positive for CIN3.

Six months after surgery, the ThinPrep® Pap smear is normal, and the HPV test is negative. Repeat endocervical curettage is negative for dysplasia.

Commentary

The colposcopic appearance of the cervix does not meet the criteria established for HSIL. Nevertheless, whenever high-grade dysplasia is suspected through cytopathology, biopsies should be obtained close to the squamocolumnar junction and/or from areas with grade 1/minor changes.

Endocervical curettage is done routinely toward the end of therapeutic resection of the cervix. If it is positive for HSIL, resection within the cervical canal may have been insufficient. However, a positive endocervical curettage does not routinely require repeat surgery. In the present scenario, the negative HPV test 6 months later is a strong indication of complete resection or cure.

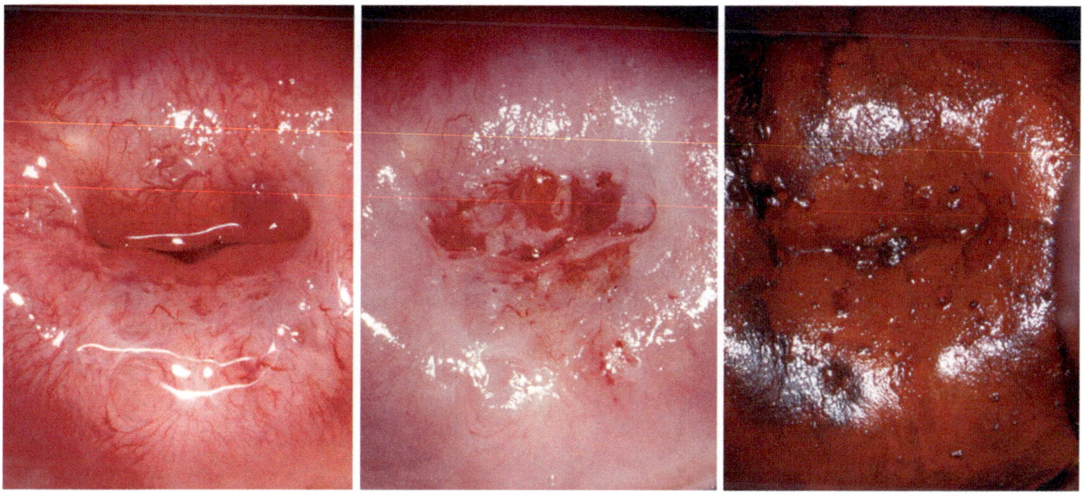

Fig. 18.27 Although colposcopic examination reveals only a minor change, the biopsy at 3 o'clock shows HSIL/CIN3

18.1.15 Diagnostic Surgery Revealing CIN3

A 30-year-old nulligravid patient has been trying to become pregnant for the past 2 years. Three months ago, a screening Pap test has been indicative of HSIL/CIN2.

Colposcopically, the squamocolumnar junction can be visualized with the Kogan speculum. After application of acetic acid, there is a large area of opaque and slightly raised acetowhite epithelium with coarse punctation (12 o'clock) and irregular mosaic (10 o'clock).

- Adequate colposcopy
- Squamocolumnar junction visible with the Kogan speculum
- T2
- Abnormal colposcopic findings: all four quadrants with opaque acetowhite areas and irregular punctation/mosaic (major change)
  Fig. 18.28

Although colposcopy shows a typical grade 2/major change, a biopsy at 4 o'clock does not reveal squamous dysplasia, and the repeat Pap smear (ThinPrep®) indicates low-grade disease only. The Hybrid capture II test is positive for HPV high-risk DNA.

Three months later, colposcopy is repeated and unchanged. A biopsy at 11 o'clock reveals CIN1 only, and the Pap test also shows cells of low-grade squamous dysplasia.

Since the patient wishes to get pregnant, she opts for surgery. The tissue around the cervical canal is removed by electrosurgical resection and the periphery is treated with CO_2 laser vaporization. Eventually, CIN3 is confirmed within the LEEP specimen.

Eight months after surgery, the Pap smear is normal, and the HPV test has become negative.

Commentary
This scenario illustrates that a single biopsy may not be representative of a suspected cervical lesion. Sometimes, a diagnostic/therapeutic intervention can be justified.

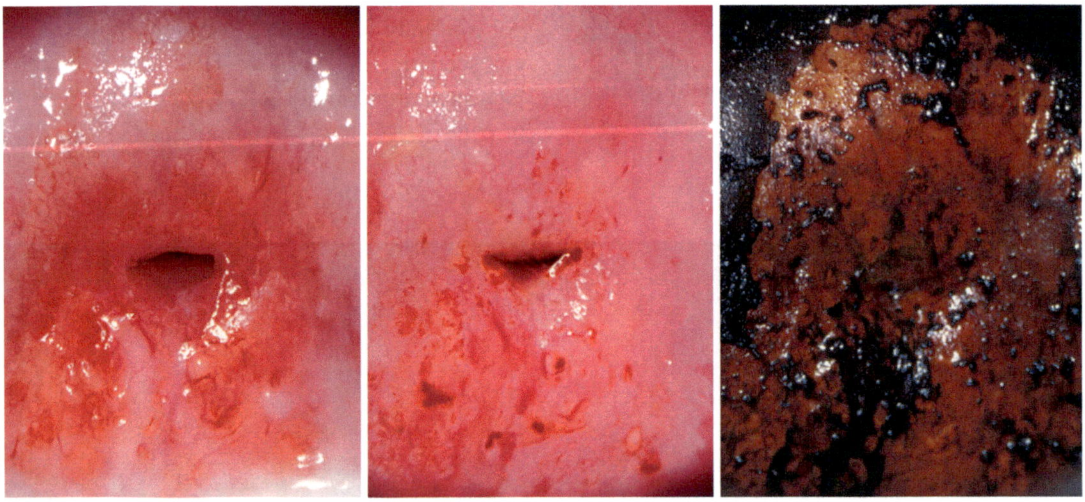

Fig. 18.28 A 30-year-old nulligravid patient with extensive opaque acetowhite changes involving all four quadrants of the cervix. Although HSIL could not be confirmed through targeted biopsy, examination of the LEEP specimen revealed HSIL/CIN3

18.1.16 CIN3 Look-Alike

A 24-year-old nulligravid patient has an HSIL Pap smear result at routine checkup. Colposcopically, a major change is identified and biopsied. Surprisingly, however, HSIL cannot be confirmed, so a second opinion is sought.

The squamocolumnar junction is clearly visible. Most of the ectocervix is acetowhite with sharply delineated borders and coarse mosaic. At 12 o'clock there is a small tissue defect at the site of the prior biopsy. Overall, colposcopy supports the suspected diagnosis of HSIL in accordance with repeat Pap smear.

- Adequate colposcopy
- Squamocolumnar junction visible
- T1
- Abnormal colposcopic findings: all four quadrants with large acetowhite area and irregular mosaic (major change) Fig. 18.29

A biopsy from 9 o'clock is obtained using a small electrosurgical loop. Again, there is no histopathologic evidence of dysplasia. The ThinPrep® Pap test suspects LSIL, and the HPV test (HC2) is negative.

Commentary

Despite the initial Pap test result and the unequivocal colposcopic picture, no cervical dysplasia could be identified. On the one hand, false-negative biopsy results are not unusual. On the other hand, biopsies had been obtained twice, the second time using an electrosurgical loop.

As the highly sensitive Hybrid capture II test is negative for HPV high-risk DNA, the presence of HPV-related intraepithelial neoplasia is indeed unlikely. Therefore, immature metaplasia may mimic the colposcopic image of high-grade squamous neoplasia.

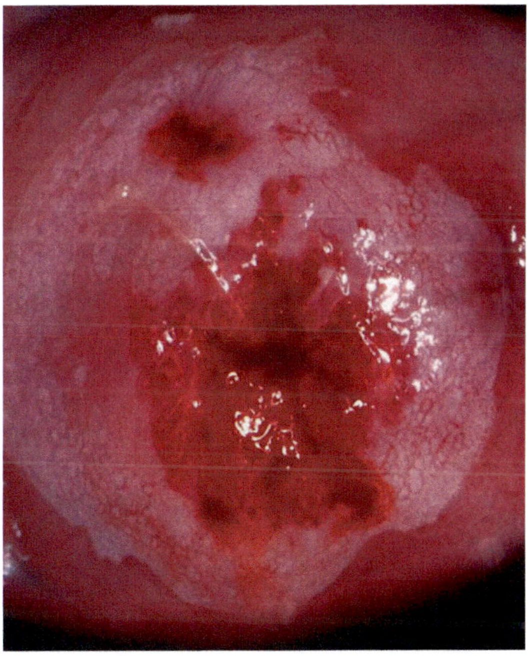

Fig. 18.29 A 24-year-old patient with large abnormal transformation zone (major change). Ultimately, squamous dysplasia could not be confirmed histologically

18.1.17 Intracervical CIN3

A 36-year-old woman has had two prior deliveries by cesarean section. Three months ago, she went for an annual checkup and was found to have an abnormal Pap smear (LSIL/HSIL). Recently, a repeat Pap test indicated HSIL/CIN3.

The entire ectocervix is normal colposcopically and stains Lugol-positive. There is a small round external cervical os, as the patient has had no vaginal delivery. The squamocolumnar junction cannot be visualized, even with the Kogan speculum.

- Adequate colposcopy
- Squamocolumnar junction not visible
- T3
- Normal colposcopic findings
  Fig. 18.30

The Pap smear (ThinPrep®) at the time of colposcopy indicates HSIL/CIN3, and the Hybrid capture II test is positive for HPV high-risk DNA. Endocervical curettage with a Stiefel® curette shows CIN3.

The patient is then treated with electrosurgical loop resection. An intracervical cylinder is obtained, which is positive for CIN3.

At follow-up 3 months later, the ThinPrep® smear is unremarkable, and the HPV test has become negative.

Commentary

The HSIL Pap smear in combination with a normal appearing and Lugol-negative ectocervix suggests endocervical dysplasia which cannot be visualized in this patient. In a scenario like this, endocervical curettage is indicated and led to the histopathological diagnosis of CIN3. Conversely, a negative curettage result would not have ruled out dysplasia. Although specificity of curettage is high, it has a very low sensitivity, especially in young patients under the age of 40.

The most likely manifestation of dysplasia had been the endocervical canal which could be verified by endocervical curettage. However, occasionally VAIN might be the reason that the Pap smear indicates HSIL and colposcopy is normal, possibly with negative curettage.

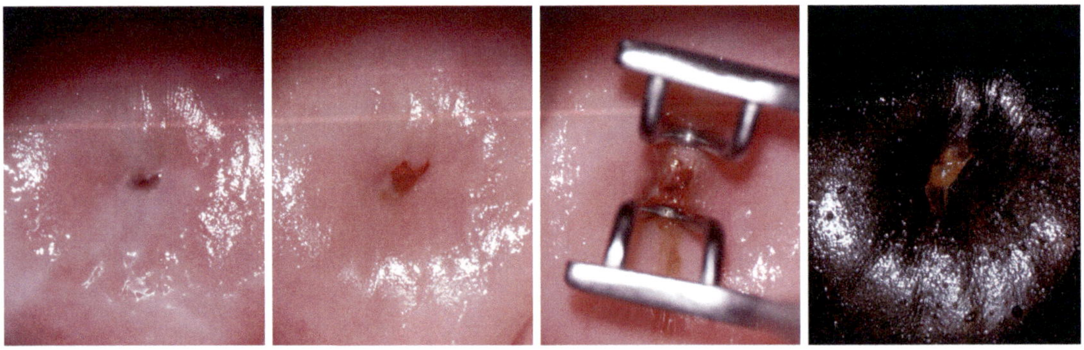

Fig. 18.30 A 36-year-old patient with intracervical HSIL/CIN3. The ectocervix is normal and Lugol-positive. The squamocolumnar junction cannot be sufficiently visualized with the Kogan speculum. Ultimately, endocervical curettage reveals HSIL/CIN3

18.1.18 CIN3 and HIV Infection

One and a half years ago, a 26-year-old patient has been diagnosed with HIV infection. Now an abnormal Pap smear (LSIL/HSIL) has been found, and the patient is referred to the colposcopy clinic. The patient desperately wants to get pregnant.

Complete visualization of the squamocolumnar junction is achieved using the Kogan speculum. Dense acetowhite epithelium is present involving all four quadrants.

- Adequate colposcopy
- Squamocolumnar junction visible with Kogan speculum
- T2
- Abnormal colposcopic findings: all four quadrants with dense and opaque acetowhite epithelium (major change) Fig. 18.31

The ThinPrep® Pap test at the time of colposcopy suggests HSIL/CIN2 with a positive HC2 test result. The cervix is biopsied at 2 o'clock and reveals HSIL/CIN3.

The abnormal tissue is removed with LEEP. On histopathologic exam, the margins are involved, whereas the endocervical curettage is negative.

Six months later, the cervix is well healed, and the entire transformation zone is still visible. Ventrally, there is a narrow acetowhite band of tissue right next to the squamocolumnar junction (Fig. 18.32). This tissue is removed completely using the Stiefel® curette. The HPV test continues to be positive, while histopathology and cytology favor CIN1.

Another 7 months later, the patient is 18 weeks pregnant. There is acetowhite tissue located within the cervical canal suggesting HSIL (Fig. 18.33).

No endocervical curettage is done, as the patient is pregnant. The ThinPrep® Pap smear is classified as ASC-US, and the HPV test is negative for HPV high-risk DNA.

Cesarean section is performed 2 weeks prior to the expected delivery date.

Another 13 months later, colposcopy is normal. The squamocolumnar junction is still visible (T2). The ThinPrep® Pap smear and the HPV test are both negative.

Commentary

This is a favorable course of disease of a patient with HIV infection, as there is a high risk of recurrence and progression of all types of intraepithelial neoplasia of the lower genital tract (Petry et al. 1994). Especially HSIL of the vulva must always be ruled out (Petry et al. 1996).

As there are no studies on a potential negative impact on pregnancy, endocervical curettage should be avoided. An endocervical Pap smear may be a viable alternative. Also, in the present scenario, histopathologic verification of dysplasia during pregnancy was not mandatory, as there was no evidence of invasive disease.

In general, immunosuppressed patients should not undergo repeat surgery within a short time interval. Also, CIN1 as diagnosed here during pregnancy does not require resection. Perhaps the pregnancy contributed to CIN regression.

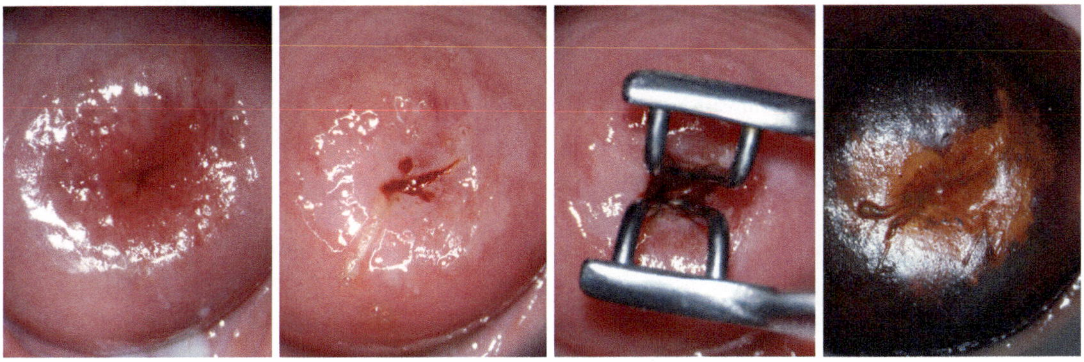

Fig. 18.31 A 26-year-old HIV-positive patient with opaque acetowhite staining in all four quadrants of the cervix (major change). The squamocolumnar junction is visible using the Kogan speculum, and a biopsy at 2 o'clock reveals HSIL/CIN3

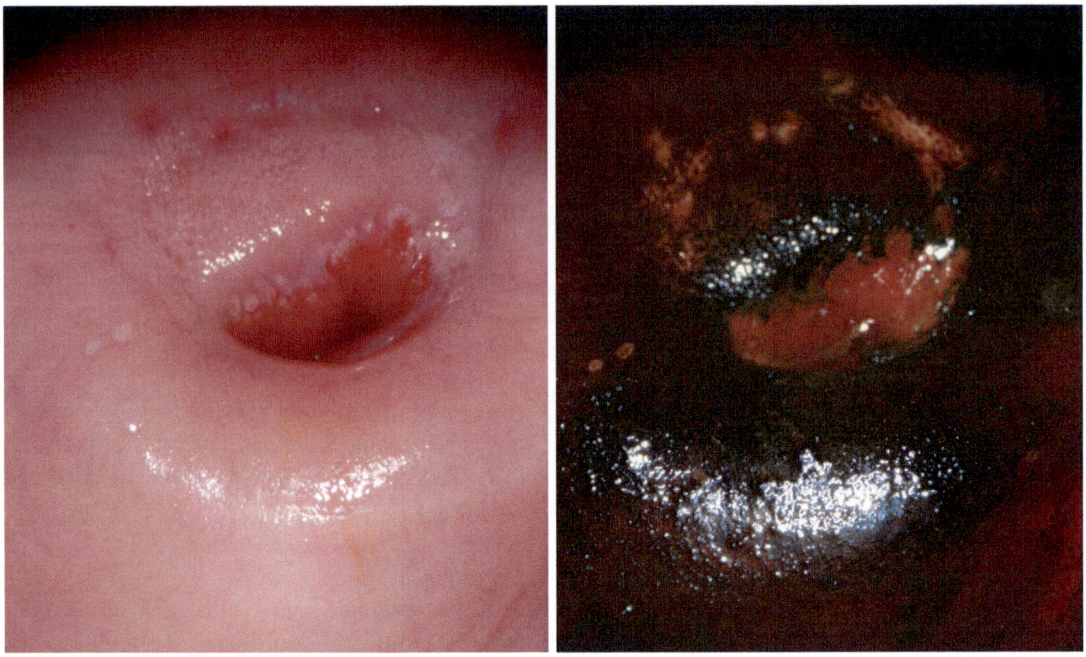

Fig. 18.32 Cervix 6 months after LEEP. The squamocolumnar junction is visible. Ventrally, a narrow acetowhite area is identified (minor change). Biopsy reveals LSIL

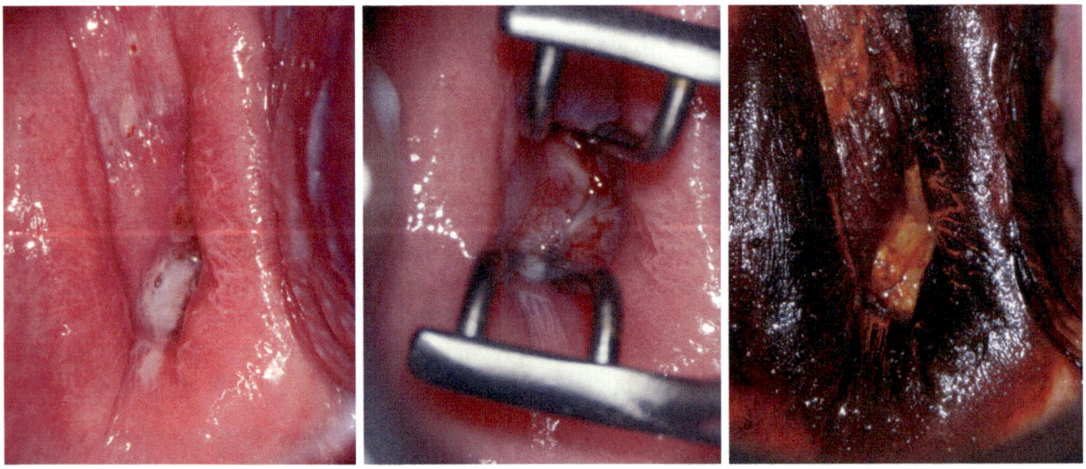

Fig. 18.33 Another 7 months later, the patient is 18 weeks pregnant. Although at the time HSIL is suspected within the cervical canal, the patient is free of disease on long-term follow-up

18.1.19 CIN3 and HIV Infection

The patient is 29 years old and nulligravid. She has an HIV infection which is not well controlled, as the number of CD4+ T lymphocytes is less than 500/µl. Otherwise she has no symptoms. A routine Pap smear shows HSIL with features suspicious for invasion, and she is referred to the colposcopy clinic.

Pronounced hyperkeratosis is seen prior to application of the acetic acid solution. After acetic acid, the aspect of the cervix remains unchanged. No features of a major change and no signs of invasion are seen.

- Adequate colposcopy
- Squamocolumnar junction visible with Kogan speculum
- T2
- Abnormal colposcopic findings: right and left dorsal quadrants with pronounced hyperkeratosis (nonspecific)
  Fig. 18.34

LEEP is performed and the entire area of abnormal tissue is removed. Histopathology shows extensive CIN3 disease with hyperkeratosis. However, there is no evidence of invasive disease.

Commentary

In this scenario, a colposcopically guided biopsy would not have been conclusive enough, since invasive disease has to be excluded with the Pap smear being classified as "HSIL with features suspicious for invasion." In addition, patients with HIV/AIDS are at a higher risk to develop cancer; hence, an early-stage diagnosis is crucial.

Carcinoma of the cervix would be considered an "AIDS-defining illness," not, however, precancerous lesions of the cervix.

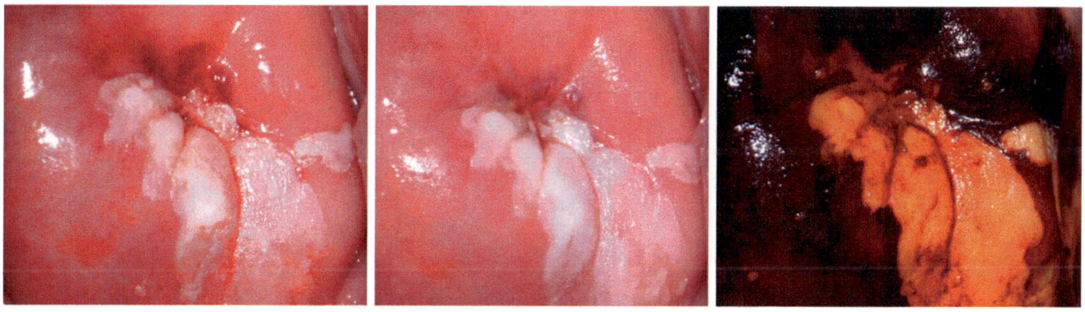

Fig. 18.34 A 29-year-old patient with HIV infection and extensive HSIL/CIN3 with hyperkeratosis

18.1.20 Ruling Out Cervical Dysplasia Through Colposcopic Triage

A 36-year-old nurse has delivered two children by cesarean section. Six and a half years prior, several abnormal Pap smears have been documented, mostly ASC-US or LSIL. Three months ago, an HPV test had been negative. Eventually, colposcopy was done showing a minor change only. A biopsy at 1 o'clock did not reveal dysplasia. At that time, the Pap test was normal.

Seven months later, the colposcopic examination is repeated. Again, no abnormal findings are recorded, and the squamocolumnar junction can be fully visualized.

- Adequate colposcopy
- Squamocolumnar junction visible with Kogan speculum
- T2
- Normal colposcopic findings
  Fig. 18.35

Again, the Pap test (ThinPrep®) is normal with a negative HPV test (HC2) (Fig. 18.36). Subsequently, further screening within the regular intervals is recommended.

Commentary

ASC-US or LSIL diagnosis on cytopathology may be an indication for colposcopy, depending on the individual circumstances. Repeated follow-up Pap tests with borderline results can lead to considerable psychological distress. Instead, colposcopic triage helps to eventually rule out the presence of a cervical lesion that requires treatment.

Also, the HC2 test for HPV high-risk DNA had been negative twice, a fact that makes any type of cervical dysplasia highly unlikely.

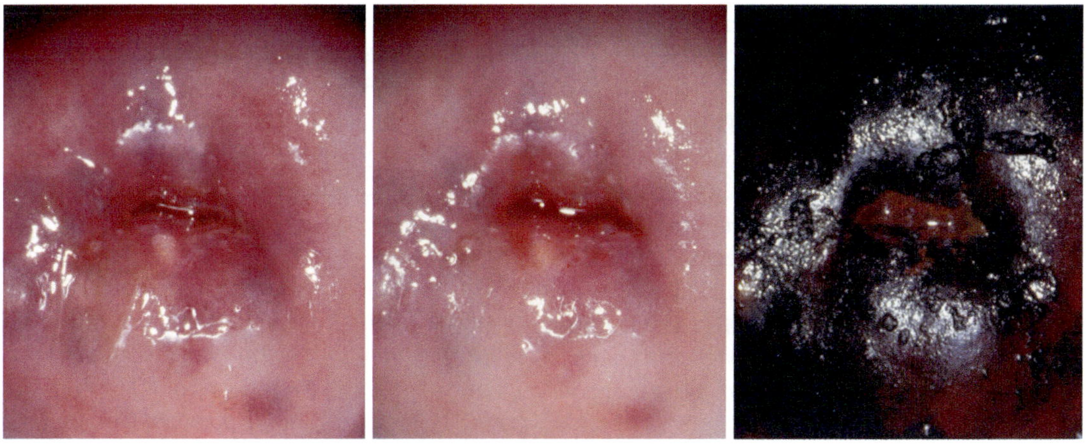

Fig. 18.35 Multiple borderline abnormal Pap smears such as ASC-US and LSIL had been documented over a long period of time. Colposcopy is normal: there is almost no difference before (left) and after (center) the application of acetic acid. The squamocolumnar junction can be visualized with the Kogan speculum. The Lugol test results in homogenous staining of the mature squamous epithelium of the transformation zone

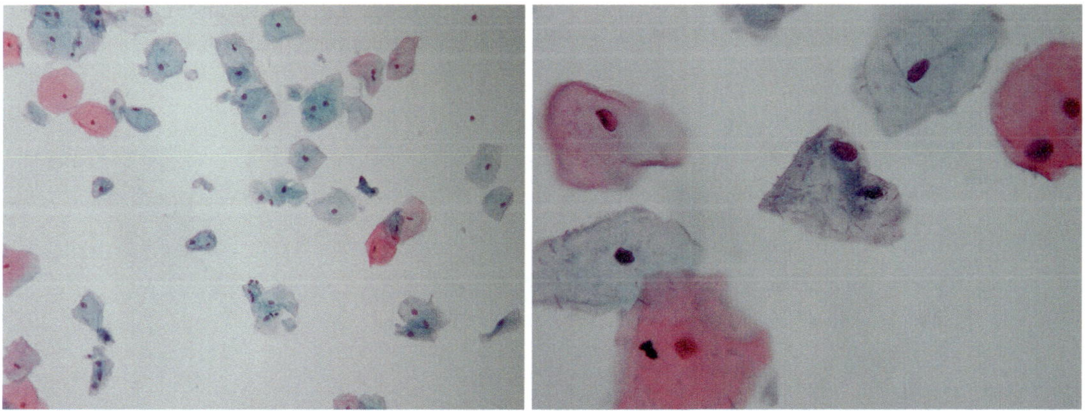

Fig. 18.36 ThinPrep® Pap test NILM (negative for intraepithelial lesion or malignancy). The background of the liquid-based cytology preparation is clear. Normal squamous cells from the superficial and intermediate layer are seen with small round or oval nuclei

18.1.21 Delayed Colposcopic Diagnosis of HSIL

A 34-year-old patient has had a Pap smear diagnosis of ASC-H (atypical squamous cells, cannot exclude HSIL) half a year before. Instead of colposcopic triage, D&C is done, and no dysplasia is found. Three months later, a repeat Pap smear is classified as AGUS (atypical glandular cells of undetermined significance). An HPV test is initiated (HPV high-risk positive) as well as a CINtec Plus® test (positive). Eventually, the patient is referred to the colposcopy clinic.

The colposcopic diagnosis is unequivocal: A typical grade 2 lesion (major change) is identified (Fig. 18.37).

- Adequate colposcopy
- Squamocolumnar junction visible
- T1
- Abnormal colposcopic findings: right dorsal quadrant with thick acetowhite area (major change)
  Fig. 18.37

CIN3 is confirmed through targeted biopsy (Figs. 18.38 and 18.39). The ThinPrep® Pap test also suggests HSIL/CIN3 (Fig. 18.40).

Finally, the abnormal tissue is removed by colposcopically guided LEEP resection in combination with CO_2 laser vaporization.

Commentary

ASC-H, i.e., the suspicion of high-grade cervical dysplasia based on screening cytology, already is a clear indication for colposcopic triage. Instead, diagnosis of CIN3 was delayed. This may not primarily be a problem of potential disease progression. However, it causes unnecessary psychological distress. Both the D&C and CINtec Plus® testing were not indicated under the circumstances described.

Colposcopy, on the other hand, was able to quickly provide a diagnosis and help to make the appropriate treatment decision.

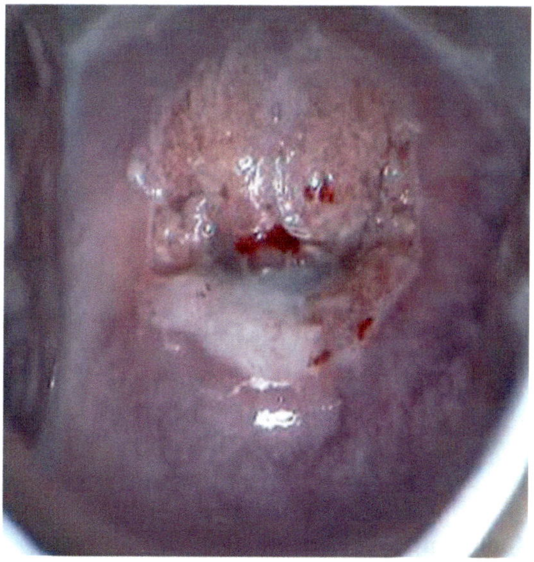

Fig. 18.37 The colposcopic diagnosis is unequivocal: there is dense and opaque acetowhite staining (major change) suggesting HSIL

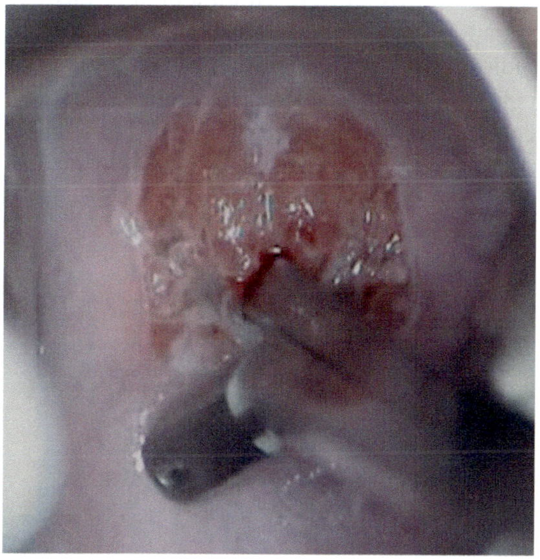

Fig. 18.38 The grade 2 lesion (major change) between 5 and 9 o'clock is well accessible for targeted biopsy, which confirms the diagnosis of HSIL (CIN3)

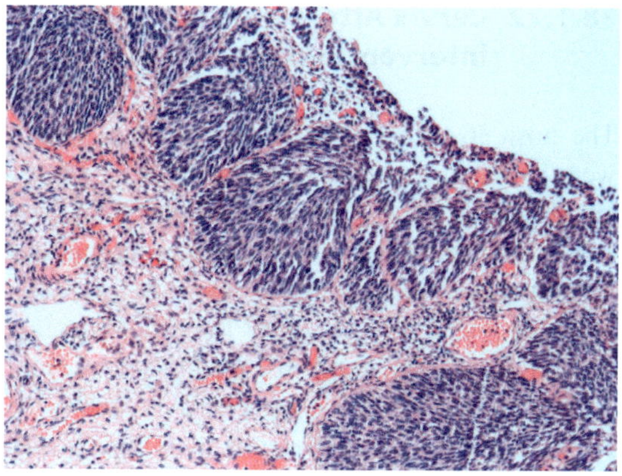

Fig. 18.39 High-grade cervical intraepithelial neoplasia (HSIL/CIN3). There are full thickness nuclear abnormalities. Characteristically for CIN3, there is no maturation across layers

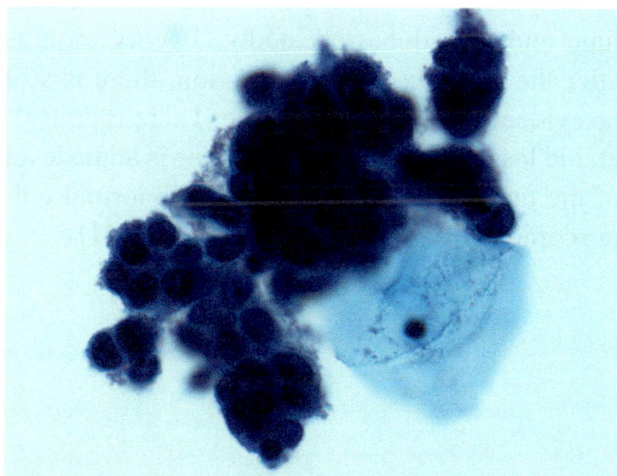

Fig. 18.40 ThinPrep® Pap smear suggesting HSIL/CIN3. Next to the basophilic intermediate cell with a small pyknotic nucleus surrounded by a dense cluster of atypical cells of the parabasal type. Typically, these cells have a high N/C ratio

18.1.22 Cervix After Three Surgical Interventions

The now 36-year-old nulligravid patient underwent cold-knife conization 5 years prior with a histologically confirmed diagnosis of CIN3. Two years prior, she underwent an electrosurgical loop resection (LEEP) in combination with CO_2 laser vaporization. This time, only low-grade disease (LSIL) was found on the histopathologic exam.

The next operation took place 1 year prior. Again, cold-knife conization was performed after the Pap smear suggested HSIL/CIN3 without prior colposcopy. Histologically, only low-grade dysplasia could be demonstrated. Four months after the third surgery, the Pap smear was abnormal again suggesting HSIL/CIN2, and the HPV test (HC2) was positive for HPV high-risk DNA. The gynecologist treating the patient at the time suggested to perform hysterectomy, and the patient seeks a second opinion.

Colposcopy is now performed for the first time and then done repeatedly. Twenty months after the third surgical intervention, there is still no evidence of recurrent disease. There is considerable loss of tissue. The cervical os is at the level of the upper vagina. However, no abnormal colposcopic findings are recorded (Fig. 18.41).

- Adequate colposcopy
- Squamocolumnar junction not visible
- T3
- Miscellaneous findings: significant loss of tissue after prior cervical resections Fig. 18.41

The ThinPrep® Pap smear is normal (NILM) (Fig. 18.42), and the Hybrid capture II test is now negative.

Another 13 months later (33 months after the third surgery), there is still no evidence of recurrent disease.

Commentary

After one surgical intervention, the risk of premature delivery (before the 37th week) is 1:9 compared to 1:24 without prior surgery (Ortoft et al. 2010). After two cervical resections, the risk is 1:3. Definitely, within a high to medium resource setting, no surgery of the cervix is indicated without prior colposcopic triage as colposcopy is considered the gold standard of cervical diagnosis. Purely diagnostic conizations, especially in women of childbearing age, are not acceptable.

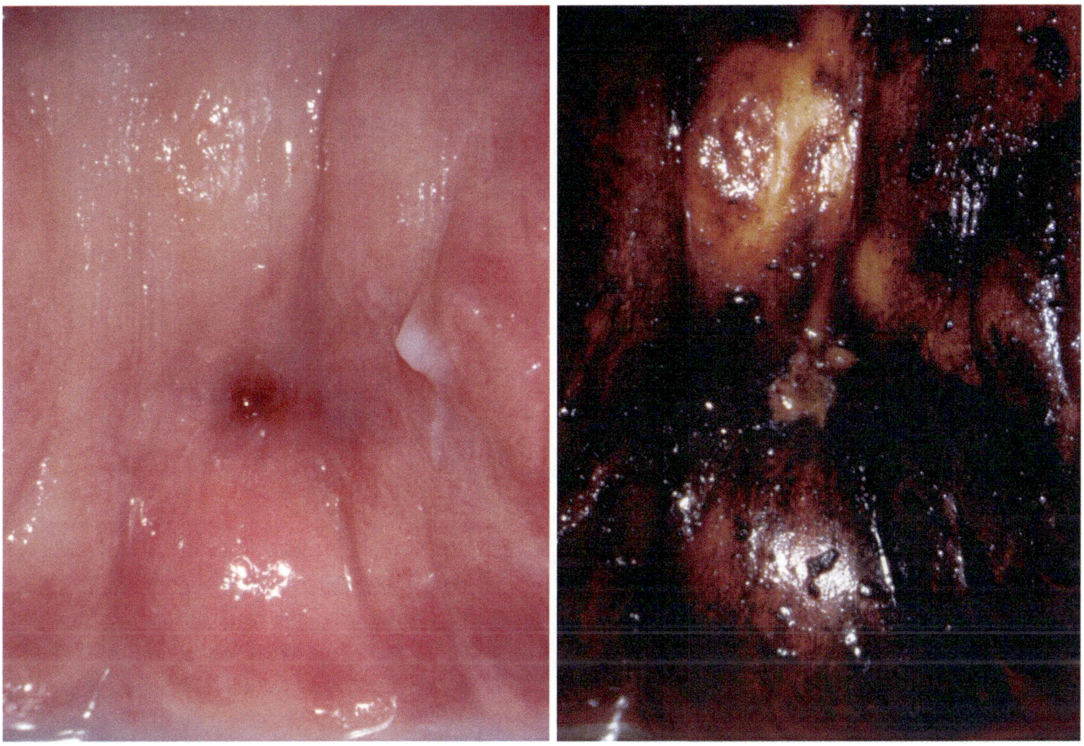

Fig. 18.41 Cervix after three surgical interventions (cold-knife conizations and LEEP/CO_2 laser treatment). The cervical os is at the level of the upper vagina. No abnormal colposcopic findings of the ectocervix are recorded. The residual cervical/upper vagina tissue is partly Lugol-negative. The squamocolumnar junction is not visible (T3)

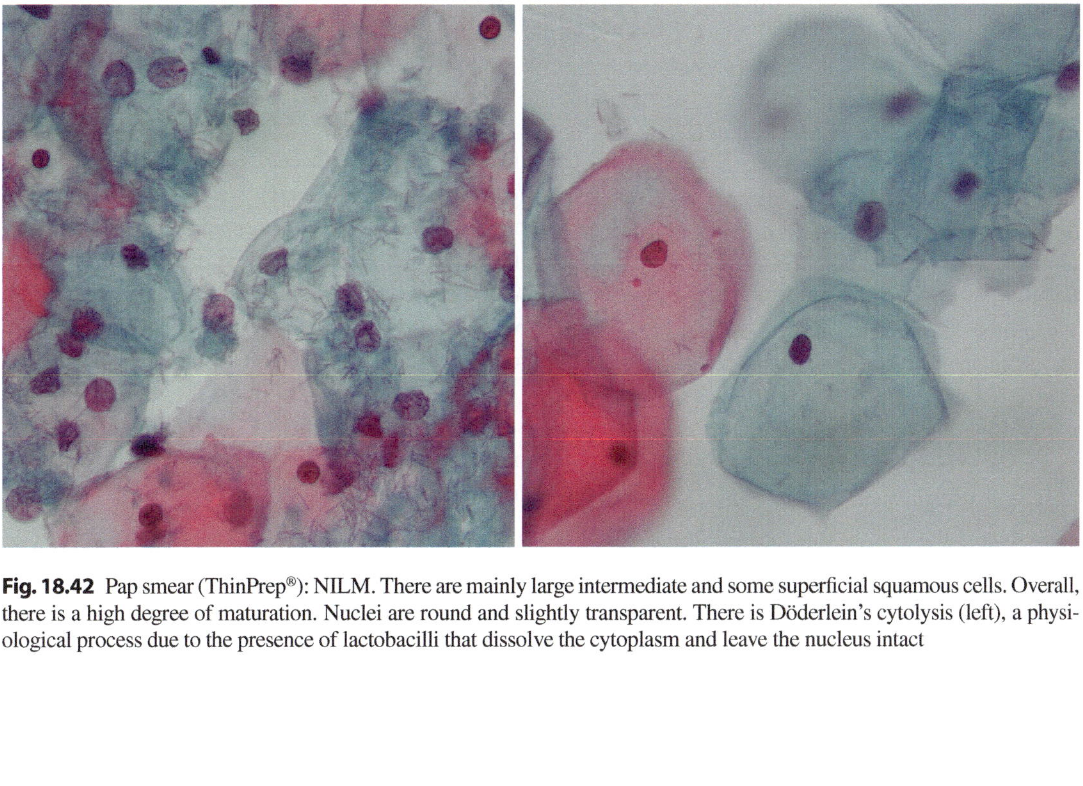

Fig. 18.42 Pap smear (ThinPrep®): NILM. There are mainly large intermediate and some superficial squamous cells. Overall, there is a high degree of maturation. Nuclei are round and slightly transparent. There is Döderlein's cytolysis (left), a physiological process due to the presence of lactobacilli that dissolve the cytoplasm and leave the nucleus intact

18.2 Recurrent Cervical Dysplasia

18.2.1 HSIL Recurrence After Conization During Pregnancy

A 31-year-old patient is 24 weeks pregnant after infertility treatment. Two months prior, a Pap test suspected HSIL/CIN3. Colposcopy and targeted biopsy confirmed the diagnosis of CIN3. However, the repeat Pap smear (ThinPrep®) is classified as "HSIL with features suspicious for invasion." Therefore, cold-knife conization with simultaneous cerclage is done in the second trimester. Hemostasis is achieved by Sturmdorf-type sutures. Histopathology shows CIN3 without evidence of invasion. The resection margins are free of dysplasia.

In the 36th week, the ectocervix is colposcopically unremarkable. However, the cervical os cannot be visualized. The ThinPrep® Pap test is classified as NILM, and the Hybrid capture II test is negative. The child is finally delivered by cesarean section. During the operation, the cervical canal is dilated.

At the first colposcopic follow-up after delivery, the cervical canal remains closed. The aspect of the ectocervix is normal with normal Pap test and negative HPV test. No cervical canal can be identified. The patient does not have a menstrual bleeding. However, amenorrhea was present earlier and had necessitated the infertility treatment.

One year after delivery, the cervical canal is opened by resecting a small amount of tissue with an electrosurgical loop. No dysplasia was detected in this specimen.

Another 6 months later, the patient presents to the colposcopy clinic again and is 9 weeks pregnant. There is a small area with a regular mosaic, which is removed with a small loop as an office procedure. Here, a recurrence (CIN3) is diagnosed. No further surgery is done as the patient is pregnant. On follow-up visits during the pregnancy, the Pap and HPV test are negative.

Seven months after the second delivery, colposcopic inspection shows a circumscribed opaque acetowhite area surrounding the cervical canal.

- Adequate colposcopy
- Squamocolumnar junction not visible
- T3
- Abnormal colposcopic findings: sharply delineated opaque acetowhite epithelium around the cervical os (major change)
  Fig. 18.43

A small cylinder is removed with the LEEP technique under local anesthesia as an office procedure. The diagnosis of recurrent HSIL/CIN3 is confirmed in concordance with the repeat Pap test and the positive HPV test result (HC2).

Colposcopy 3 years later shows no recurrence (Fig. 18.44) with a normal Pap smear (ThinPrep®) and a negative HPV test.

Commentary

Usually, conization during pregnancy can be avoided. However, in the present scenario, invasive disease had been suspected because of the Pap smear result. Cold-knife conization was performed in combination with cerclage. However, LEEP is feasible during pregnancy (see Sect. 10.3). As the blood flow within the pregnant cervix is greatly increased, hemostasis may be difficult. In this scenario, hemostasis could only be achieved through Sturmdorf-type sutures. This may have contributed to the subsequent occlusion of the cervical canal.

The present scenario also shows that circumscribed manifestations of cervical dysplasia can be safely removed under local anesthesia as an office procedure.

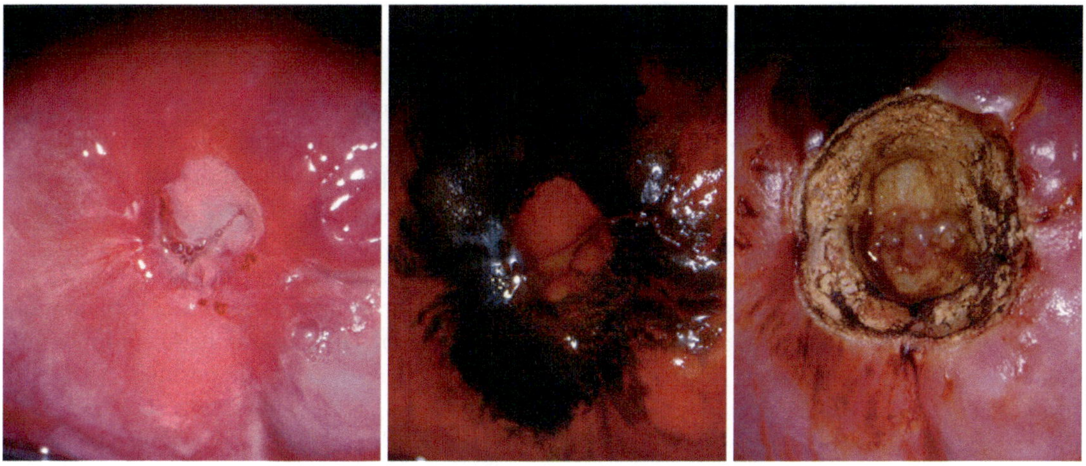

Fig. 18.43 Recurrent HSIL/CIN3 after LEEP during pregnancy. The opaque acetowhite and Lugol-negative area is removed with a small loop under local anesthesia as an in-office procedure

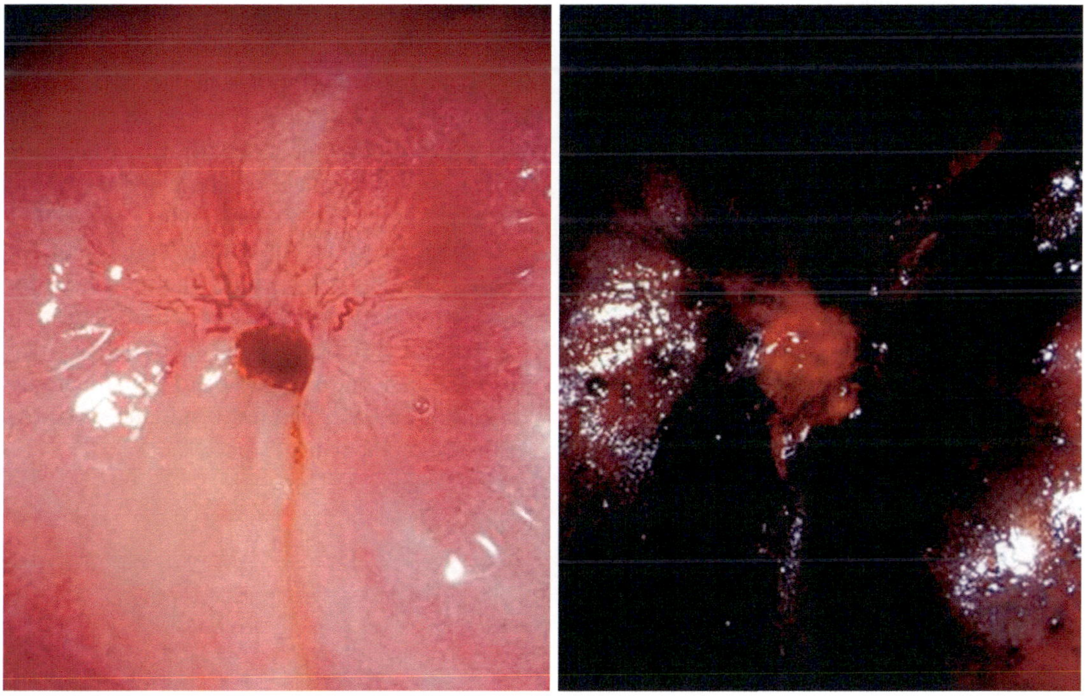

Fig. 18.44 Three years after LEEP, which had been performed as an office-based procedure, the patient remains free of disease

18.2.2 Suspected Recurrence After LEEP/CO_2 Laser Treatment

About 2 years prior, a 27-year-old nulligravid patient was diagnosed with an abnormal Pap smear (LSIL). Four follow-up smears were obtained, all classified as ASC-US. One year ago, the HC2 test was positive for HPV high-risk DNA.

Colposcopic examination shows a large ectopy partially covered by metaplastic squamous epithelium. The cervix is bleeding on touch. There is a clearly delineated delicate acetowhite area within the left ventral quadrant, which is Lugol-negative.

- Adequate colposcopy
- Squamocolumnar junction visible
- T1
- Abnormal colposcopic findings: left ventral quadrant with delicate acetowhite and epithelium with sharp borders (minor change)
  Fig. 18.45

Targeted biopsy shows HSIL/CIN2 in accordance with the ThinPrep® Pap smear. The Hybrid capture II test is positive for HPV high-risk DNA.

The patient is treated with a combination of LEEP (resection of the left ventral quadrant) and CO_2 laser (vaporization of the remaining transformation zone).

Eleven months later, the ectocervix has healed well. The squamocolumnar junction is visible and a new ectopy has formed. Overall, the colposcopic exam is unremarkable (Fig. 18.46). However, the ThinPrep® Pap test shows cells of low-grade intraepithelial neoplasia with morphologic signs of HPV infection. Accordingly, the Hybrid capture II test is still positive.

Another 14 months later, the cervix is unchanged (Fig. 18.47) as are Pap smear and HPV test results. Colposcopic inspection of the vagina shows no evidence of intraepithelial neoplasia. Further follow-up visits are scheduled.

Commentary

The fact that the cervix bleeds on touch is by no means a reliable criterion for preneoplasia or even invasive disease. However, bleeding can make the colposcopic assessment more difficult or lead to "inadequate" colposcopy as per the definition of the Rio nomenclature.

Low-grade squamous intraepithelial neoplasia (LSIL) should no longer be interpreted as disease requiring treatment, and repeat surgery in a patient of childbearing age should be avoided. Nevertheless, one should not underestimate the impact of an LSIL Pap test result and a positive HPV test on the patient's psyche.

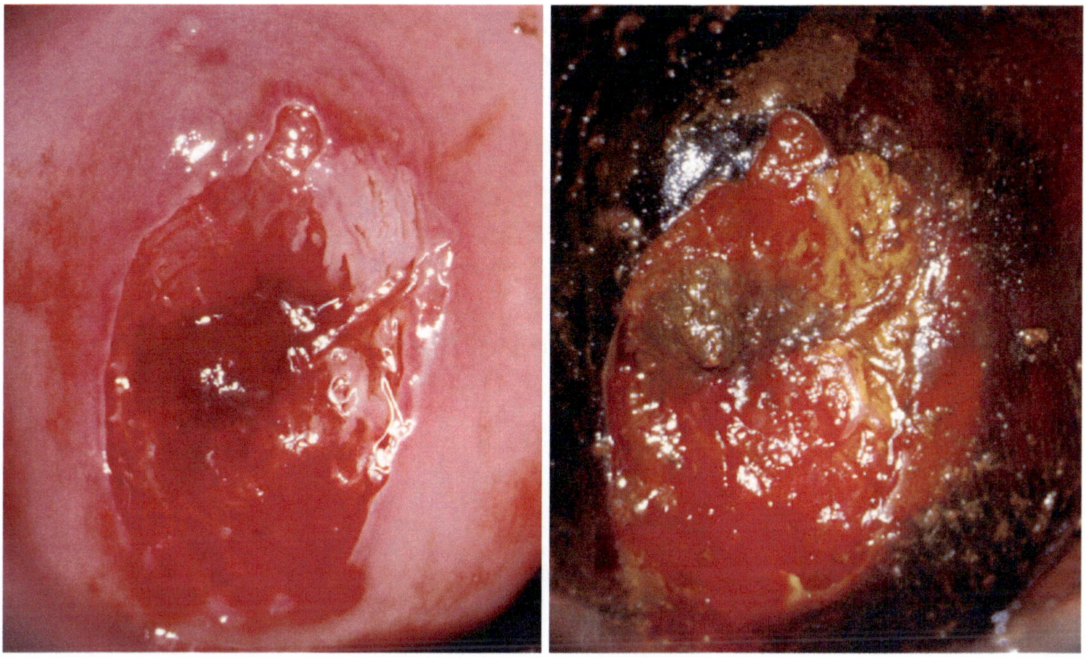

Fig. 18.45 A 27-year-old nulligravid patient with a minor change lesion within the left ventral quadrant of the cervix

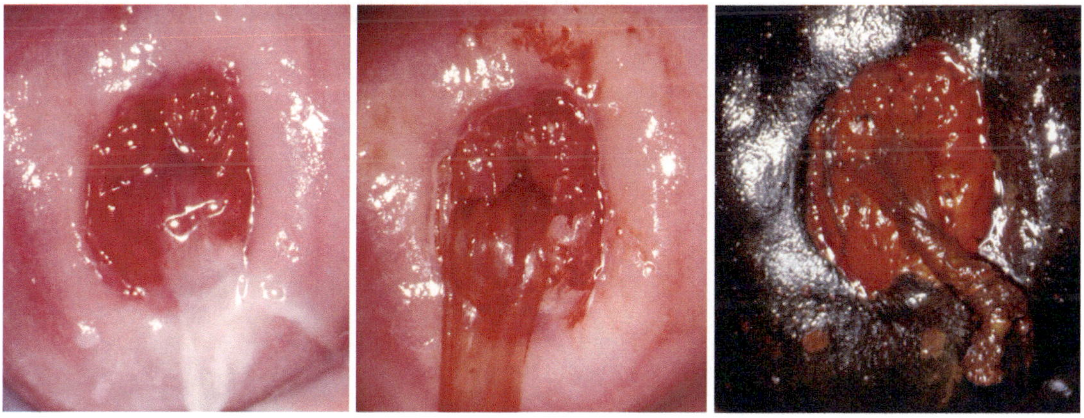

Fig. 18.46 Eleven months after LEEP and CO_2 laser treatment, the colposcopic appearance of the cervix is normal

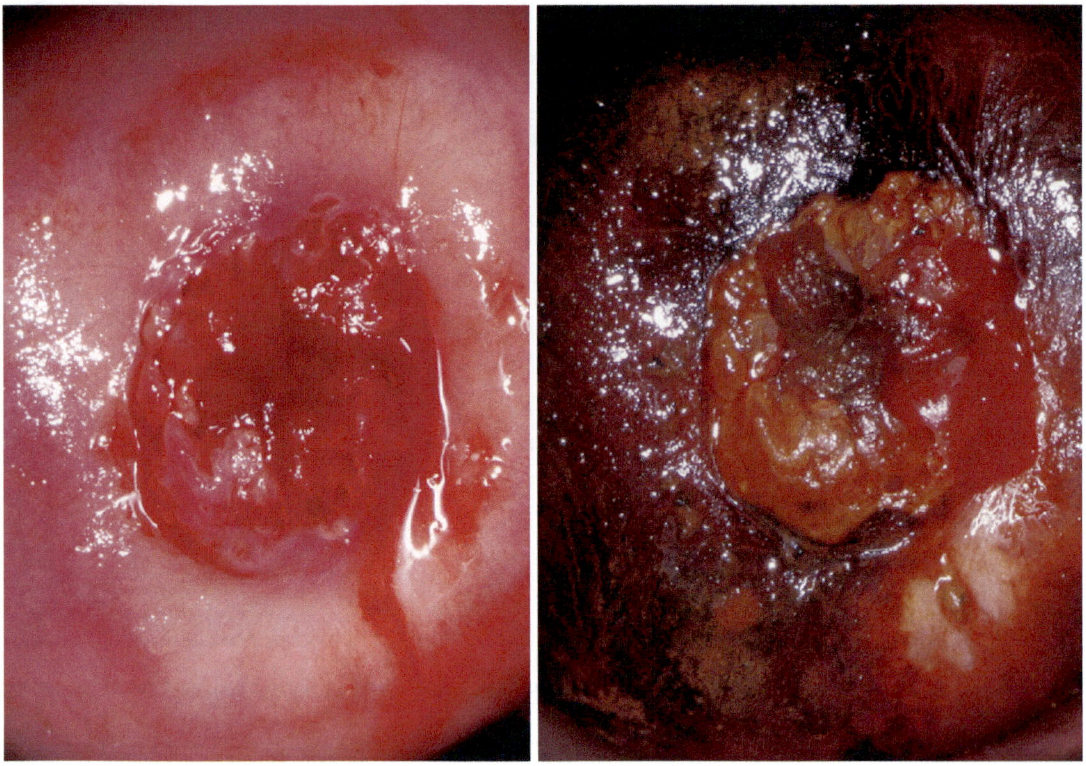

Fig. 18.47 Another 14 months later, colposcopy is still normal. However, the Pap smear is positive for LSIL, and the HPV test (HC2) remains positive for high-risk HPV

18.2.3 Recurrence 16 Months After LEEP

At the age of 33, moderate cervical dysplasia (CIN2) is verified by colposcopic biopsy during pregnancy. The baby is delivered by cesarean section as amniotic infection is suspected.

Postpartum, high-grade intraepithelial neoplasia is reconfirmed by targeted biopsy, and the dysplastic tissue is removed with a medium-sized electrosurgical loop. At the time, moderate to severe dysplasia extends to the endocervical resection margins. The endocervical curettage is negative.

On two follow-up examinations, the Pap smear is indicative of LSIL.

Sixteen months after LEEP surgery, the squamocolumnar junction can be visualized with the Kogan speculum. Within a newly formed transformation zone, small opaque sharply delineated acetowhite areas are seen.

- Adequate colposcopy
- Squamocolumnar junction visible with Kogan speculum
- T2
- Abnormal colposcopic findings: opaque, sharply delineated acetowhite epithelium around the cervical os (major change) Fig. 18.48

A biopsy at 12 o'clock shows HSIL/CIN2.

The abnormal tissue is removed with the electrosurgical loop with a final histopathologic diagnosis of CIN3.

Over the following three and a half years, Pap smears are normal. Eventually, the patient is treated in another hospital and again undergoes conization for recurrent disease. At the time, the patient is 39 years old. Hysterectomy is discussed.

Commentary

The scenario described poses a considerable psychological burden on the patient. Eventually, hysterectomy has been suggested. This may be justified in selected cases of recurrent intraepithelial neoplasia of the cervix. However, the patient has to be made aware that there is a significant risk of subsequent vaginal intraepithelial neoplasia (VAIN) after removal of the uterus for preneoplastic disease.

If a patient wishes to maintain fertility, alternatives to hysterectomy should be pointed out, such as repeat loop/laser treatments, cervical amputation, or trachelectomy.

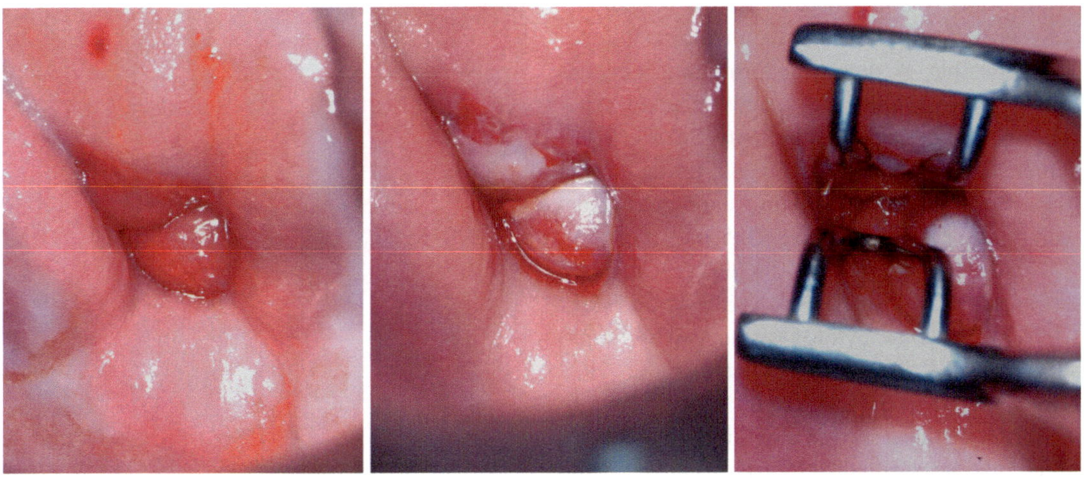

Fig. 18.48 Recurrent HSIL/CIN2 disease 16 months after LEEP

18.2.4 Recurrence After Positive Endocervical Curettage

A 30-year-old patient is referred for colposcopic evaluation with a Pap test diagnosis of HSIL/CIN3. The HPV test (HC2) is positive.

The squamocolumnar junction is visible with the endocervical speculum. Application of acetic acid reveals the typical aspect of high-grade dysplasia. The entire transformation zone is covered by acetowhite epithelium with irregular mosaic. The major change is well demarcated toward the periphery.

- Adequate colposcopy
- Squamocolumnar junction visible with Kogan speculum
- T2
- Abnormal colposcopic findings: all four quadrants with sharply delineated acetowhite epithelium with irregular mosaic (major change)
  Fig. 18.49

A biopsy at 12 o'clock confirms CIN3 disease. Subsequently, the patient undergoes surgery (LEEP). A large loop is used to resect a cylinder-shaped piece of tissue. The resection margins are free of dysplasia. However, the endocervical curettage specimen contains fragments of high-grade squamous intraepithelial neoplasia.

Six months after surgery, follow-up colposcopy is performed. The squamocolumnar junction is visible. A new transformation zone has formed which again shows a major change, especially within the ventral quadrants. Schiller's test demonstrates that the peripheral tissue of the transformation zone is mature enough to react with the Lugol solution (Fig. 18.50).

A biopsy is obtained at 12 o'clock close to the opening of the cervical canal, which shows HSIL/CIN2, whereas the cytologic smear (ThinPrep®) suggests HSIL/CIN3. Surprisingly, the HC2 HPV test is negative at the time.

Subsequently, a second operation is performed to remove the residual dysplastic tissue by using a small loop under colposcopic guidance. This time, the endocervical curettage is negative.

Three months later, colposcopy reveals a minor change with a fine regular mosaic (Fig. 18.51). Biopsy confirms immature metaplasia. The ThinPrep® Pap smear is normal, and the Hybrid capture II test is still negative.

Commentary

Endocervical curettage is routinely done in conjunction with LEEP. However, first the LEEP specimen(s) is removed and subsequently the curettage tissue is obtained from the remaining endocervical canal, and this order should not be reversed.

Endocervical curettage is also indicated if the entire transformation zone is visible. In the present scenario, the positive curettage preceded the diagnosis of recurrent or rather persistent disease 6 months later.

Endocervical curettage may also be useful to identify adenocarcinoma in situ, which is frequently associated with squamous intraepithelial lesions.

It is noteworthy that the Hybrid capture II test had been negative at the time of dysplasia diagnosis. This demonstrates that a negative HPV test is not the perfect "test of cure," even though false-negative results are relatively rare. For the Hybrid capture II test, Negri et al. (2007) found a false-negative test rate of 1.81% for ≥CIN2 lesions.

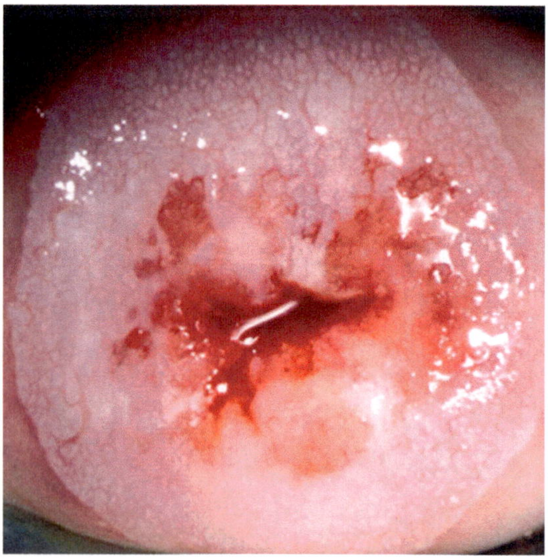

Fig. 18.49 HSIL/CIN3 confirmed by biopsy from the dense acetowhite tissue at 12 o'clock (major change)

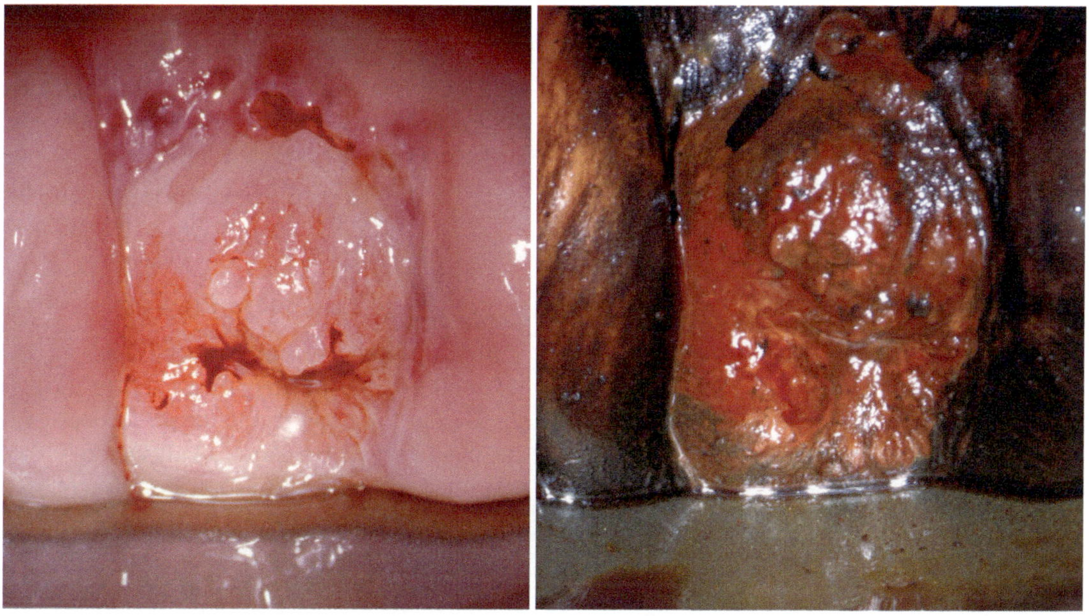

Fig. 18.50 Six months after loop resection with persistent or recurrent HSIL/CIN2 within the ventral quadrants

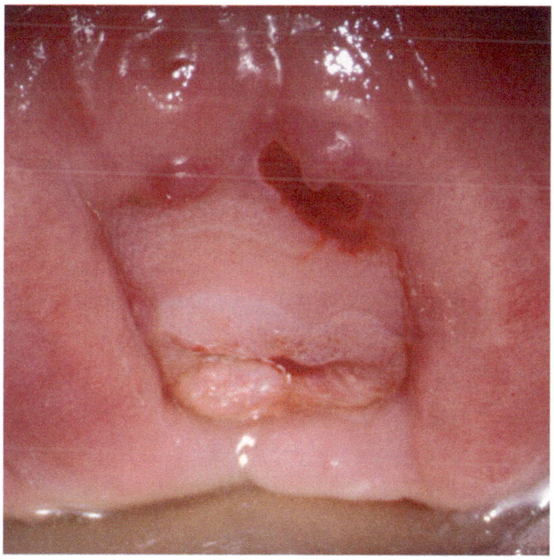

Fig. 18.51 Cervix 3 months later after a second loop resection has been performed. Biopsy from the ventral acetowhite area (minor change) reveals immature metaplasia only

18.2.5 Large Recurrence 4 Months After Conization

A 34-year-old patient undergoes conization for HSIL/CIN2 disease. The margins of the specimen are free of dysplasia.

Four months later, the patient undergoes follow-up colposcopy. Now the entire ectocervix is covered by small and slightly raised patches which are confluent and are reminiscent of flat condylomata. Lugol staining shows a mixed pattern and delineates the Lugol-negative patchy areas.

- Adequate colposcopy
- Squamocolumnar junction visible with Kogan
- T2
- Abnormal colposcopic findings: all four quadrants covered with slightly raised opaque acetowhite patches (major change)
  Fig. 18.52

The abnormal tissue corresponds to HSIL/CIN2/CIN3 on biopsy and is removed by LEEP under colposcopic guidance.

Five months later, colposcopy still shows a major change. Surrounding the opening of the cervical canal, there is a slightly raised opaque acetowhite epithelium which again has a patchy aspect toward the periphery (Fig. 18.53).

A biopsy, however, shows LSIL only. Therefore, the decision is made to wait and see. Subsequently, the patient becomes pregnant, and delivery is done by cesarean section. Fourteen months later, colposcopy is normal as well as the ThinPrep® Pap test, and the HPV test is now negative.

Commentary

Diffuse recurrences, or rather persistence of disease shortly after treatment for cervical dysplasia, are rare. The fact that in the present scenario the margins had been free of dysplasia is not uncommon, as the correlation between margin status and risk of recurrence is weak.

In patients who still desire to become pregnant, restraint is required with regard to repeat surgery of the cervix. However, when such operations cannot be avoided, the tissue loss should be kept as small as possible using the smallest loop available or by performing CO_2 laser vaporization. Of course, all surgical interventions have to be done under colposcopic guidance as this leads to smaller specimens without compromising margin status (Hilal et al. 2018).

In the scenario described here, re-operation did not completely eliminate the dysplastic tissue. The fact that ultimately HSIL had been eliminated completed may be due to the pregnancy as it is well established that spontaneous regression may occur, both after vaginal delivery as well as after cesarean section.

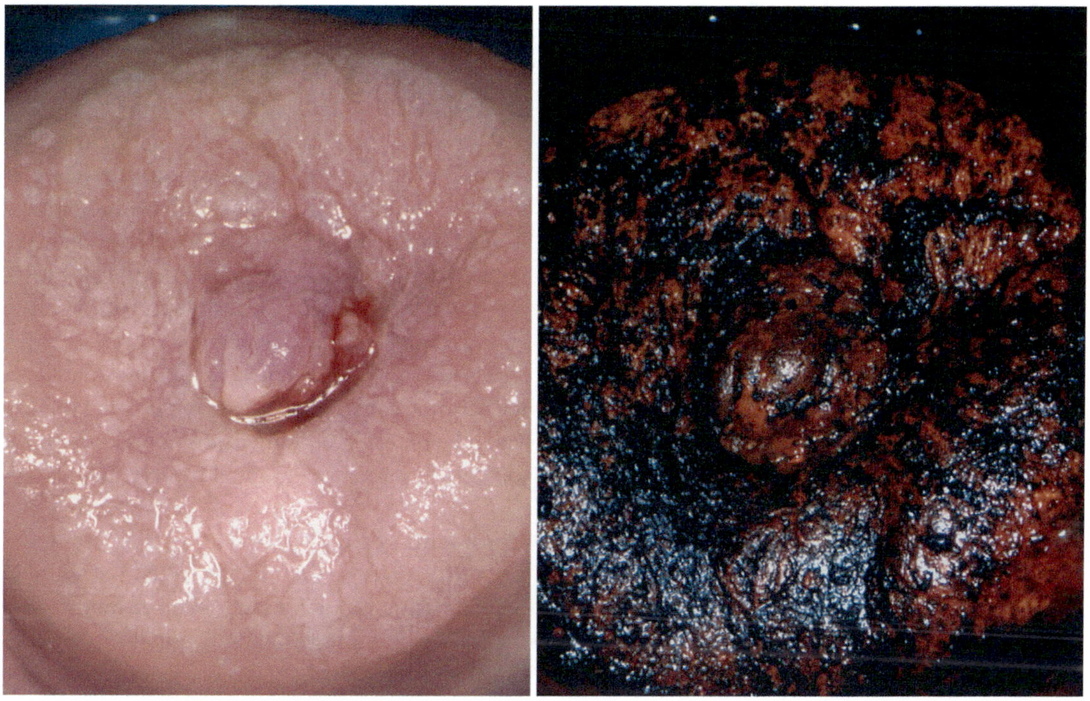

Fig. 18.52 Four months after conization for HSIL/CIN2; the cervix is covered by multiple acetowhite areas which are diagnosed histopathologically as HSIL/CIN3 disease

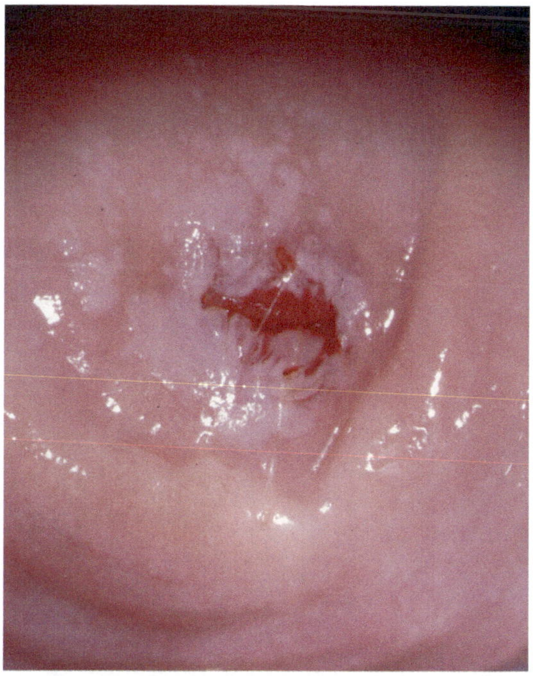

Fig. 18.53 After repeat loop resection, areas of acetowhite epithelium are still present (major change)

18.2.6 Recurrence After Two Prior Conizations

Five years ago, the patient, who is now 45 years old, underwent a cone biopsy for CIN3, labeled "carcinoma in situ" at the time. One and a half years ago, she underwent a second conization. The indication for surgery had been based on a cytological diagnosis, and no colposcopy prior to surgery had been done. Histopathologically, no dysplasia could be verified. Subsequent Pap smears were still abnormal, so the patient is now referred to the colposcopy clinic.

The cervical os is located at the level of the vagina, i.e., most of the ectocervix has been removed. The opening of the cervical canal is narrowed and the squamocolumnar junction cannot be visualized. However, the cytology brush can be inserted without problems. At 7 o'clock an area of thin acetowhite epithelium is visible. Lugol staining is only partly positive.

- Adequate colposcopy
- Squamocolumnar junction not visible
- T3
- Abnormal colposcopic findings: significant loss of tissue, right dorsal quadrant with delicate acetowhite epithelium (minor change)
  Fig. 18.54

The ThinPrep® Pap test suggests HSIL/ CIN3, and the Hybrid capture II test is positive for HPV DNA. A biopsy at 4 o'clock close to the cervical os shows HSIL/CIN2.

Now, the patient undergoes cervical tissue resection for the third time. An intracervical cylinder is removed using a small electrosurgical loop. The remaining ectocervical tissue and the upper vagina, which are partly Lugol-negative, are treated with CO_2 laser vaporization. The endocervical curettage is negative.

Follow-up exams shows significant stenosis of the cervical canal, so adequate monitoring for cervical dysplasia is no longer possible. Eventually, the patient undergoes vaginal hysterectomy.

Commentary

Both the colposcopic image after acetic acid application and the image after staining with the iodine solution resemble vaginal intraepithelial neoplasia. Most of the ectocervix has been removed in the prior two conizations, so the vagina may already be involved.

Ultimately, the decision was made to remove the uterus as detection of intracervical recurrence would have been close to impossible due to narrowing of the cervical os.

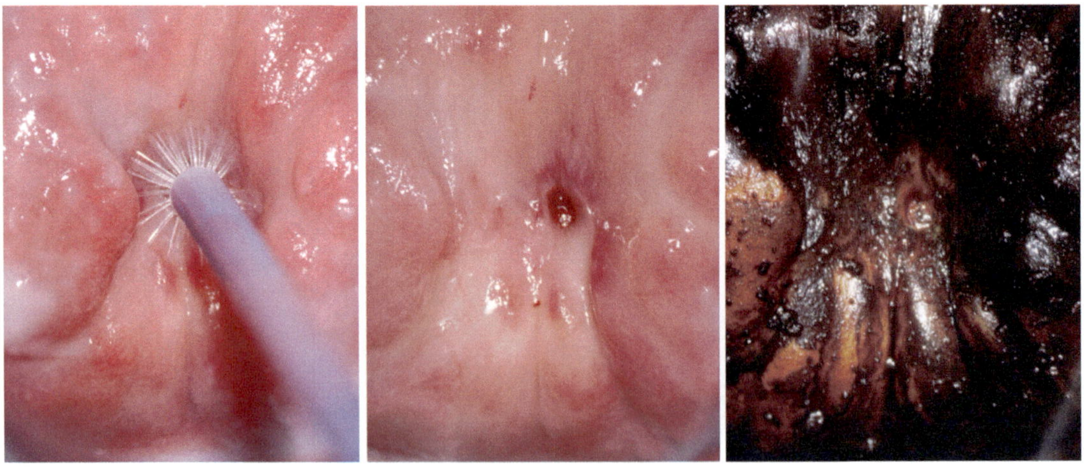

Fig. 18.54 Cervical tissue defect in a 45-year-old patient after two prior conizations. A biopsy of the transparent acetowhite and Lugol-negative area at 4 o'clock reveals HSIL/CIN2

18.2.7 Atrophy and Intracervical Recurrence

Seven months prior, conization has been performed for HSIL/CIN3 in a 57-year-old patient. The endocervical curettage also contained fragments of severe dysplasia.

When the patient presents for follow-up colposcopy, the cervix is atrophic with characteristic petechial bleeding caused by the blades of the speculum. The opening of the cervical canal is located within the plane of the upper vagina. The cervix and upper vagina are Lugol-negative.

- Adequate colposcopy
- Squamocolumnar junction not visible
- T3
- Normal colposcopic finding: atrophy Fig. 18.55

The ThinPrep® Pap smear is difficult to interpret due to atrophic and inflammatory changes (ASC-US). The Hybrid capture II test is positive for HPV high-risk DNA. The scanty endocervical curettage material is suspicious for dysplasia.

The patient undergoes repeat cervical surgery (LEEP), and intracervical CIN3 is found.

Commentary

The endocervical curettage, which had been positive at the time of conization 7 months prior, suggests an increased probability of disease persistence, as has been the case in the present scenario.

Atrophy of the squamous epithelium significantly interferes with the quality of both cytopathologic and histopathologic evaluations. According to the official colposcopy nomenclature (Bornstein et al. 2012a, b), the examination is called "inadequate" when "the cervix is obscured by inflammation, bleeding, or scarring." Although the cervix is not obscured, colposcopy should be considered "inadequate" as severe atrophy is present. Whenever feasible, topical estrogen treatment should be administered 10–14 days prior to colposcopy.

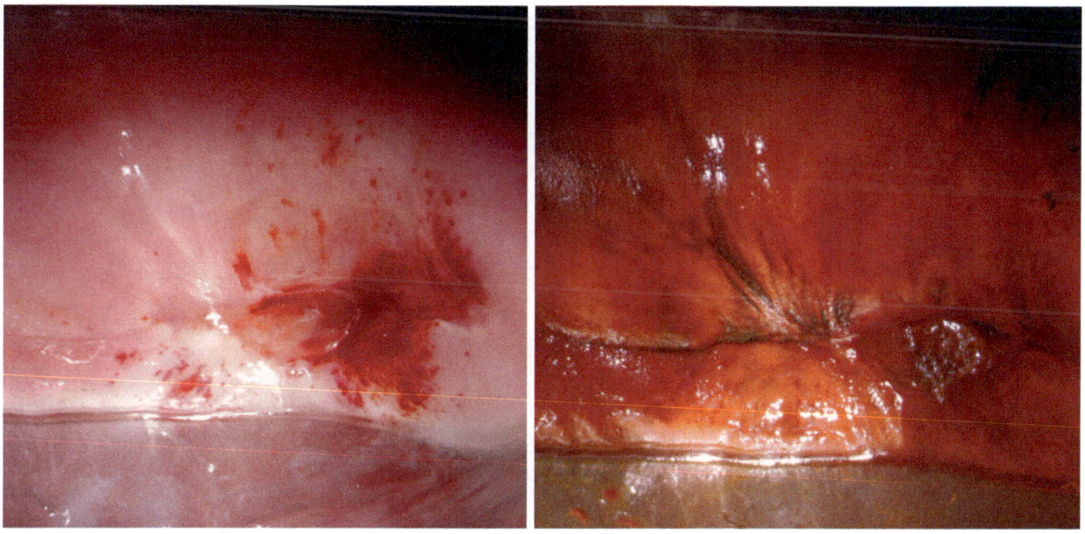

Fig. 18.55 A 57-year-old patient who underwent cone biopsy for HSIL/CIN3 3 months prior with persistent intracervical disease. Due to atrophy and scarring, colposcopic diagnosis is limited

18.2.8 Cervical Stenosis After Two Conizations

A 46-year-old patient had been treated for tubal infertility but did not become pregnant. Before the age of 20, the first conization for cervical dysplasia had been performed. Five years later, she underwent conization for the second time. Now, there is stenosis of the cervical canal, and no endocervical Pap smear is possible any more. No endocervical cells are present in the recent smear, which otherwise had been normal. The Hybrid capture II test is negative for HPV high-risk DNA.

The colposcopic exam shows severe scarring and stenosis of the cervical canal. Otherwise, the ectocervical squamous epithelium is normal and reacts Lugol-positive.

- Adequate colposcopy
- Squamocolumnar junction not visible
- T3
- Miscellaneous findings: stenosis of the cervical os
  Fig. 18.56

A small endocervical cylinder is removed by means of a small electrosurgical loop and endocervical curettage is performed. No dysplasia is detected in the specimens.

The patient was then lost to follow-up.

Commentary

Severe cervical stenosis after surgical dysplasia treatment, which prevents an adequate Pap smear, may obscure recurrent dysplasia (or cancer) in the area of the intracervical transformation zone (see Sect. 18.4.4). However, there are no guidelines on how to manage patients with cervical stenosis.

If the cervix is re-opened surgically as in this scenario, there is a high likelihood that stenosis recurs. In some patients, hysterectomy may be necessary (see Sect. 18.2.6).

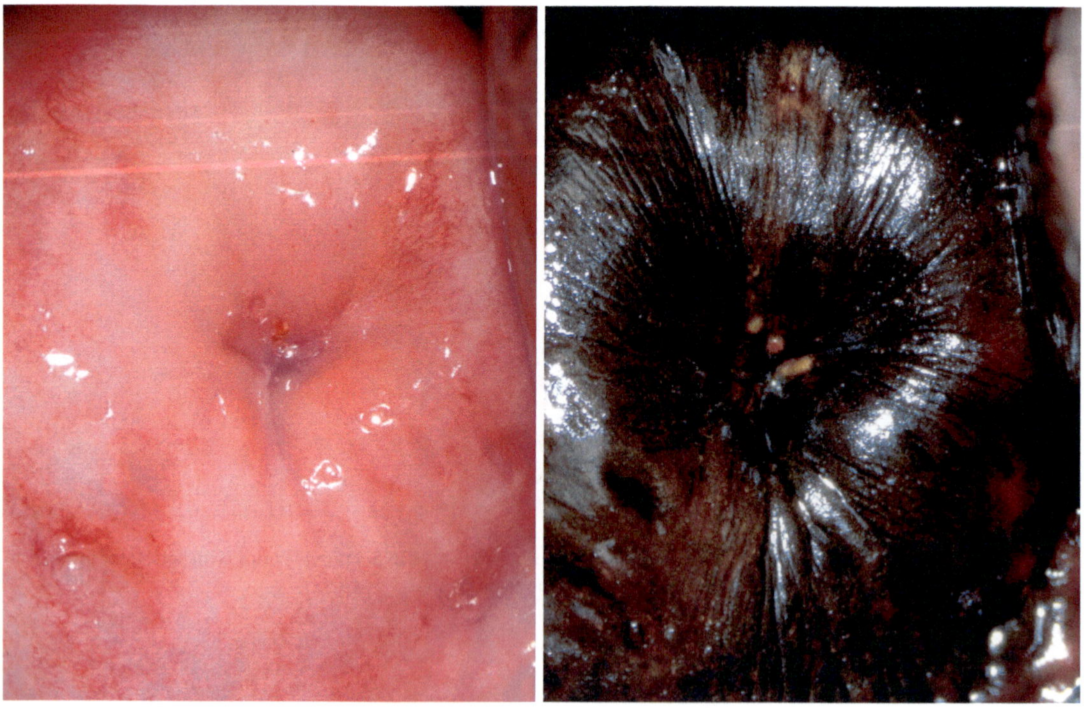

Fig. 18.56 A 46-year-old patient who underwent conization twice resulting in cervical stenosis. Intracervical cell collection is no longer feasible

18.3 Vaginal Intraepithelial Neoplasia

18.3.1 VAIN After Hysterectomy for HSIL/CIN3

A 27-year-old patient has had two prior conizations, most recently for CIN3 labeled "carcinoma in situ." Five months after the second conization, abdominal hysterectomy is performed despite the fact that she is nulligravid. Histological examination of the uterus reveals low-grade intraepithelial neoplasia of the cervix with condylomatous changes. Resection margins are free of disease.

One year after hysterectomy, the Pap test suggests HSIL/VAIN3. The ThinPrep® smear shows koilocytes as well as immature dyskaryotic cells with a high N/C ratio (Fig. 18.57).

Colposcopic examination reveals multiple raised leukoplakic areas in the upper third of the vagina. These lesions are more pronounced after application of acetic acid and stain Lugol-negative.

- Adequate colposcopy
- Abnormal colposcopic findings: the upper one third of the vagina with dense acetowhite and Lugol-negative areas (major change)
  Fig. 18.58

Biopsies shows LSIL and HSIL/CIN2, i.e., VAIN1 and VAIN2.

The patient is then treated by CO_2 laser vaporization of the upper vagina. In the following years, laser treatment is repeated twice due to persistent or recurrent VAIN.

Commentary

Recurrent cervical intraepithelial neoplasia is not an indication for hysterectomy and certainly not if the patient is of childbearing age.

There had been no colposcopic examination before hysterectomy, and ultimately only LSIL with condylomatous changes had been found on histopathology. This also calls into question the decision to remove the uterus. After adequate colposcopic evaluation, recurrences of HSIL of the cervix can usually be treated more conservatively by preserving the uterus. Das et al. (2005) recommend hysterectomy for recurrent dysplasia only if there is no sufficient tissue left that can be resected with the electrosurgical loop. In 33 hysterectomies performed on such an indication, vaginal intraepithelial neoplasia occurred in four cases (12%).

As an alternative to hysterectomy, amputation of the ectocervix or partial trachelectomy is recommended. Jeng et al. (2006) treated 20 patients with recurrent, high-grade cervical dysplasia and did not experience recurrences within a 2-year follow-up.

CO_2 laser vaporization is the preferred treatment that will not interfere with vaginal function. A treatment depth of 1.5 mm is sufficient (Benedet et al. 1992). However, long-term studies show that the success rate of CO_2 laser vaporization is only 69% (Rome and England 2000).

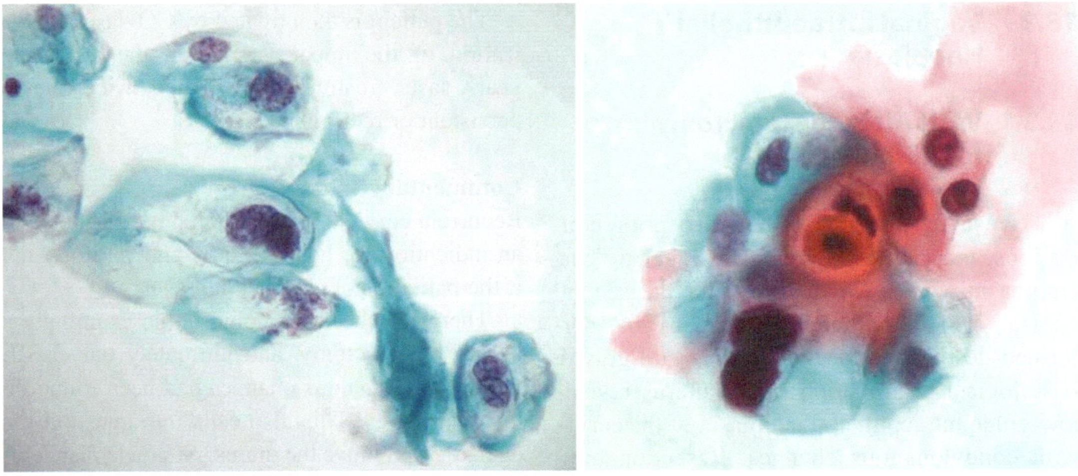

Fig. 18.57 ThinPrep® smear of the vagina with koilocytes (left) as well as immature dyskaryotic cells with a high N/C ratio (right)

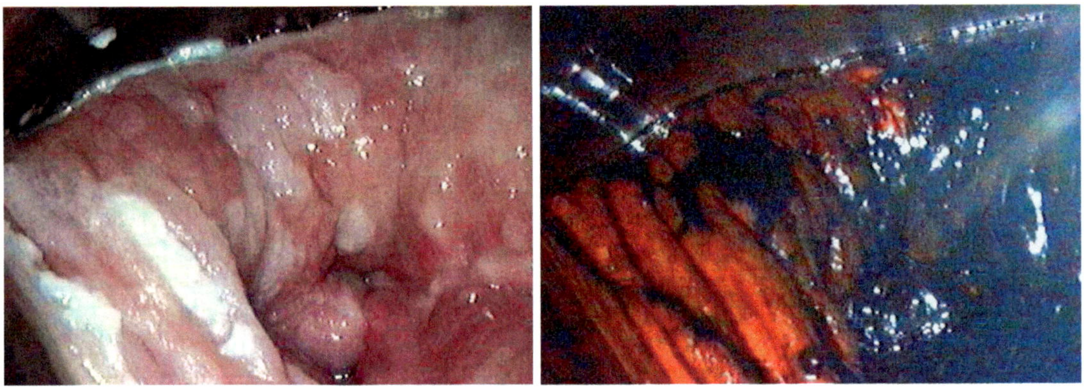

Fig. 18.58 Dense acetowhite and Lugol-negative epithelium of the upper vagina. Biopsies reveal VAIN1 and VAIN2

18.3.2 VAIN3 and HSIL of the Vulva in a Liver Transplant Patient

A 68-year-old patient underwent abdominal hysterectomy 30 years prior because of fibroids and bleeding. Eight years prior, she received a liver transplant because of biliary cirrhosis. Under immunosuppressive treatment, she then developed both vulvar and vaginal intraepithelial neoplasia.

Within the vagina, there are several sharply delineated thick acetowhite plaques of a condyloma-like appearance, which stain Lugol-negative.

- Adequate colposcopy
- Abnormal colposcopic findings: the upper and middle one third of the vagina with raised opaque acetowhite plaques, which are Lugol-negative (major change)
  Fig. 18.59

The vulva has the typical multiform appearance of vulvar intraepithelial neoplasia with white, gray, pink, reddish, and dark brown skin areas, as hyperpigmentation is alternating with hyperkeratosis (Fig. 18.60).

Ten weeks after CO_2 laser vaporization, the skin of the vulva is fully healed, and there is no evidence of HSIL (Fig. 18.61).

Whereas HSIL of the vulva has been successfully treated by laser surgery, vaginal intraepithelial neoplasia subsequently recurs several times requiring repeated surgical interventions. Three and a half years after the initial diagnosis of VAIN, squamous cell carcinoma of the vagina develops, and primary radiation therapy is initiated. Another 2 years later, the patient is free of recurrence with a normal colposcopy exam, normal Pap smear, and negative HC2 test.

Commentary

Vaginal intraepithelial neoplasia has a high relapse rate, more so than HSIL of the vulva. Drug-induced immunosuppression as in the present scenario further complicates matters. Overall, both vaginal and vulvar precancerous lesions are more difficult to control as they tend to be more extensive, will frequently relapse, and may become malignant.

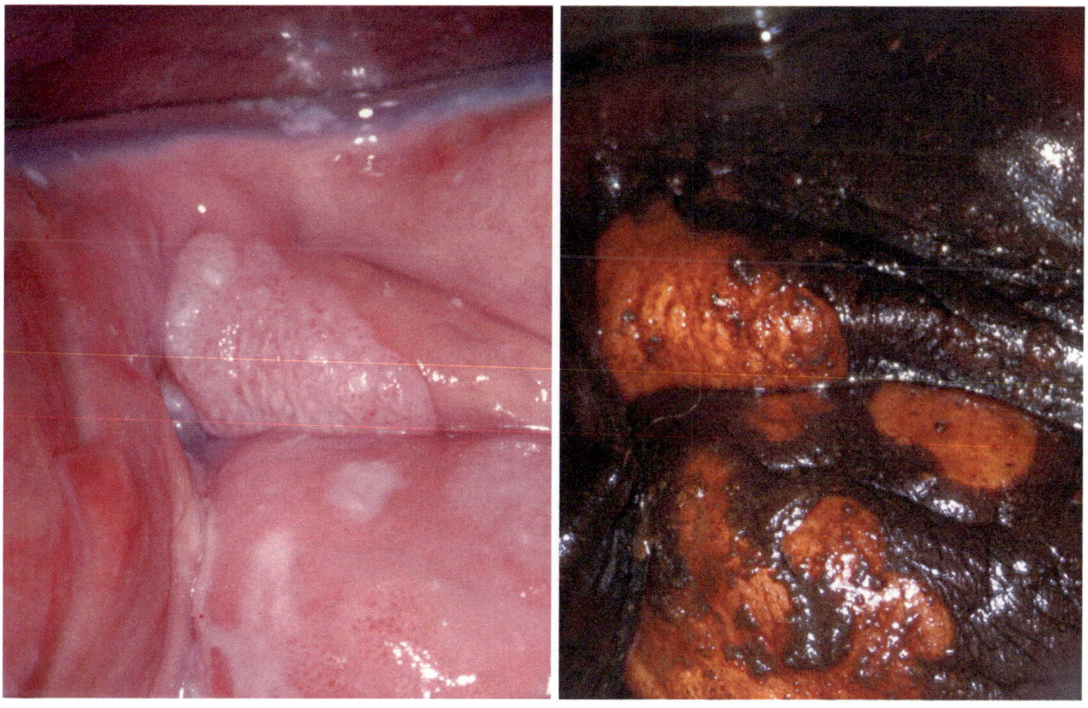

Fig. 18.59 A 68-year-old patient under immunosuppressive treatment following liver transplant surgery with VAIN3 presenting as thick opaque acetowhite areas which are Lugol-negative with well-defined borders

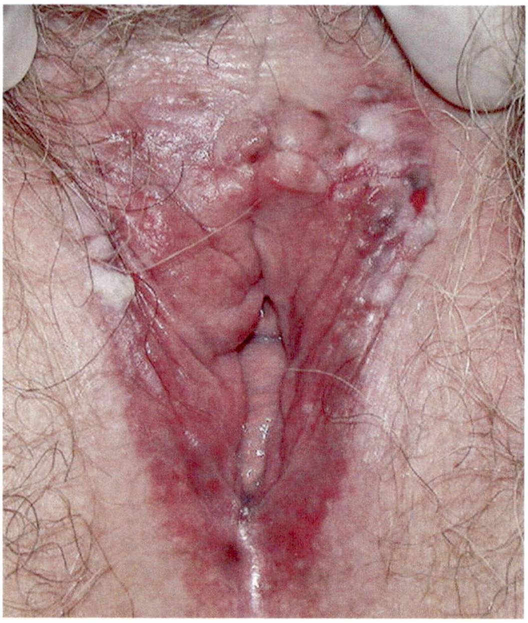

Fig. 18.60 Extensive HSIL of the vulva of a 68-year-old liver transplant patient

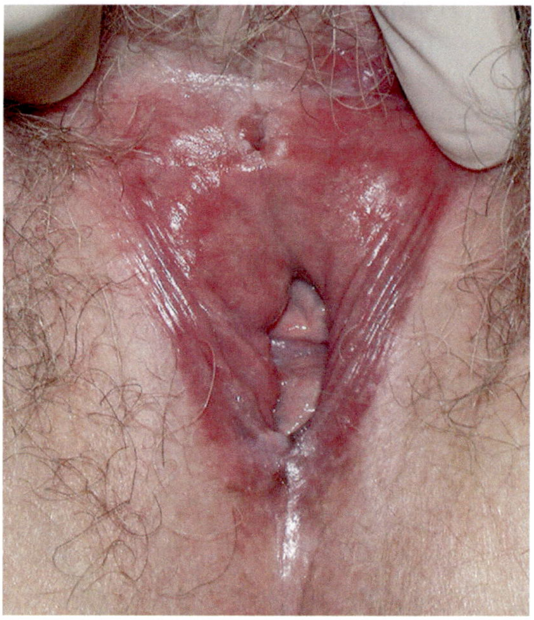

Fig. 18.61 Ten weeks after CO_2 laser vaporization, there is no evidence of HSIL of the vulva

18.3.3 VAIN3 Misdiagnosed as CIN3

The patient is 28 years old. Her mother had "the uterus removed because of cancer." Two sisters have been treated for cervical dysplasia. The patient is referred to the colposcopy clinic 7 months after conization for HSIL/CIN3. Two months after surgery, the Pap smear indicates HSIL/CIN2.

There is a considerable cervical defect. However, the squamocolumnar junction is clearly visible with no sign of grade 2 epithelial changes, only a narrow border of thin acetowhite epithelium adjacent to the squamocolumnar junction.

- Adequate colposcopy
- *Cervix*
  - Squamocolumnar junction visible
  - T1
  - Abnormal colposcopic findings: a small band of thin acetowhite epithelium close to the squamocolumnar junction (minor change)

  Fig. 18.62
- *Vagina*
  - abnormal colposcopic findings: upper one third of the vagina, right lateral wall, several Lugol-negative areas with sharp borders (major change)

  Fig. 18.63

The ThinPrep® Pap smear obtained from the cervix at the time of colposcopy suggests HSIL/CIN3. A biopsy from the vaginal wall confirms the colposcopic diagnosis of vaginal intraepithelial neoplasia (VAIN3). Eventually, CO_2 laser vaporization of the vaginal intraepithelial neoplasia is performed.

Commentary

The patient's history suggests some kind of genetic component with an increased risk of HPV related disease.

Mutations in the p53 gene or in the human leukocyte antigens (HLA) are among the genetic factors discussed (de Araujo Souza and Villa 2003).

In the case of cervical dysplasia, examination of the vulva as well as the vagina is an essential part of the colposcopic examination in order to rule out VIN and VAIN, respectively.

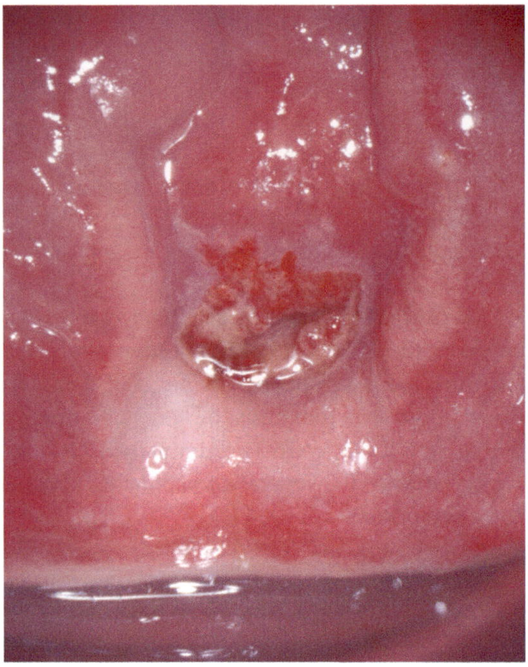

Fig. 18.62 A 28-year-old patient underwent conization. Seven months later, the Pap smear still indicates HSIL. The squamocolumnar junction is visible with a small band of acetowhite epithelium ventrally (minor change)

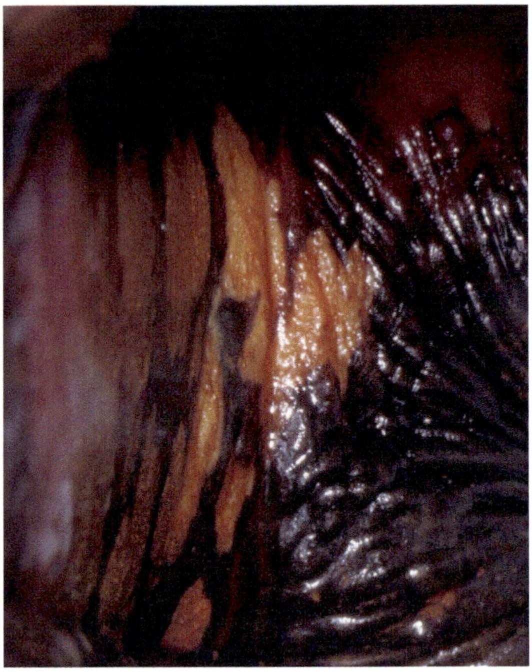

Fig. 18.63 Adjacent to the cervix, at the right vaginal wall VAIN3 is identified

18.4 Squamous Cell Carcinoma of the Cervix

18.4.1 Squamous Cell Carcinoma of the Cervix

A 65-year-old woman has been diagnosed with chronic lymphocytic leukemia 13 years ago. A year prior she underwent surgery for squamous cell carcinoma of the head. Now she has had an abnormal Pap smear and is referred for colposcopic examination.

The cervix bleeds on touch. Prior to the application of acetic acid, atypical vessels within the ventral quadrants are visible. When touching the dorsal quadrant with the cotton swap, the epithelium comes off. There is a strong acetowhite reaction. The surface of the atypical epithelium is irregular. The upper vagina is also involved (FIGO stage IIA).

- Adequate colposcopy
- Squamocolumnar junction not visible
- T3
- Suspicious for invasion: atypical vessels, bleeding on touch, irregular surface, detachment of the epithelium
  Fig. 18.64

When trying to obtain a tissue sample, the biopsy forceps slides off the surface of the cervix. Therefore, the ectocervix is held in place with a Schroeder tenaculum forceps.

The ThinPrep® Pap smear suggests squamous cell carcinoma, and the Hybrid capture II test is positive for high-risk DNA. Histopathology confirms HSIL/CIN3 as well as moderately differentiated keratinizing squamous cell carcinoma.

As the pre-existing leukemia still requires chemotherapy and as the vagina is also involved, primary radiation therapy (teletherapy as well as brachytherapy) is initiated. Unfortunately, 1 year later, the patient develops a local recurrence, which is then treated with palliative irradiation.

Commentary
If cervical cancer is suspected, this needs to be confirmed histopathologically. In most scenarios, no anesthesia is required, and multiple biopsies are obtained within an office setting. Bleeding can be controlled by vaginal packing.

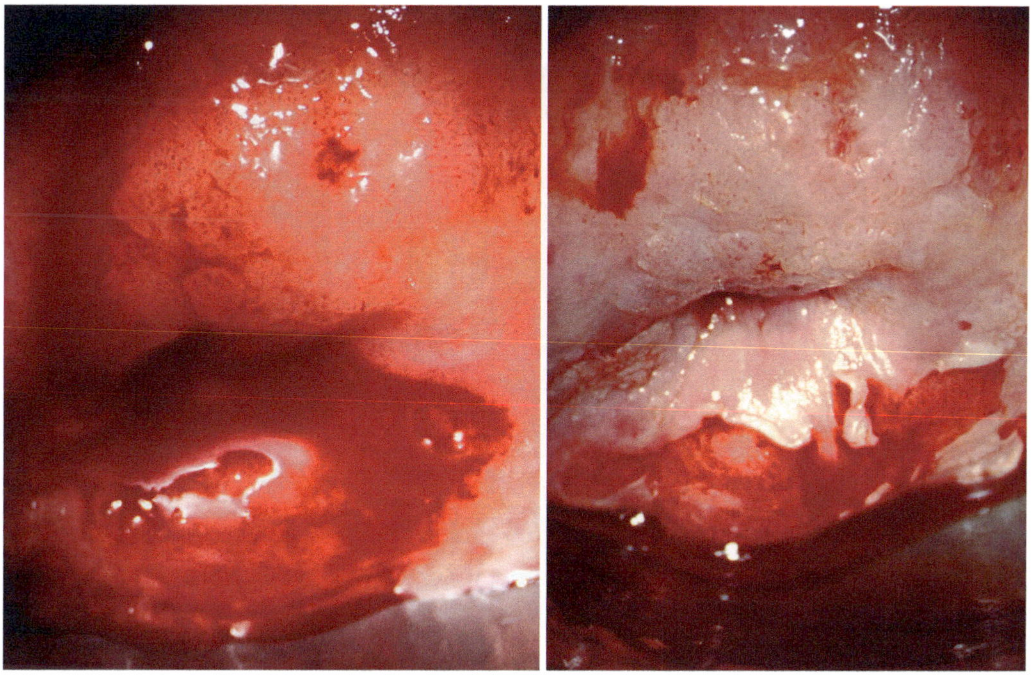

Fig. 18.64 Squamous cell carcinoma of the cervix with atypical vessels seen prior to application of acetic acid (left) and detachment of the abnormal epithelium (right)

18.4.2 Squamous Cell Carcinoma of the Cervix

For the last 6 months, a 47-year-old woman has had irregular bleeding including metrorrhagia. The Pap smear suggests HSIL. However, cervical biopsy reveals invasive squamous cell carcinoma of the cervix.

The colposcopic exam shows atypical vessels at 12 o'clock. These vessels are still visible after acetic acid has been applied. The epithelium is very vulnerable. In the dorsal quadrants of the cervix, small sheets of epithelium have become detached (rag sign). In addition to the overall impression of malignancy, there is an irregular mosaic as in HSIL. The squamocolumnar junction is not visible. There may be a significant amount of tumor within the cervical canal.

- Adequate colposcopy
- Squamocolumnar junction not visible
- T3
- Suspicious for invasion: atypical vessels, bleeding on touch, detachment of the epithelium
  Fig. 18.65

The ThinPrep® Pap smear indicates squamous cell carcinoma. The tumor is clinically staged as FIGO IB1.

Radical hysterectomy is performed as well as pelvic lymphadenectomy. The final pathology report shows moderately differentiated keratinizing squamous cell carcinoma. There is bilateral involvement of the obturator lymph nodes, so percutaneous irradiation in combination with cisplatin chemotherapy is recommended.

Commentary

Unfortunately, the early stages of carcinoma of the cervix are either free of symptoms or, as presented in this scenario, symptoms are nonspecific such as bleeding disorders.

The initial Pap test from the invasive cervical cancer indicated high-grade intraepithelial neoplasia only. In the present scenario, colposcopy and targeted biopsies have been crucial for the diagnosis of cervical carcinoma.

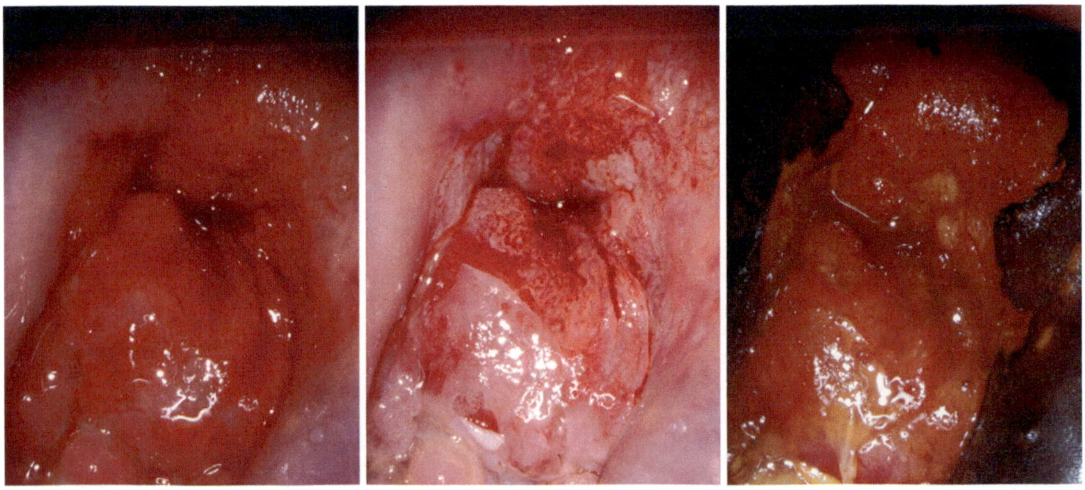

Fig. 18.65 Squamous cell carcinoma of the cervix with atypical vessels, which are most pronounced after the application of acetic acid (center)

18.4.3 Squamous Cell Carcinoma of the Cervix

A 50-year-old, morbidly obese patient presented to the department of internal medicine 4 weeks prior. She had collapsed several times, and cancer-related anemia was suspected. Initially, she refused a gynecological examination. Computer tomography showed a large pelvic mass leading to right ureteral obstruction. The pelvic lymph nodes were enlarged, and nodal metastases were suspected.

Eventually, the gynecological examination is performed, and an apple-sized cervical tumor dilating the vagina is identified. The tumor tissue is soft and friable and is bleeding on touch.

- Adequate colposcopy
- Squamocolumnar junction not visible
- T3
- Suspicious for invasion: cervix replaced by friable tumor tissue, bleeding on touch Fig. 18.66

The ThinPrep® Pap smear does not yield a conclusive diagnosis (ASC-US). Biopsy shows poorly differentiated squamous cell carcinoma.

The tumor stage is determined as FIGO IIIB, and the patient is treated with primary radiation therapy. Concomitant chemotherapy with cisplatin is not given due to poor renal function.

Commentary

If there is any suspicion of cervical cancer either through inspection with the naked eye or colposcopy, multiple biopsies should be obtained, whereas cytological diagnosis is not appropriate and may be false negative, even in scenarios with overt cancer as in the patient presented here. As pointed out earlier, Pap smears, whose results are mentioned here, have usually been obtained for educational purposes.

Especially in advanced tumors such as this, tissue biopsies are not painful for the patient, and sufficiently large tissue samples should be obtained to unequivocally prove invasion. Necrotic tissue biopsies should be avoided. Bleeding can be controlled by vaginal packing, which should not be too tight in order not to compress the urethra.

Without histopathologic confirmation of the suspected malignancy, no further treatment planning is possible.

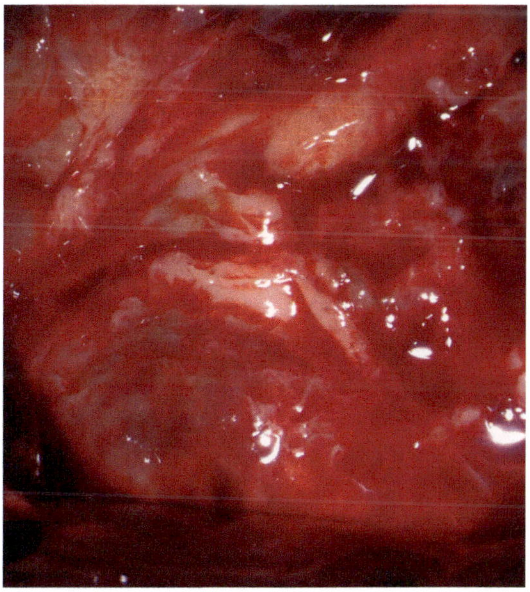

Fig. 18.66 Squamous cell carcinoma of the cervix. The cervix is replaced by fragile tumor tissue

18.4.4 Hidden Cervical Carcinoma After Prior Conization

Fifteen years prior, a 62-year-old patient underwent conization for HSIL/CIN3. In recent years, no gynecologic screening examinations have been done. When the patient experiences a strong postmenopausal bleeding, D&C is performed, which reveals moderately differentiated squamous cell carcinoma of the cervix.

Colposcopic examination shows a considerable cervical tissue defect in an otherwise normal appearing cervix. The squamocolumnar junction is not visible. The cytological brush narrowly passes the opening of the cervical canal. Obviously, the cancer does not extend to the ectocervix.

- Adequate colposcopy
- Squamocolumnar junction not visible
- T3

- Normal colposcopic findings: significant loss of cervical tissue after prior conization
  Fig. 18.67

Clinical examination shows FIGO stage IB1 disease. Radical hysterectomy is aborted when exploratory laparotomy reveals paraaortic lymph node metastases. Primary chemoradiation with cisplatin is initiated.

Commentary

The present scenario is a typical example of intracervical carcinoma which is not accessible to colposcopic examination and is diagnosed eventually when the patient develops severe postmenopausal bleeding. Both squamous cell carcinomas and adenocarcinomas may be hidden within the cervical canal.

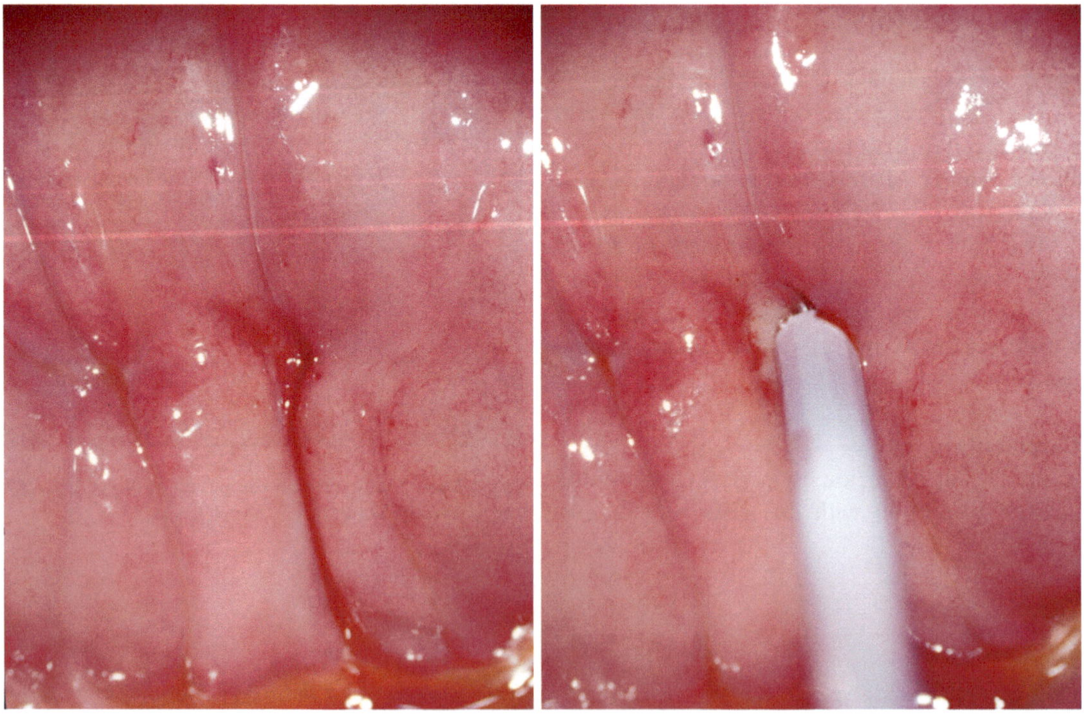

Fig. 18.67 Intracervical squamous cell carcinoma of the cervix after prior conization for HSIL/CIN3 with subsequent narrowing of the cervical canal. However, a cervical brush can still be inserted (right)

18.4.5 Microcarcinoma of the Cervix

A 33-year-old patient plans to get pregnant. However, several Pap smears have been obtained suggesting low to moderate squamous dysplasia of the cervix. The two most recent Pap smears are classified as ASC-US. Around this time, the patient consults a new gynecologist. Based on the prior cytopathology, the gynecologist now performs colposcopy and diagnoses a grade 1/ minor change. Biopsy of this lesion yields not only HSIL/CIN3 ("carcinoma in situ") but also early invasive disease. The patient is then scheduled for conization to determine the stage of the disease.

Surprisingly, preoperative colposcopy is normal without evidence of a grade 2 or grade 1 change and no colposcopic signs of invasion.

- Adequate colposcopy
- Squamocolumnar junction cannot be visualized completely
- T3
- Normal colposcopic findings: no evidence of preinvasive or invasive disease (as diagnosed histopathologically) Fig. 18.68

The cytological smear at this time is classified as ASC-H. High-grade squamous dysplasia is suspected. However, there is no cytological evidence of invasive carcinoma (Fig. 18.69).

After applying Lugol's solution, the tissue is resected using a medium-sized electrosurgical loop, yielding a well-preserved cone-shaped piece of tissue (Figs. 18.70 and 18.71). The volume of the resected tissue is measured using Archimedes' principle (Fig. 18.72), which is 3 cm^3. Histopathology reveals CIN3 ("carcinoma in situ") with a depth of invasion of 1.5 mm and a horizontal spread of 4 mm (FIGO stage IA1). The resection margins are free of invasive disease, while the dysplastic epithelium reaches the cervical resection margin (Fig. 18.73).

Commentary

In the present scenario, colposcopy indications were based on the presence of repeatedly abnormal Pap smears. Colposcopy did not give rise to the suspicion of cancer. Not even a major change was visible. The gynecologist made the correct decision and carried out a biopsy of the minor change. Surprisingly, this biopsy was able to establish not only the diagnosis of HSIL/CIN3 but also early invasion.

In this particular patient, preservation of the uterus is justifiable as no additional risk factors such as lymphovascular space invasion are present.

Re-conization must be considered if there is evidence of persistent pre-invasive disease during the first colposcopic follow-up exam after 3 months. However, it has to be kept in mind that a second conization will lead to a significantly higher complication rate of future pregnancies. Also, Reich et al. (2001) found that 78% of patients who underwent re-conization did not have any residual disease.

Close follow-up exams including colposcopy, endocervical curettage, endocervical cytology, and biopsy of any abnormal areas including grade 1 are required if the uterus is preserved.

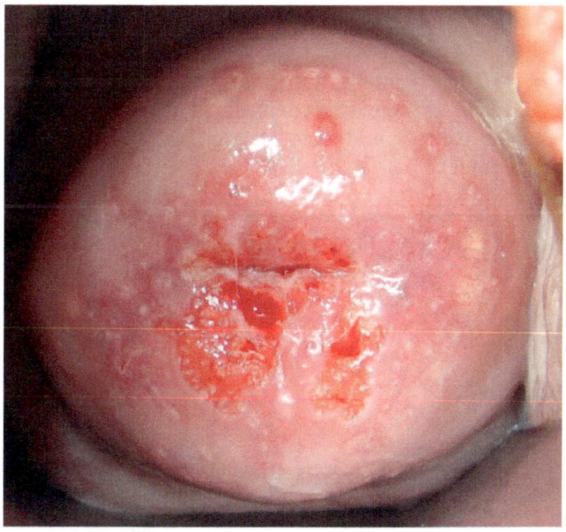

Fig. 18.68 Squamous cell carcinoma of a FIGO stage IA1 cervix. Colposcopic examination does not show any abnormality

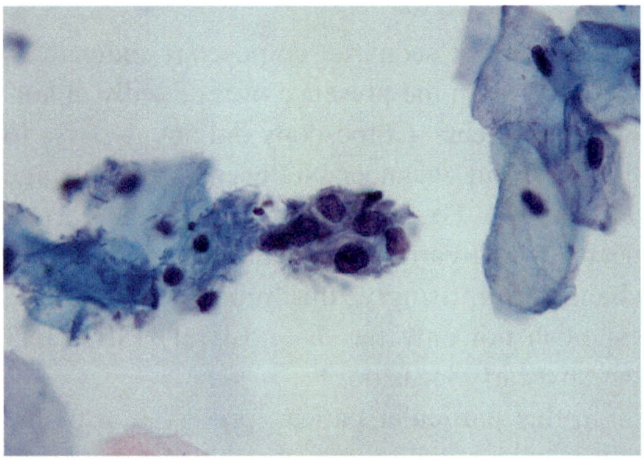

Fig. 18.69 Squamous cell carcinoma of a FIGO stage IA1 cervix. The ThinPrep® Pap smear is classified as ASC-H. The background is clean (no tumor diathesis). There is a small group of parabasal-type cells with an increased nucleus-cytoplasm ratio

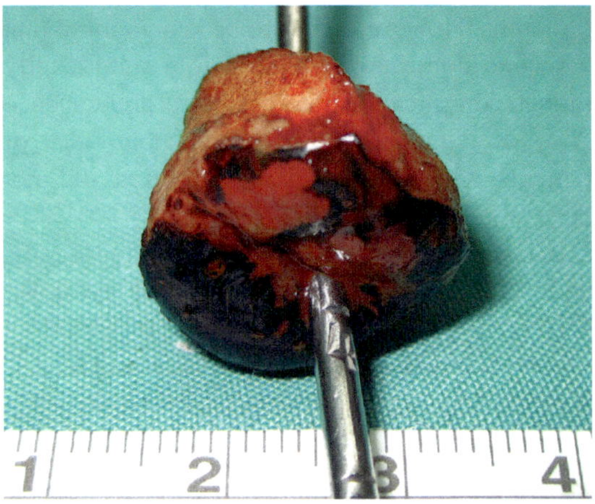

Fig. 18.70 Squamous cell carcinoma of a FIGO stage IA1 cervix. A cone-shaped piece of cervical tissue is removed using a mid-sized electrosurgical loop ("one-pass technique")

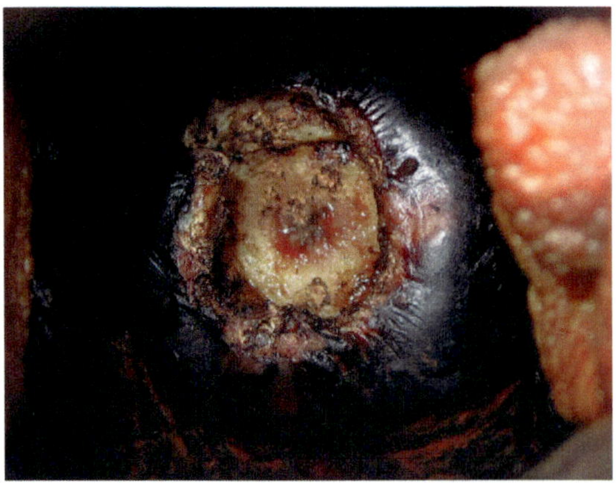

Fig. 18.71 Squamous cell carcinoma of a FIGO stage IA1 cervix. The ectocervix immediately after removal of a cone-shaped piece of tissue through LEEP

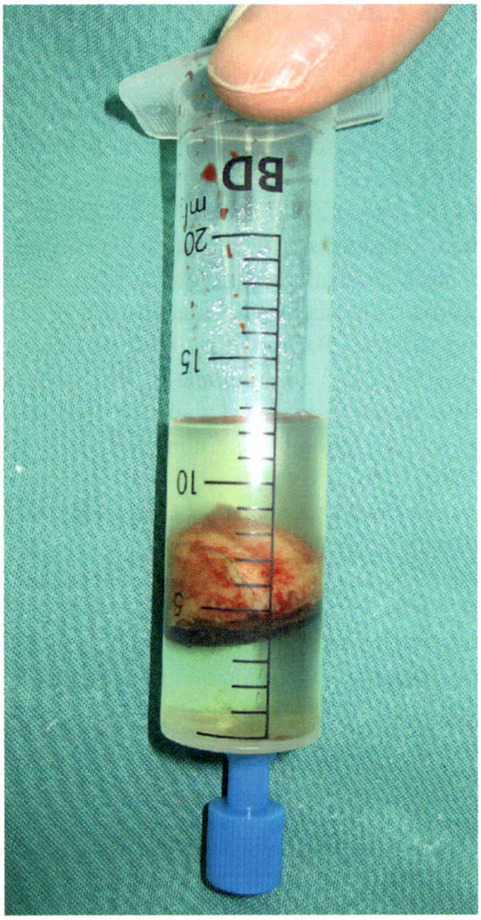

Fig. 18.72 Squamous cell carcinoma of the cervix FIGO Stage IA1. A resection volume of 3 cm^3 is determined using Archimedes' principle

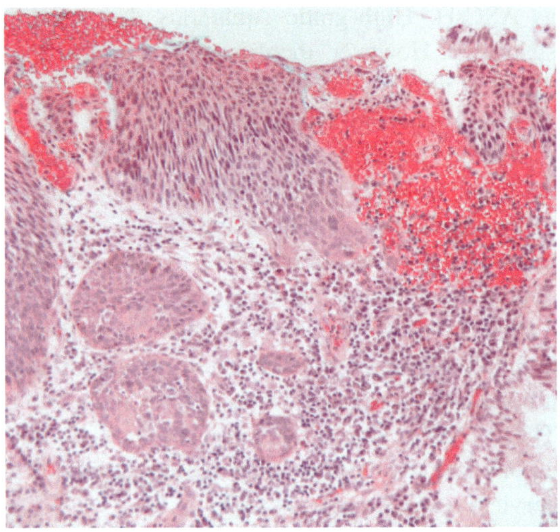

Fig. 18.73 Microcarcinoma of the cervix. While the surface is covered by CIN3, several small nests of squamous cell carcinoma invade the cervical stroma

18.4.6 Long-Term Outcome of Cervical Carcinoma Treated by Conization

A 33-year-old patient, nulligravida, has an abnormal Pap test result on routine screening suggesting HSIL/CIN3 (Fig. 18.74). Colposcopy shows dense acetowhite areas with mosaic at 1 o'clock which is biopsied and reveals CIN3. The endocervical curettage is negative.

LEEP resection is done, and surprisingly invasive cancer is found within the high-grade squamous lesion (Figs. 18.75 and 18.76). The squamous cell carcinoma is classified as microinvasive with a depth of invasion of 1 mm and a horizontal spread of 5 mm. Resection margins are free of invasive and pre-invasive disease. However, the endocervical curettage specimen contains fragments of CIN3. Therefore, re-conization is done 8 weeks later. There is no residual disease. Also, both the repeat Pap and HPV tests (HC2) are negative.

The patient is then observed for more than 12 years. Ultimately, the patient opts not to have children for reasons unrelated to the prior cancer diagnosis. Follow-up Pap tests are always normal. Three years after the cancer diagnosis, the HPV test is temporarily positive without evidence of recurrence.

At the age of 40, she has breast cancer which is considered low risk.

Figure 18.77 shows the colposcopic findings 12 years after the diagnosis of microcarcinoma of the cervix.

- Adequate colposcopy
- Squamocolumnar junction not visible
- T3
- Normal colposcopic findings: scarring after two prior conizations
  Fig. 18.77

At the time of colposcopy, the Pap test is normal and the HPV test is negative.

Commentary

It is not uncommon for microinvasion located within an area of CIN3 to be diagnosed only after LEEP, as usually no colposcopic signs suspicious for invasion are seen. Therefore, it is rather by chance that microcarcinoma is found on targeted biopsy (see 18.4.5). Up to a depth of invasion of 3 mm, cervical cancer is staged as microcarcinoma FIGO IA1 (Bhatla et al. 2018). Compared to the prior version of FIGO staging (Pecorelli 2009), the lateral extent of the lesion is no longer considered.

At this very early stage, metastases into the lymph nodes are very unlikely; if no lymphovascular space invasion is present, lymph node resection is not required.

If the patient wants to maintain fertility, LEEP or cold-knife conization is acceptable, if free margins are achieved. A prophylactic hysterectomy after completion of childbearing is not required in a patient with long-term follow-up as presented here.

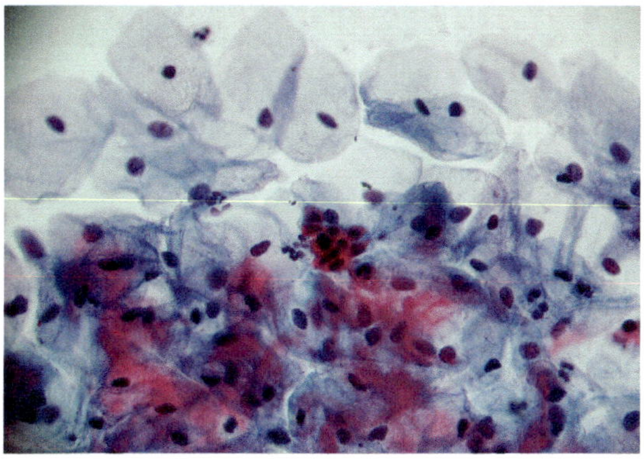

Fig. 18.74 ThinPrep® Pap smear suggesting HSIL/CIN3. In the center of the image, there is a small group of basal-type cells with hyperchromatic and polymorphic nuclei surrounded by eosinophilic cytoplasm. The N/C ratio is high. This small cluster of abnormal cells is surrounded by normal intermediate cells. There is no tumor diathesis

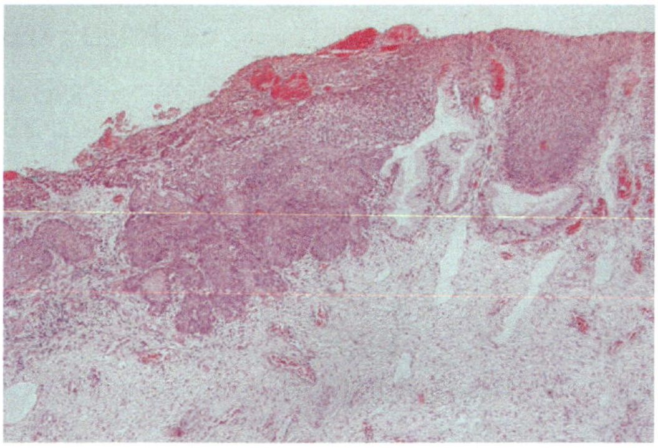

Fig. 18.75 There is full-thickness basal cell-type atypia (HSIL/CIN3) extending into the endocervical glands (right) with infiltrating nests of squamous cell carcinoma (left)

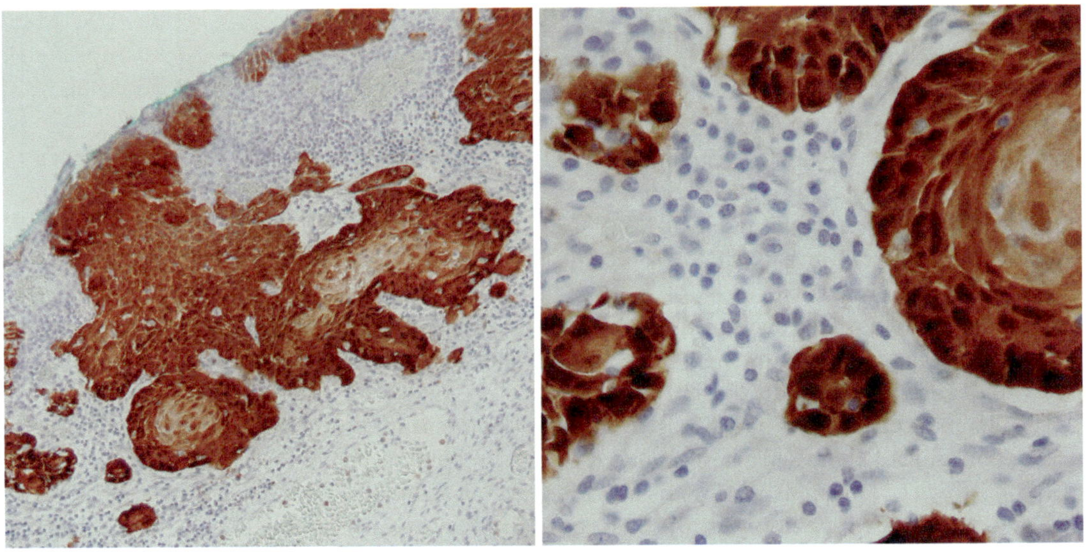

Fig. 18.76 Immunostaining with p16 in microinvasive squamous cell carcinoma of the cervix. The tumor cells are all p16 positive

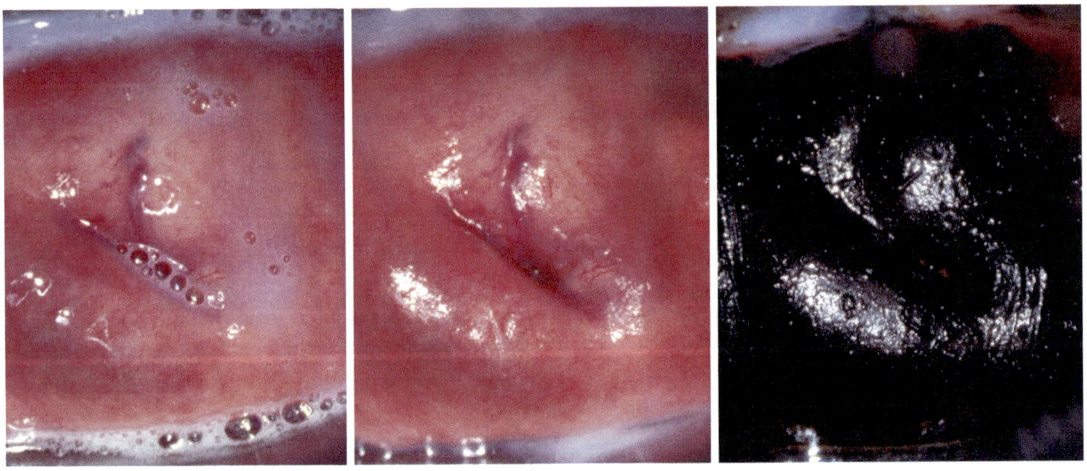

Fig. 18.77 Colposcopy 12 years after LEEP for FIGO stage IA1 cervical carcinoma. The squamocolumnar junction is not visible (T3), and the opening of the cervical canal is distorted due to scarring from two prior conizations. The ectocervix is homogeneously Lugol-positive

18.5 Cervical Adenocarcinoma

18.5.1 Adenocarcinoma of the Cervix

A 40-year-old patient is asymptomatic. Twice, the Pap test had been positive for HSIL/CIN2, and the patient is eventually referred to colposcopic triage.

The squamocolumnar junction is not visible. The cervical os is surrounded by exophytic polyp-like structures with an irregular surface. Colposcopically, these findings are suspicious for invasion.

- Adequate colposcopy
- Squamocolumnar junction not visible
- T3
- Suspicious for invasion: irregular surface with exophytic polyp-like appearance Fig. 18.78

The repeat Pap smear shows atypical glandular cells and tumor diathesis, suspicious for adenocarcinoma of the cervix (Fig. 18.79).

A biopsy taken at 12 o'clock is also suspicious for adenocarcinoma. However, for definitive histopathological diagnosis, a conization is required, which ultimately confirms the diagnosis of a moderately differentiated adenocarcinoma. Subsequently, the patient undergoes radical hysterectomy.

Commentary

Invasive cervical carcinomas originating from the endocervical glandular epithelium as well as its precursor, adenocarcinoma in situ, are more difficult to diagnose than HSIL and squamous cell carcinoma. This applies to all diagnostic modalities: cytopathology, colposcopy, and sometimes even histopathology.

Usually, the colposcopic appearance of overt adenocarcinoma of the cervix is not different from that of squamous cell carcinoma. However, in the present scenario, the peculiar polyp-like appearance may lead to the suspicion of adenocarcinoma.

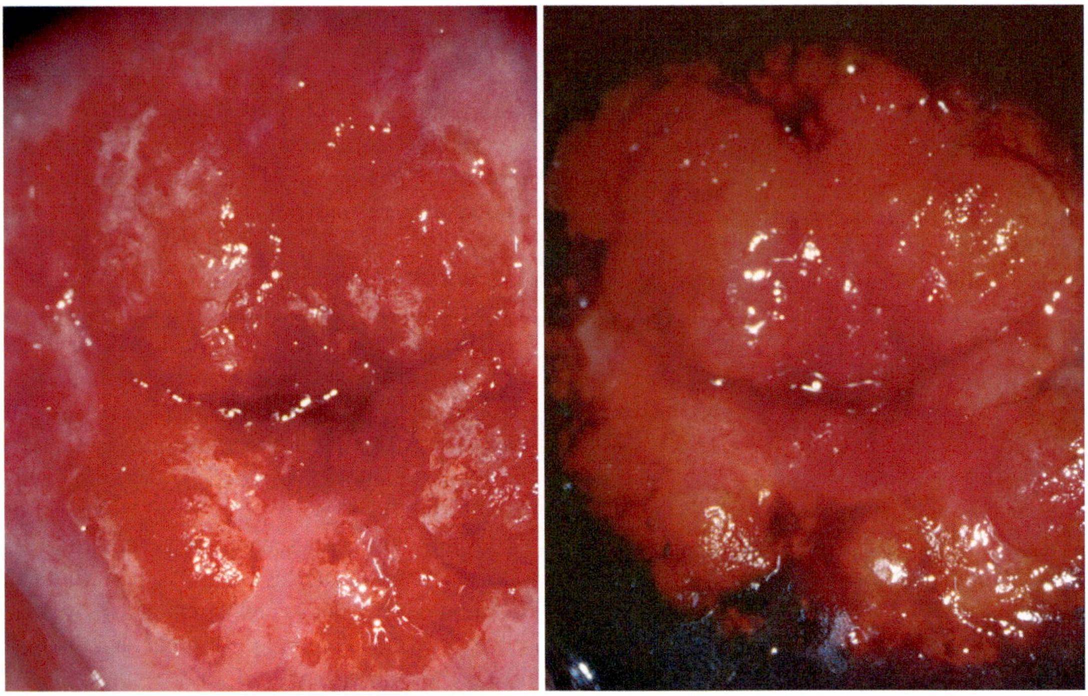

Fig. 18.78 Adenocarcinoma of the cervix with irregular surface and an exophytic polyp-like appearance

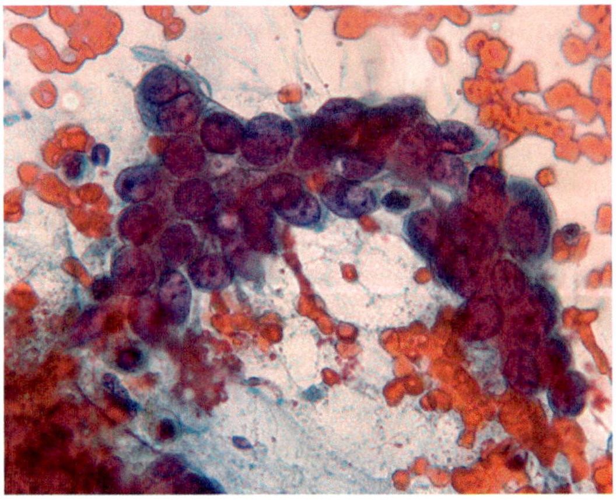

Fig. 18.79 Pap smear from cervical adenocarcinoma with a cluster of atypical glandular cells on a "dirty background" (so-called tumor diathesis)

18.5.2 Adenosquamous Carcinoma of the Cervix

Two and a half years ago, a 47-year-old patient has been treated for irregular menstrual bleeding. Recently, the bleeding problem re-occurred.

Colposcopy is performed. The squamocolumnar junction is visualized with the Kogan speculum. There is a small tissue defect within the left ventral quadrant beginning close to the squamocolumnar junction with a small island of intact squamous epithelium toward the periphery.

- Adequate colposcopy
- Squamocolumnar junction visible with Kogan speculum
- T2
- Suspicious for invasion: left ventral quadrant with small ulceration
  Fig. 18.80

The Hybrid capture II test is positive for HPV high-risk DNA, and the Pap smear (ThinPrep®) is suspicious for endocervical adenocarcinoma. The image shows a three-dimensional cluster of atypical cells, most likely originating from the endocervical glandular epithelium with a background consistent with tumor diathesis typical for ThinPrep® preparations (Fig. 18.81).

Biopsy confirms the clinical cancer diagnosis. The tumor shows partly squamous and partly glandular differentiation (adenosquamous carcinoma). LEEP is performed and confirms FIGO stage IB1 disease, so the patient is treated by radical hysterectomy and pelvic lymph node dissection. Lymph nodes are negative.

Commentary

The small tissue defect is due to malignant growth causing an ulceration. Though still small, this must be interpreted as suspicious for invasion.

By using all diagnostic modalities available (colposcopy, cytopathology, targeted biopsy), there is a high probability that even such a small lesion will be diagnosed correctly.

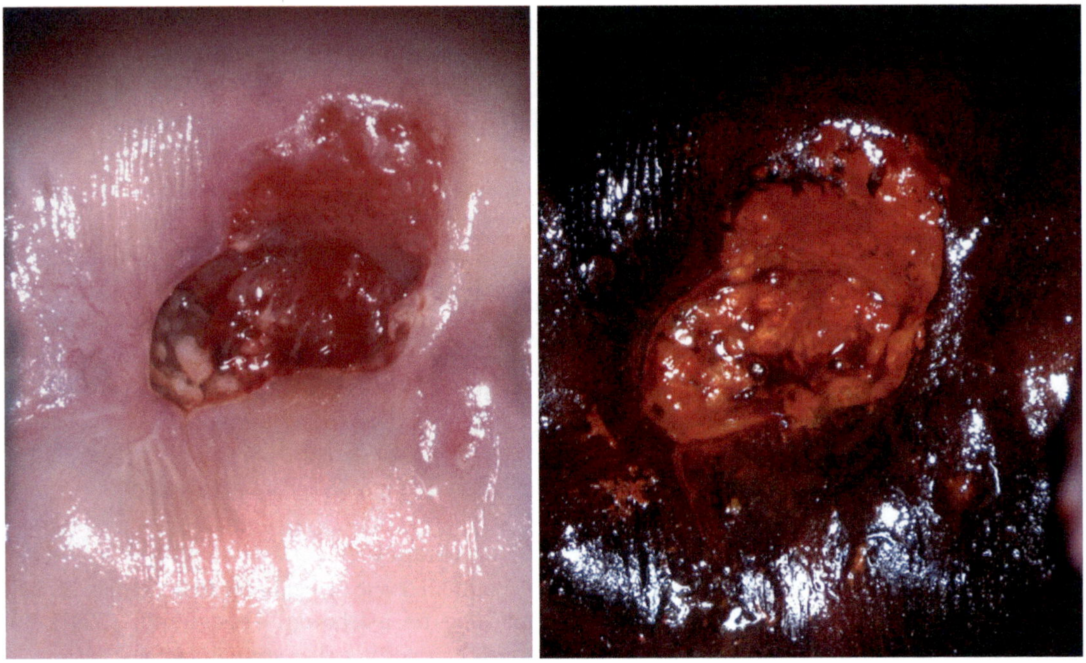

Fig. 18.80 Adenosquamous carcinoma of the cervix with a small ulceration between 1 and 2 o'clock

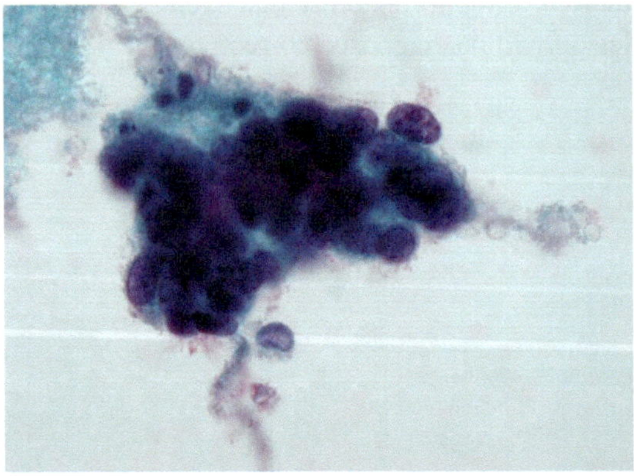

Fig. 18.81 Pap smear (ThinPrep®) of adenosquamous carcinoma of the cervix with a dense group of glandular tumor cells

18.5.3 Villoglandular Carcinoma of the Cervix

A 45-year-old patient (G0) is free of symptoms. The screening Pap test is normal (NILM). However, the attending gynecologist refers the patient to the colposcopy clinic because of the unusual appearance of the cervix.

Colposcopic examination shows an unusual amount of mucus. After application of the acetic acid solution, villous-like transformation of the entire ectocervix is visible.

- Adequate colposcopy
- Squamocolumnar junction not visible
- T3
- Suspicious for invasion: villous-like transformation of the ectocervix
  Fig. 18.82

Biopsy reveals villoglandular carcinoma of the cervix. The patient is treated by modified radical hysterectomy (Piver type II). The pelvic lymph nodes are not involved.

Commentary
Villoglandular carcinoma is a rare manifestation of adenocarcinoma of the cervix (Lellé et al. 2000). Mostly younger women under the age of 40 are affected. Prognosis is considered favorable. While it has previously been assumed that villoglandular carcinoma does not metastasize to the lymph nodes, Utsugi et al. (2002) reported a patient with bulky lymph node metastases.

According to the WHO classification of female cancer of 2020 (WHO Classification of Tumours Editorial Board 2020), the villoglandular variant is part of the group of HPV-associated adenocarcinoma of the uterine cervix and is classified as a rare variant of usual type adenocarcinoma. Characteristically, tumor cells show only mild atypia, and invasion of the cervical stroma is minimal or absent. In the case of stromal invasion, prognosis is probably similar to that of other HPV-associated adenocarcinomas.

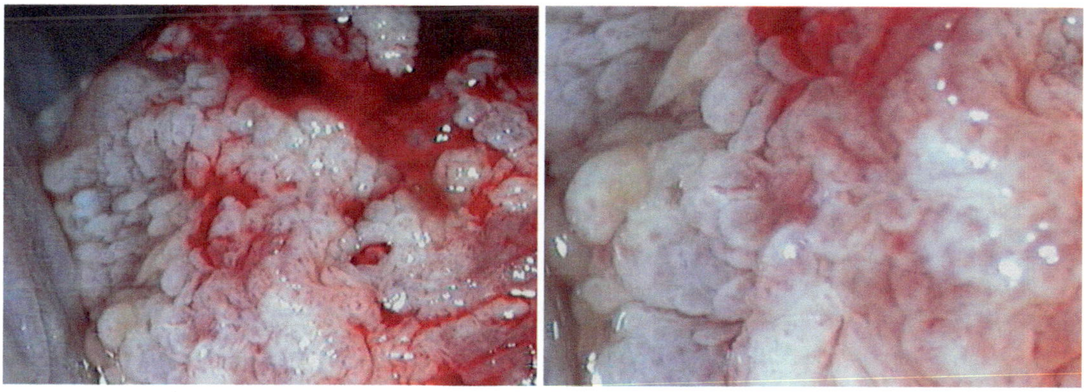

Fig. 18.82 Villoglandular carcinoma of the cervix with villous-like transformation of the ectocervix

18.6 Pregnancy

18.6.1 CIN3 at Tenth Week of Gestation with Postpartum Diagnosis of Microcarcinoma

A 32-year-old patient has had two prior vaginal deliveries. Also, several spontaneous abortions and a tubal pregnancy have occurred. Prior Pap smears have been normal. Now, in the seventh week of gestation, the Pap smear suggests HSIL/CIN3.

The squamocolumnar junction can be visualized with the Kogan speculum, as the cervical canal can be spread easily due to pregnancy-related tissue changes. The mature transformation zone is densely acidowhite. At 6 and 11 o'clock (outside the image frame), there is an irregular punctation. From this area, two biopsies are obtained. Overall, the cervical surface is slightly irregular but does not raise the suspicion of cancer.

- Adequate colposcopy
- Squamocolumnar junction visible with Kogan speculum
- T2
- Abnormal colposcopic findings: almost the entire ectocervix with dense and opaque acetowhite staining (major change)
  Fig. 18.83

The ThinPrep® Pap smear suggests HSIL/CIN3, and the Hybrid capture II test is positive for HPV high-risk DNA. In accordance with these cytological and clinical findings, the two tissue samples reveal HSIL/CIN3 ("carcinoma in situ").

In the 25th week, colposcopy is repeated. Again, the Pap smear indicates HSIL/CIN3. At 3 o'clock, a small tissue defect is biopsied using a small electrosurgical loop. Again, only preinvasive disease (CIN3) is detected.

Ten months after spontaneous delivery, colposcopy still suggests extensive high-grade dysplasia without any suspicion of invasion. The abnormal cervical tissue is eventually removed with an electrosurgical loop requiring several passes. Within the CIN3 lesion, focal microinvasion is detected, which reaches the resection margins. Endocervical curettage is positive for CIN3.

Ultimately, the patient chooses hysterectomy. No residual disease is detected within the uterus. Six months later, the vagina is examined colposcopically to rule out vaginal intraepithelial neoplasia. The ThinPrep® Pap test is normal, and the Hybrid capture II test has turned negative.

Commentary

The microcarcinoma of the cervix which had been diagnosed 10 months after delivery either had developed during pregnancy or afterwards or had been hidden during prior colposcopic exams and biopsies. As pregnancy-related changes further complicate colposcopic assessment, it is not unusual to miss concomitant microinvasion.

The prior Pap smears were re-assessed after the diagnosis of invasion had been established and found to be correct.

Despite the fact that microcarcinoma of the cervix might be missed during pregnancy, this does not justify LEEP or cold-knife conizations with its significant concomitant morbidity if no cytological or other findings suggest invasive disease. Also, vaginal delivery in a patient with an unrecognized microinvasive lesion is unlikely to have any negative effects on the mother or the baby.

After informed consent, the patient decided to undergo hysterectomy. However, a more conservative surgical approach with preservation of fertility would also have been acceptable.

Following hysterectomy for HSIL and microinvasion, a follow-up colposcopy to rule out VAIN should be done.

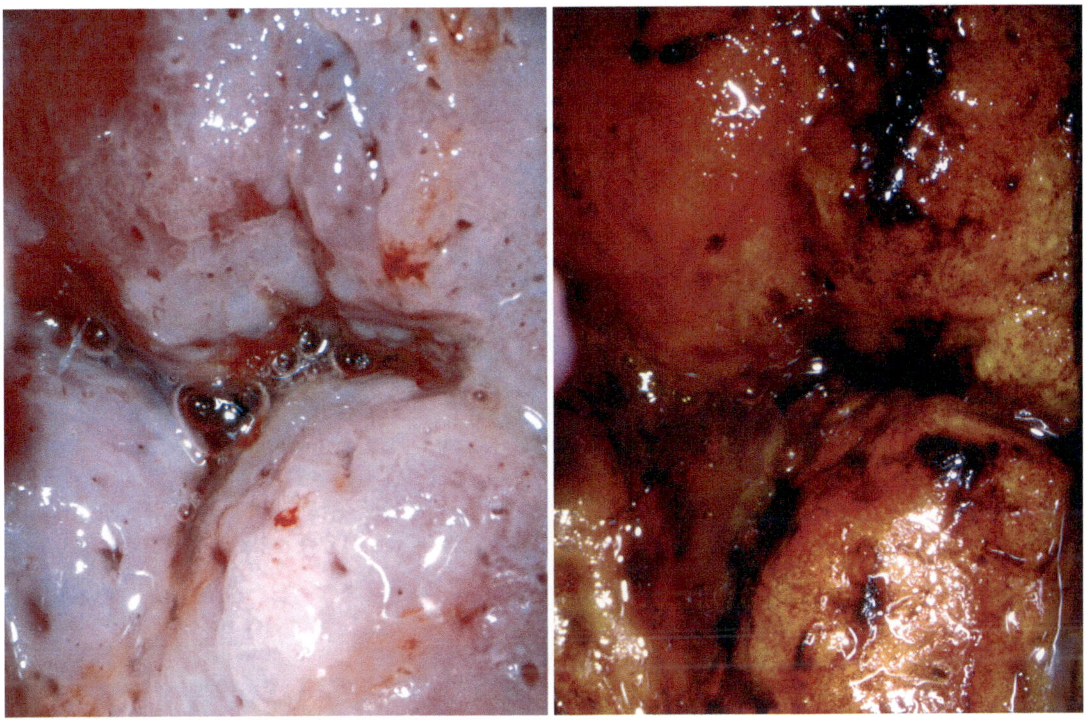

Fig. 18.83 Cervix at the tenth week of gestation with opaque acetowhite staining (major change) encompassing the entire ectocervix. Postpartum loop resection revealed microinvasive squamous cell carcinoma

18.6.2 CIN3 at 14th Week of Gestation

A 28-year-old female patient, gravida II, is now 14 weeks pregnant. Four weeks ago, the screening Pap test showed HSIL/CIN3, and the patient is sent for colposcopy.

The squamocolumnar junction cannot be visualized within the dorsal quadrants. Acetic acid application produces an opaque white reaction within the ventral quadrants.

- Adequate colposcopy
- Squamocolumnar junction partially visible
- T3
- Abnormal colposcopic findings: ventral quadrants with opaque acetowhite color (major change)
  Fig. 18.84

A biopsy is obtained from the acetowhite area described above, and HSIL/CIN3 is confirmed.

In the 24th week, the patient presents for a follow-up examination. The ventral acetowhite tissue is now more pronounced and limited to an area at 12 o'clock (Fig. 18.85). There is significantly more mucus production. However, the squamocolumnar junction is now visible (T1). No repeat biopsies are obtained.

At this time, the ThinPrep® Pap smear shows no dysplasia. Both in the 14th and 24th weeks, the Hybrid capture II test is positive for HPV high-risk DNA.

Twelve weeks after spontaneous delivery, thin acetowhite tissue can be seen which extends into the cervical canal. The white area of the dorsal cervix is mucus which has reacted with the acetic acid solution (Fig. 18.86).

Endocervical curettage is now positive for LSIL/CIN1, while the ThinPrep® Pap smear shows HSIL/CIN3, and the HPV test continues to be positive.

Subsequently, the patient undergoes LEEP surgery. Histologically, CIN3 is still present.

Another 16 weeks later, the squamocolumnar junction is not visible. However, the ectocervix is normal and stains uniformly Lugol-positive (Fig. 18.87).

The Pap smear (ThinPrep®) is NILM, and the Hybrid capture II test is now negative.

Commentary

When the squamocolumnar junction cannot be visualized completely in the early weeks of pregnancy, it is likely to become visible later on, as the cervix enlarges due to pregnancy-related fluid retention.

The more advanced the pregnancy, the more difficult colposcopic assessment becomes. As illustrated by these images, the postpartum colposcopic appearance correlates only weakly with the findings during pregnancy, and the dysplastic area appears to have partially regressed. However, the biopsy still revealed HSIL/CIN3.

The normal Pap smear result in the 24th week cannot be interpreted as spontaneous regression of CIN as cytology is frequently false negative, and the colposcopic appearance still suggested HSIL.

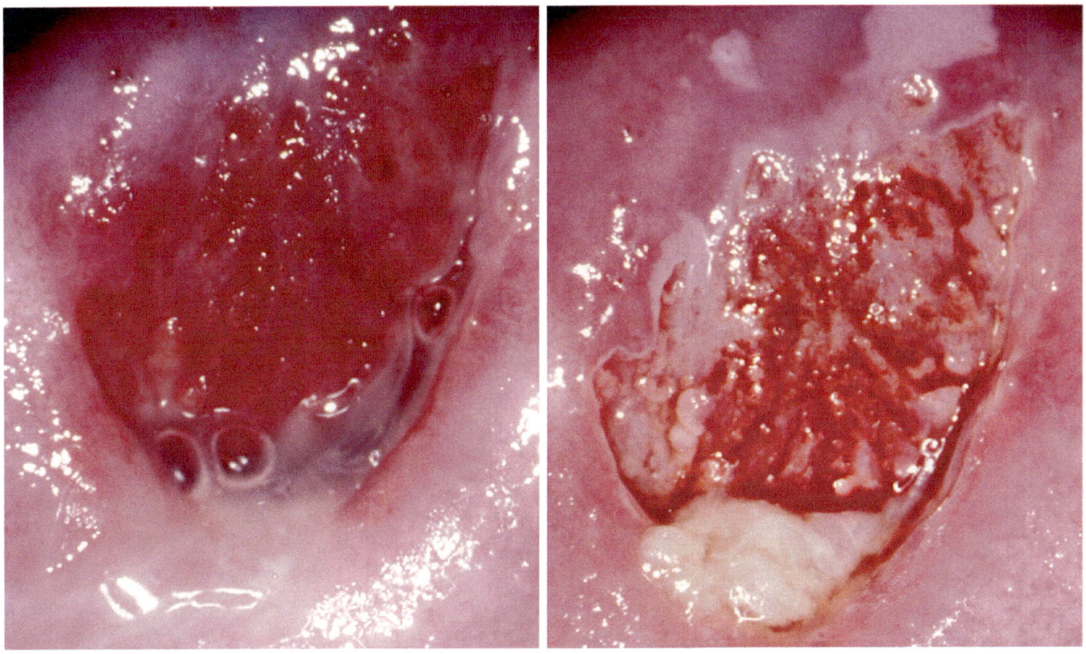

Fig. 18.84 HSIL/CIN3 at 14th week of gestation

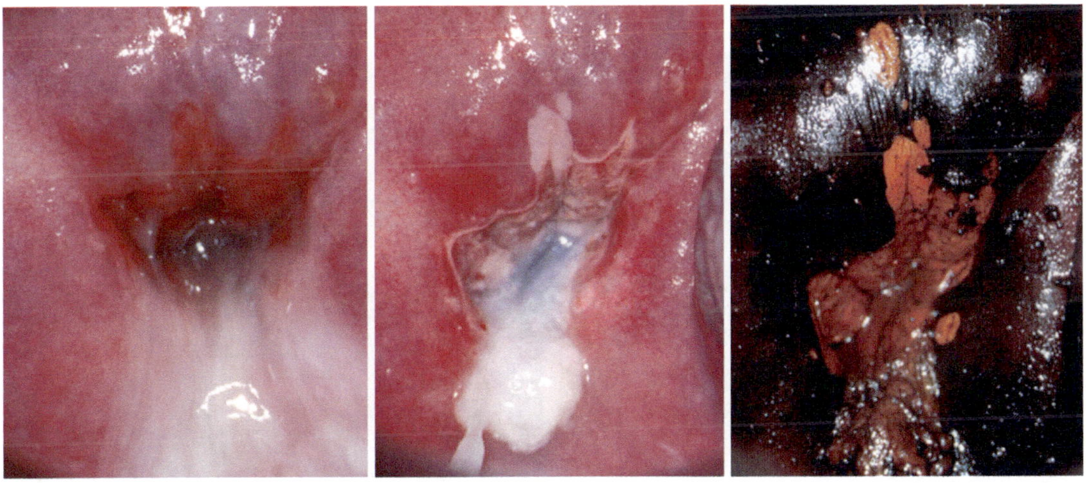

Fig. 18.85 HSIL/CIN3 at 24th week of gestation

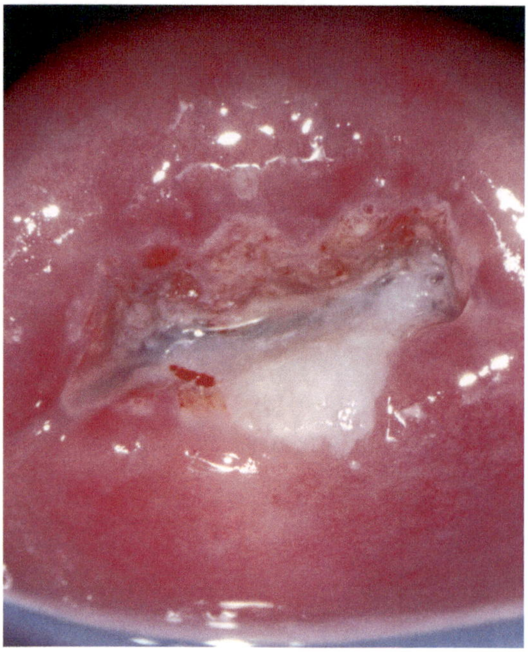

Fig. 18.86 HSIL/CIN3 12 weeks after spontaneous vaginal delivery

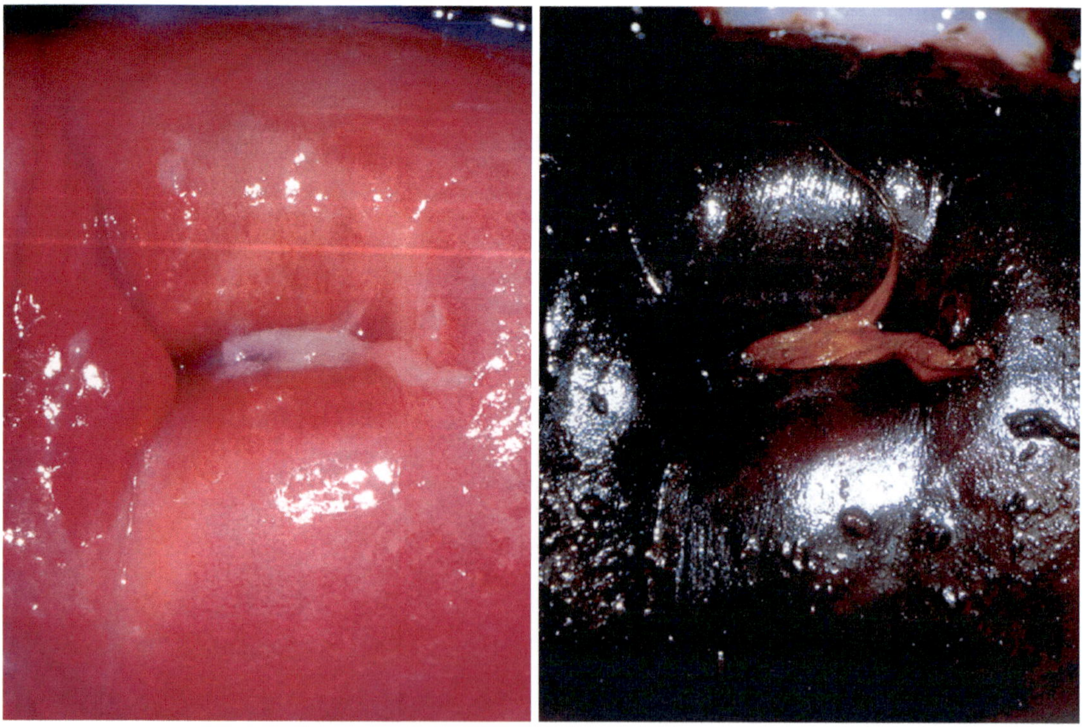

Fig. 18.87 16 weeks after LEEP for HSIL/CIN3

18.6.3 CIN3 at 17th Week of Gestation with 40 Months Colposcopic Follow-Up

A 33-year-old patient is expecting her first child. She is in her 17th week of pregnancy. Two months ago, the Pap test showed HSIL/CIN3. The Pap test had then been repeated twice, suggesting only ASC-US and LSIL, respectively.

The squamocolumnar junction can be visualized (T2). The increased mucus production is pregnancy related. Ventrally, within the transformation zone, several small slightly raised opaque acetowhite patches can be seen.

- Adequate colposcopy
- Squamocolumnar junction partially visible
- T3
- Abnormal colposcopic findings: ventral quadrant patches of opaque acetowhite appearance (major change)
  Fig. 18.88

The ThinPrep® Pap smear again shows cells indicating HSIL/CIN3. As expected, the Hybrid capture II test is positive for HPV high-risk DNA. The biopsy at 12 o'clock reveals partly moderate and partly severe dysplasia (HSIL/CIN2/CIN3).

Around the estimated date, the baby is delivered with vacuum assistance, and 2 months later, colposcopic exam is repeated and found to be normal (Fig. 18.89). The ThinPrep® Pap test indicates LSIL/CIN1, and the HPV test is still positive for high-risk DNA. At the patient's request, an intrauterine device (IUD) (copper) is inserted.

Seven months after delivery, the squamocolumnar junction can be visualized with a cotton swab, and mature metaplasia is seen ventrally (Fig. 18.90). Overall, colposcopy is normal. The ThinPrep® Pap smear is normal, whereas the HPV test is still positive.

Fourteen months after delivery, metaplastic transformation has progressed further (Fig. 18.91). At 12 o'clock, a random biopsy is taken, which is free of dysplasia. However, the ThinPrep® Pap smear again suggests HSIL/CIN2 with a still positive HPV test.

These findings are discussed with the patient who opts for diagnostic/therapeutic LEEP. The IUD is left in place. Histopathology shows both LSIL/CIN1 and HSIL/CIN2. The endocervical curettage is negative.

Twenty months after this operation, a newly formed ectopy is seen, which bleeds on touch, so colposcopic assessment is limited (Fig. 18.92). However, the ThinPrep® Pap test is now normal, and the HPV test has become negative.

Commentary

If a cervical smear suggests HSIL/CIN3, cytopathologic follow-up is not indicated neither during nor outside of pregnancy. A negative Pap test or a Pap test indicating a less severe lesion does not change clinical management and might occur due to the low sensitivity of Pap screening. On the other hand, the specificity of cervical cytopathology for the detection of high-grade squamous intraepithelial lesions is as high as 96.8%, whereas repeat Pap tests do have a sensitivity of only 55.4% when repeated within a short period of time (Mayrand et al. 2007).

The endocervical glandular cells, especially when an ectopy is present, secrete abundant cervical mucus under the influence of a rising level of estrogen as the pregnancy progresses. Sometimes, cervical tissue that is densely acetowhite during pregnancy may only be due to mild dysplasia, as pregnancy-related changes may look like high-grade dysplasia. However, in the present scenario, histological examination confirms the presence of CIN3.

If a diagnosis of high-grade squamous dysplasia is made during pregnancy, colposcopic diagnosis should be confirmed again postpartum, as spontaneous regression of intraepithelial neoplasia through the birth mechanism is possible, regardless of whether it is a spontaneous delivery or a cesarean section.

Eventually, HSIL was diagnosed 14 months after delivery. It remained unclear whether this was persistent disease or recurrence.

An intrauterine device should only be used if dysplasia treatment has been completed. This applies especially to the expensive hormone-secreting IUDs. However, frequently it is feasible to perform LEEP and endocervical curettage without having to remove the IUD.

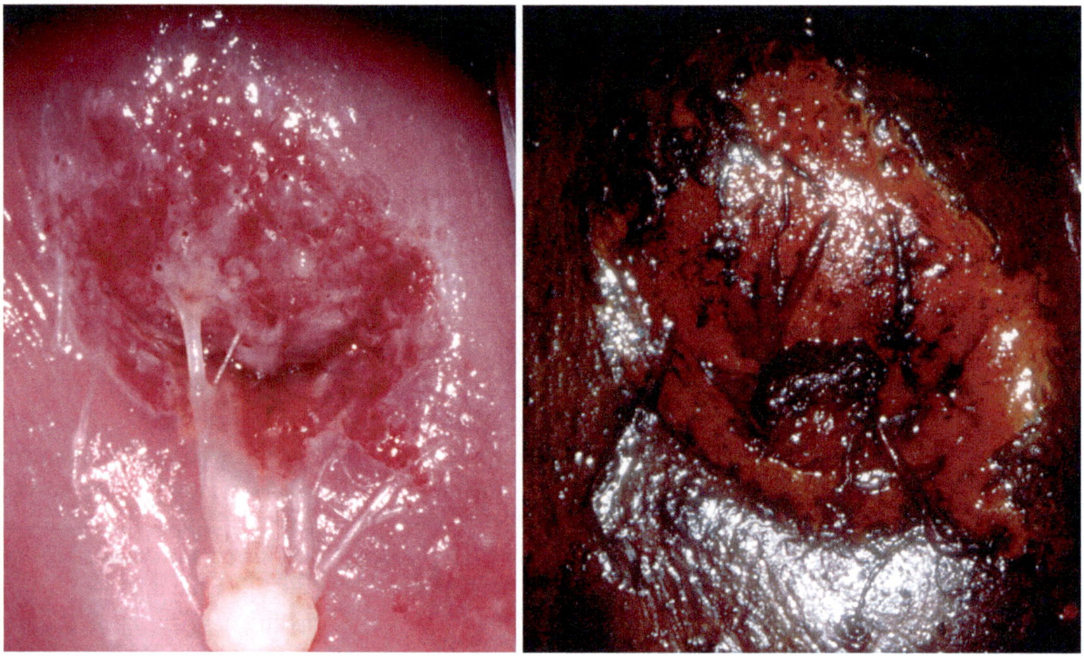

Fig. 18.88 HSIL/CIN3 at 17th week of gestation

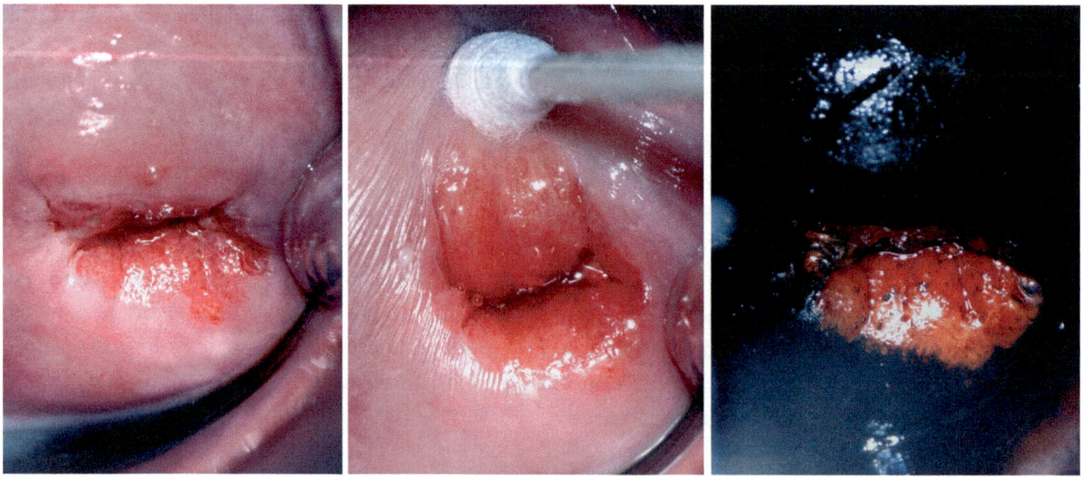

Fig. 18.89 HSIL/CIN3 8 weeks after vaginal delivery

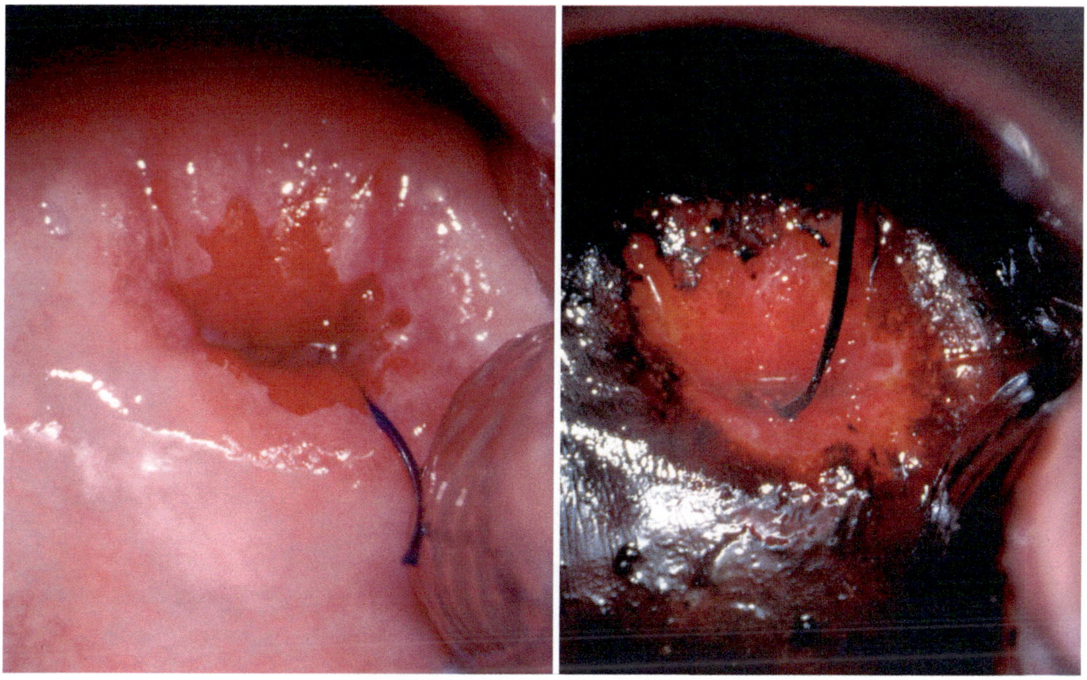

Fig. 18.90 HSIL/CIN3 7 months after delivery

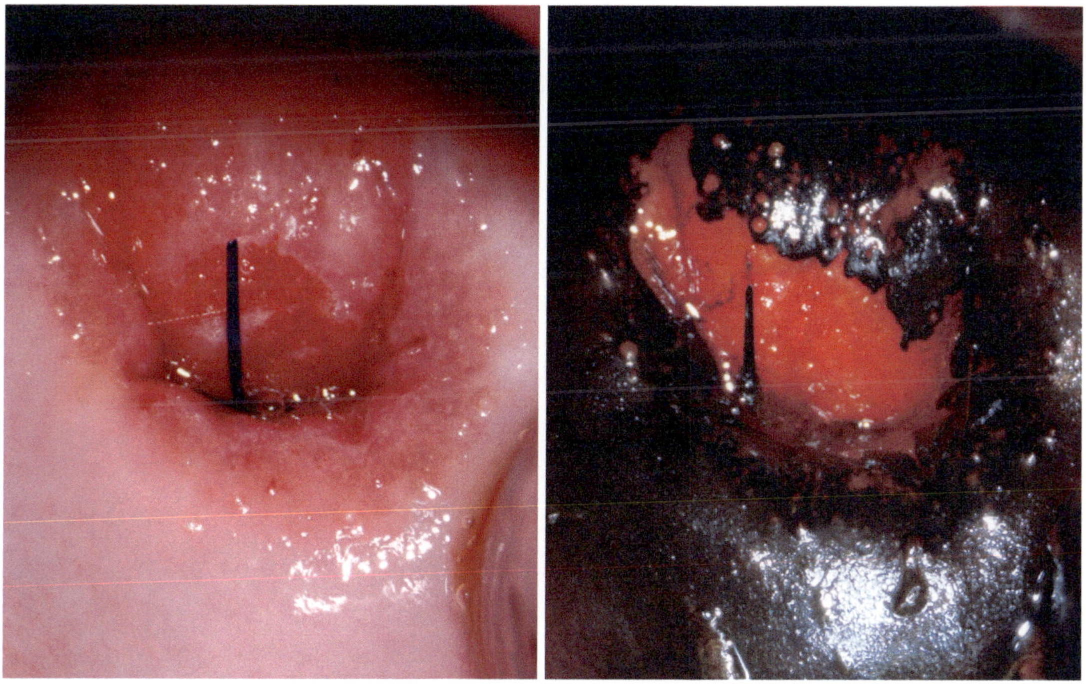

Fig. 18.91 HSIL/CIN3 14 months after delivery

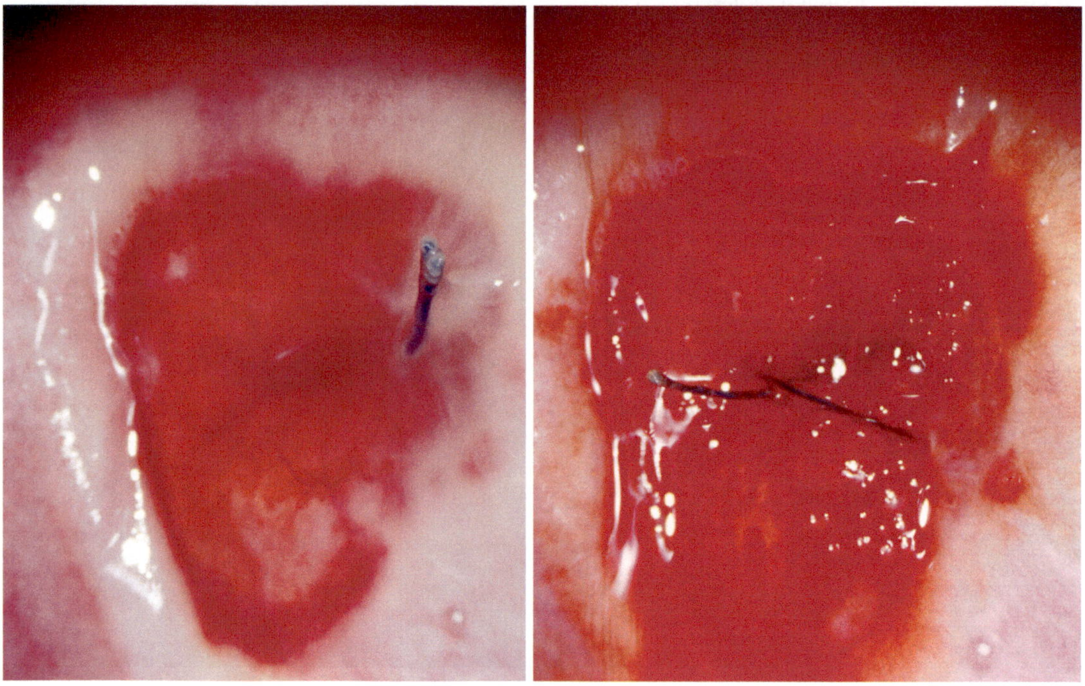

Fig. 18.92 Twenty months after LEEP revealing both LSIL/CIN1 and HSIL/CIN2

18.6.4 CIN3 at 29th Week of Gestation

Within the past 2 years, a 26-year-old female patient, who is in her 29th week of pregnancy, has repeatedly had abnormal Pap smears, initially suspecting LSIL. More recently, HSIL/CIN2 was suspected.

The cervix is bluish and very soft. The inside of the distal cervical canal can be inspected with the help of the Kogan speculum. Thus, an acetowhite area with irregular mosaic becomes visible. Although not obvious in the image, the upper limit of the acetowhite area can be seen.

- Adequate colposcopy
- Squamocolumnar junction visualized with Kogan speculum
- T2
- Abnormal colposcopic findings: inside the cervical canal acetowhite area with irregular mosaic (major change)
  Fig. 18.93

The ThinPrep® Pap smear shows HSIL/CIN2, and the Hybrid capture II test is positive for HPV high-risk DNA. Targeted biopsy reveals HSIL/CIN3.

In the 40th week of pregnancy, the baby is delivered spontaneously.

The patient returns to the colposcopy clinic 3 months later. The dense acetowhite area described intracervically during pregnancy is now visible on the outside, and the squamocolumnar junction can be visualized (Fig. 18.94).

ThinPrep® Pap smear suggests high-grade dysplasia: HSIL/CIN2. The HPV test has remained positive. The biopsy at 12 o'clock close to the squamocolumnar junction verifies the persistence of CIN3, and removal by LEEP is recommended. However, the patient declines and wants to postpone the surgery.

One year after delivery, the acetowhite lesion is still present. Compared to the earlier image, the lesion appears to have partially regressed (Fig. 18.95). However, it is more likely that part of the dysplastic epithelium has been removed by the prior biopsy.

Cytology (HSIL/CIN3) and the positive HPV test both indicate the persistence of high-grade squamous dysplasia.

Eventually, the patient undergoes surgery, and persistent disease is confirmed histopathologically. Endocervical curettage is negative.

Commentary

In the present scenario, the patient should have undergone colposcopy prior to pregnancy as the screening Pap test had already indicated high-grade squamous dysplasia. Delaying the diagnostic workup of an abnormal Pap smear until the patient is pregnant makes colposcopic evaluation more difficult. But above all, the psychological burden for the pregnant patient is significantly higher.

In patients with HSIL/CIN3 confirmed by biopsy and without any evidence of invasive disease, vaginal delivery is still the preferred method of delivery. When the follow-up colposcopy is done 3 months postpartum, all pregnancy-related changes will have disappeared, and the diagnosis of CIN should be verified again as spontaneous regression sometimes occurs.

Partially intracervical lesions can be visualized better in the second or third trimester, as the squamocolumnar junction will slowly shift toward the distal part of the cervical canal or the ectocervix as the cervix enlarges and the tissue becomes softer. There are no objections to obtain an intracervical biopsy under direct colposcopic vision. However, blind curettage of the endocervix carries the risk of injury to the amniotic sac.

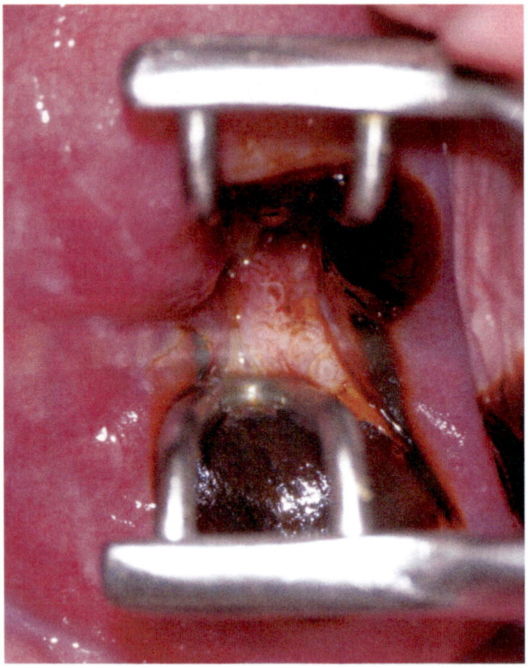

Fig. 18.93 HSIL/CIN3 at the 29th week of gestation

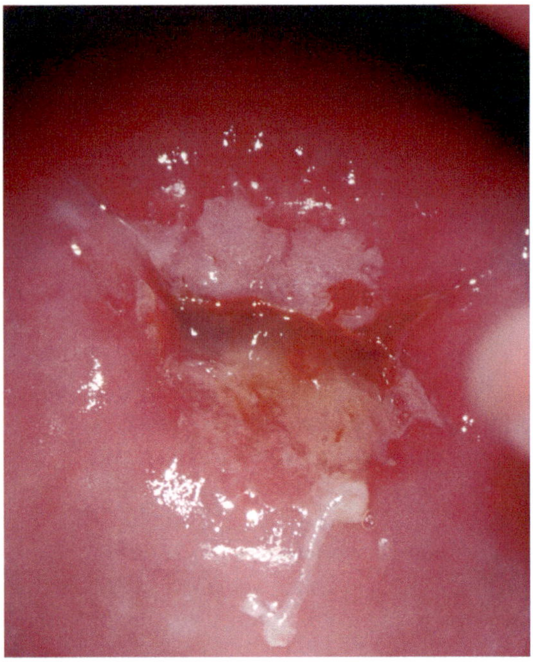

Fig. 18.94 HSIL/CIN3 12 weeks after spontaneous vaginal delivery

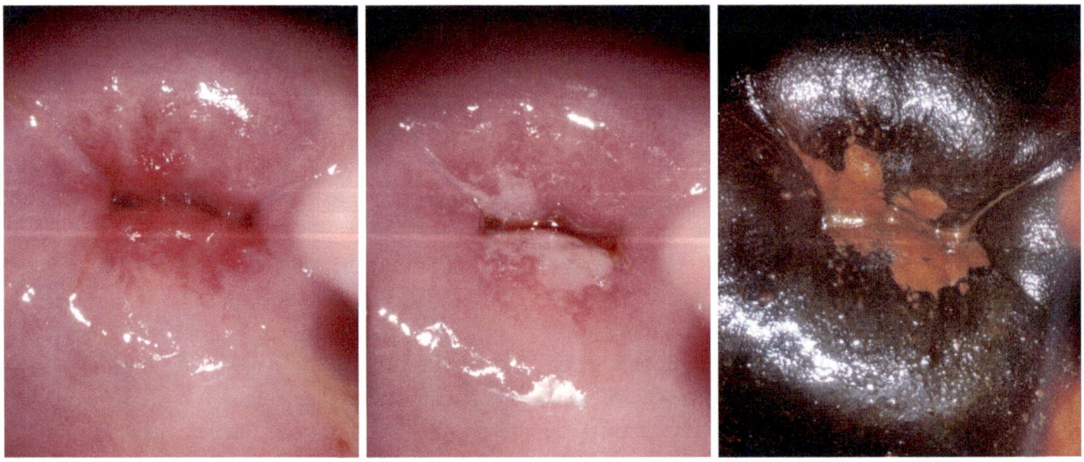

Fig. 18.95 HSIL/CIN3 1 year after delivery

18.6.5 Suspected Cervical Cancer at Eighth Week of Gestation

The patient is 36 years old. She has had two spontaneous deliveries in the past. Six years ago, her third child had been born by cesarean section. Since then, no Pap test has been done until now when she presents in the eighth week of gestation. The Pap test is suspicious for squamous cell carcinoma of the cervix, and she is referred to the colposcopy clinic.

Colposcopy does not reveal advanced invasive disease. However, extensive dense acetowhite epithelium around the opening of the cervical canal is seen (major change) suggesting HSIL/CIN3. In addition, there is a small epithelial defect at 6 o'clock, possibly due to early invasive disease.

- Adequate colposcopy
- Squamocolumnar junction visualized with Kogan speculum
- T2
- Suspicious for invasion: around the cervical os, an opaque acetowhite staining with small tissue defect at 6 o'clock Figs. 18.96 and 18.97

Another Pap smear (ThinPrep®) obtained at the time of colposcopy is suspicious for cancer (Fig. 18.98). The tissue samples both at 12 and 6 o'clock show HSIL/CIN3, which extends into the endocervical glands. However, no invasion is detected (Figs. 18.99 and 18.100).

Ultimately, the decision is made to operate. In the ninth week, a cerclage is placed, and the cervical tissue is removed with the electrosurgical loop. The final histopathology also shows extensive HSIL/CIN3 with endocervical gland involvement, but no cancer.

Unfortunately, in the 11th week, the patient has a spontaneous abortion.

Commentary

The most important task of colposcopy in pregnancy is to rule out invasive disease. In the present case, cervical carcinoma was suspected based on two consecutive Pap test results and also on the colposcopic assessment which at the time was influenced strongly by the cytological diagnosis.

Ultimately, an invasive lesion needs to be ruled out. LEEP in pregnancy is feasible (Mitsuhashi and Sekiya 2000). Cerclage is helpful to both manipulate the cervix during surgery and to facilitate hemostasis which is a major concern in pregnancy. From an obstetrical point of view, there is no evidence as to whether a cerclage is useful or not.

When doing LEEP in pregnancy, it is usually necessary to resect the anterior and posterior part of the ectocervix separately, as the cervix is enlarged. With such a surgical procedure, it is possible to clarify whether there is invasive disease or not. However, it is usually not possible to achieve free margins.

The fact that a spontaneous abortion occurred just 2 weeks later may of course be related to the surgical intervention. Schaefer et al. (2012) observed one miscarriage (3.7%) in 27 LEEP between the 9th and 10th week of gestation. On the other hand, the spontaneous abortion rate during the first trimester is high. Among parous women, 43% have experienced one or more first trimester miscarriages (Cohain et al. 2017).

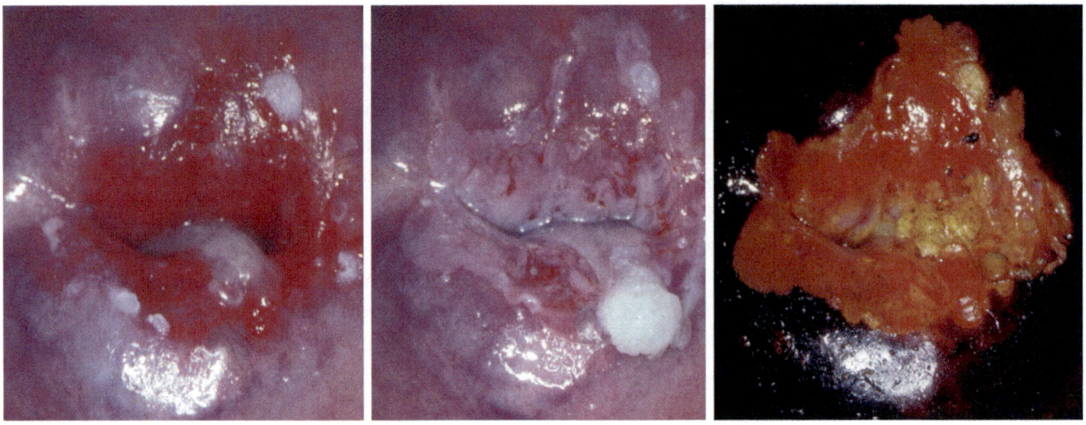

Fig. 18.96 Colposcopy in the eighth week of pregnancy after the cytological diagnosis of invasive disease. After application of acetic acid, almost the entire transformation zone turns white. Toward the periphery of the ectocervix, there is a more delicate aceto-whitening (minor change). Closer to the cervical os, opaque areas with irregular mosaic are seen (major change). A small tissue defect at 6 o'clock is identified

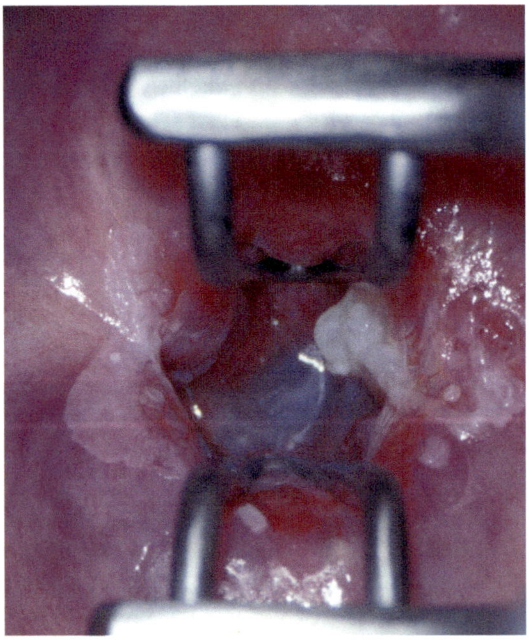

Fig. 18.97 Colposcopy in the eighth week of pregnancy after the cytological diagnosis of invasive disease. The squamocolumnar junction can be completely visualized with the Kogan speculum

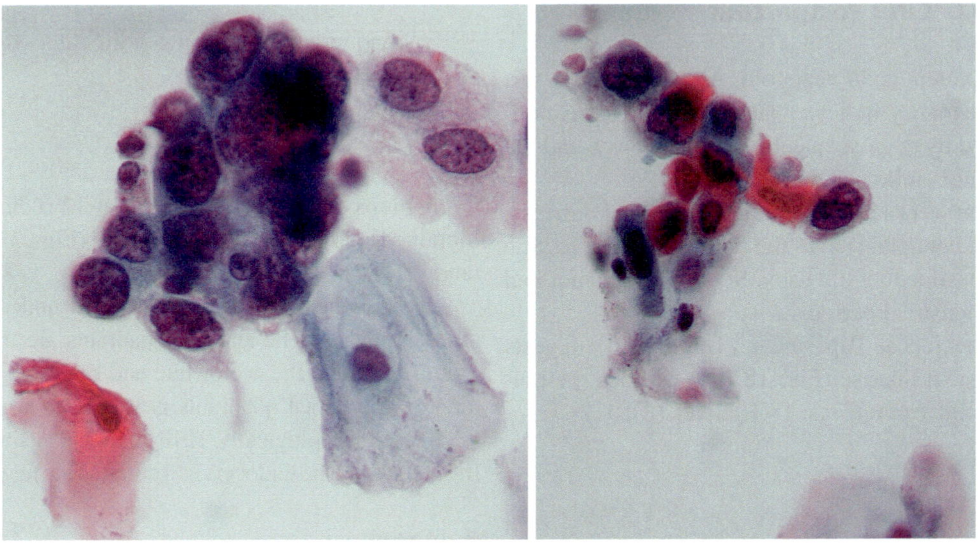

Fig. 18.98 ThinPrep® Pap smear suspicious for squamous cell carcinoma in the eighth week of pregnancy. Compared to the large intermediate cell to the right of the image, the group of atypical cells has large hyperchromatic nuclei with only minimal cytoplasm. In addition, atypical basal-type cells show signs of keratinization with marked polymorphism of the partially eosinophilic cytoplasm. Cells like this may also occur in keratinizing squamous cell carcinoma

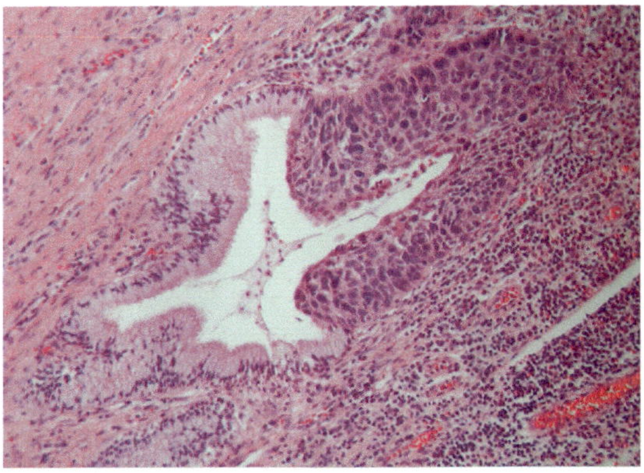

Fig. 18.99 HSIL/CIN3 at eighth week of pregnancy. The dysplastic epithelium extends into a cervical gland. This may not be confused with true stromal invasion

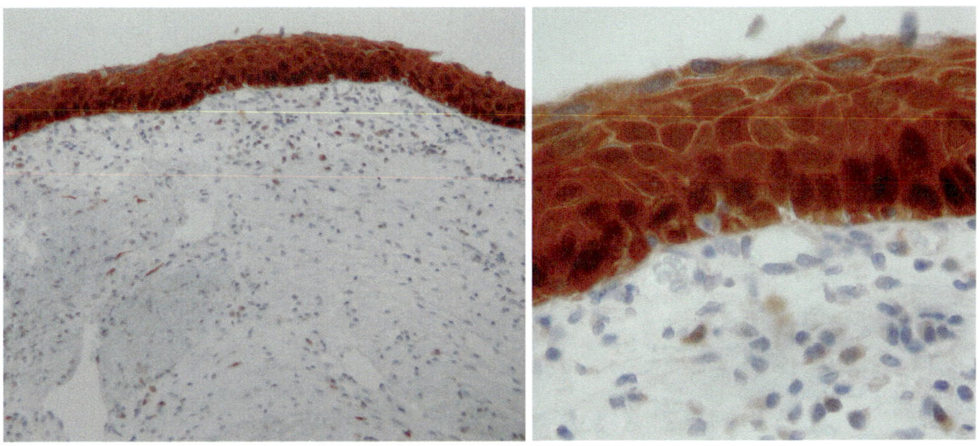

Fig. 18.100 Immunocytochemical staining with p16 of HSIL/CIN3 at the eighth week of pregnancy. The entire squamous cell epithelium is p16 positive. The basal membrane is intact

18.6.6 CIN3 Postpartum

The patient is 34 years old. A screening Pap test in pregnancy indicates HSIL/CIN3. This is confirmed by colposcopically guided biopsy, and the patient is followed during pregnancy.

Ten weeks after spontaneous vaginal delivery, the patient presents to the colposcopy clinic. She is breastfeeding the baby. So far, she has not had her menstrual period.

The repeat Pap smear (ThinPrep®) suggests persistent disease (Fig. 18.101) as does the colposcopic exam (Figs. 18.102 and 18.103).

- Adequate colposcopy
- Squamocolumnar junction visible
- T1
- Abnormal findings: dorsal quadrants, slightly transparent acetowhite epithelium (minor change); ventral quadrants, opaque acetowhitening with ridge sign (major change)

Figs. 18.102 and 18.103

A biopsy from the ridge sign at 12 o'clock is obtained, and HSIL/CIN3 is verified (Figs. 18.104 and 18.105).

Subsequently, surgery is performed under general anesthesia. The anterior quadrants are treated with LEEP, and the acetowhite and Lugol-negative area of the dorsal quadrants is vaporized with the CO_2 laser. Histologically, HSIL/CIN3 is again confirmed, while the endocervical curettage is negative.

Commentary

During pregnancy, squamous high-grade dysplasia of the cervix is not treated surgically unless invasion is suspected. After delivery, the diagnosis must be verified again, because spontaneous regression is possible, regardless whether it is a vaginal delivery or a cesarean section.

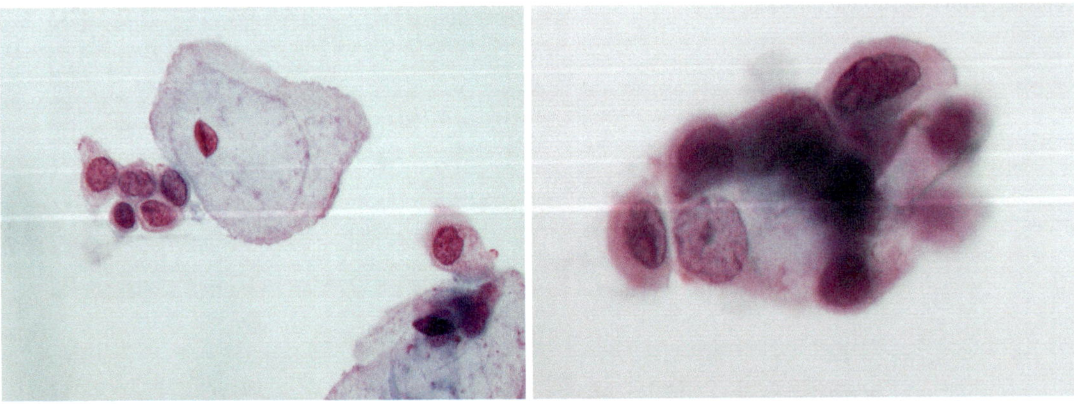

Fig. 18.101 ThinPrep® Pap smear indicating HSIL/CIN3. On the left, next to a normal intermediate cell with a small nucleus, there is a group of basal-type cells with altered chromatin structure and an increased N/C ratio. The chromatin changes with macronucleoli and folding and indentations of the nuclear membrane are particularly evident in thin-layer preparation such as ThinPrep® or SurePath®

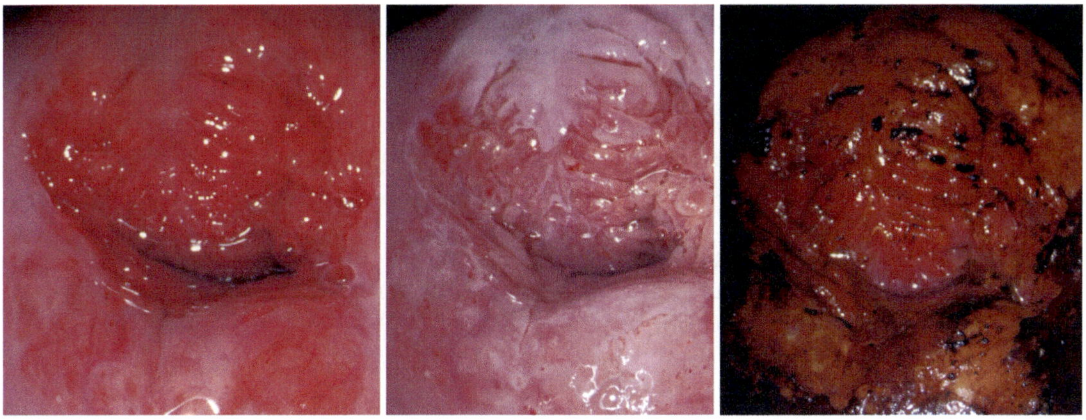

Fig. 18.102 Persistent HSIL/CIN3 10 weeks postpartum. Before the application of acetic acid (left), the cervix looks normal. After acetic acid (center), the transformation zone is visible (T1), and there is an opaque acetowhite area ventrally (major change). The more transparent epithelium dorsally may represent LSIL or immature metaplasia (minor change)

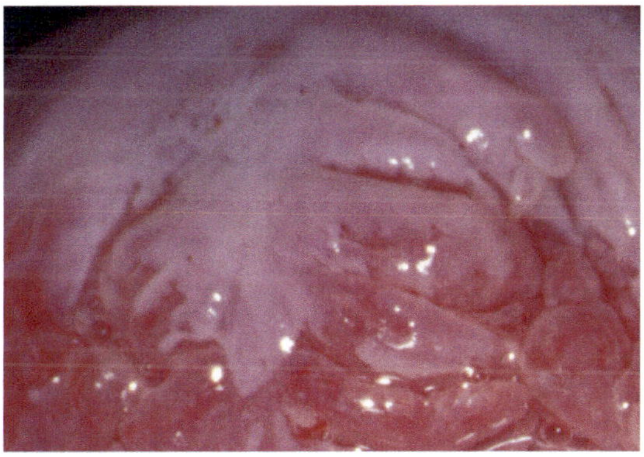

Fig. 18.103 Persistent HSIL/CIN3 10 weeks postpartum. The opaque, raised acetowhite epithelium on the ventral part of the cervix represents a typical ridge sign, one of the pathognomonic colposcopic signs of HSIL

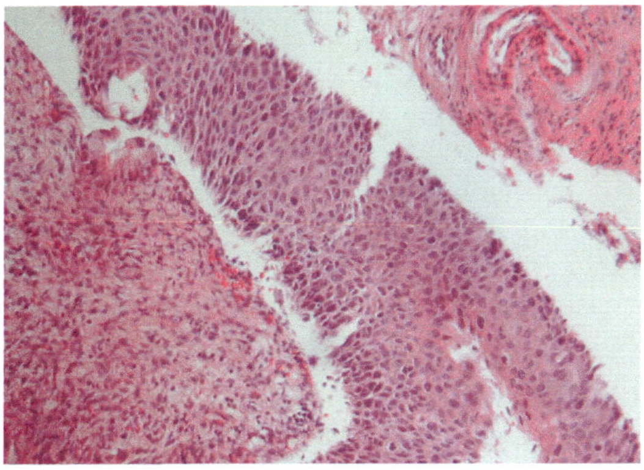

Fig. 18.104 Cervical biopsy from 12 o'clock (ridge sign). The abnormal cells with increased N/C ratio involve the entire thickness of the epithelium

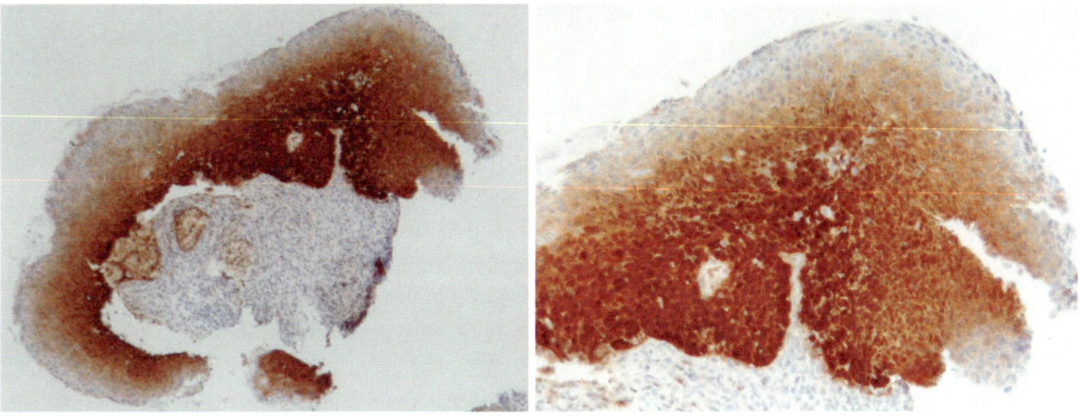

Fig. 18.105 p16 immunostaining of HSIL/CIN3. The p16-positive cells reach the upper third of the atypical squamous epithelium

18.6.7 Persistent CIN3 in Pregnancy and Postpartum

A 29-year-old patient consults her gynecologist because of amenorrhea and finds out that she is 5 weeks pregnant. A Pap smear is obtained, which is positive for HSIL/CIN3.

In the 16th week, the patient presents to the colposcopy clinic. The squamocolumnar junction can be visualized by spreading the soft cervical os, and opaque acetowhite staining involving all four quadrants is identified (Figs. 18.106 and 18.107).

- Adequate colposcopy
- Squamocolumnar junction visible with Kogan
- T2
- Abnormal findings: all four quadrants with opaque acetowhite color (major change)
  Figs. 18.106 and 18.107

A biopsy is obtained at 4 o'clock and confirms HSIL/CIN3. As there is no evidence or suspicion of cancer, the patient is just further monitored throughout her pregnancy. She has an uncomplicated spontaneous delivery and comes back to the colposcopy clinic three and a half months later.

- Adequate colposcopy
- Squamocolumnar junction visible with Kogan
- T2
- Abnormal findings: all four quadrants with opaque acetowhite color (major change)
  Fig. 18.108

The ThinPrep® Pap smear still shows HSIL/CIN3 (Fig. 18.109), which is verified by a biopsy taken at 6 o'clock (Figs. 18.110 and 18.111). The patient is then treated surgically with the LEEP technique.

Commentary
Early on, in the 16th week of gestation, invasive disease had been ruled out through colposcopically guided biopsy, and the patient could be treated conservatively. Three and a half months postpartum, the abnormal colposcopic finding was less prominent. However, targeted biopsy confirmed the persistence of high-grade squamous dysplasia, so that the dysplastic tissue had to be removed by the LEEP technique.

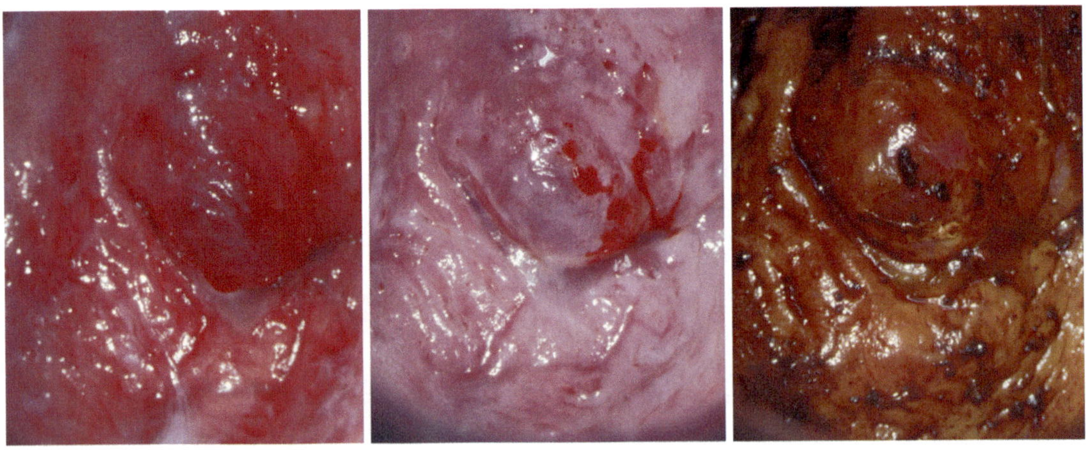

Fig. 18.106 HSIL/CIN3 at 16 weeks of gestation. After applying the acetic acid solution (center), a rapid and only slowly receding opaque acetowhite staining is observed (major change). As expected, the acetowhite epithelium is Lugol-negative

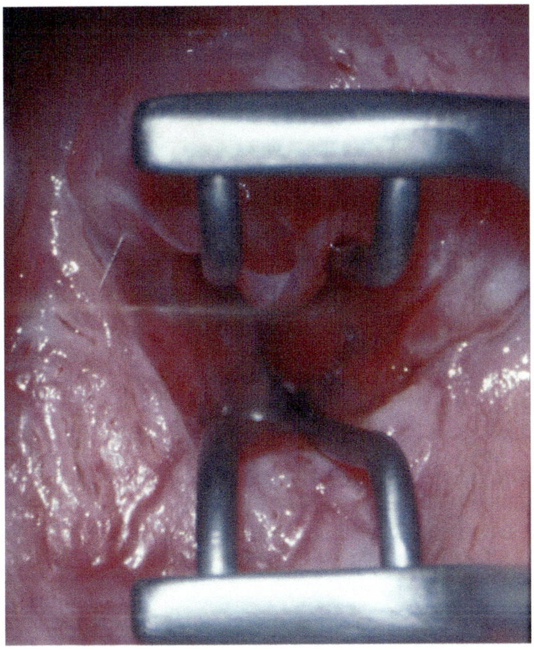

Fig. 18.107 HSIL/CIN3 at 16 weeks of gestation. Using the Kogan speculum, the soft cervical canal is gently opened. Now the squamocolumnar junction can be visualized (T2)

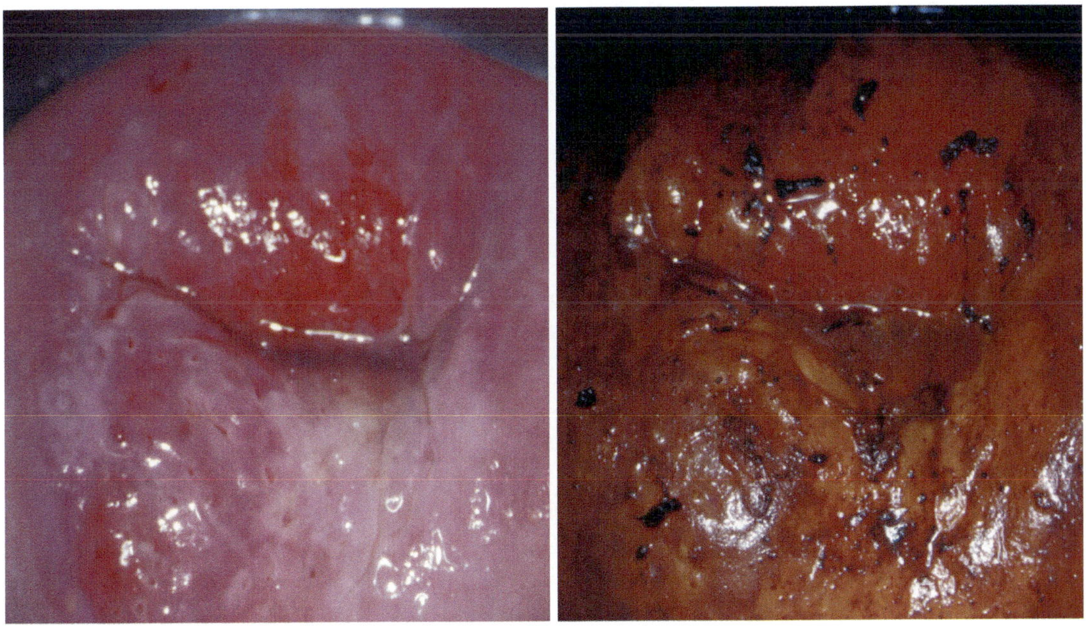

Fig. 18.108 Persistence of HSIL/CIN3 three and a half months postpartum. Compared to Fig. 18.106, the intensity of the acetowhite stain has receded anteriorly as it has become more transparent. Dorsally, there are grade 2/major epithelial changes. Schiller's test is still negative both dorsally and ventrally

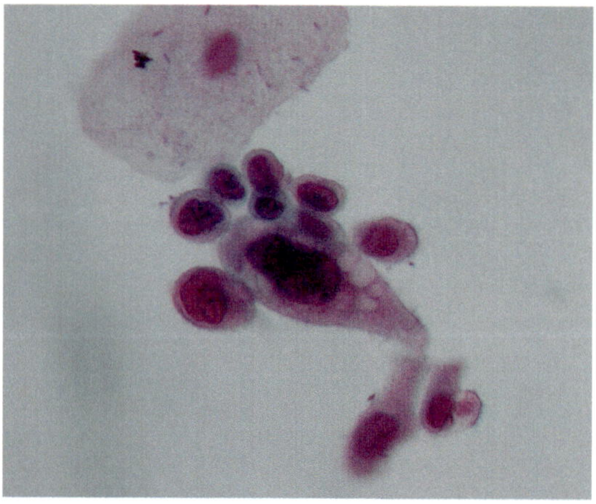

Fig. 18.109 ThinPrep® Pap smear with HSIL/CIN3. There is a marked pleomorphism of this group of small cells with increased N/C ratio. In the center, a large irregular hyperchromatic nucleus is seen with cytoplasmic vacuolation

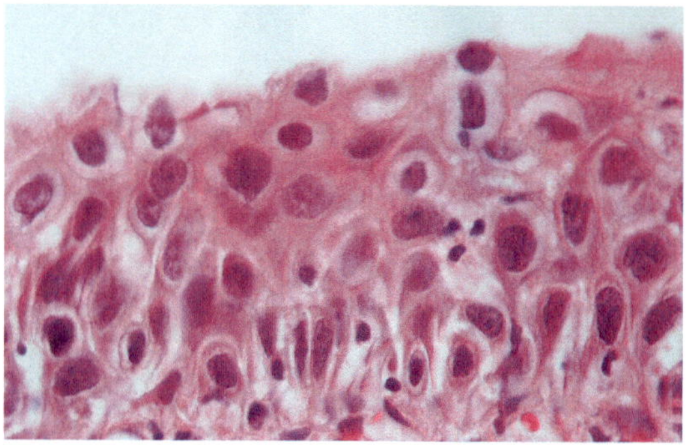

Fig. 18.110 HSIL/CIN3 postpartum. The squamous epithelium shows atypical nuclear changes including the upper third. The epithelium is flat due to postpartum atrophy. The patient is still breastfeeding and her menstrual period has not returned yet

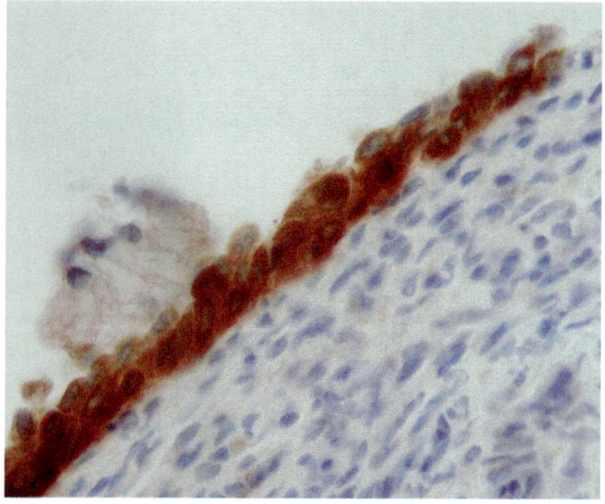

Fig. 18.111 p16 immunostaining of HSIL/CIN3 postpartum. p16 immunostaining may greatly facilitate the histopathologic diagnosis if atrophy is present

18.6.8 Regression of CIN3 After Miscarriage at 10 Weeks of Pregnancy

Recently, a 31-year-old patient has spent 1 year in South America. One and a half years earlier, the cervical smear had been abnormal (ASC-US and AGUS), but no colposcopy had been done. After returning from abroad, the Pap test is repeated and shows atypical endocervical cells suspecting adenocarcinoma in situ (AGC endocervical favor neoplastic), and the patient is referred to the colposcopy clinic.

At the time of the consultation, the patient is 6 weeks pregnant. According to the colposcopic assessment, there is no indication of a high-grade lesion (squamous or glandular).

- Adequate colposcopy
- Squamocolumnar junction visible using a cotton swab
- T2
- Abnormal findings: circumferential thin acetowhite staining (minor change)
  Fig. 18.112

However, a biopsy at 6 o'clock from this grade 1 lesion is positive for HSIL/CIN3 without evidence of AIS (Fig. 18.113). No endocervical curettage is done because of the pregnancy. The ThinPrep® Pap smear indicates HSIL/CIN2 without the presence of abnormal glandular cells (Fig. 18.114).

The patient is asked to return for colposcopy 8 weeks later. However, at 10 weeks, she has a spontaneous abortion, and curettage is performed.

Surgery (LEEP) is delayed by several weeks and is eventually scheduled 11 weeks after the miscarriage. At this time, the Pap test is classified as NILM, and the HPV test (HC2), which had been positive for HPV high-risk DNA at the time of the initial HSIL/CIN3 diagnosis, is now negative. Colposcopy is also normal, and the squamocolumnar junction is visible. Thus, the surgery is canceled and the patient told to return for follow-up after 6 months.

At this time, she is already 26 weeks pregnant again. Colposcopy is normal.

- Adequate colposcopy
- Squamocolumnar junction visible with Kogan
- T2
- Normal findings: ectocervix Lugol-positive
  Fig. 18.115

The ThinPrep® Pap test is normal, and the HPV test still negative.

Commentary

There has been a considerable delay between the cytologically suspected diagnosis of adenocarcinoma in situ and consultation of the colposcopy clinic. When the patient finally presented to colposcopy, she was already pregnant preventing endocervical curettage, which would have been an important diagnostic element for the diagnosis of a glandular lesion. A grade 1/minor change was biopsied instead which revealed HSIL/CIN3. However, this does not rule out concurrent AIS, as half to three-quarters of all AIS patients have concomitant CIN (Wright 1999).

AIS is difficult to diagnose both cytologically as well as colposcopically. Therefore, in the scenario presented here, AIS could only be ruled out during follow-up, especially when the HPV test had become negative, as this is the strongest indicator of cure available to date.

In principle, the persistence of high-grade cervical intraepithelial neoplasia diagnosed during pregnancy should be verified after any kind of pregnancy and delivery including (spontaneous) abortion or cesarean section.

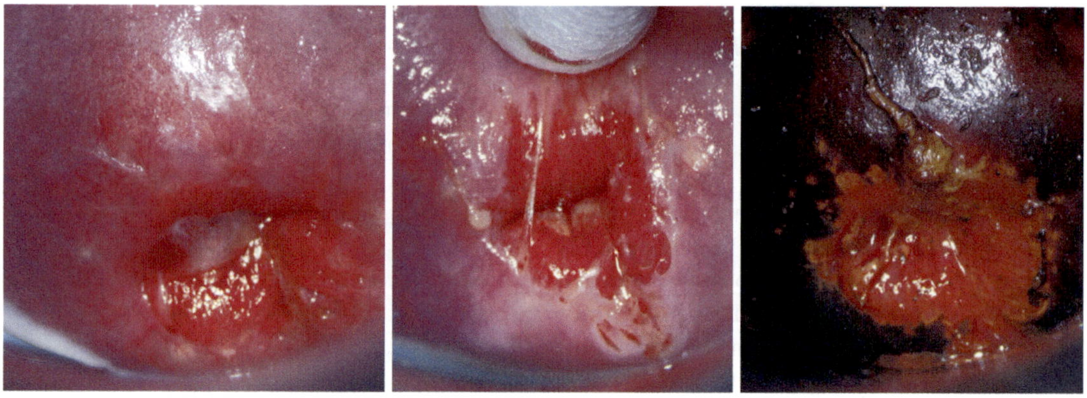

Fig. 18.112 Suspected adenocarcinoma in situ at 6 weeks of pregnancy. The squamocolumnar border can be visualized (center). The squamous cell epithelium next to it turns acetowhite but stays slightly translucent. Nevertheless the biopsy at 6 o'clock revealed HSIL/CIN3

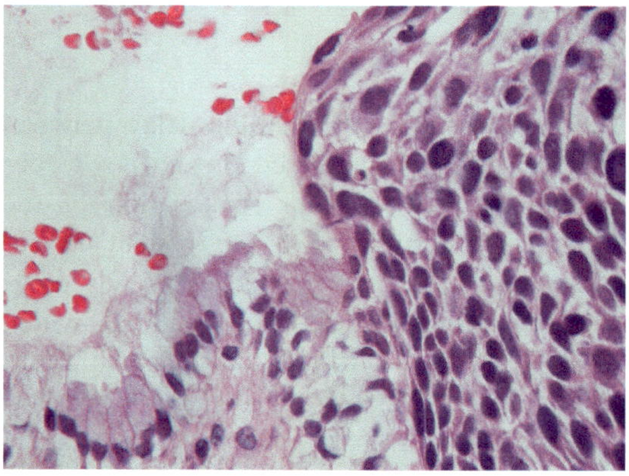

Fig. 18.113 The tissue sample at 6 o'clock shows HSIL/CIN3 with an abrupt transition from normal endocervical gland cells, which are in palisade arrangement

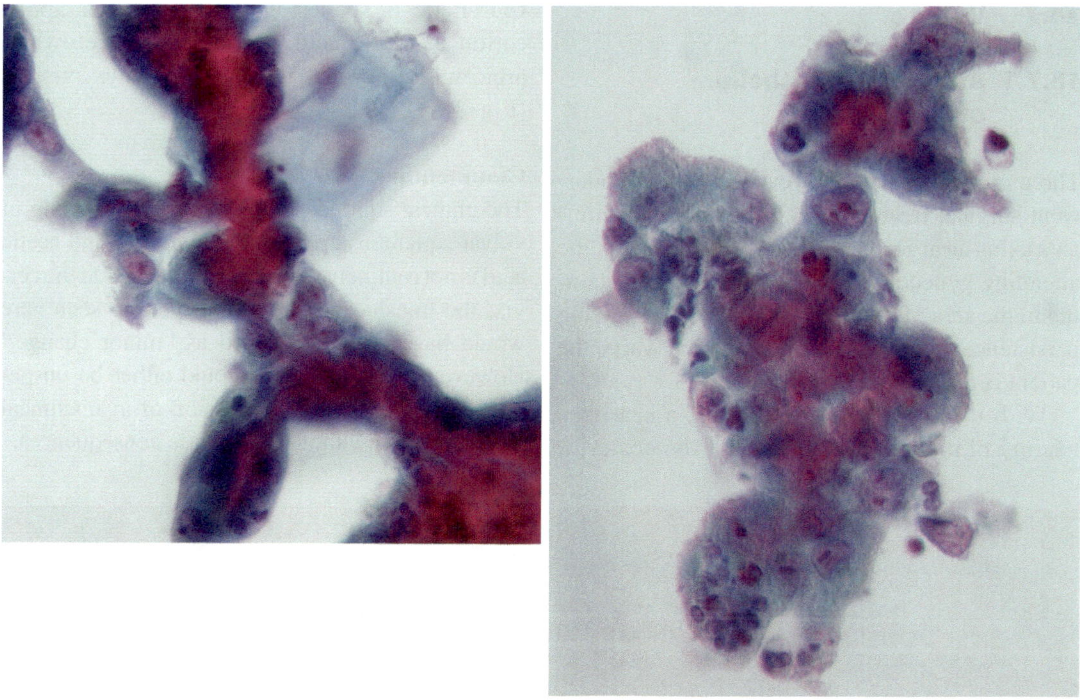

Fig. 18.114 ThinPrep® Pap smear positive for HSIL/CIN2. The nuclei are enlarged and have conspicuous macronucleoli. The arrangement of these abnormal cells is reminiscent of glandular cells. However, similar patterns occur in squamous cell neoplasia when these cells extend into cervical glands. The decision to classify the squamous lesion as CIN2 (and not CIN3) is based on the observed N/C ratio as there is still a certain amount of cytoplasm left surrounding the abnormal nuclei

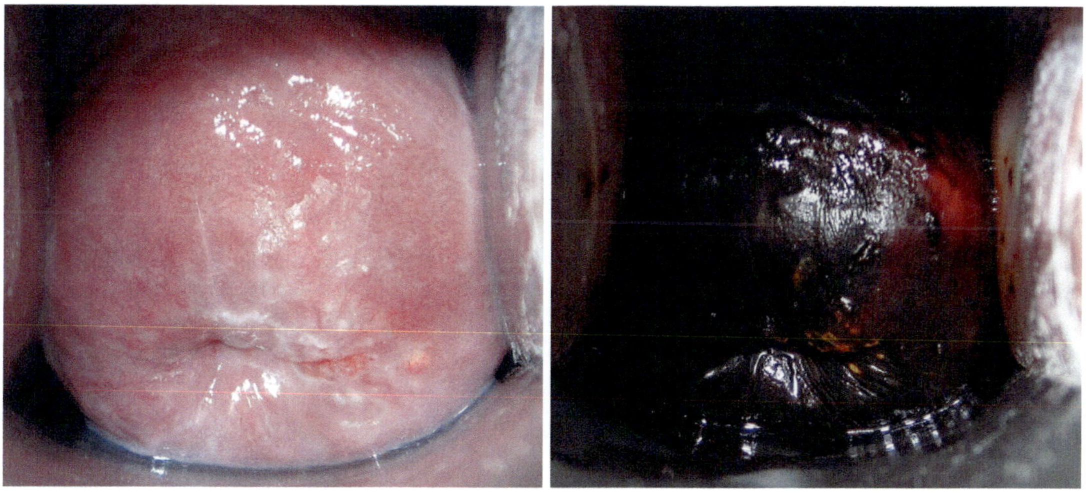

Fig. 18.115 Follow-up colposcopy 10 months after diagnosis of HSIL/CIN3. The patient is pregnant again at 25 weeks. The inside of the cervical canal can be visualized with the Kogan speculum as the tissue is soft due to pregnancy-related changes. The entire ectocervix is normal as it is homogeneously Lugol-positive. The normal Pap test and especially the now negative HPV test confirm the spontaneous regression of CIN3

18.7 Vulva

18.7.1 Acetowhite Epithelium of the Vulva

Three months prior, a 21-year-old patient underwent surgical treatment for condylomata acuminata using an argon beamer. During follow-up, the attending gynecologist noticed acetowhite staining in the area of posterior fourchette. Suspecting persistence or recurrence of the genital warts, the patient is referred for repeat surgery.

With the aid of the colposcope, a scar-free healing of the treated skin area of the posterior fourchette is seen (Fig. 18.116). After application of acetic acid, a translucent acetowhite area with distinct borders becomes visible (Fig. 18.117).

Commentary

The clinical significance of acetowhite staining of vulvar squamous epithelium is unclear, and acetic acid is not routinely applied to the vulva. On the cervix, the translucent acetowhite staining seen here would have been interpreted as "minor change." However, in this patient it could either be unspecific or possibly be an expression of a subclinical HPV infection without therapeutic consequences.

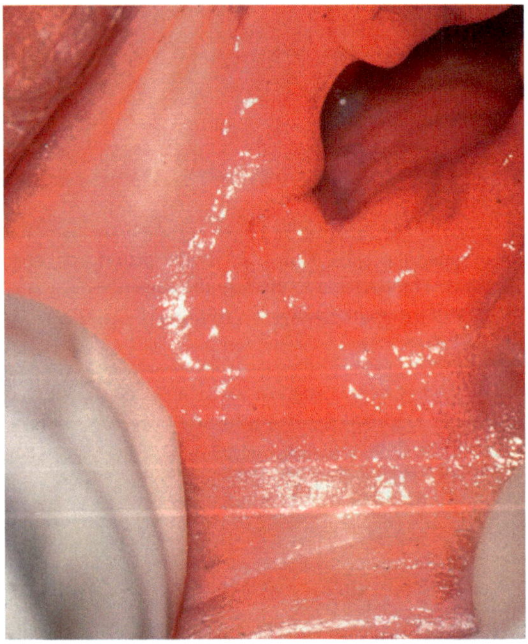

Fig. 18.116 Posterior fourchette prior to application of acetic acid

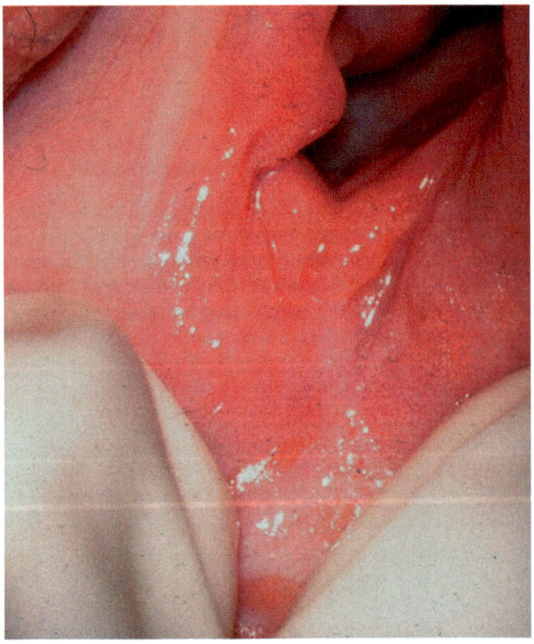

Fig. 18.117 Posterior fourchette following application of acetic acid. A transparent acetowhite staining with well-defined borders is visible

18.7.2 Paget's Disease

Eight years prior, at the age of 84, a right hemivulvectomy had been performed for Paget's disease of the vulva without evidence of invasion. All resection margins were found to be positive. No further treatment was done. For the last 2 years, the patient complained of vulvar discomfort.

Now, at the age of 92, she is referred to the colposcopy clinic. There is a marked erythema of the keratinizing squamous epithelium involving almost the entire vulva, which is more pronounced on the left side. No tissue defects or ulcerations are seen (Fig. 18.118).

Close colposcopic inspection of the left labium majus shows a slightly raised papillary surface with small islands of leukoplakia. Again, there are no skin defects (Fig. 18.119).

The diagnosis of extramammary Paget's disease of the vulva is confirmed histologically by punch biopsy. The patient is treated with 60 Gy of external radiation in 24 fractions. Three months after completion of radiotherapy, the erythema is less pronounced. However, the skin changes from Paget's disease have not resolved completely.

Commentary

Extramammary Paget's disease of the vulva typically has a high rate of recurrence. When a macroscopically or colposcopically free margin is achieved, margins are usually still positive histologically. Therefore, less radical surgery may be chosen with subsequent topical imiquimod treatment, when local recurrence occurs.

Invasive Paget's disease of the vulva is rare compared to Paget's disease of the breast. In a study by Borghi et al. (2018), 10 out of 79 patients with Paget's disease of the vulva (12.7%) presented with invasive or microinvasive disease either at first diagnosis or at follow-up.

Paget's disease of the vulva appears to be radiation sensitive (Moreno-Arias et al. 2003). According to a meta-analysis by Snast et al. (2020), apart from surgery, imiquimod and radiation therapy are the most appropriate treatment modalities.

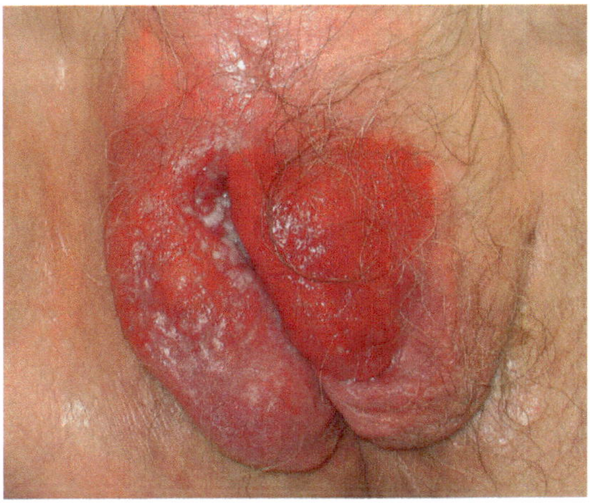

Fig. 18.118 Recurrent Paget's disease of the vulva

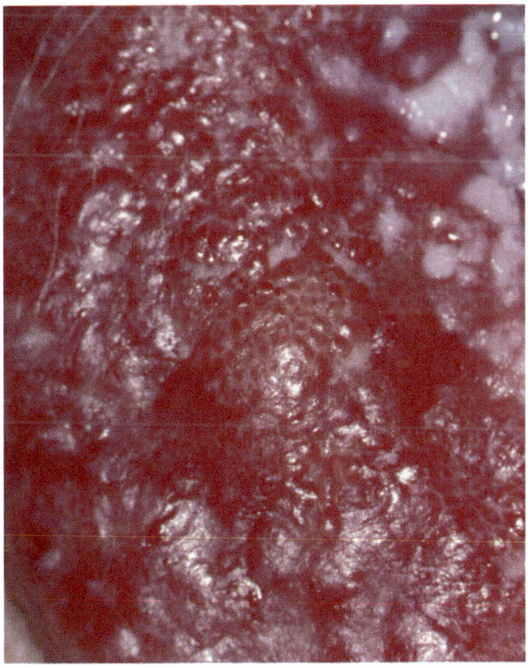

Fig. 18.119 Colposcopic aspect of recurrent Paget's disease of the vulva

18.7.3 HSIL of the Vulva with Microcarcinoma Mimicking Condyloma Acuminata

A 38-year-old patient is referred by her gynecologist for treatment of condylomata. During the last 2 years, she has noticed a slowly growing “wart” in the area of the posterior fourchette. Recently, she is uncomfortable sitting.

The patient did not have yearly check-up exams. However, all exams so far have been normal.

Inspection with the aid of the colposcope reveals a 3 × 1 cm tumor of the perineum close to the anus, which is pedunculated with a slender stalk (Fig. 18.120). Initially, HSIL of the vulva is suspected.

However, after application of acetic acid, a tiny ulcer (upper part of the image) is identified, so invasive disease cannot be ruled out (Fig. 18.121).

The pedunculated tumor can be excised easily, and the clinical diagnosis is confirmed by histopathology. There is extensive HSIL of the vulva, but also a localized area of microinvasion is detected (depth of invasion <1 mm). Resection margins are free.

Commentary

The slow course of this condition over a period of 2 years is typical. On closer inspection, the lesion does not have any of the features of condylomata acuminata. For diagnosis and management, no colposcope would have been necessary. However, it may allow a more accurate diagnosis as, in the present scenario, the clinical diagnosis of incipient invasive disease.

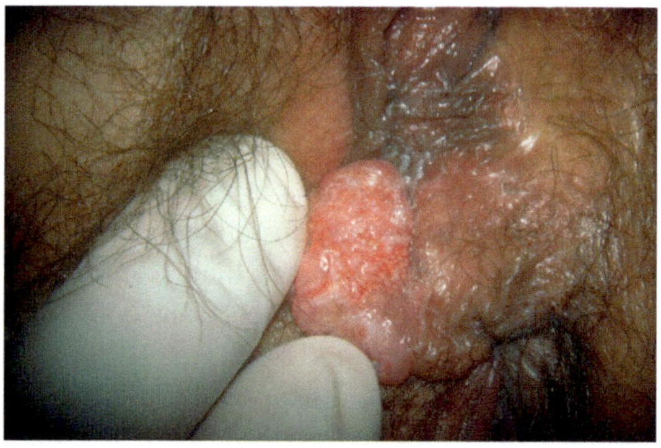

Fig. 18.120 HSIL of the vulva with microinvasion

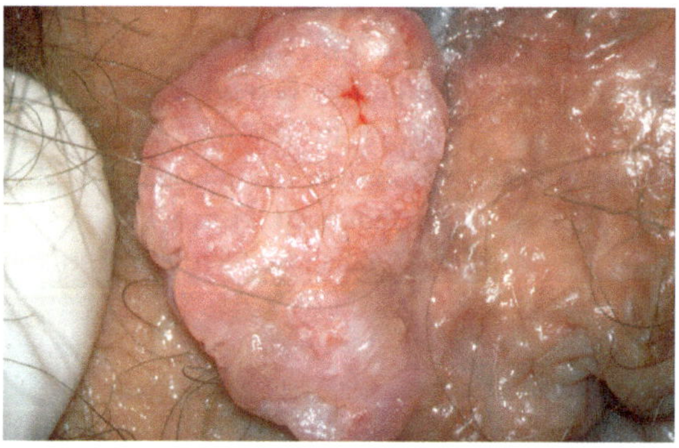

Fig. 18.121 Colposcopic aspect of HSIL of the vulva with microinvasion

18.7.4 HSIL of the Vulva with Microcarcinoma

For the last 8 weeks, a 57-year-old patient has been treated for a small ulcer of the vulva. The patient complains of vulvar discomfort, especially in the subclitoral region. Several topical treatments have been tried including clotrimazole and panthenol ointments. When there is still no improvement, the patient is referred to a specialized clinic.

The vulva is atrophic. Spreading of the small labia breaks the skin of the anterior commissure. Below the clitoris, a large erythroplakic area is identified with a central ulceration and atypical vessels (Fig. 18.122).

After application of acetic acid, a 4 × 4 cm area with coarse granular acetowhite epithelium is visible (Fig. 18.123).

The entire abnormal skin area is excised using a focused CO_2 laser beam, conserving the clitoris and the urethra. The suspected diagnosis of HSIL is confirmed including focal microcarcinoma (depth of invasion <1 mm).

Commentary

Unfortunately, vulvar cancer, especially in younger women, is frequently not diagnosed properly by obtaining a biopsy, sometimes with serious consequences for the further course of the disease and its prognosis.

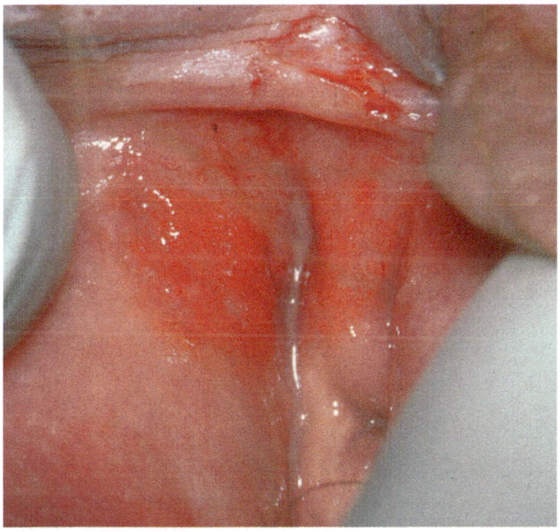

Fig. 18.122 HSIL of the vulva with microinvasion in the subclitoral region

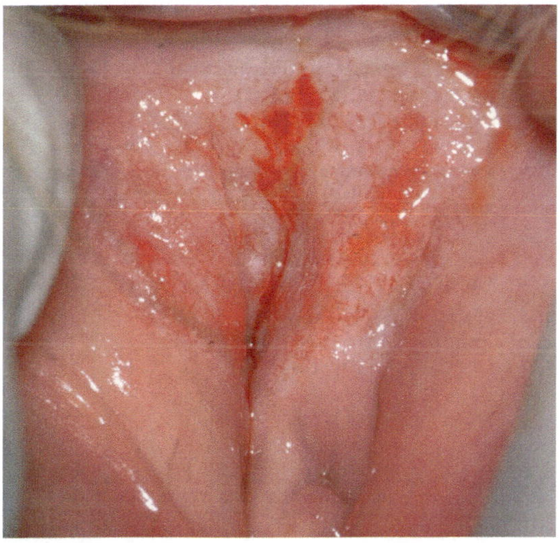

Fig. 18.123 HSIL of the vulva with microinvasion. When a lesion is located within the non-keratinizing squamous epithelium of the vulva close to the vagina, application of acetic acid may be helpful during colposcopic inspection

18.7.5 HSIL of the Vulva Associated with Vulvar Cancer

The patient is 38 years old. She has suffered from recurrent genital warts for a decade. However, she never underwent adequate treatment, neither appropriate topical creams nor any kind of surgery. Now, sitting has become increasingly uncomfortable. The note from her attending gynecologist reads: "Request treatment of Condylomata acuminata."

Examination of the vulva shows leukoplakia as well as hyperpigmentation within the right interlabial fold (Fig. 18.124). Overall, this would be consistent with HSIL of the vulva.

However, when the right labium minus is turned to the other side, a 2 cm ulceration with a raised border becomes apparent, and the colposcopic diagnosis is vulvar carcinoma, possibly associated with HSIL (Fig. 18.125).

The lesion is excised by laser surgery with the focused CO_2 laser beam together with a safety margin. The surrounding tissue is vaporized with the laser. Histological examination reveals keratinizing squamous cell carcinoma of the vulva, which is 2 cm in diameter with a depth of invasion of 5 mm. Subsequently, bilateral inguinal lymph node dissection is performed. Fortunately, lymph nodes are negative.

Eight years after this diagnosis, the patient is still free of disease.

Commentary

Surprisingly, the 2 cm ulcerating carcinoma had been overlooked during previous gynecological exams. Possibly, it had been obscured by the vaginal speculum.

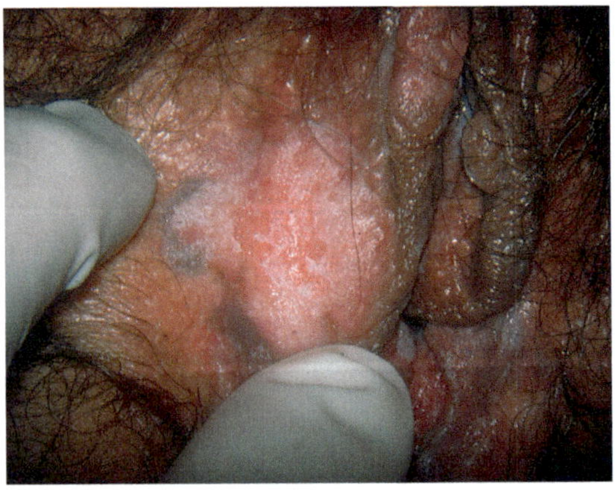

Fig. 18.124 HSIL of the vulva within the right interlabial fold

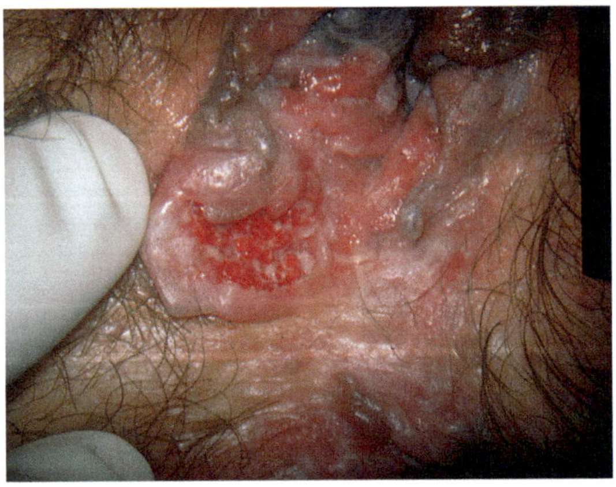

Fig. 18.125 Ulceration of the inner aspect of the right labium minus which is suspicious for cancer

18.7.6 Malignant Melanoma of the Vulva and Vagina

A 48-year-old patient is referred to the colposcopy clinic because of a "pigment disorder" of the vulva. The patient is free of symptoms.

The examination reveals extensive hyperpigmentation on the inner aspect of the right side of the labium minus as well as around the urethra. The epithelium is raised compared to the surrounding tissue (Fig. 18.126).

In addition, several small pigmented areas are found on the vaginal wall (Fig. 18.127).

These clinical findings suggest malignant melanoma rather than melanosis vulvae. This is confirmed by punch biopsies from both the periurethral and the vaginal lesion (Clark level III).

Subsequently, radical vulvectomy with inguinofemoral lymphadenectomy and a colectomy are performed. The lymph nodes are not affected. Despite adjuvant systemic therapy, the patient develops liver and lung metastases 6 months later.

Commentary

The images shown should at least raise suspicion that this may be malignant melanoma and that biopsy is required. One should always be aware that melanoma is the second most common type of cancer of the vulva following squamous cell carcinoma. There is no contraindication for incisional biopsy.

Murzaku et al. (2014) suggest a systematic diagnostic approach to distinguish vulvar nevi or melanosis from melanoma. The following criteria favor malignant melanoma:

- Patient age >50 years
- Irregular coloration
- Asymmetric borders
- Diameter >7 mm
- Elevated lesion
- Associated bleeding
- Pruritus
- Discharge

If the diagnosis of malignant melanoma is confirmed, the patient must be treated by an interdisciplinary team led by the oncologic dermatologist who will decide about the extent of surgery as well as the appropriate medical treatment.

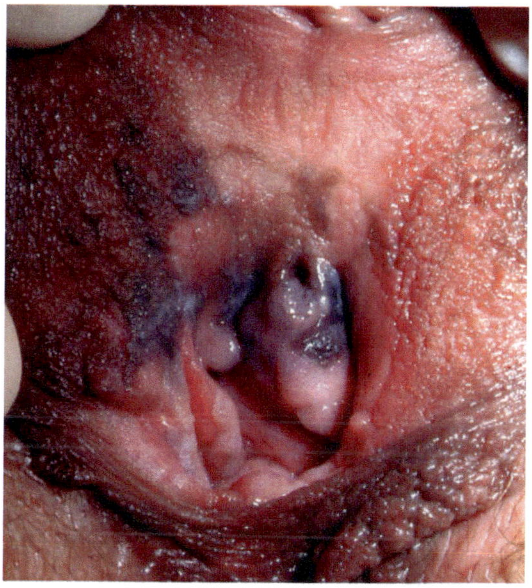

Fig. 18.126 Malignant melanoma of the introitus of the vulva involving the distal urethra

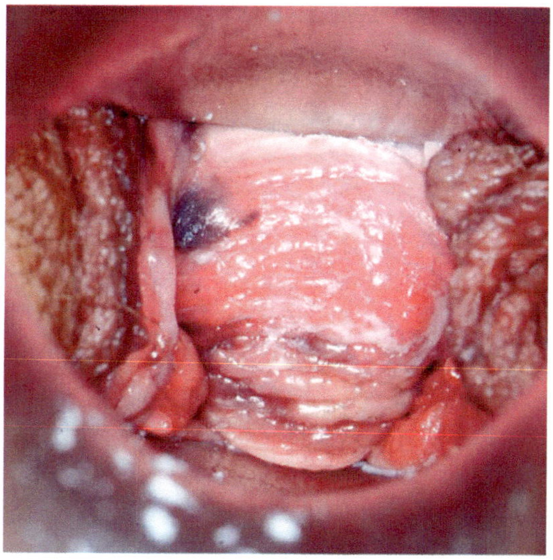

Fig. 18.127 Malignant melanoma located on the vaginal wall

18.7.7 Vulvar Manifestation of Primary Syphilis

A 45-year-old patient complains of vulvar pain. She describes a burning sensation. The first symptoms started about two and a half weeks ago. Temporarily, the patient had a fever and chills. She has already been treated with acyclovir as herpes simplex infection had been suspected. However, there was no improvement.

On the inside of the labia minora, flat ulcerations of about 2 cm in diameter can be seen (Fig. 18.128).

Ultimately, the fluorescent treponemal antibody absorption (FTA-ABS) test establishes the diagnosis of a *Treponema pallidum* infection. Thus, the patient suffers from syphilis, and the ulceration is a vulvar manifestation of primary syphilis.

Apparently, the patient's partner only showed minor symptoms and had not consulted a physician.

Commentary

The vulvar lesion shown here is also called "chancre" and is typically found during the primary stage of syphilis, about 3 weeks after the infection. As these lesions contain treponema bacteria, the disease can be transmitted through direct contact sexual contact.

When syphilis is diagnosed at the primary stage, penicillin is the treatment of choice, and cure rates are high.

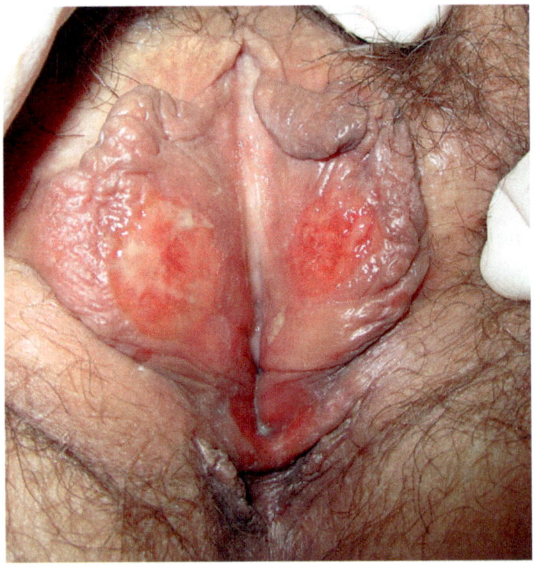

Fig. 18.128 Syphilis of the vulva. The flat ulcerations contain *Treponema pallidum* and can be sexually transmitted. This so-called chancre is a typical manifestation of primary syphilis

18.7.8 Condylomata Acuminata of the Vulva in the 33rd Week of Gestation

A 30-year-old patient is expecting her second child after a cesarean section 3 years earlier. Now she would like to give birth by vaginal delivery.

In the 33rd week of pregnancy, she presents to the colposcopy clinic with genital warts. These lesions are limited to the labia majora and the posterior commissure (Fig. 18.129). The warts are a few millimeters in size and flat (Fig. 18.130). The clinical diagnosis of condylomata acuminata is made.

Under general anesthesia the condylomata acuminata are treated by CO_2 laser vaporization. In the 40th week of pregnancy, the patient has an uncomplicated vaginal delivery. At the time of delivery, no condylomata are visible.

Commentary

Vulvar lesions are usually biopsied in order to establish a definitive diagnosis. However, there are a few exceptions, when the clinical picture is unequivocal. This may be the case for lichen sclerosus of the vulva or for condylomata acuminata as in the present scenario.

During pregnancy, topical imiquimod treatment is not allowed. If there is only a small skin area to be treated, trichloroacetic acid (TCA) can be applied. This is usually done in the gynecologist's office. If a larger area is affected, CO_2 laser vaporization under general anesthesia is necessary. The 33rd week of pregnancy is an opportune time to eliminate condyloma of the vulva prior to vaginal delivery.

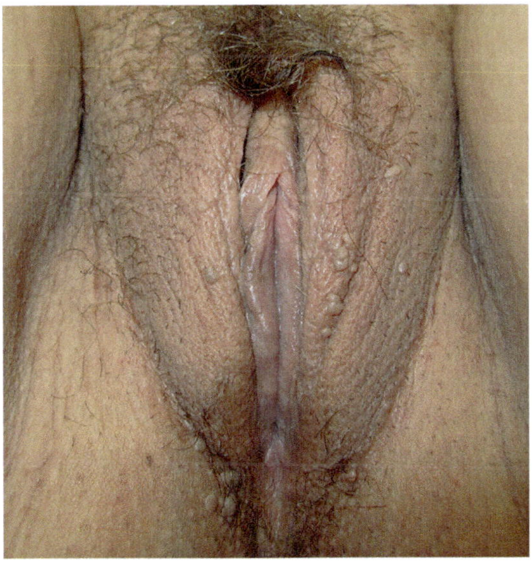

Fig. 18.129 Condylomata acuminata of the vulva in the 33rd week of pregnancy. Only the external vulva and the posterior commissure are affected

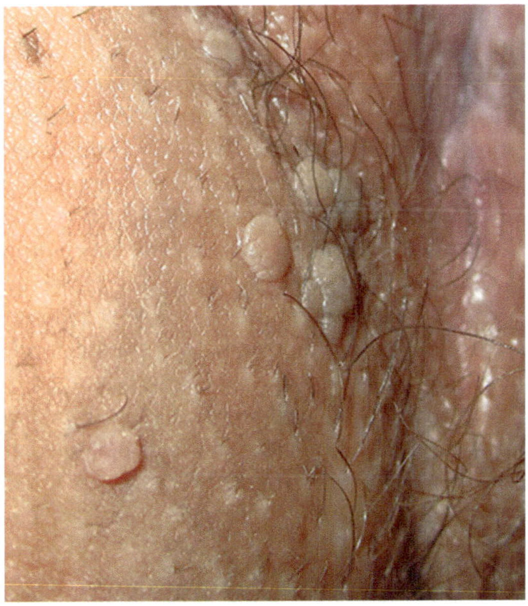

Fig. 18.130 Condylomata acuminata of the vulva in the 33rd week of pregnancy. The warts are flat. Using the colposcope, visual inspection suffices to establish the diagnosis without the need for biopsies

18.7.9 Lichen Planus with Complete Vulvar Synechia

A 49-year-old patient has been suffering from a vaginal stenosis for at least 16 years. No definitive diagnosis has been established so far. Sixteen years ago, she had delivered her first child vaginally. In addition to an episiotomy, there had been extensive tears in the vaginal area due to incipient stenosis. The second child was born by cesarean section a year later because of stenosis of the vulva and vagina. After delivery, an attempt was made to correct the constriction; however, the effect was not long term.

At the time of presentation in the colposcopy clinic, there is complete synechia of the vulva. The clitoris and urethra are not recognizable. Only dorsally, there is still a very small opening. Here a small cotton swab can be inserted into the vagina. Surprisingly, the patient has no micturition problems. The characteristic plaque-shaped erythema of lichen planus is currently absent (Figs. 18.131 and 18.132).

With the focused CO_2 laser beam, the synechiae are cut step by step under colposcopic guidance. At the end, the structures of the external vulva are visible again. The vagina appears to be normal and is not stenotic (Fig. 18.133).

Biopsies at the time of surgery can not confirm the clinical diagnosis of lichen planus. However, 1 year later, the patient presents with changes of the oral mucosa. Biopsy confirms the diagnosis of lichen planus.

Despite topical cortisone treatment, the vulva slowly closes up again. Seven years later, the urethral opening is also affected (Fig. 18.134), and the now 56-year-old patient undergoes laser surgery again.

Besides the recurring vulvar stenosis, which now also involves the lower vagina, the patient has no symptoms in the genital area, whereas the lesions of the oral mucosa repeatedly cause discomfort (Fig. 18.135).

Commentary

Lichen planus of the genital area can be associated with synechia, either of the vulva or of the vagina. At the time of the first visit to the colposcopy clinic, the disease had already persisted for many years without being diagnosed correctly. In the non-acute phases of lichen planus, no skin lesions may be visible.

Unfortunately, only the symptoms of lichen planus can be treated. In particular, the stenotic form described here proved to be resistant to treatment.

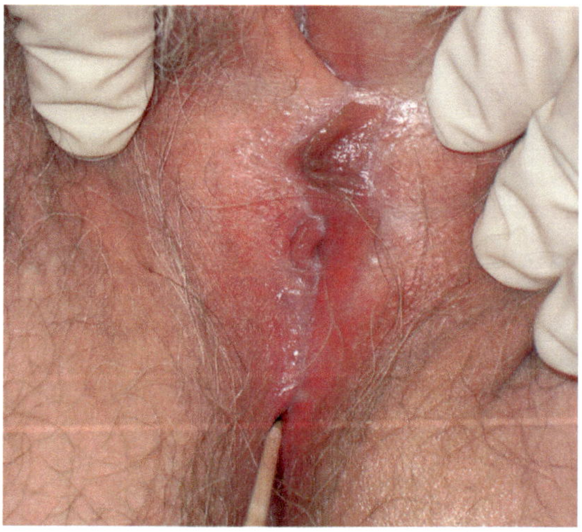

Fig. 18.131 Lichen planus of the vulva. In this non-active stage of the disease, there is complete synechia of the labia majora and minora. Micturition is still possible through a very small vaginal opening

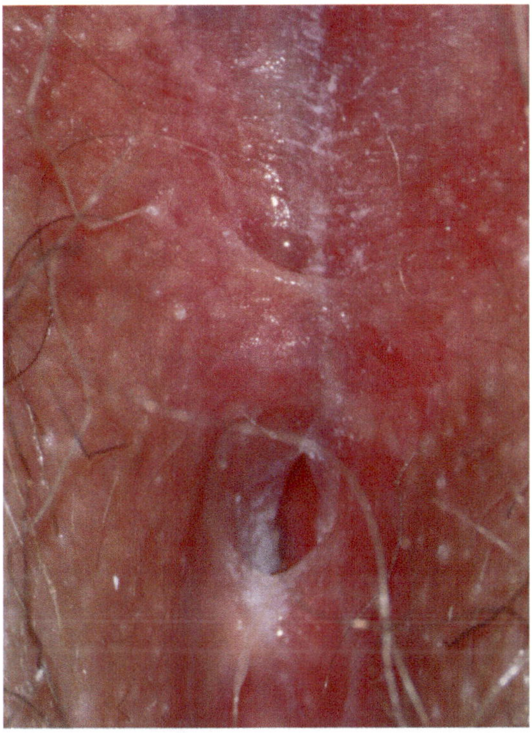

Fig. 18.132 Synechia of the vulva in lichen planus. The vulvar introitus is almost completely closed

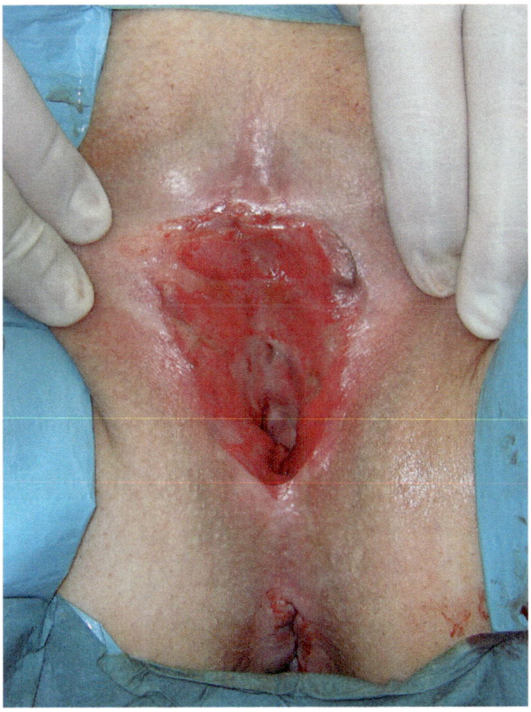

Fig. 18.133 Synechia of the vulva immediately after CO_2 laser surgery. The labia minora are completely atrophic. The clitoris, urethra, and vaginal opening are now visible again

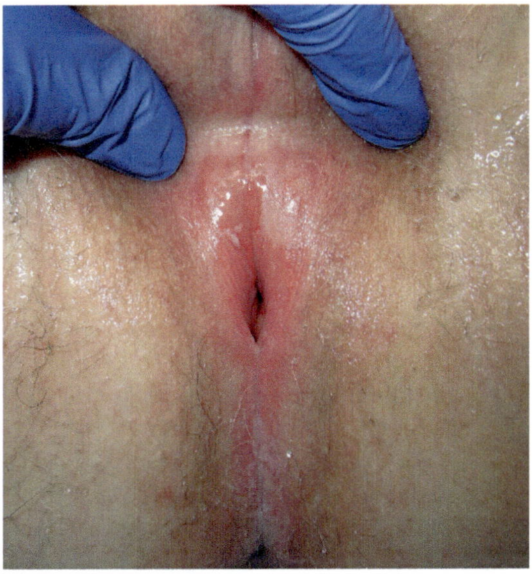

Fig. 18.134 Recurrence of vulvar synechia 7 years later. The vulvar introitus is almost completely closed again and the patient complains of urinary retention

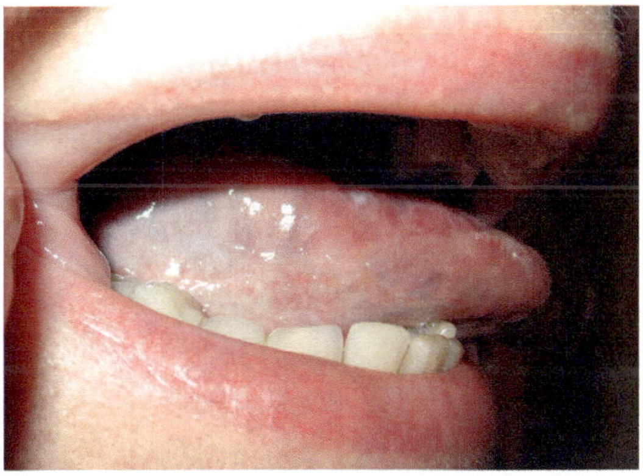

Fig. 18.135 Lichen planus of the oral mucosa. The lateral aspect of the tongue has a fine reticular pattern

18.7.10 Circumscribed HSIL of the Vulva

Seven years prior, a 56-year-old woman underwent bone marrow transplantation for treatment of chronic myeloid leukemia. She quit smoking 13 years ago.

To the left of the vaginal opening and lateral to the labium minus, a 1.5 × 1.5 cm slightly prominent lesion is seen with small red and white (leukoplakia) areas (Figs. 18.136 and 18.137).

A punch biopsy is performed revealing HSIL of the vulva (Fig. 18.138). ThinPrep® cytology is obtained by scraping the abnormal skin with a scalpel and is also positive (Fig. 18.139).

Eventually, the HSIL lesion is resected completely using the focused CO_2 laser beam.

Commentary

The nomenclature of preinvasive lesions of the vulva has undergone many changes during recent years. Besides the expression "HSIL of the vulva" suggested by ISSVD, the 2020 WHO nomenclature favors "squamous intraepithelial lesion of the vulva, HPV-associated" (WHO Classification of Tumours Editorial Board 2020).

When there is no suspicion of invasive disease, HSIL of the vulva can either be resected or vaporized by CO_2 laser. Electrocautery or other types of laser are not recommended as this causes scarring. A small circumscribed lesion as in this scenario is removed by using the focused laser beam like a scalpel.

HSIL of the vulva does not require wide resection margins, as HSIL by definition is not cancer. Therefore, a combination of CO_2 laser resection and vaporization of the margins is acceptable.

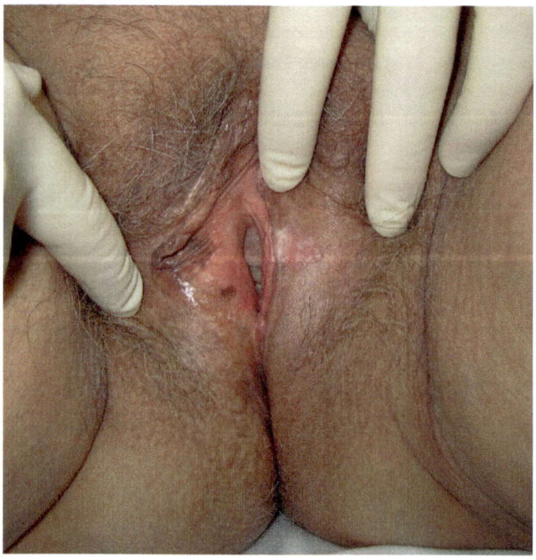

Fig. 18.136 HSIL of the vulva. The slightly prominent lesion is located lateral to the atrophic left labium minus. The pigmentation disorder on the right side of the vagina can be considered benign

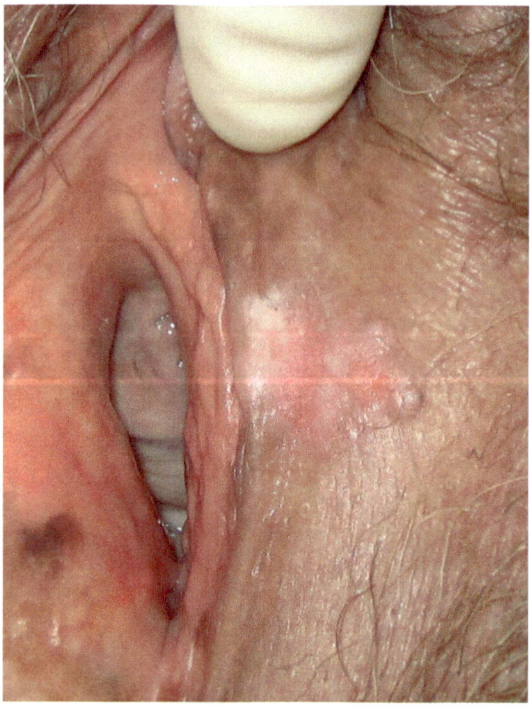

Fig. 18.137 HSIL of the vulva. The lesion has sharp borders with a characteristic irregular surface of reddish and white color

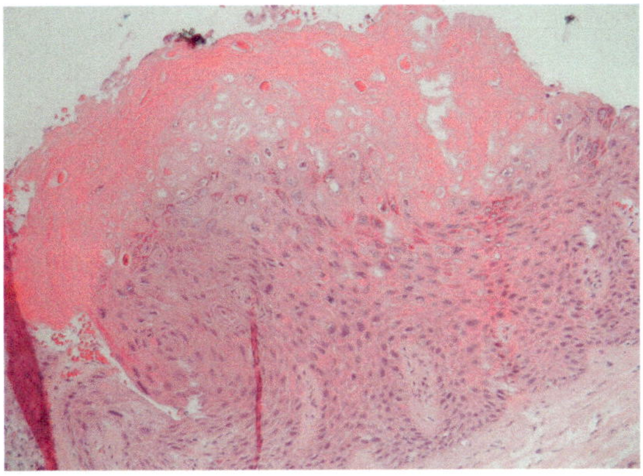

Fig. 18.138 HSIL of the vulva. There is prominent hyperkeratosis, and normal squamous epithelium is replaced by immature cells with pleomorphic nuclei and increased N/C ratio

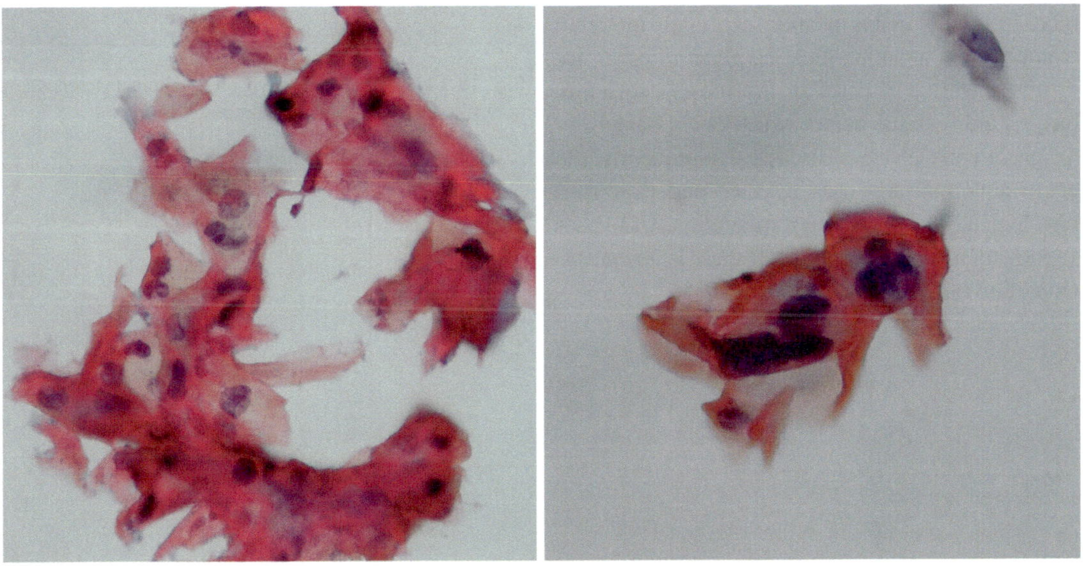

Fig. 18.139 ThinPrep® cytology with numerous dyskeratocytes indicating HSIL of the vulva. These cells can not be distinguished from those of well-differentiated squamous cell carcinoma

18.7.11 Subclitoral HSIL

The patient is 43 years old and free of symptoms. During her annual gynecologic exam, a small area with hyperkeratosis and a tiny ulcer of the vulva are identified. The lesion is located close to the midline between the urethra and clitoris (Figs. 18.140 and 18.141).

A 4 mm punch biopsy reveals HSIL of the vulva. The entire lesion is removed by CO_2 laser resection. Final histology does not show invasive disease (Fig. 18.142).

Commentary

The lesion described here is very small. However, it is located very close to the midline between the urethra and clitoris. As vulvar cancer has been observed more frequently in this location, especially in young women, close attention must be given in order not to miss invasive disease. In the present scenario, there is a tiny tissue defect which could have been a sign of early invasive disease. Consequently, the entire abnormal area was resected and examined histologically to rule out microinvasion. CO_2 laser vaporization is not acceptable, if there is any suspicion of invasive disease.

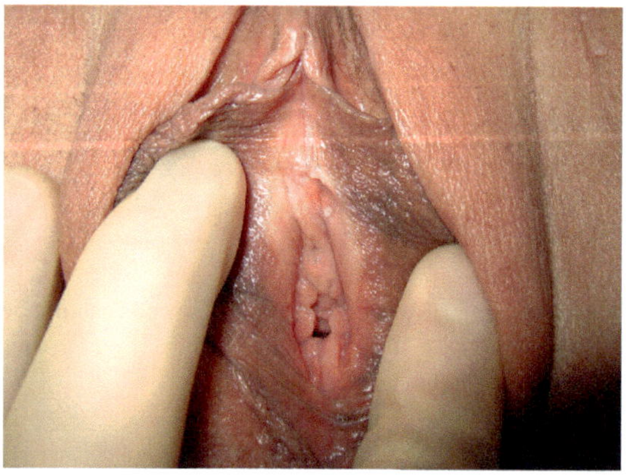

Fig. 18.140 Subclitoral HSIL. This small lesion in a 43-year-old patient may easily be missed on routine gynecologic examination

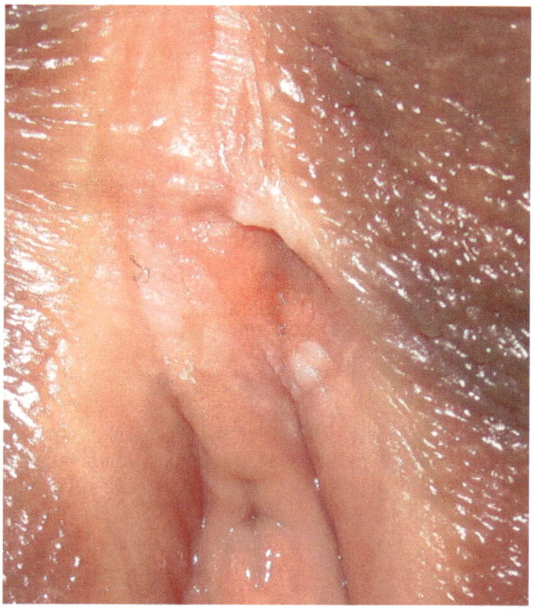

Fig. 18.141 Subclitoral HSIL. The clinical diagnosis is confirmed by a 4 mm punch biopsy

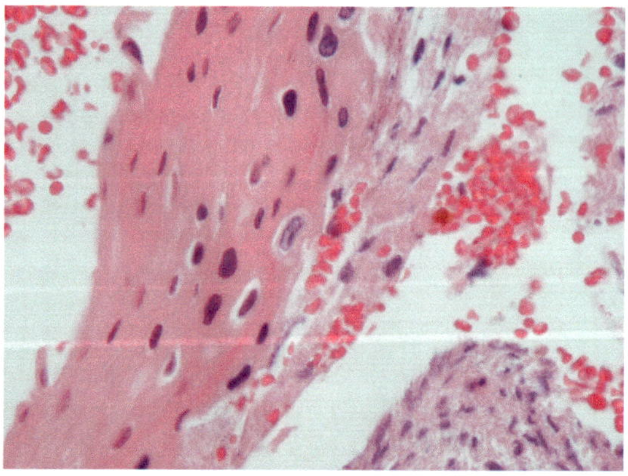

Fig. 18.142 Subclitoral HSIL. There is hyperkeratosis with retention (parakeratosis) of abnormal nuclei

18.7.12 Periurethral HSIL

A 35-year-old patient is a heavy smoker. Four months earlier, she complained of itching and burning pain of the vulva. A vulvar biopsy revealed a "carcinoma in situ." The biopsy had been done 4 days after a spontaneous abortion. Subsequently, local resections around both labia minora were performed. Histology revealed HSIL. Resection margins were positive.

The colposcopic exam shows an erythematous lesion, located between the clitoris and urethra involving also the urethral orifice. The surface of the epithelium is irregular and rugged with possible ulceration bilaterally close to the urethra. Clinically, invasive disease cannot be ruled out (Fig. 18.143).

The abnormal tissue is excised with the focused CO_2 laser beam. Part of the distal urethral is also removed, whereas the clitoris is preserved.

The histological exam eventually shows HSIL without evidence of invasion (Fig. 18.144).

Commentary

As in previous scenarios, the vulvar lesion is located in the midline around the anterior commissure, and the patient is only 35 years old. Special attention should be paid because midline carcinomas of young women in this particular localization are on the rise.

HSIL of the vulva may be treated via CO_2 laser vaporization. However, in the present scenario, invasive disease cannot be ruled out. Therefore, surgical resection is performed.

Initially, the histopathology read "carcinoma in situ." Terminologies such as "carcinoma in situ," "squamous carcinoma in situ," "Morbus Bowen," etc. should not be used any more.

The patient is a heavy smoker. There is a relation between HSIL of the vulva and smoking; the majority of these patients smoke or have smoked heavily in the past.

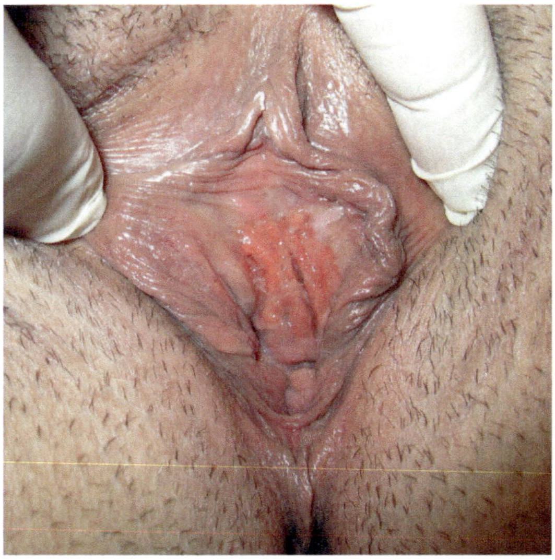

Fig. 18.143 HSIL of the vulva involving the urethra. The skin between the clitoris and the urethra is erythematous with an irregular almost polypoid surface. An invasive lesion cannot be ruled out clinically

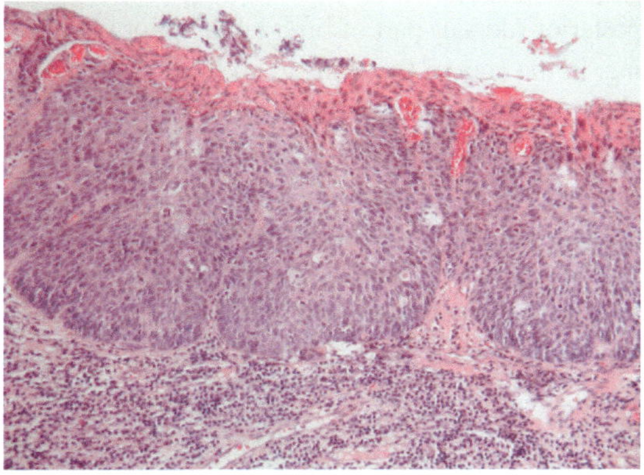

Fig. 18.144 HSIL of the vulva. The squamous epithelium is thickened and replaced by small atypical cells with increased N/C ratio. Also, there is parakeratosis

18.7.13 Long-Term Follow-Up of Recurrent HSIL of the Vulva

The patient is 46 years old when she first presents to the colposcopy clinic. Four years earlier, she underwent vaginal hysterectomy for recurrent CIN. In the same year, she was treated with CO_2 laser for HSIL of the vulva. After that, another three operations were performed in quick succession, also because of HSIL of the vulva.

The patient now complains of itching and a stinging pain of the vulva. Also, the vulva is very sensitive to touch. She is worrying that she might develop cancer and that the clitoris might have to be removed. She wants to preserve sexual functions and sexual sensation. Presently, she has no partner. For many years, she has been smoking heavily.

Now (point in time 0) a thorough examination of vulva and vagina is performed. Colposcopically and cytologically, there is no evidence of intraepithelial neoplasia. The anatomy of the vulva is well preserved despite three prior interventions (Fig. 18.145). The posterior (dorsal) part of both labia minora is missing. In the area of the glans as well as the frenulum clitoridis, the characteristic skin changes of HSIL of the vulva such as discrete swelling and depigmentation can be seen (Fig. 18.146).

The patient then undergoes surgery (fourth vulvar operation) under general anesthesia. The lesion close to the clitoris is vaporized with the CO_2 laser. At the same time, a tissue sample from a similar lesion located at the posterior commissure is obtained, and the posterior vulva is also treated with the laser. The biopsy confirms the clinical HSIL diagnosis.

Subsequently, a treatment with imiquimod cream (Aldara®) is initiated. Nevertheless, the patient has a recurrence and is operated again 1 year later (fifth vulvar operation). Intraoperative biopsy reveals high-grade anal intraepithelial neoplasia (AIN3; Fig. 18.147).

Subsequently, the patient is again treated with topical imiquimod for 18 weeks. Initially she is asked to apply the cream three times a week. However, due to local side effects, she can tolerate treatment only once a week.

Seven months after laser surgery, she is again seen in the colposcopy clinic (point in time 0 + 16 months). Again, there is clinical manifestation of HSIL of the clitoris (Fig. 18.148). Two months later (point in time 0 + 18), this lesion has increased in size and also affects the right labium minus (Fig. 18.149) as well as the perianal region at 12 o'clock (Fig. 18.150).

The patient consults a proctologist, who excises the lesion that extends into the anal canal. In addition, the surrounding anal tissue and the vulvar manifestations are laser treated (sixth vulvar operation). Histopathology confirms AIN3. Margins are positive.

Eight months after this operation (point in time 0 + 29 months), the vulva appears to be normal apart from a small area of leukoplakia at the right labium minus (Fig. 18.151). The perianal and anal regions are also free of disease (Fig. 18.152).

At 0 + 37 months, the patient complains of vulvar itching. The aforementioned area on the right labium minus has become more prominent (Fig. 18.153). At this point in time, the patient does not want to have another operation, especially as her birthday is due in a few days. In the following months, the patient still declines surgery and is monitored at short intervals. At 0 + 38 months (Fig. 18.154) and 0 + 40 months (Fig. 18.155), the lesion has changed little. Eventually, CO_2 laser vaporization is performed (0 + 41 months; seventh vulvar operation).

Figure 18.156 presents the vulva at 0 + 48 months. For the first time, the vulva and perianal region are clinically free of disease.

Commentary

In order to treat recurrent HSIL of the vulva and AIN3 without the need of mutilating cold-knife tissue resections, the patient had to undergo seven vulvar or anal/perianal operations over a period of 8 years. Despite the numerous CO_2 laser treatments, it has been possible to preserve the vulvar anatomy without significant scarring.

Topical application of imiquimod (van Seters et al. 2008; Terlou et al. 2011) would be the treatment of choice for this patient. However, almost all patients develop local or systemic side effects which limits its use in HSIL of vulva and anus.

According to Wallbillich et al. (2012), two-thirds of patients with HSIL of the vulva are active or former smokers. However, most patients will not be able to quit smoking, even though they are well aware of the detrimental association with vulvar HSIL.

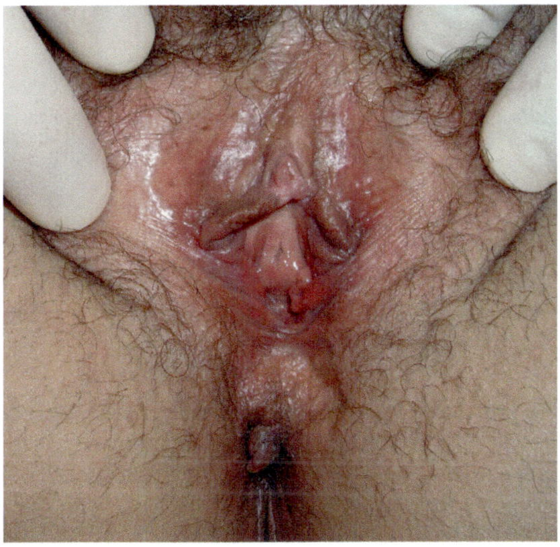

Fig. 18.145 Point in ime 0. Except for a small HSIL lesion of the clitoris, the vulva is normal. Due to three previous operations, part of the labia minora is missing

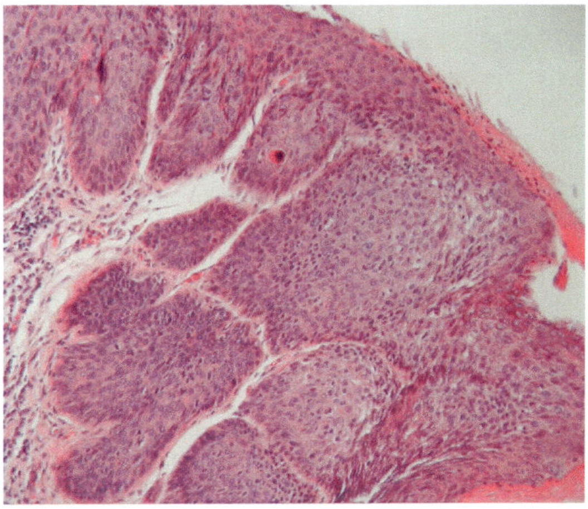

Fig. 18.147 Grade 3 anal intraepithelial neoplasia (AIN3). The biopsy was taken at the time of the fifth vulvar operation and shows a disorganized atypical basal-type epithelium with overlying parakeratosis

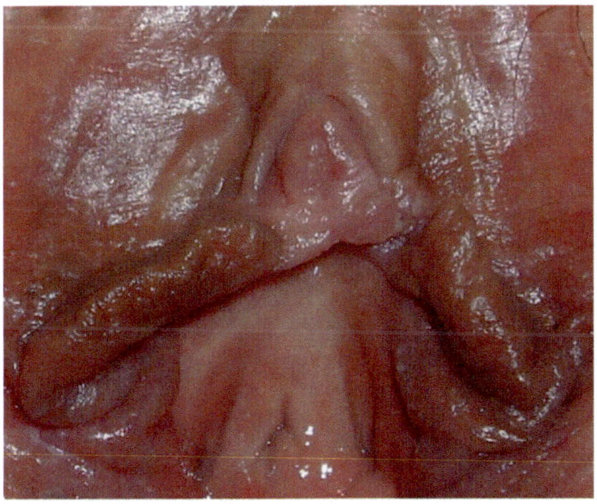

Fig. 18.146 Point in time 0. The glans and the frenulum clitoridis show depigmentation and an irregular surface. The glans itself has an irregular surface. The clitoral prepuce is not affected

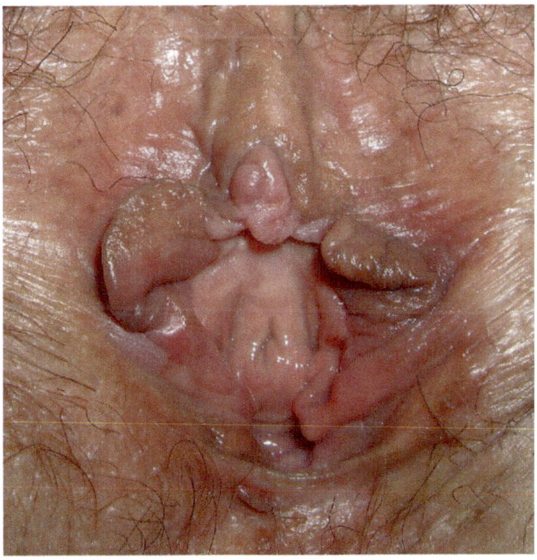

Fig. 18.148 0 + 16 months. Despite several prior CO_2 laser treatments, the clitoris again shows characteristic HSIL changes. At the right labium minus, there is a small area of leukoplakia

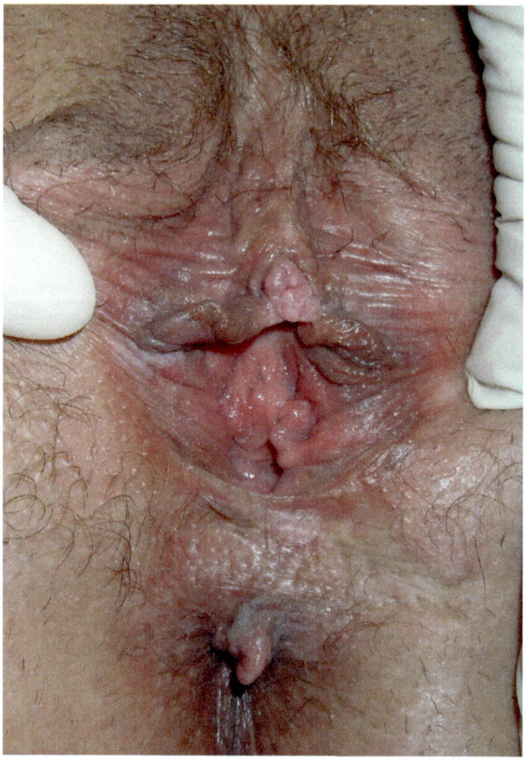

Fig. 18.149 0 + 18 months. Dysplastic changes are more pronounced, now affecting not only the clitoris but also the right labium minus and the ventral perineum

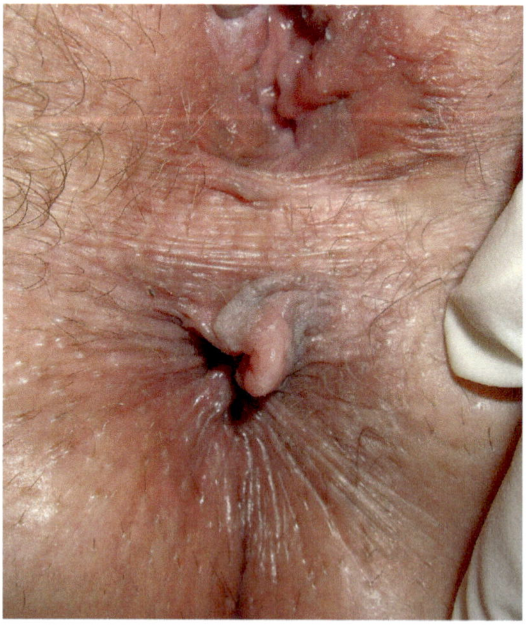

Fig. 18.150 0 + 18 months. At the perineum (12 o'clock), pigment disorders and hypertrophy of the skin are seen. Biopsy confirms grade 3 anal intraepithelial neoplasia (AIN3)

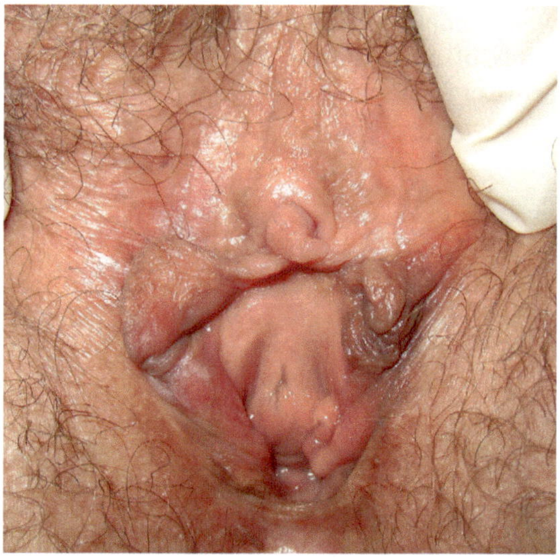

Fig. 18.151 0 + 29 months. Eight months prior, surgery had been performed again. There is a small area of leukoplakia on the right labium minus. Otherwise, the vulva is unremarkable

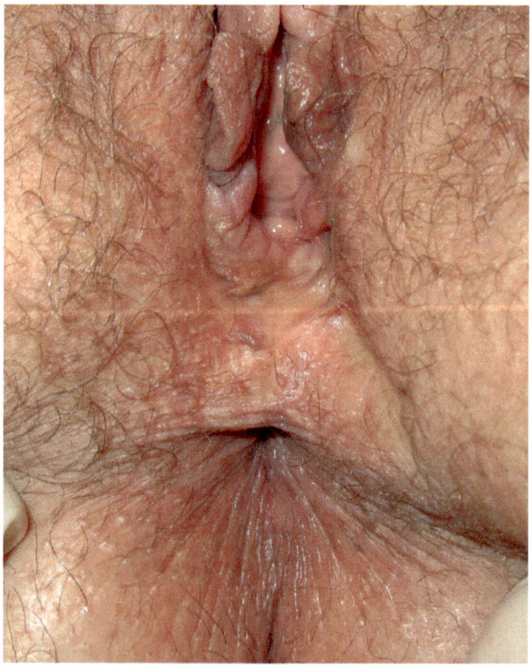

Fig. 18.152 0 + 29 months. The perianal region at 12 o'clock is free of dysplasia

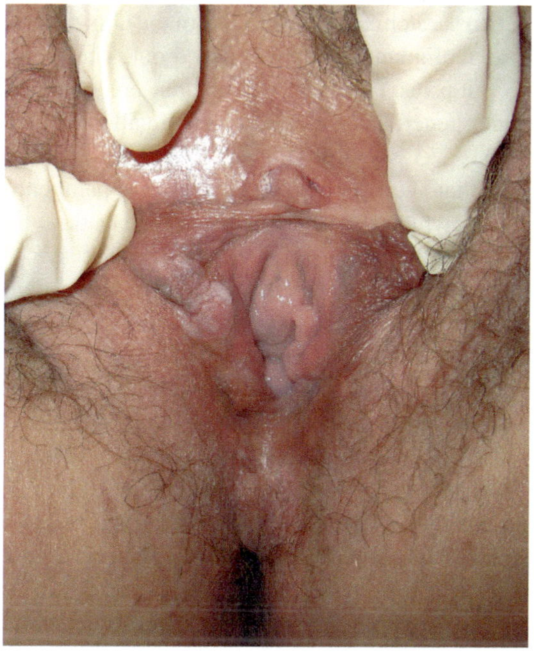

Fig. 18.153 0 + 37 months. At the right labia minus, there is a circumscribed area with hypertrophy, hyperkeratosis, and abnormal pigmentation representing a new manifestation of HSIL

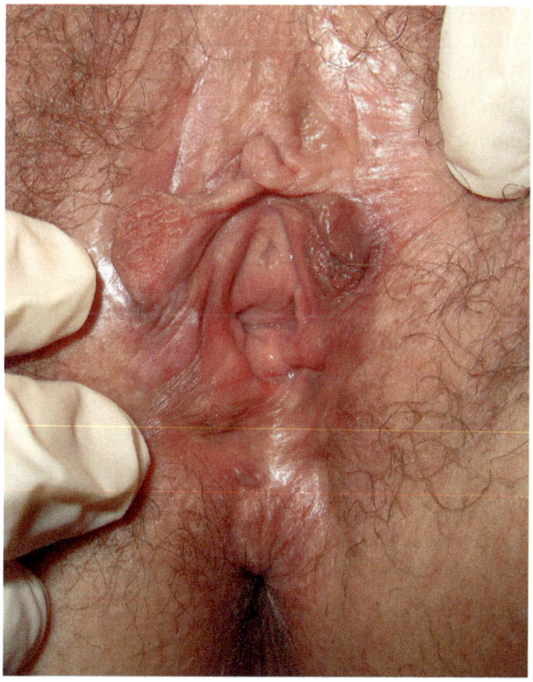

Fig. 18.154 0 + 38 months. Short-term follow-up shows no change compared to Fig. 18.153

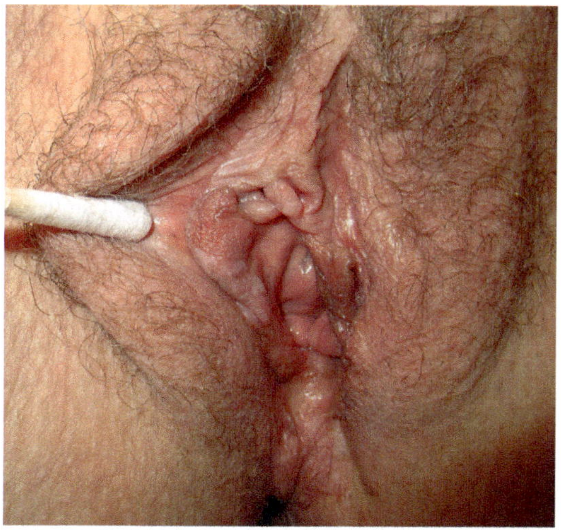

Fig. 18.155 0 + 40 months. Again, there is no significant change compared to Figs. 18.153 and 18.154

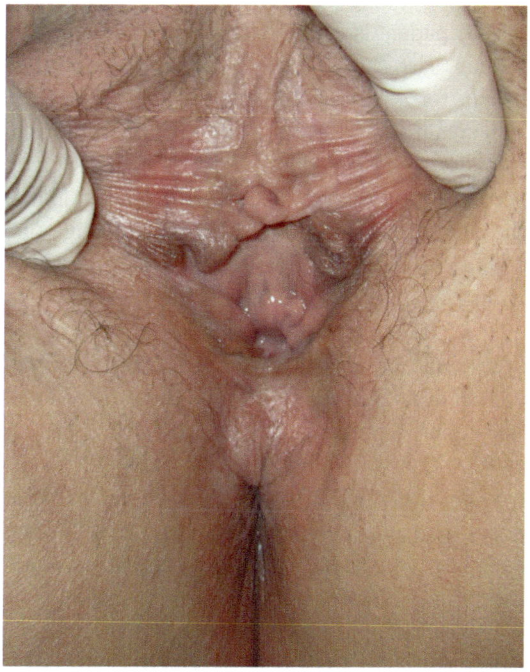

Fig. 18.156 0 + 48 months. After CO_2 laser vaporization 7 months earlier, the vulva and perianal regions are free of recurrence from HSIL

18.7.14 Vulvar Carcinoma Associated with Lichen Sclerosus

At the age of 54, a patient presents to the colposcopy clinic for the first time. She complains of vulvar discomfort, such as pain and itching, especially at night. She has had these symptoms off and on for about 20 years. Lately, these problems have gotten worse.

The patient is using an estrogen cream which brings some relief. In the past, she has tried a testosterone-containing ointment as well as panthenol cream, and she has applied black tea. Hydrocortisone-containing ointments have been applied with varying degrees of success.

Based on the clinical image, the diagnosis of lichen sclerosus of the vulva is made (point in time 0; Fig. 18.157). Up to now, no biopsies have been taken.

The patient is told to stop all prior treatments. Instead, she should apply clobetasol, a cortisol cream, for a period of 3 months and use a basic skin cream several times a day to prevent the skin from drying out. In addition, she should be seen by her private gynecologist biannually and is told that she can return to the colposcopy clinic at any time.

Subsequently, the patient is seen six times within a period of 7 years.

0 + 22 months: Presently, there are only minor symptoms, mainly vulvar itching. Examination of the vulva reveals no suspicious areas. Physiogel AI® cream is prescribed twice a day.

0 + 43 months (Fig. 18.158): The symptoms have increased. The patient is unhappy with the poor therapeutic effect of Physiogel AI® cream and has consistently used a hydrocortisone-containing ointment for the past 6 months. A 4 mm punch biopsy is obtained from a tissue defect close to the clitoris, which is negative. Again, a clobetasol cream is recommended, and the patient is asked to return for a follow-up exam after 3 months.

0 + 46 months (Fig. 18.159): The symptoms are now described as "bearable." However, clobetasol had been applied only briefly. Another short-term follow-up appointment is scheduled.

0 + 49 months (Fig. 18.160): The patient has moderate symptoms. The skin lesions appear to be more severe with superficial erosions possibly due to scratching. However, from the clinical picture, malignancy cannot be ruled out. Therefore, six biopsies from the vulvar area are obtained under general anesthesia, which are all negative.

0 + 53 months (Fig. 18.161): The patient says that she is coping. She favors the panthenol cream, which she applies several times a day.

0 + 72 months (Fig. 18.162): Vulvar symptoms are more severe now. Recently, the patient has noticed a vulvar swelling. On the left side close to the vagina, an approximately 2 cm exophytic tumor has formed. Two 4 mm punch biopsies confirm the diagnosis of a well-differentiated squamous cell carcinoma of the vulva (Fig. 18.163). The direct Pap smear obtained from the surface of the tumor is also suspicious for cancer (Fig. 18.164).

Radical tumor resection is performed (Fig. 18.165), and the defect is covered by a VY advancement flap from the pubis (Moschella and Cordova 2000) (Fig. 18.166). The sentinel lymph nodes from the left inguinal are free of tumor.

Commentary

Histomorphologically, lichen sclerosus is not a precancerous lesions in contrast to HSIL of the vulva. Nevertheless, there is an increased risk of cancer of about 4% (Buckley and Fox 1988). Therefore, patients with lichen sclerosus should undergo regular checkups. The frequency of these exams depends on the age of the patient, the duration of the disease, and especially the severity of lichen sclerosus. Usually, biannual examinations are advisable.

If any abnormality is seen, a punch biopsy is recommended to rule out invasive disease. Unfortunately, cytological smears have a high false-negative rate and cannot be a substitute for histopathology-based diagnosis.

The patient was reluctant to use class I or II topical steroids. However, presently, maintenance treatment with cortisone creams is recommended for long-term symptomatic relief but also in the hope of preventing cancer.

As itching is a major symptom of lichen sclerosus, long-term use of Physiogel AI® cream may be helpful as it improves regulation of the endocannabinoid system, which plays a role in the etiology of itching (Staender et al. 2006).

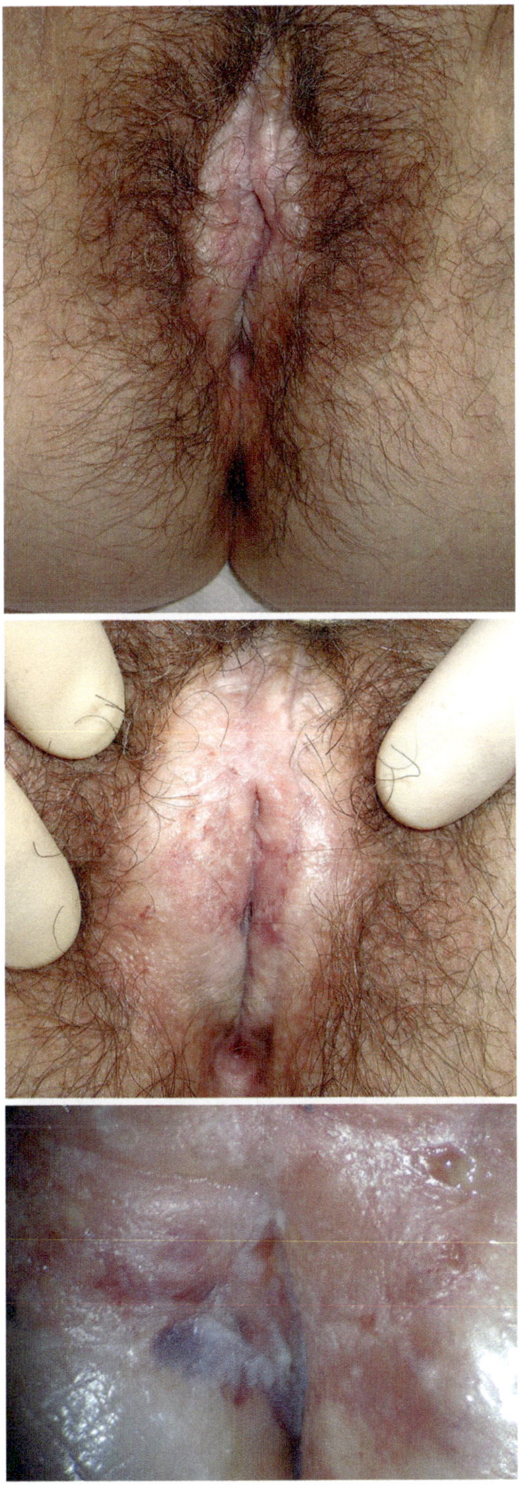

Fig. 18.157 Lichen sclerosus of the vulva (point in time 0). Mainly the anterior (ventral) vulva is involved with atrophy and hyperkeratosis. The perianal region is not affected. The colposcopic exam shows a bluish discoloration which is due to subcutaneous hemorrhage

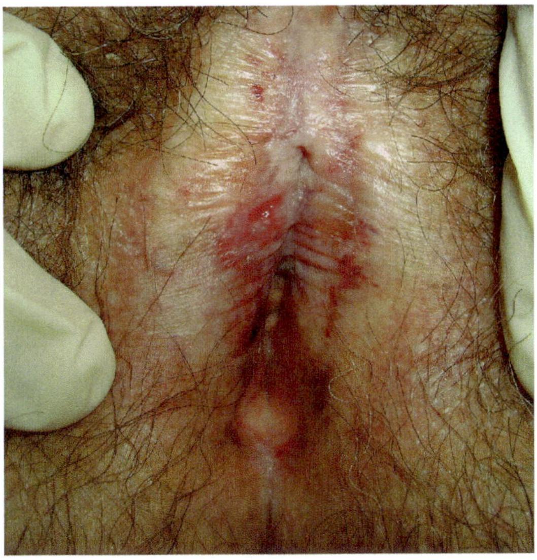

Fig. 18.158 Lichen sclerosus of the vulva (point in time 0 + 43 months). The tissue defect located on the right laterodorsal side of the atrophic clitoris could be a scratching artifact. However, invasive disease had to be ruled out by punch biopsy

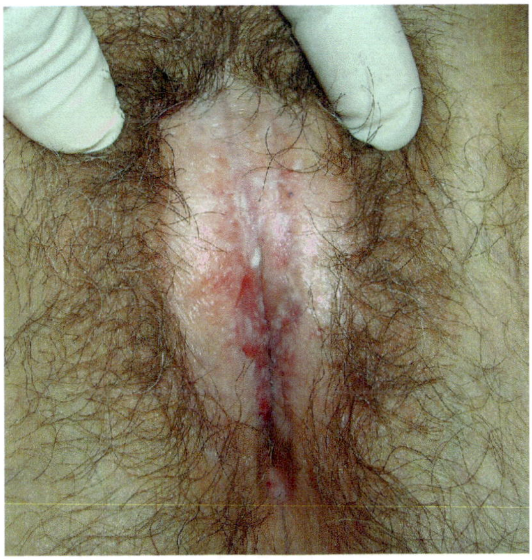

Fig. 18.159 Lichen sclerosus of the vulva (point in time 0 + 46 months). There are no epithelial defects. Nevertheless, short-term follow-up is needed

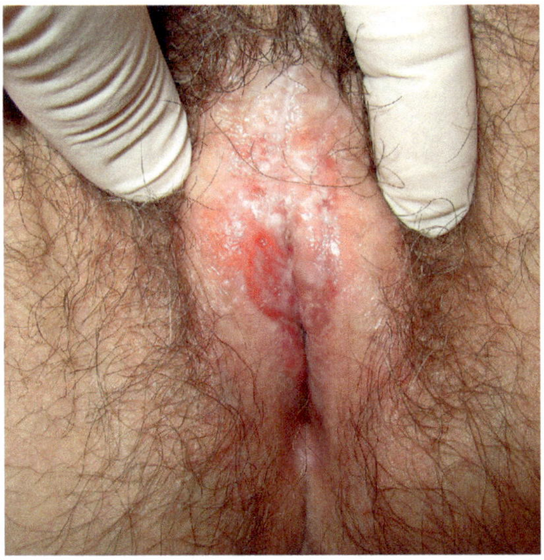

Fig. 18.160 Lichen sclerosus of the vulva (point in time 0 + 49 months). The circumscribed area of erythema has increased in size, and epithelial defects have developed. Under general anesthesia, six biopsies are obtained to rule out malignancy

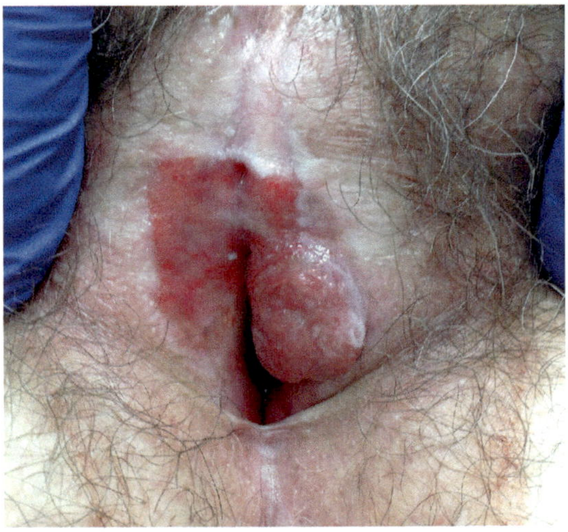

Fig. 18.162 Squamous cell carcinoma of the vulva after a long history of lichen sclerosus (point in time 0 + 72 months). On the left side, there is now a 2 cm exophytic tumor

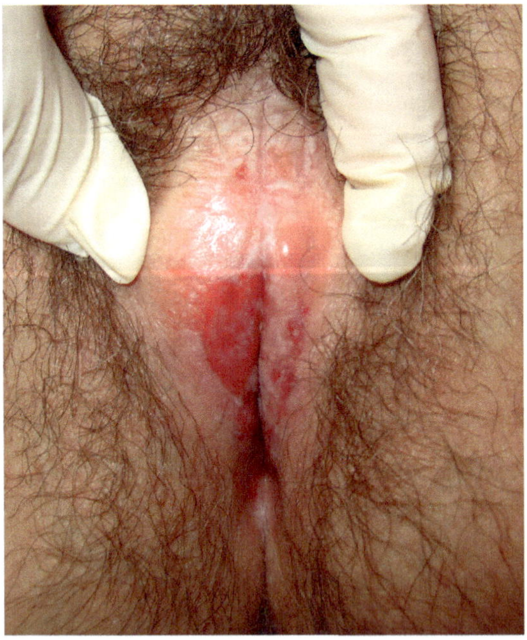

Fig. 18.161 Lichen sclerosus of the vulva (point in time 0 + 53 months). The erythema is more pronounced compared to 3 months earlier. However, it has not increased in size

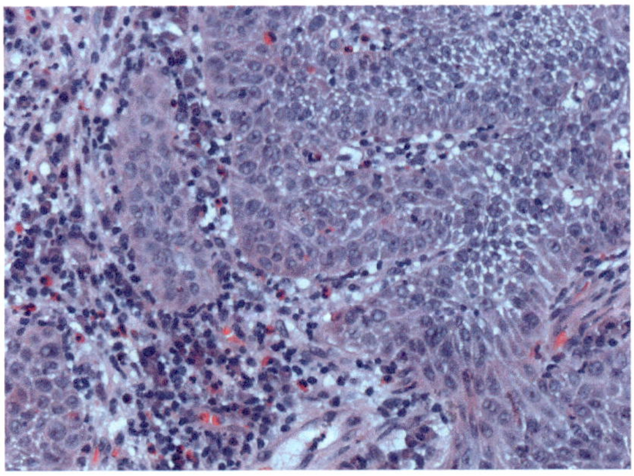

Fig. 18.163 Punch biopsy from a well-differentiated squamous cell carcinoma of the vulva. The tumor cell aggregates advance into the stroma (With kind permission of Prof. Dr. H.U. Kasper, Münster, Germany)

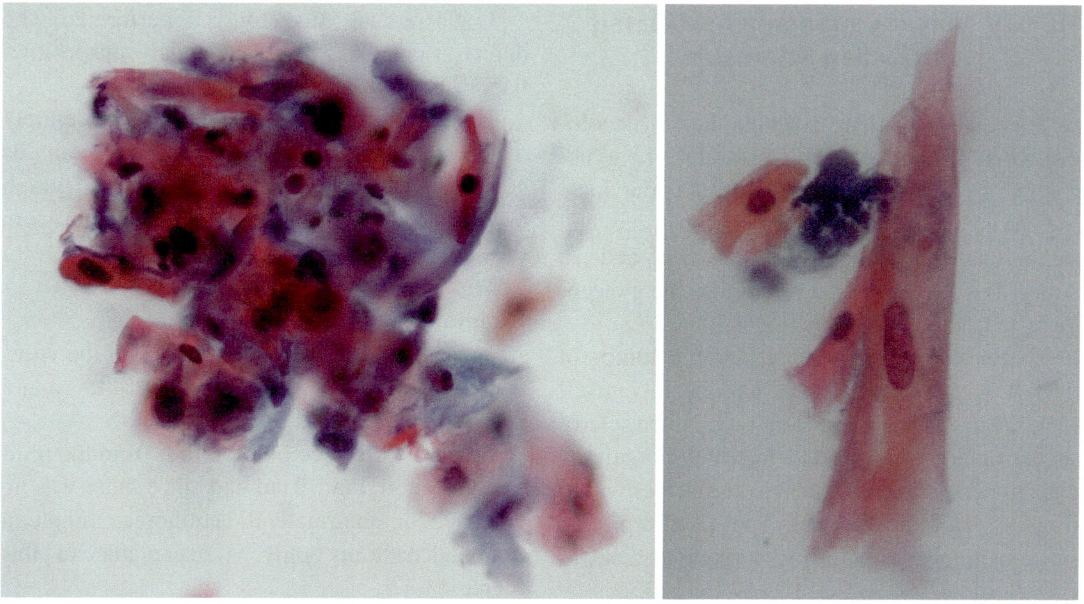

Fig. 18.164 ThinPrep® Pap smear suspicious for squamous cell carcinoma of the vulva. Numerous dyskeratocytes are seen. There is no tumor diathesis. As cytological smears from the vulva have a high false-negative rate, Pap tests are no alternative to histopathology-based diagnosis

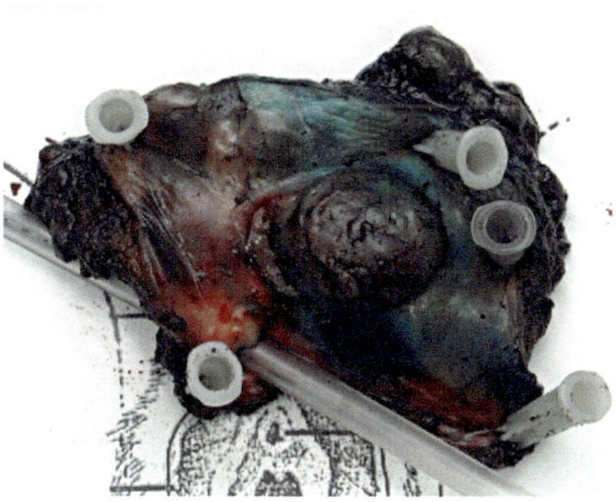

Fig. 18.165 The vulvar tumor has been removed with a 2 cm resection margin. The distal urethra has also been resected (marked with a catheter). The discoloration is due to injection of methylene blue, which together with technetium-99 m is used for sentinel lymph node labeling

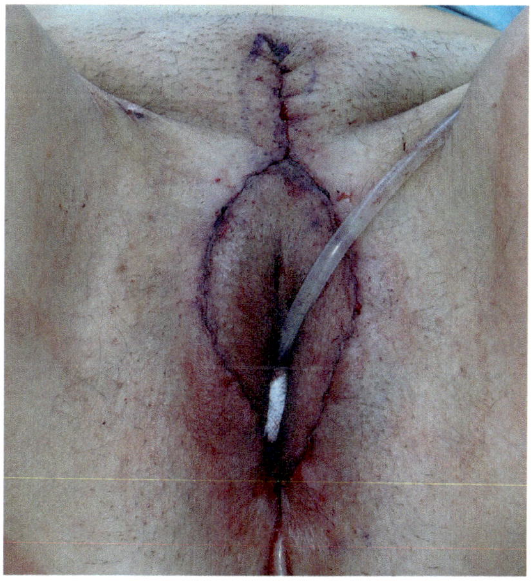

Fig. 18.166 After radical tumor resection, the resulting defect is covered with a VY advancement flap from the pubis. The sentinel lymph nodes of the left groin have been removed through the vulvar incision

18.7.15 Vulvar Carcinoma Associated with Lichen Sclerosus

A 75-year-old patient consults her gynecologist when she notices a vulvar tumor. The gynecologist performed a punch biopsy under local anesthesia which is positive for squamous cell carcinoma with a depth of invasion of at least 3 mm. The patient is then referred to the gynecologic cancer center for treatment.

There is a conspicuous exophytic tumor of the left vulva close to the vagina. The vulva itself shows skin changes consistent with lichen sclerosus (atrophy of the clitoris and both labia minora with hyperkeratosis of the vulva and perineum) (Figs. 18.167 and 18.168). The ThinPrep® Pap smear is highly suspicious for squamous cell carcinoma of the vulva (Fig. 18.169).

Local radical vulvectomy is performed. The defect is covered with a pudendal transposition flap.

Histopathology shows a 2.7 cm moderately differentiated partially keratinizing squamous cell carcinoma (Fig. 18.170). The inguinal lymph nodes on the left are not involved. Biopsies from the right introitus are free of tumor.

Commentary

As mentioned earlier, cytopathology of the vulva is much inferior to histopathology and cannot rule out invasive or preinvasive disease.

Since the distance of the tumor from the midline was more than 1 cm and since there was no evidence of contralateral carcinoma, unilateral lymphadenectomy only is acceptable in this scenario.

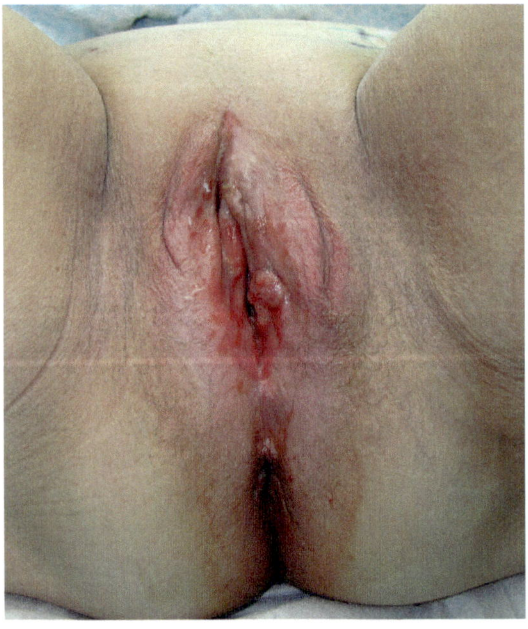

Fig. 18.167 Vulvar carcinoma associated with lichen sclerosus. Thin hyperkeratosis encompasses the vulva and the perineum with prominent atrophy. The perianal region is not affected by lichen sclerosus. The vulva is asymmetric due to tumor formation on the left side

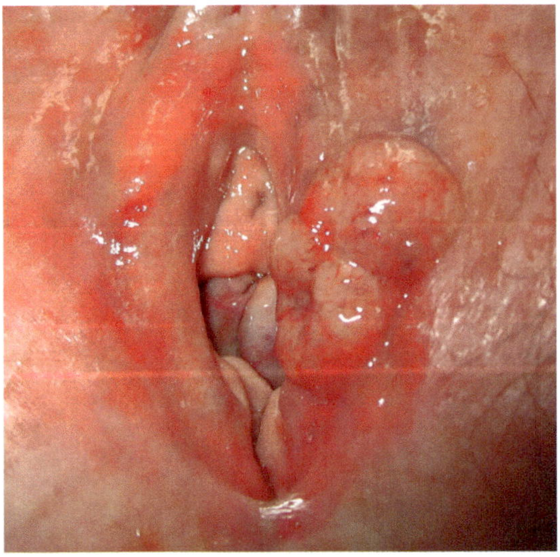

Fig. 18.168 Vulvar carcinoma associated with lichen sclerosus. The clitoris and the labia minora are completely atrophied. The vulvar carcinoma has an exophytic growth pattern with atypical vessels

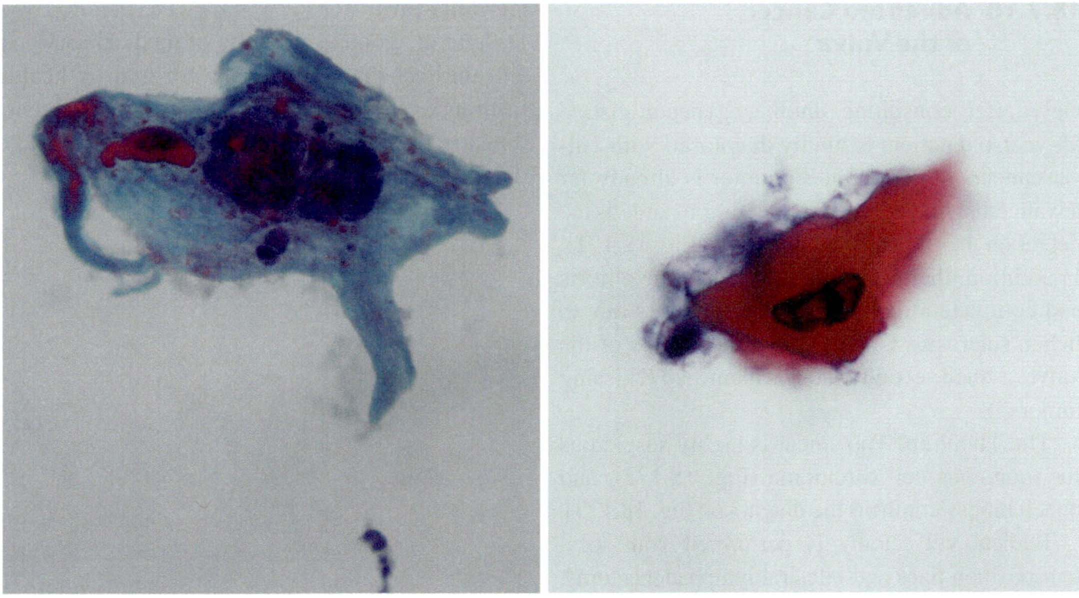

Fig. 18.169 ThinPrep® smear from vulvar carcinoma. Compared to squamous carcinoma of the cervix, the cells of vulvar carcinoma usually have a markedly different morphology and can be more difficult to diagnose (Nauth 2002). The dyskeratocytes shown here do not have an increased N/C ratio. Although the nuclei are enlarged, there is also more cytoplasm with a bizarre appearance

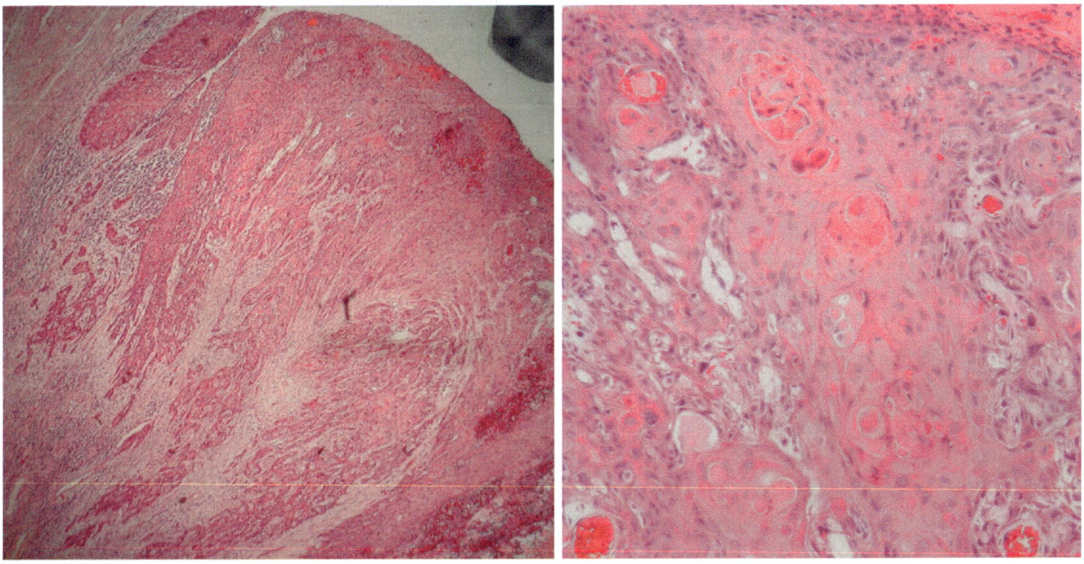

Fig. 18.170 Squamous cell carcinoma of the vulva. There is diffuse infiltration of the stroma by squamous cell carcinoma which form keratin pearls

18.7.16 Advanced Cancer of the Vulva

Only after consulting another gynecologist, a 55-year-old patient is finally diagnosed with vulvar cancer. At this point the tumor is already far advanced with significant ulceration and tissue defect on the right side of the vulva (Fig. 18.171). In addition, there is major atrophy of the clitoris and complete atrophy of the labia minora due to lichen sclerosus. On the contralateral side of the vulva, a small second cancer is identified ("kissing tumors").

The ThinPrep® Pap smear is highly suspicious for squamous cell carcinoma (Fig. 18.172), and punch biopsy confirms the diagnosis (Fig. 18.173).

Radical vulvectomy is performed with local transposition flaps and bilateral lymphadenectomy. The carcinoma of the right side is 4.6 cm in diameter with a depth of invasion of 5 mm, while on the left, a 2 mm microcarcinoma is identified with a depth of invasion of 1 mm. There is a single lymph node metastasis in the right groin which is 1 cm in diameter. Subsequently, the patient undergoes adjuvant radiation therapy of the inguinal and pelvic region.

Commentary

Despite the good availability of medical services and the fact that patients are covered by health insurance within a high-resource environment, diagnosis of vulvar carcinoma is still frequently delayed.

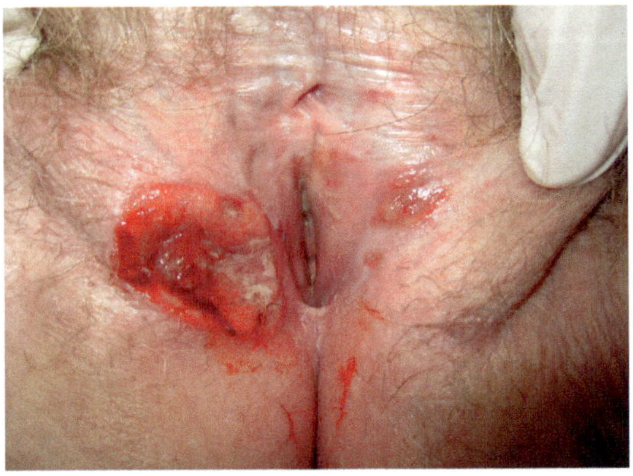

Fig. 18.171 Advanced carcinoma of the vulva associated with lichen sclerosus. The 55-year-old patient has pronounced atrophy of the clitoris and complete atrophy of both labia minora. There is a large ulcerating carcinoma on the right side and a small also malignant lesion on the left side

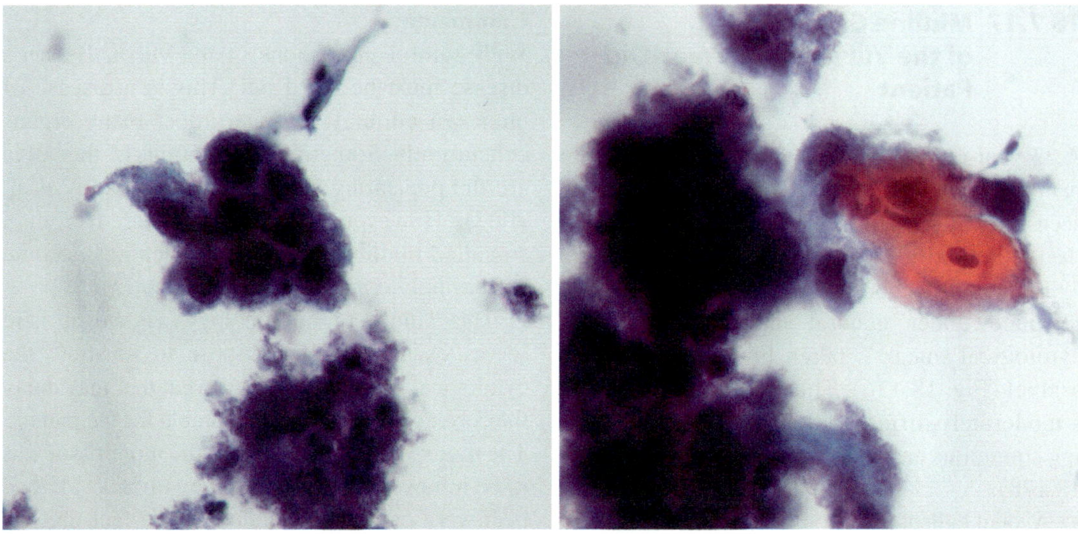

Fig. 18.172 ThinPrep® Pap smear of vulvar carcinoma. The tumor cell clusters are predominantly from non-keratinizing epithelium. The N/C ratio is increased

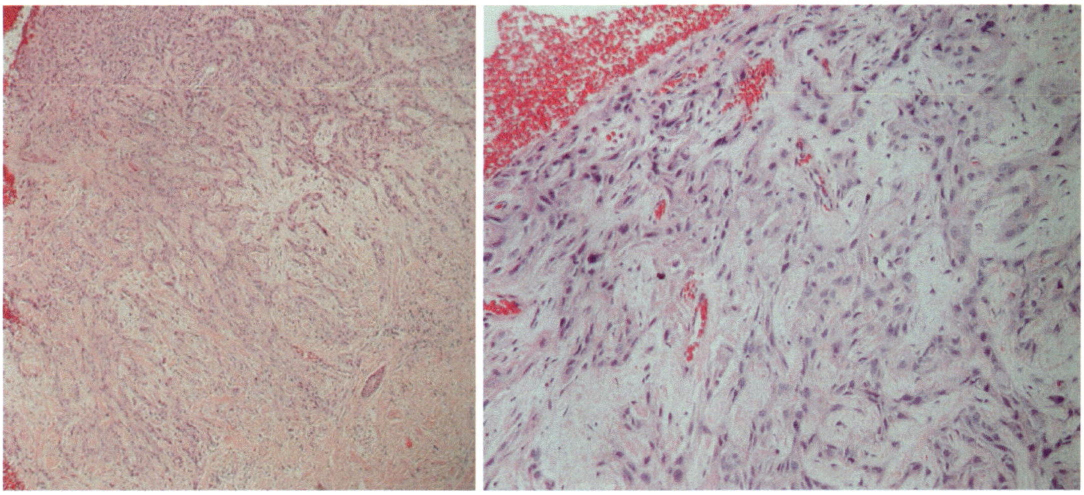

Fig. 18.173 Vulvar carcinoma. The atypical epithelial cells have penetrated the stroma. The cancer is a non-keratinizing, moderately differentiated squamous cell carcinoma

18.7.17 Midline Carcinoma of the Vulva in a 33-Year-Old Patient

A 33-year-old patient complains of an extremely painful subclitoral lesion. Two small ulcers are seen halfway between the glans of the clitoris and the urethral orifice (Figs. 18.174 and 18.175).

Because of the pain, the punch biopsy is obtained under general anesthesia. Also, a cytological smear is taken by scraping with a scalpel (Fig. 18.176). The punch biopsy shows a moderately differentiated partially keratinizing squamous cell carcinoma (Figs. 18.177 and 18.178).

A local radical resection is performed including the distal part of the urethra (Fig. 18.179). The clitoris is preserved. Histopathology shows a 9 mm carcinoma with a depth of invasion of less than 1 mm (microcarcinoma). In a subsequent operation, the sentinel lymph nodes are removed from both inguinofemoral areas. These lymph nodes are negative.

Commentary

With painful ulcerations of the vulva, Behçet's disease must be ruled out. This is a disease of unknown etiology that can affect many organs concurrently. Sometimes ulcerations of the vulva are the presenting symptom (Haidopoulos et al. 2002). However, the patient suffered from a so-called midline carcinoma, which has become increasingly common in young women.

The ThinPrep® morphology as shown here serves exclusively the purpose to illustrate the cytological morphology. Any event that may delay the correct diagnosis is unfavorable for the patient. The more extensive the tumor, the more tissue has to be removed. The fact that the vulvar lesion had been very painful contributed to the fact that the cancer had been diagnosed at an early stage.

At a depth of invasion of less than 1 mm, vulvar cancer is considered a microcarcinoma. Lymph node metastases are unlikely and inguinofemoral lymphadenectomy is usually not required. However, sentinel lymph node resection may be considered (Sidor et al. 2006).

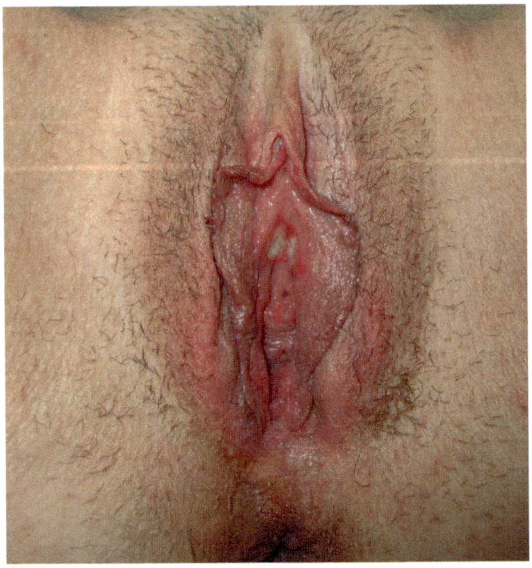

Fig. 18.174 Midline carcinoma of the vulva. Initially, the 33-year-old patient consulted her gynecologist because of a painful vulvar lesion located between the clitoris and urethra

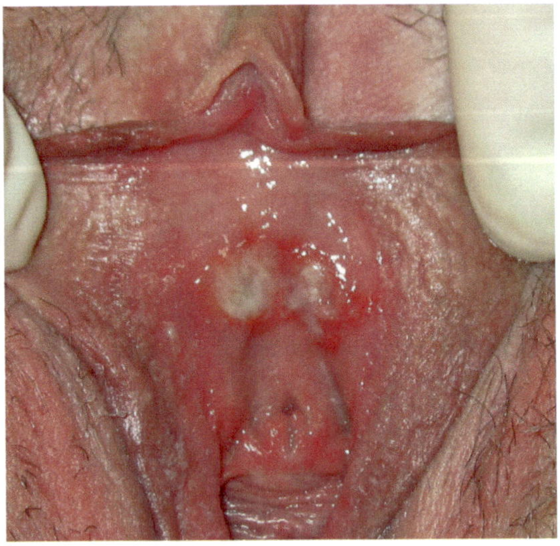

Fig. 18.175 Midline carcinoma of the vulva

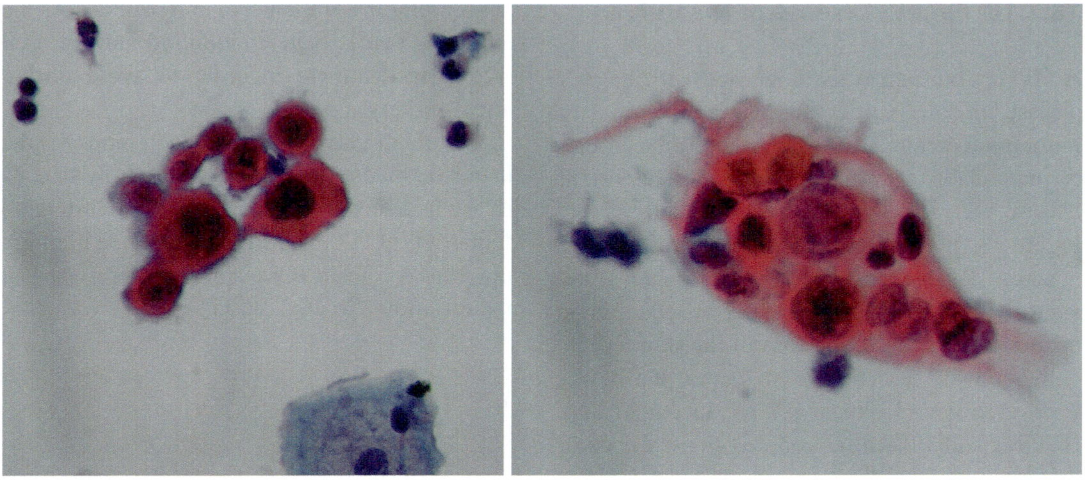

Fig. 18.176 ThinPrep® cytology of vulvar carcinoma. Groups of keratinizing atypical cell with hyperchromatic or enlarged pleomorphic nuclei are seen

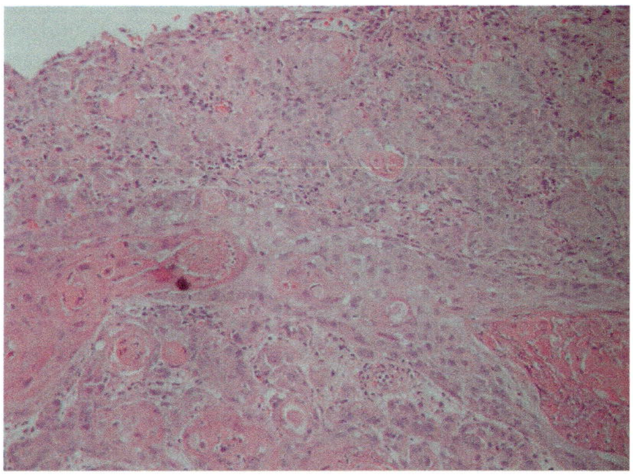

Fig. 18.177 Squamous cell carcinoma of the vulva. The stroma is invaded by well-differentiated keratinizing squamous cell carcinoma

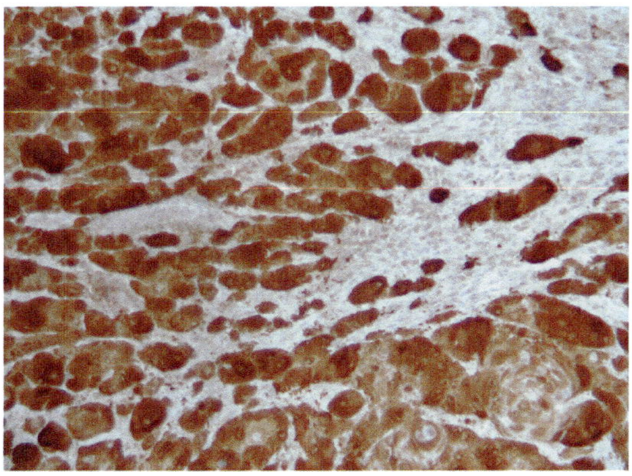

Fig. 18.178 p16 immunostaining in vulvar carcinoma. Cancer cells invading the stroma are all p16 positive

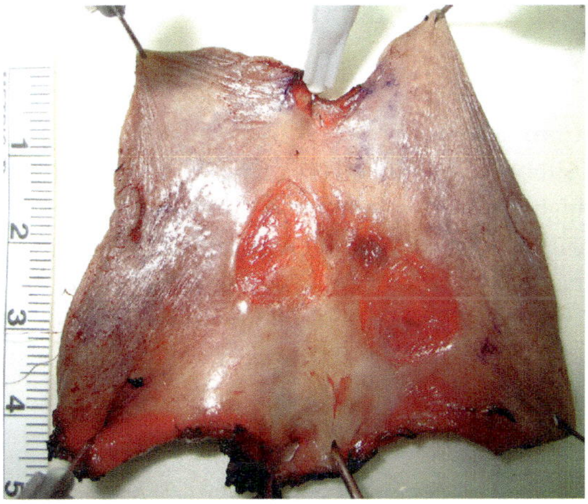

Fig. 18.179 The vulvar carcinoma was removed with a resection margin of 1.5–2 cm. The clitoris could be preserved. The distal part of the urethra has been removed

18.7.18 Paget's Disease of the Vulva

A 60-year-old patient is diagnosed with Paget's disease of the vulva. Topical application of imiquimod cream is chosen as the primary treatment modality. However, because of persistent disease, surgical resection is eventually done. Figure 18.180 shows the macroscopically visible extent of Paget's disease. On the left side of the vagina, there is a 7 × 7 cm area of leukoplakia mixed with small excoriations of the skin.

After wide resection of this area, the defect is covered with a gluteal VY advancement flap. Histologically, the resection margins are free of disease.

The so-called Paget cells within the squamous epithelium can be seen both cytologically using a Rovers Vulvar Sampler® (van den Einden et al. 2012; Fig. 18.181) as well as histologically (Fig. 18.182).

Commentary

Although imiquimod cream has been found to be highly effective in Paget's disease of the vulva, surgical resection is preferable as primary treatment, as invasive disease has to be ruled out. Fanning et al. (1999) found invasive Paget's disease in 12 of the 100 patients examined and also adenocarcinoma of the vulva in 4 patients. As the recurrence rate is high, imiquimod may be used for further treatment in order to avoid further radical surgery.

As with all vulvar lesions, punch biopsy is the diagnostic method of choice. Only rarely Paget's disease is detected by cytopathology (Castellano Megias et al. 2002). However, cytopathology may play a role in the event of a rare cervical manifestation (Gu et al. 2005).

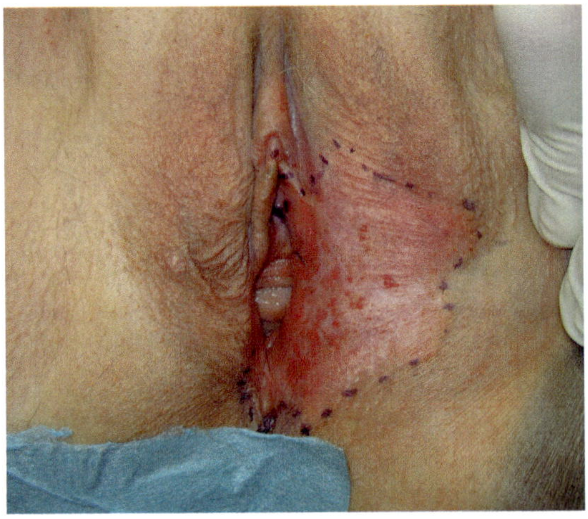

Fig. 18.180 Paget's disease of the vulva. The skin of the left introitus shows numerous small excoriations as well as discrete leukoplakia

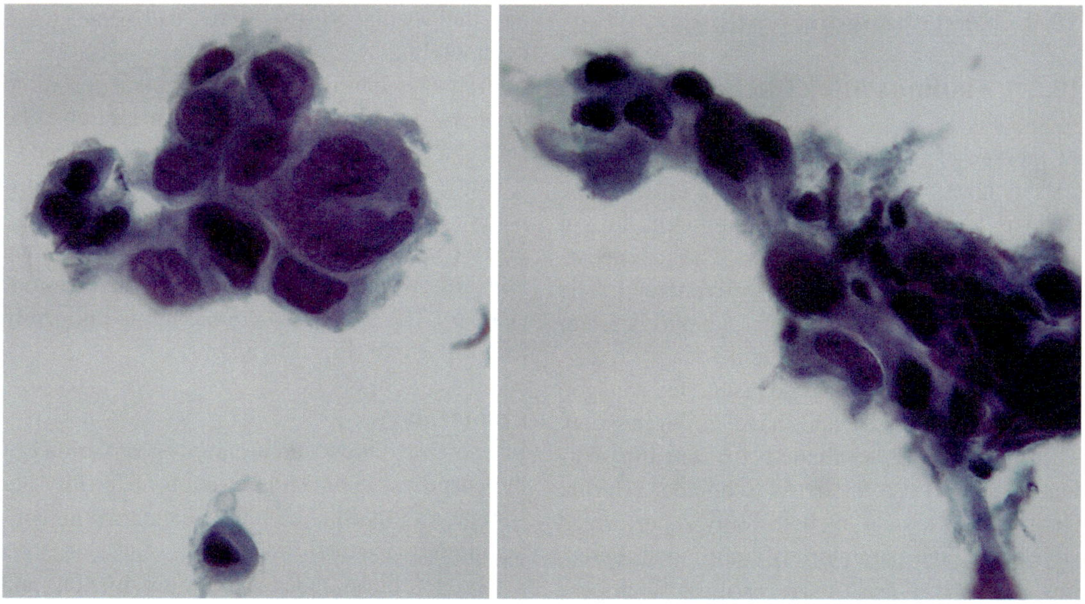

Fig. 18.181 ThinPrep® cytology of Paget's disease of the vulva. The direct swab was taken using a Rovers Vulvar Sampler®. Groups of atypical pleomorphic cells with high N/C ratio are seen

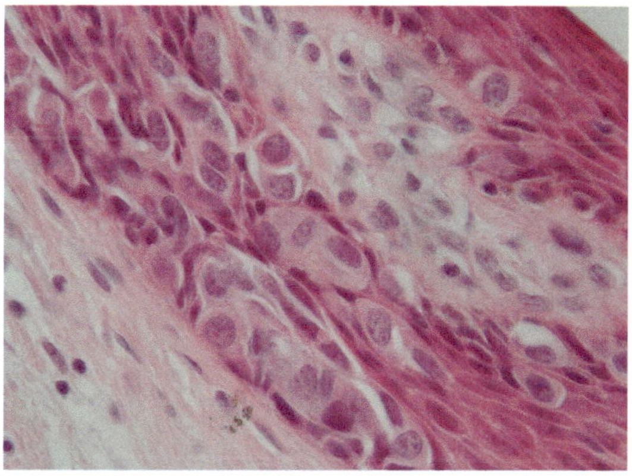

Fig. 18.182 Paget's disease of the vulva. Large round Paget cells are seen with pale cytoplasm within the basal layers of the epidermis

18.8 Miscellaneous Findings

18.8.1 Findings After Trachelectomy

At the age of 29, the nulligravid patient undergoes conization. Surprisingly, not only HSIL/CIN3 is found but also adenocarcinoma in situ and invasive adenocarcinoma. The adenocarcinoma is described as well differentiated. The horizontal extension of the invasive part is 3 mm with a depth of invasion of 2 mm.

At the time, the patient had just gotten engaged and wants to marry and have children soon. Therefore, she is evaluated for fertility-sparing surgery by Professor A. Schneider (Berlin, Germany). A radical trachelectomy is performed with pelvic and parametrial lymph node dissection. No further preinvasive or invasive disease is found in the uterus, and the lymph nodes are not involved.

Three months after trachelectomy, she presents to the colposcopy clinic for the first follow-up exam. In the upper vagina, there is a flat cervix-like structure. Within the ventral left quadrant, the tissue is acetowhite with regular punctation (minor change) (Fig. 18.183).

A biopsy from this area is normal, and the ThinPrep® Pap smear is classified as NILM. The HPV test (HC2) is negative.

One year after trachelectomy, the patient is 15 weeks pregnant (Fig. 18.184). In the 12th week of pregnancy, cerclage had been performed, and the opening to the uterus had been closed completely.

At the beginning of the 40th week of gestation, the baby is delivered by cesarean section. The cerclage is removed, and the cervix is reopened.

Another 11 months later, colposcopy examination shows ectocervix-like tissue protruding into the vagina. A circular area of glandular tissue is visible which reacts to the acetic acid (minor change). The squamous epithelium is uniformly Lugol-positive (Fig. 18.185).

Commentary

In cervical adenocarcinoma, preservation of the corpus uteri and preservation of fertility are sometimes possible. Usually, treatment with conization only is not sufficient.

By definition, adenocarcinoma in situ and invasive adenocarcinoma originate within or close to the endocervical canal. Therefore, special care must be taken to completely remove the lesion proximally when doing a trachelectomy. In the trachelectomy series presented by Hertel et al. (2006), 31% of patients had adenocarcinomas, and three out of four patients with recurrence had cervical adenocarcinoma.

Furthermore, follow-up exams for glandular cervical neoplasms can be a challenge as cytopathology may be less reliable. In the present scenario, the negative HPV test is the most reliable indicator that the patient is free of recurrence (Costa et al. 2007).

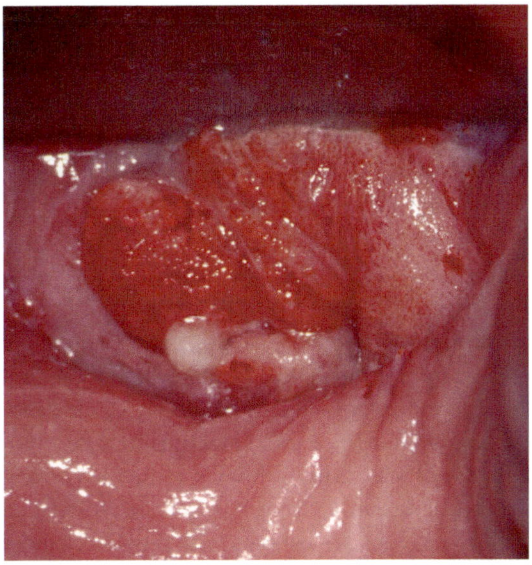

Fig. 18.183 Distal vagina 3 months after successful treatment for adenocarcinoma of the cervix by radical trachelectomy

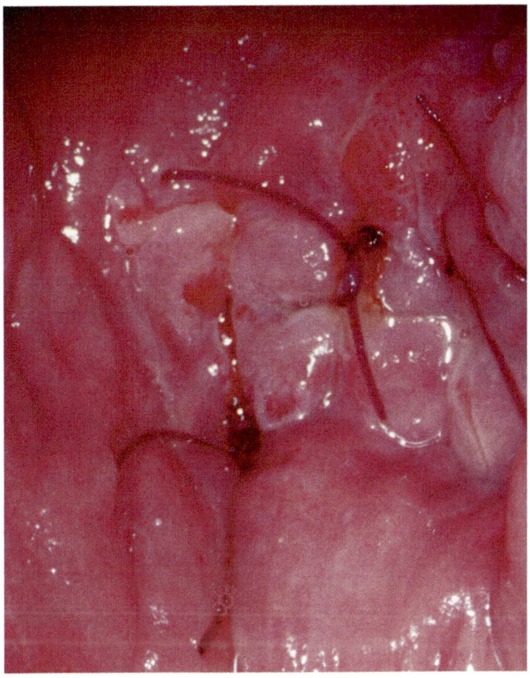

Fig. 18.184 One year after trachelectomy, the patient is 15 weeks pregnant. The opening of the uterus has been closed by cerclage

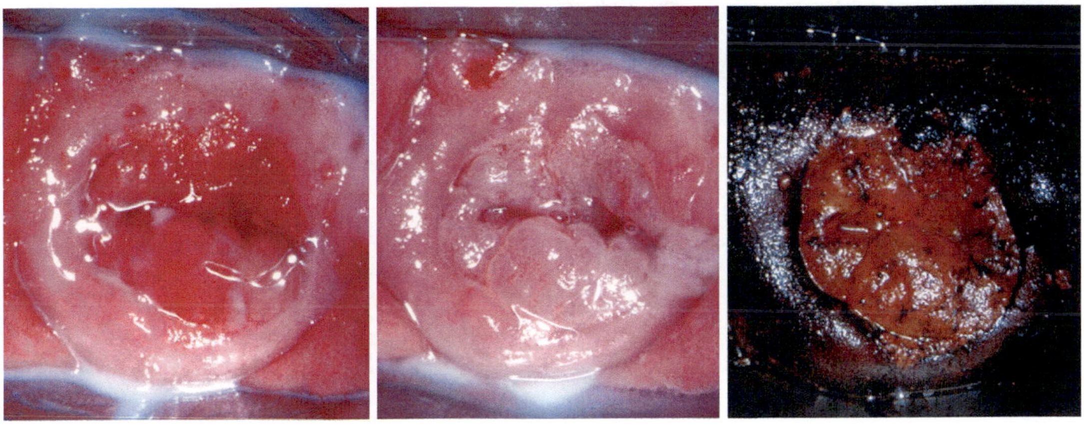

Fig. 18.185 Eleven months after cesarean section and prior trachelectomy for invasive adenocarcinoma of the cervix

18.8.2 Radiation-Induced Changes of the Vagina

A 37-year-old patient underwent a radical hysterectomy 5 years ago for a 5 cm keratinizing squamous cell carcinoma of the cervix (FIGO stage IB3). Pelvic lymph nodes were not involved. At the time, brachytherapy of the vagina was deemed appropriate due to the large tumor mass. A total dose of 21 Gy of iridium was administered in three fractions.

The colposcopy exam of the upper vagina shows a thin and translucent epithelium with numerous prominent vessels with strong variations in size. However, these vessels are not atypical (Fig. 18.186).

On the inner aspect of the left labium minus as well as on the vaginal wall, vascular changes are even more pronounced with dilated corkscrew-shaped capillaries (Fig. 18.187).

The ThinPrep® Pap smear from the vagina is interpreted as ASC-US with HPV-induced cell changes. The Hybrid capture II test is HPV high-risk DNA positive.

Postoperatively, HPV testing (HC2) had been done multiple times. Five months and 17 months after initial surgery, the HPV test had been negative. After 25 months, the HPV test was positive again.

Commentary

Clinically and cytologically there is no suspicion of recurrence. A histological biopsy is therefore not required. Minor and sometimes major cytological abnormalities following radiation therapy are not unusual. Cytology is not an established follow-up exam for patients with previous cancer of the cervix.

The significance of a positive HPV test result during follow-up is also unclear.

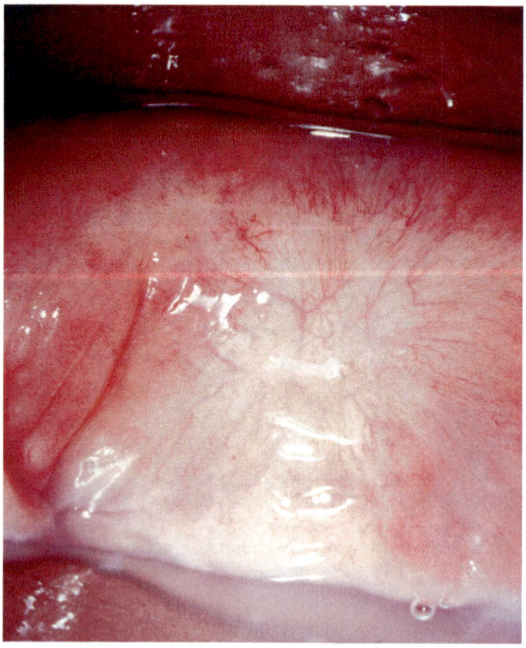

Fig. 18.186 A 37-year-old patient 5 years after radical hysterectomy and postoperative brachytherapy with radiation-induced vascular changes of the distal vagina

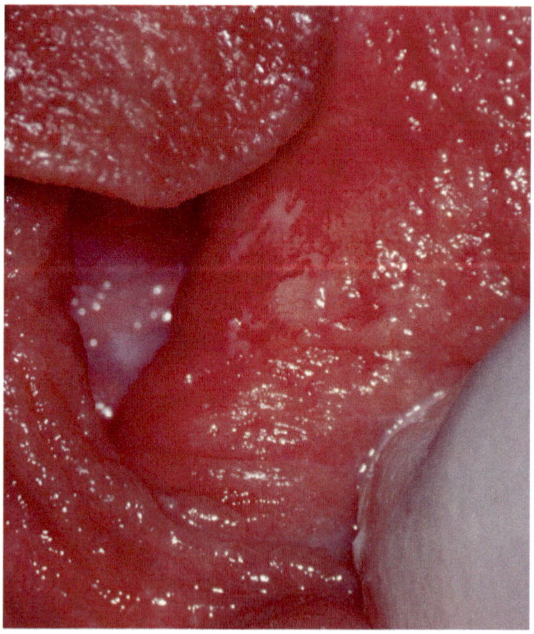

Fig. 18.187 Vascular changes of the vulvar introitus 5 years after brachytherapy

18.8.3 Bicornuate and Bicollis Uterus

The patient is 32 years old. So far, she has not tried to conceive. A routine speculum exam reveals a vaginal septum reaching the middle one third of the vagina. In the upper vagina, two small equal-sized cervices are visible (Figs. 18.188 and 18.189).

Pap smears are obtained separately from the right and left cervix, both classified as NILM. The HPV test (HC2) is negative.

Commentary

This malformation of the uterus is called Uterus bicornis et bicollis. When diagnosed, each cervix should be evaluated independently. Pinto et al. (2004) described the synchronous development of high-grade cervical dysplasia in a patient with a double cervix. Different types of HPV were identified: HPV 33 on one cervix and HPV 35 on the other.

According to Zong et al. (2019), patients with genital tract malformations, especially when associated with urinary malformations, are at an increased risk to develop adenocarcinoma of the cervix and/or vagina.

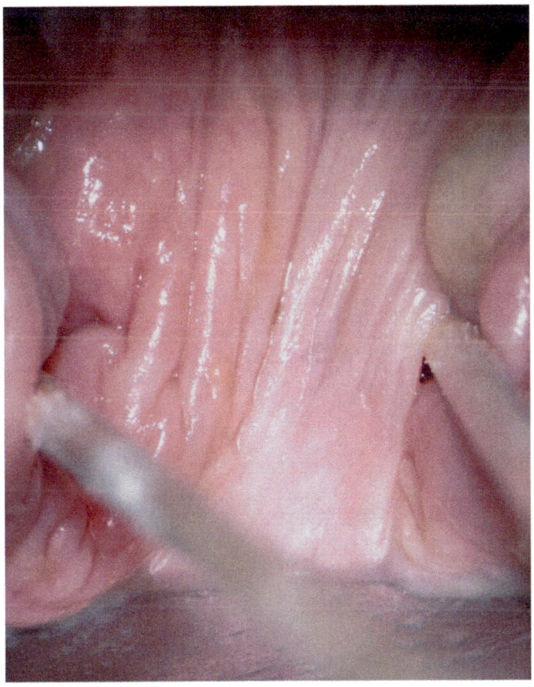

Fig. 18.188 Uterus bicornis et bicollis. The two cervices are marked by cotton swabs

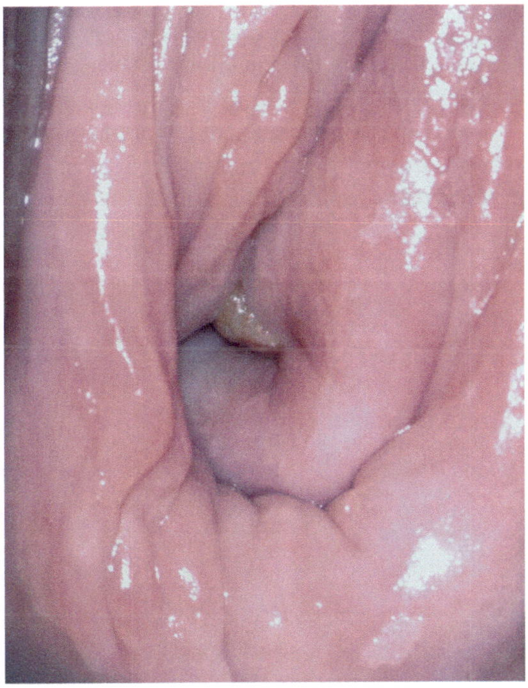

Fig. 18.189 Uterus bicornis et bicollis. One of the two cervices is visualized colposcopically

18.8.4 Colposcopic Triage of Irradiation-Induced Tissue Changes

A 78-year-old patient suffered from cancer of the urinary bladder 24 years ago. Transurethral resection had been followed by telecobalt irradiation. Five years earlier, the right kidney and ureter had been removed for urothelial carcinoma. At the same time, uterus and bladder were resected, again followed by radiation therapy. In the following years, her gynecologist continued to obtain Pap smears the vagina. These were from classified as ASC-US suspecting "radiation dysplasia."

Repeatedly, she has developed a suburethral ulcer. A Pap smear from this lesion is classified as suspicious for squamous cell carcinoma (Fig. 18.190).

The colposcopic examination of the vagina shows atrophic epithelium without evidence of recurrent disease (Fig. 18.191). A tissue sample from the upper vagina is also normal (Fig. 18.192).

Commentary

Cervical cytopathology, which has been originally developed by Papanicolaou (Pap test), should be used for screening of cancer of the cervix and its high-risk precursors. Other indications are less clear and may be misleading either through underdiagnosis, for example, of vulvar lesions, or overdiagnosis as is the case in the present scenario. The pelvic area had been irradiated twice. Therefore, the likelihood of a false-positive Pap test is very high, as cellular radiation changes can not be distinguished reliably from cancer. Also, early diagnosis of recurrent disease can not be achieved through cytopathology.

If despite all of this a Pap smear were obtained and were abnormal (ASC-US or higher), colposcopy and targeted biopsy are suitable for clarification of the diagnosis.

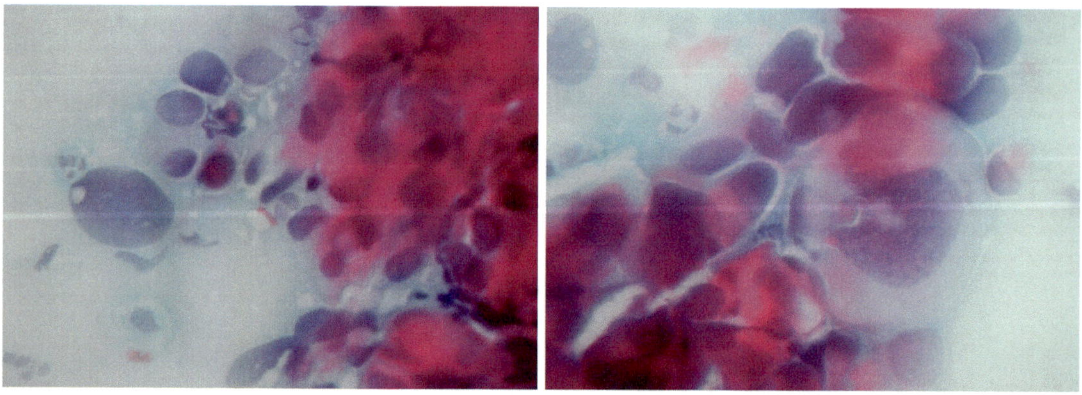

Fig. 18.190 Pap smear from a suburethral ulcer after radiation therapy. The nuclei are significantly enlarged with anisokaryosis and pleomorphism. The chromatin structure is blurred due to degenerative changes. As the background suggests tumor diathesis, the Pap smear was classified as suspicious for squamous cell carcinoma. (With kind permission of Dr. Jürgen Schulz, Osnabrück, Germany)

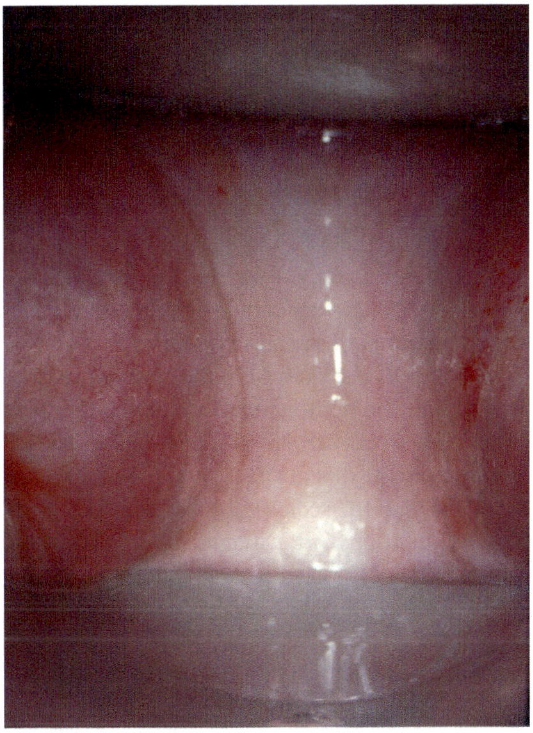

Fig. 18.191 After a Pap smear result suggesting squamous cell carcinoma, colposcopy is done. The upper vagina is atrophic without any tissue defects. On the right side of the image, there is a small tear of the epithelium due to stretching of the vagina with the speculum

Fig. 18.192 The tissue sample of the vagina at the time of colposcopy shows atrophic but normal squamous epithelium otherwise

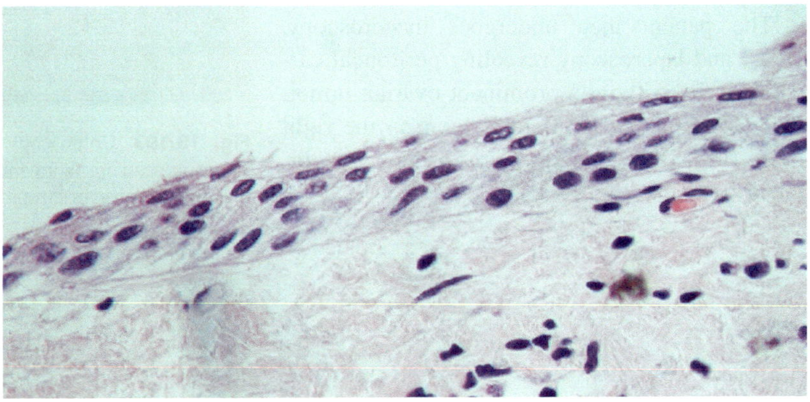

18.8.5 Advanced Ovarian Carcinoma Misdiagnosed as CIN

The routine Pap smear from a 53-year-old patient is positive for HSIL/CIN3. Conization is done without prior colposcopy. The histopathology report comes back negative for cervical dysplasia. Subsequently, the Pap test is still positive (ASC-US), and 6 months after conization the patient is referred to the colposcopy clinic.

The cervix has significant scarring from the previous surgery, and there is minor bleeding from the atrophic epithelium.

- Adequate colposcopy
- Squamocolumnar junction not visible
- T3
- Normal findings: atrophy and scarring Fig. 18.193

The cytological smear (ThinPrep®) shows abnormal glandular cells, which are suspicious for invasive disease, possibly originating from endometrial or ovarian neoplasm (Fig. 18.194). The Hybrid capture II test is negative for HPV high-risk DNA.

The patient then undergoes hysteroscopy, D&C, and laparoscopy revealing peritoneal carcinomatosis without a prominent ovarian tumor. A small peritoneal implant is seen on the right ovary (Fig. 18.195), and there is ascites containing tumor cells (Fig. 18.196).

In the course of the subsequent radical tumor surgery, further tumor deposits on the right diaphragm are identified and removed. The final diagnosis is high-grade serous carcinoma of the peritoneum, FIGO stage IIIB.

Commentary

Nwanodi et al. (2008) report on 24 patients with abnormal cervical cytology leading to the diagnosis of ovarian cancer and another five cases with carcinoma of the peritoneum.

When cells are shed from the endometrium or from inside the peritoneum through the fallopian tubes, they frequently show degenerative changes that complicate diagnosis.

In the present scenario, conization had been done without any prior diagnostic investigation, which is clearly not acceptable any more.

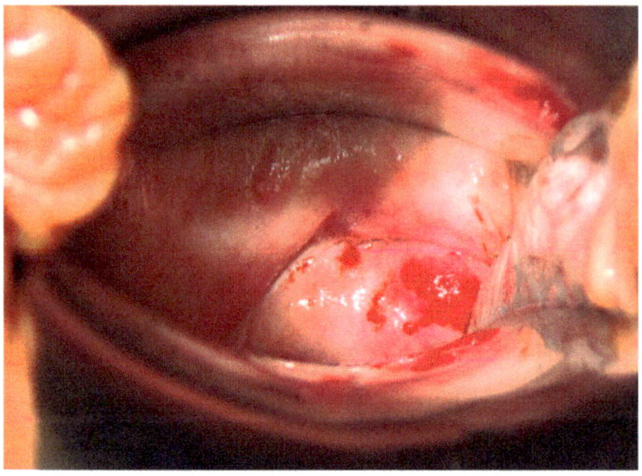

Fig. 18.193 Colposcopy 6 months after conization. There is scarring from the previous surgery and minor bleeding because of atrophy

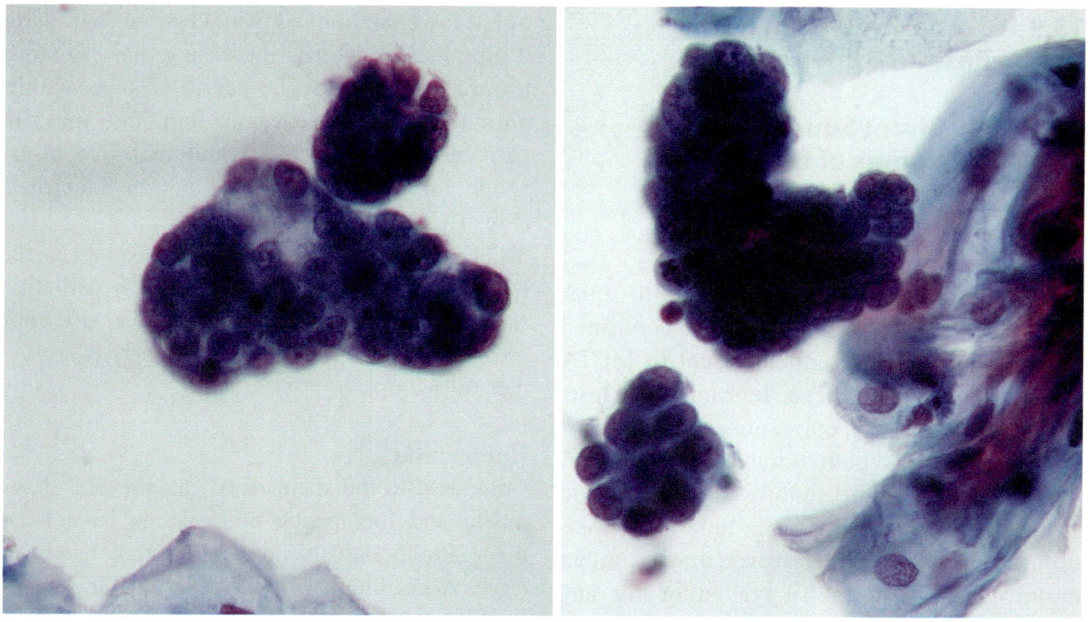

Fig. 18.194 ThinPrep® Pap smear indicating glandular carcinoma originating either from the endometrium or the ovary. Three-dimensional cell clusters are seen with so-called common borders or community borders

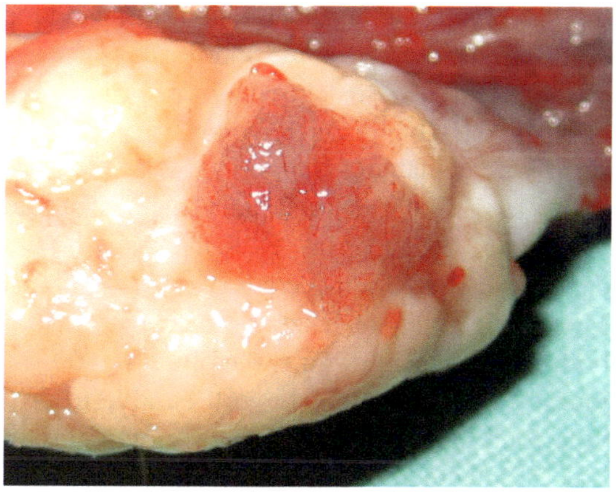

Fig. 18.195 The right ovary shows a small tumor implant which is ultimately diagnosed as high-grade serous carcinoma of the peritoneum

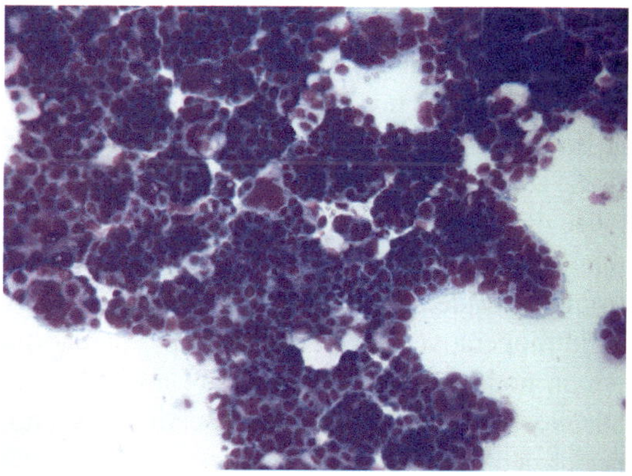

Fig. 18.196 Cytopathology of ascites in high-grade serous carcinoma of the peritoneum. Morphology is similar to the cell clusters found in the cervical smear (Fig. 18.194)

18.9 Scenarios Within a Low-Resource Environment

18.9.1 Recurrent Squamous Cell Carcinoma of the Cervix 19 Months After Limited Radical Surgery

A 52-year-old patient is diagnosed with squamous cell carcinoma of the cervix confirmed by biopsy. She is subsequently sent to META Referral Hospital in Mbeya, Tanzania. HIV tests are negative. On clinical exam, a large cervical mass invades both parametria. However, the uterus is still are mobile, and the pelvic sidewalls not involved, so the tumor is classified as FIGO stage IIB. However, due to limited resources, no intravenous pyelogram nor any other imaging studies are performed to rule out hydronephrosis.

Exploratory laparotomy through a lower midline incision is done and a modified radical hysterectomy with bilateral salpingo-oophorectomy performed (Figs. 18.197 and 18.198). Intraoperatively, no hydronephrosis is present. A double ureter is identified on the right side (Fig. 18.199). The cervix is enlarged to about twice the size of the corpus of the uterus with the tumor growing within the cervix and extending it from the inside.

Intraoperatively, pelvic and paraaortic lymph nodes are palpated and are not enlarged. Diagnostic lymph node dissection is not performed.

The patient returns to META Referral Hospital for regular follow-up exams and is doing well 19 months later she is complaining of left lower abdominal pain. Over the following 2 months, the pain is increasing and radiating toward the left leg. The pelvic exam is within normal limits. However, an immobile mass is palpable in the left lower abdomen. On ultrasound, an 11 x 9 cm complex mass is identified (Fig. 18.200).

The patient is referred to Ocean Road Cancer Institute (ORCI) in Dar es Salaam for palliative radiation therapy. However, the patient does not present at the cancer hospital and there is no further follow-up.

Commentary

Compared to the standard of care, several diagnostic and therapeutic concessions have been made. Preoperatively, no imaging study had been done. According to FIGO rules, an intravenous pyelogram needs to be obtained to rule out stage IIIB disease. Furthermore, no lymph node dissection was performed. As it was highly unlikely at the time of the procedure that the patient would be able to obtain adjuvant radiation therapy in the event of positive nodes, the additional morbidity of lymph node dissection could not be justified. For example, no bipolar electrocautery for hemostasis was available.

In Tanzania, Ocean Road Cancer Institute in the capital city of Dar es Salaam is the only cancer hospital in the country. Patients from Mbeya in Tanzania need to be able to afford both travel expenses for the more than 800 km journey and someone who will be able to provide food and housing for the 3-month stay in Dar es Salaam.

The patient developed a large recurrence, most likely from a lymph node recurrence.

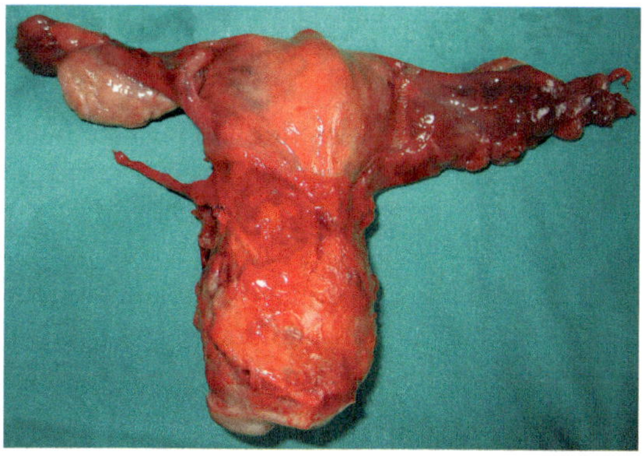

Fig. 18.197 Squamous cell carcinoma of the cervix FIGO stage IIB. The hysterectomy specimen shows a massively enlarged cervix which is about twice the size of the corpus of the uterus. Clinically, the tumor invades both parametria but does not reach the pelvic sidewall

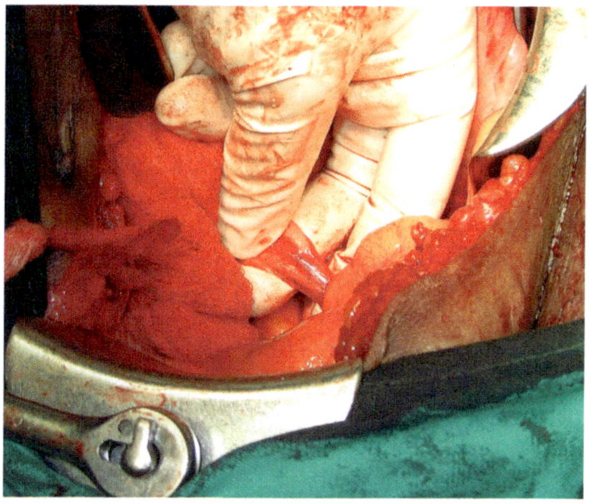

Fig. 18.199 No preoperative imaging has been done. Intraoperatively, a double ureter is identified on the left side

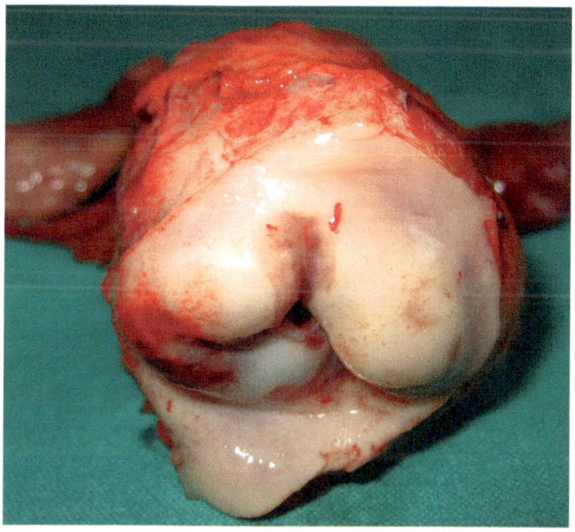

Fig. 18.198 Squamous cell carcinoma of the cervix FIGO stage IIB. Part of the vagina has been removed. The tumor is located mostly within the cervix

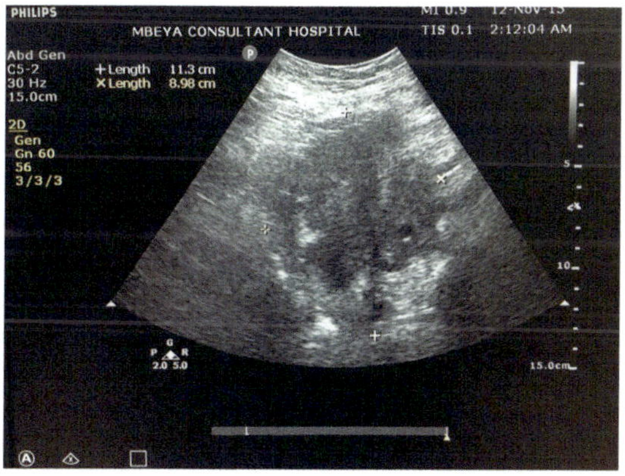

Fig. 18.200 Nineteen months after limited radical surgery, an 11 x 9 cm mass is identified in the left lower abdomen

18.9.2 Advanced-Stage Carcinoma of the Vulva in a 29-Year-Old HIV-Positive Patient

A 29-year-old patient presents to Matema Lutheran Hospital in the south of Tanzania with soft tissue destruction of almost the entire vulva (Fig. 18.201). The anterior sphincter is involved. However, the patient does not complain of stool incontinence. The urethra is still intact. Peripherally, there is wart-like thickening of the skin especially at the remaining perineum and around the anus.

The patient suffers from AIDS with a very low CD4 count of 156 cells/ul. Biopsy confirms squamous cell carcinoma of the vulva. Due to advanced-stage disease, only palliative treatment can be offered.

Commentary

The young patient had surprisingly few symptoms despite almost complete destruction of the soft tissue of the vulva. As she is severely immunocompromised, the differential diagnosis includes infectious gangrene such as streptococcal gangrene or gangrenous cellulitis (Brook 2008); the clinical picture does not reveal any inflammatory signs. Furthermore, the surrounding tissue suggests HPV-related vulvar intraepithelial neoplasia.

The emergence of anterior midline carcinoma of the vulva in young women has been reported in Germany (Hampl et al. 2008). In addition, a cluster of VIN as well as vulvar carcinoma has been identified in Australian indigenous women (Condon et al. 2009); no increase in vulvar carcinoma in sub-Saharan Africa has yet been reported.

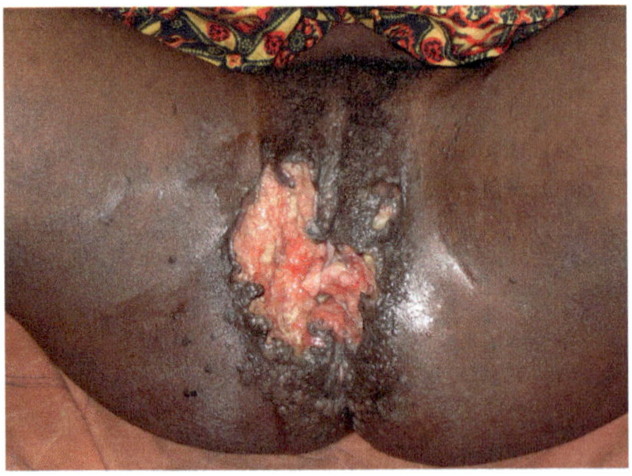

Fig. 18.201 A 29-year-old HIV-positive patient with advanced squamous cell carcinoma of the vulva

18.9.3 Advanced but Operable Adenocarcinoma of the Cervix

A 51-year-old patient presents to META Referral Hospital, Mbeya, Tanzania, with biopsy-confirmed moderately differentiated adenocarcinoma of the cervix. She is HIV negative.

On speculum exam (Fig. 18.202), the cervix is only partially visible as there is abundant bleeding from the cervix. Vaginal and rectal examination shows enlargement of the cervix with an estimated diameter of more than 4 cm. However, the parametrial tissue does not appear to be involved. Despite the fact that no imaging studies are available to rule out ureteral involvement, the cervical cancer is classified as FIGO stage IB2 and seems operable.

A lower midline incision is made and the abdominal cavity explored. On palpation, pelvic and paraaortic lymph nodes are not enlarged. Intraoperatively, there is no evidence of tumor extension beyond the cervix. A radical hysterectomy and bilateral salpingo-oophorectomy are performed (Fig. 18.203). On macroscopic inspection of the surgical specimen (Figs. 18.204 and 18.205), the extent of the cervical tumor becomes visible: there is a large exophytic mass protruding from the ventral aspect of the cervix, whereas the posterior cervix is free of disease. The tumor tissue extends into the distal half of the cervical canal.

Cytopathology points toward a glandular origin of the cancer (Figs. 18.206 and 18.207) and is confirmed by histopathology (Figs. 18.208 and 18.209).

Commentary

Approximately 10–20% of cervical carcinomas arise from glandular epithelium (Hopkins and Morley 1991a, b; Benedet et al. 2003). The percentage of adenocarcinomas in sub-Saharan Africa or Tanzania is unknown. Definitely, the majority of cervical carcinomas are of the squamous type. In the case presented here, the clinical features are not different from squamous cell carcinoma. The tumor is mostly located on the outside of the cervix with limited extension into the cervical canal (Fig. 18.210).

Management of adenocarcinoma of the cervix is not different from treatment of squamous cell carcinoma. In this case, no lymph node dissection has been performed because at the time it was considered highly unlikely that the patient would be able to receive adjuvant radiation therapy in the event of lymph node involvement. Bilateral salpingo-oophorectomy had also been performed. According to Shimada et al. (2006), ovarian metastases are significantly more likely in patients with cervical adenocarcinoma than patients with squamous cell carcinoma (5.3% versus 0.8%, respectively).

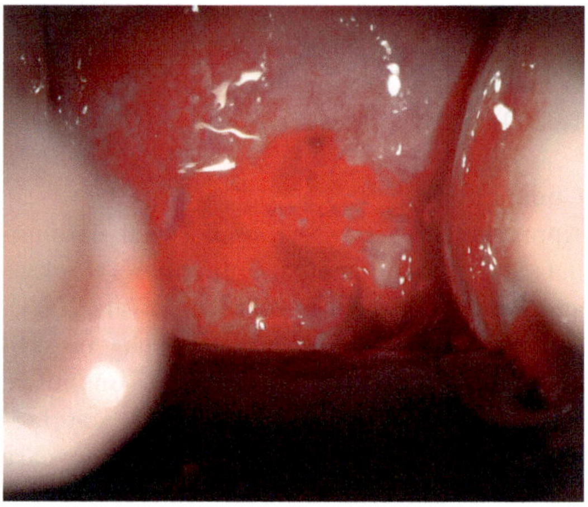

Fig. 18.202 Adenocarcinoma of the cervix. Due to profuse bleeding, the cervix is only partially visible. On colposcopic exam, the surface of the ventral part of the cervix appears is irregular

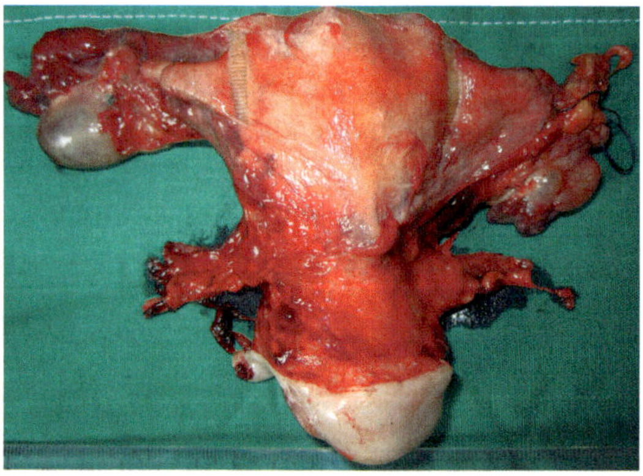

Fig. 18.203 Adenocarcinoma of the cervix. Radical hysterectomy with bilateral salpingo-oophorectomy has been performed and macroscopically the tumor has been removed completely with a sufficient safety margin

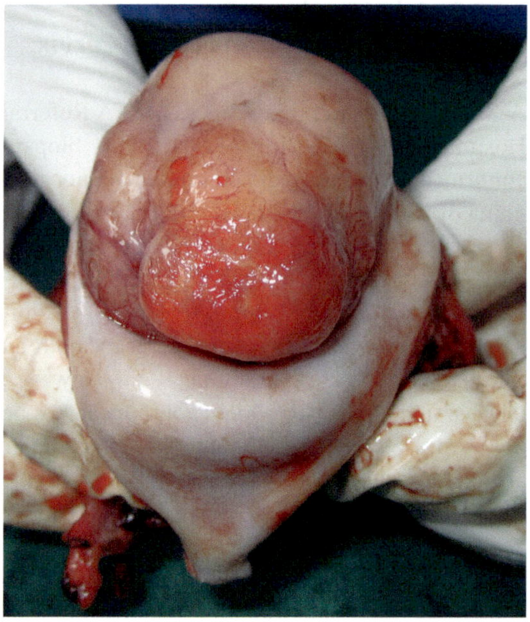

Fig. 18.204 Adenocarcinoma of the cervix. The large tumor is situated at the anterior (ventral) aspect of the cervix

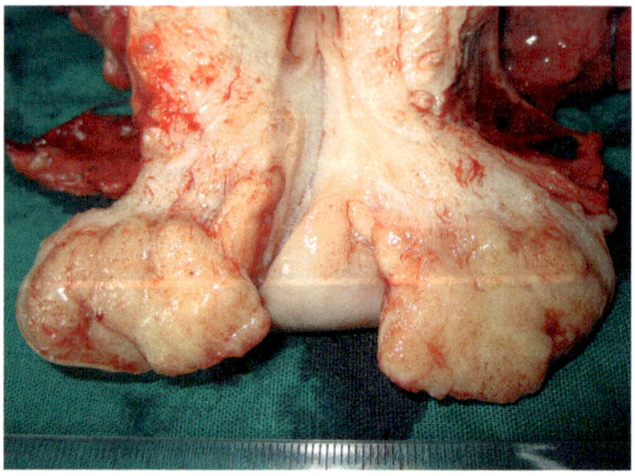

Fig. 18.205 Adenocarcinoma of the cervix. The cervix has been cut longitudinally at the 12 o'clock position. The cervical tumor has well-defined margins and extends into (or arises from) the distal part of the cervical canal. The dorsal part of the cervix appears to be free of disease

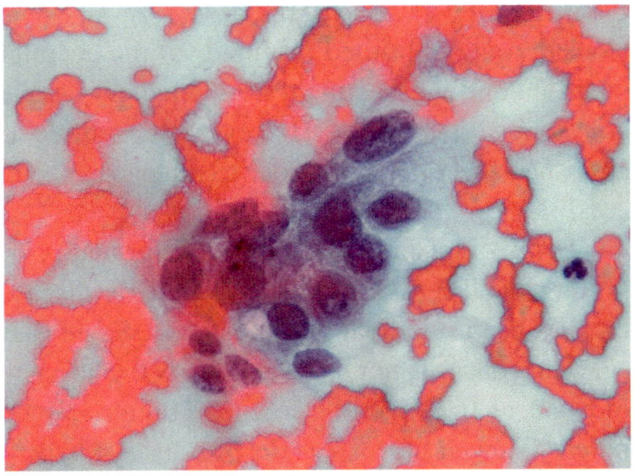

Fig. 18.206 Cytopathology of adenocarcinoma of the cervix. There is a cluster of atypical cells almost devoid of cytoplasm with red blood cells in the background

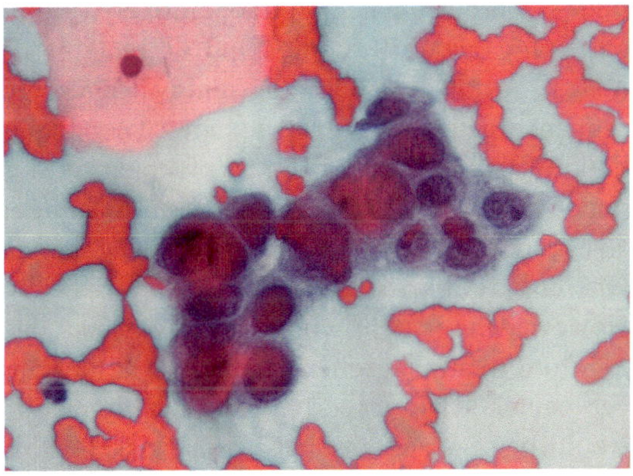

Fig. 18.207 Cytopathology of adenocarcinoma of the cervix. A superficial squamous cell is located in the upper left part of the image. The tumor cells exhibit pronounced variation in size

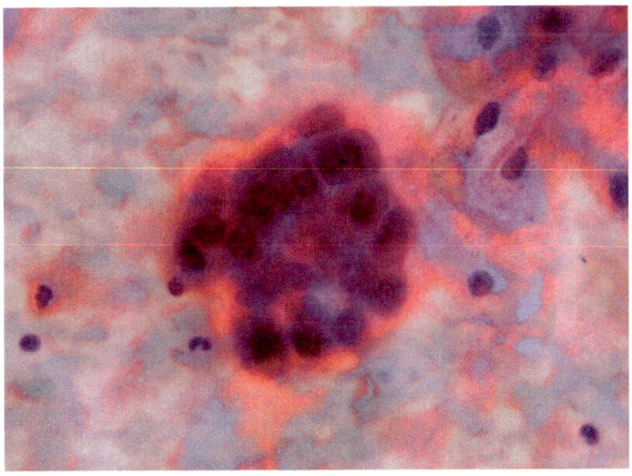

Fig. 18.208 Cytopathology of adenocarcinoma of the cervix. The tumor cells are arranged in a glandular pattern

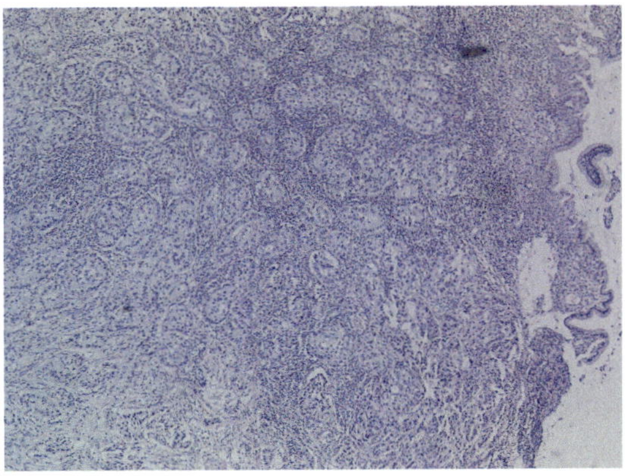

Fig. 18.209 Adenocarcinoma of the cervix. The cervix is infiltrated by a tumor with glandular differentiation

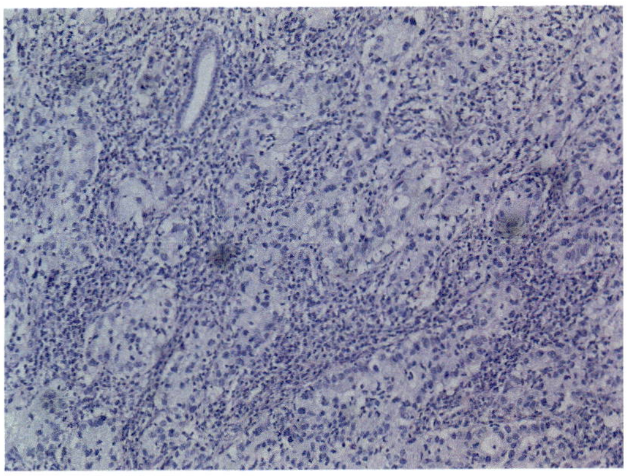

Fig. 18.210 Adenocarcinoma of the cervix. The glandular origin is clearly visible

18.9.4 FIGO Stage IB1 Squamous Cell Carcinoma of the Cervix

A 41-year-old patient presents to META Referral Hospital in Mbeya, Tanzania, with biopsy-confirmed squamous cell carcinoma of the cervix. Her HIV test is positive. On gynecological exam, a friable mass which is bleeding on touch is seen at the anterior and the posterior aspect of the cervix (Figs. 18.211 and 18.212). This lesion is estimated to be less than or equal to 4 cm in diameter. The cancerous growth does not involve the vagina. On transvaginal and transrectal palpation, the parametria are free of disease.

Although no imaging studies are available to evaluate the kidneys and the ureters the tumor is classified as FIGO stage IB1 disease and the patient is scheduled for radical surgery.

An exploratory laparotomy is performed through a lower midline incision. There are no enlarged pelvic or paraaortic lymph nodes. The pararectal and paravesical spaces are opened. No macroscopic tumor involvement is visible. The bladder is then mobilized from the anterior aspect of the cervix. Again, there is no evidence of the tumor extending beyond the cervix. Eventually, a Piver type III (Piver et al. 1974) radical hysterectomy and a bilateral salpingo-oophorectomy are performed (Fig. 18.213).

On macroscopic inspection, the cervical tumor does not reach beyond the confines of the cervix (Fig. 18.214). The Pap smear obtained prior to surgical treatment shows the typical morphology of squamous cell carcinoma (Figs. 18.215 and 18.216).

The patient is discharged on postoperative day 5 without any immediate complications following surgery.

Commentary

Considering the limited resources of the hospital environment, the treatment of this patient can be considered successful. However, several decisions had been made in order to adapt to special conditions:

No imaging studies had been performed prior to surgery. Therefore, FIGO stage IIIB disease had not been ruled out preoperatively. Stage IIIB cervical cancer is not only defined as the absence of a cancer-free space between the tumor and the pelvic sidewall but also as the presence of hydronephrosis or a nonfunctioning kidney (Pecorelli 2009).

No pelvic or paraaortic lymph node dissection had been performed. Although no enlarged nodes were palpated intraoperatively, clinical exam (as well as any kind of imaging of nodes) is not as reliable as removal and subsequent histopathological exam. The likelihood of pelvic lymph node involvement in this patient would be around 23% based on tumor size according to a prospective Gynecologic Oncology Group study (Delgado et al. 1989). However, the patient would not have been able to afford treatment (chemoradiation) at the cancer center. Therefore, lymph node dissection would have posed an unnecessary risk for this particular patient.

Both ovaries have been removed in this 41-year-old patient. Traditionally, organ preservation is not a priority in a country like Tanzania, as there will be only a single opportunity for the patient to receive any kind of surgical treatment. Nevertheless, the probability of ovarian metastases from FIGO stage I or II squamous cell carcinoma of the cervix is low: 0.79% according to Shimada et al. (2006).

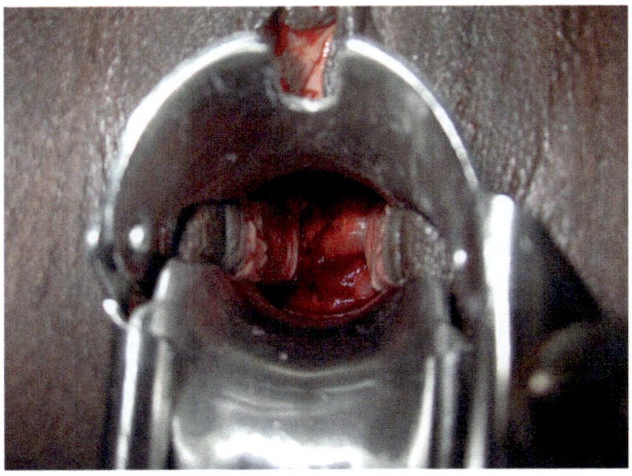

Fig. 18.211 Squamous cell carcinoma of the cervix presenting as an ulceration encompassing most of the cervix, and bleeds upon touch

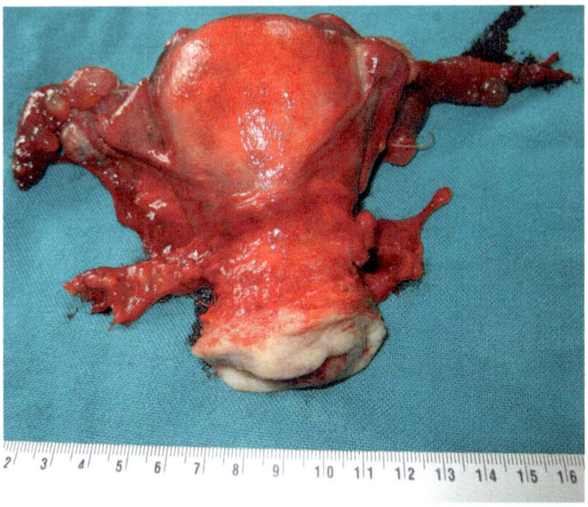

Fig. 18.213 Radical hysterectomy specimen of a Piver class III procedure with transection of the parametria at the pelvic sidewall. Part of the upper vagina has been removed as well as both ovaries and fallopian tubes

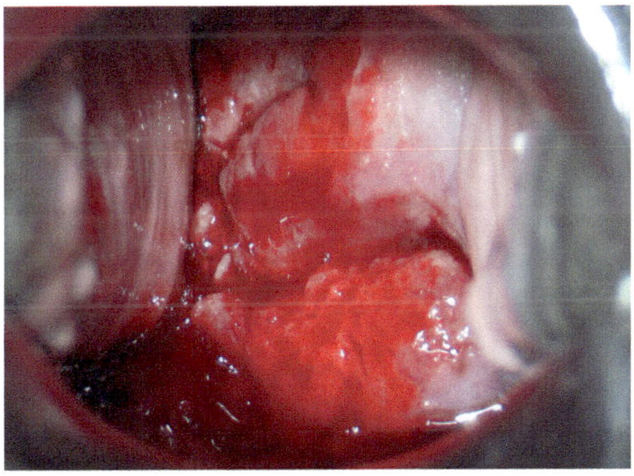

Fig. 18.212 Squamous cell carcinoma of the cervix. Colposcopically, only a small area of the cervix is covered by intact epithelium. Most of the cervix consists of tumor tissue with blood pooling in the posterior speculum

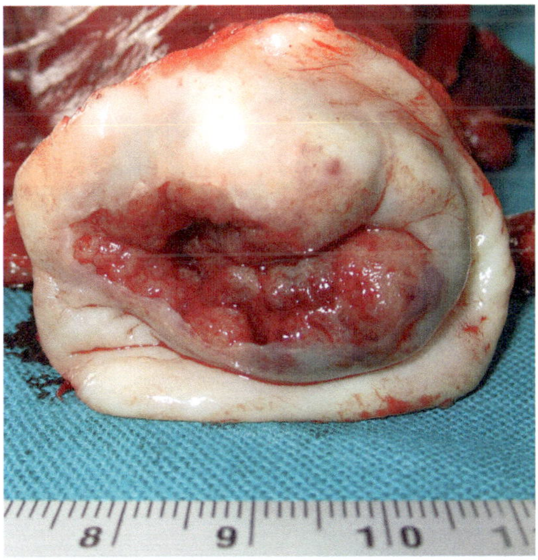

Fig. 18.214 Cervical aspect of the surgical specimen. The cancerous ulceration is limited to the cervix without involvement of the vagina

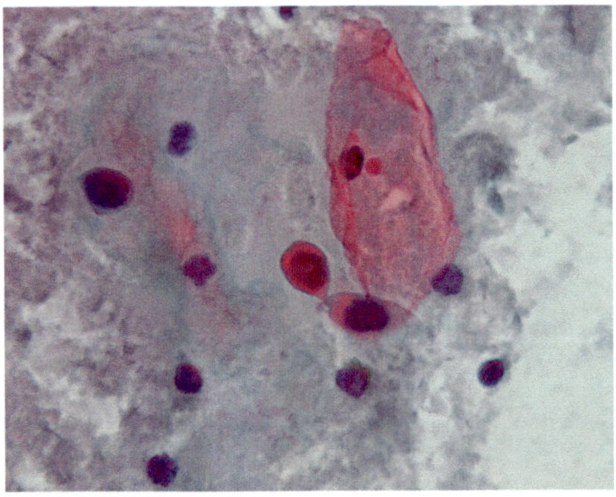

Fig. 18.215 Pap smear from squamous cell carcinoma of the cervix. A large superficial squamous cell is lying next to two tumor cells with enlarged nuclei with only a small rim of cytoplasm remaining. There is dense protein precipitation visible around the cells

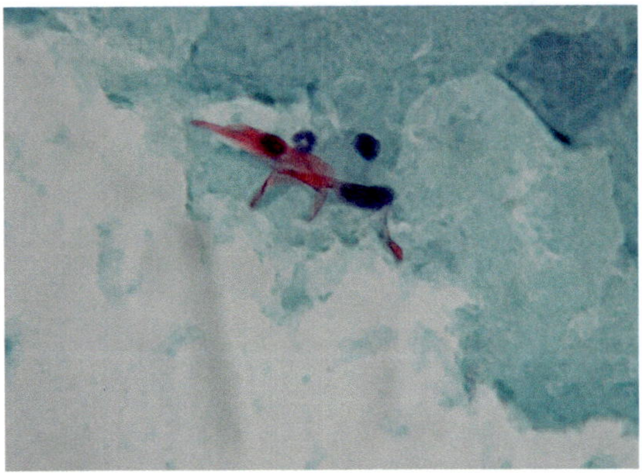

Fig. 18.216 Pap smear from squamous cell carcinoma of the cervix. There are two spindle cells with dense nuclei which are suggestive of keratinizing squamous cell carcinoma. In addition, there is significant protein precipitation in the background

18.9.5 Fifteen Months of Treatment Delay in a Patient with Cancer of the Cervix

A 38-year-old patient had been diagnosed with moderately differentiated squamous cell carcinoma of the cervix 15 months previously in a hospital in the Southern Highlands of Tanzania. At that time, surgical treatment was not considered and the patient was counseled to present to the sole Tanzanian cancer hospital, the Ocean Road Cancer Institute, at the nation's capital, Dar es Salaam, for primary radiation therapy. However, the patient could not afford the travel expenses and did not receive any treatment for the ensuing 15 months. She now presents to META Referral Hospital, Mbeya, Tanzania, and is again evaluated clinically. HIV testing is negative. On clinical exam, there is a cauliflower-like tumor growth visible at the cervix (Fig. 18.217). Both on colposcopy as well as vaginal and rectal exam, the tumor appears to be still limited to the cervix and the cancer is staged as FIGO IB1.

Subsequently, radical hysterectomy and bilateral salpingo-oophorectomy is performed. Macroscopically, the tumor is removed completely and is less than 4 cm in diameter (Figs. 18.218, 18.219, and 18.220), thus confirming the preoperative clinical staging. No enlarged pelvic or paraaortic lymph nodes are palpated. However, there is an enlarged right parametric lymph node, which is removed together with the radical hysterectomy specimen (Fig. 18.221).

Commentary

The vast majority of cervical cancer patients within a low-resource environment such as Tanzania will not receive any medical support. Tragically, the patient and her family could not afford the travel expenses to the cancer hospital and the additional living expenses during their stay in the large city. Thus, the biopsy-confirmed cervical carcinoma remained untreated until the disease was re-evaluated 15 months later. Surprisingly, it was still early-stage disease amenable to surgery. It might have been possible to treat the patient by simple hysterectomy when the cancer had been first diagnosed. However, the circumstances and medical details of the initial diagnosis have remained unclear.

The slow rate of cancer progression in this patient is certainly remarkable. As is the case in most types of cancer, there are no data available on clinical growth rate. Once a patient is diagnosed with cervical cancer, she will usually undergo treatment. However, there are data available on deliberate treatment delay in pregnancy. From a small number of patients ($n = 8$), Duggan et al. (1993) concluded that planned treatment delay in order to achieve fetal maturity appears to be an acceptable option in patients with stage I disease. However, there is no doubt that treatment delay will lead to disease progression in a considerable number of patients (Kantelhardt et al. 2014), thus worsening treatment outcomes.

As the patient's treatment has been compromised by not performing lymphonodectomy and the lack of an adjuvant treatment option in the case of positive parametrial and/or pelvic lymph nodes, the treatment performed might be palliative only.

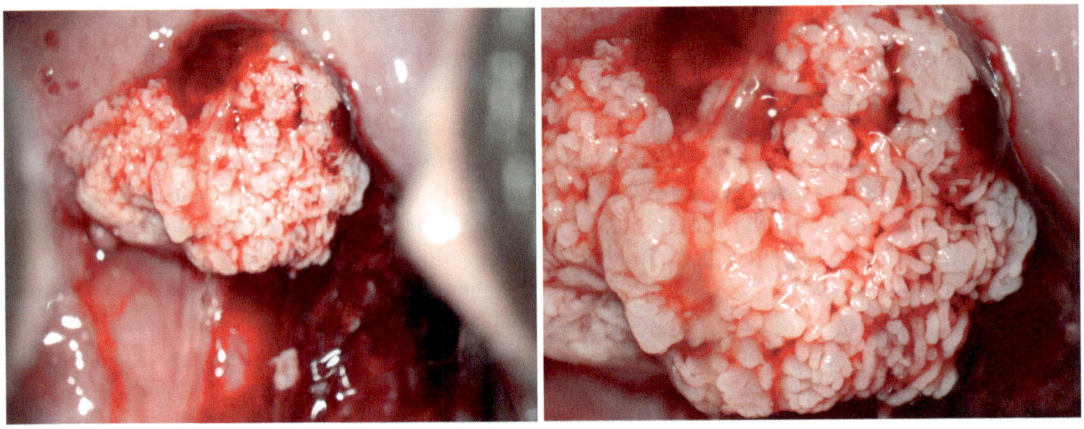

Fig. 18.217 Moderately differentiated squamous cell carcinoma of the cervix. A cauliflower-like exophytic growth extends from the cervix

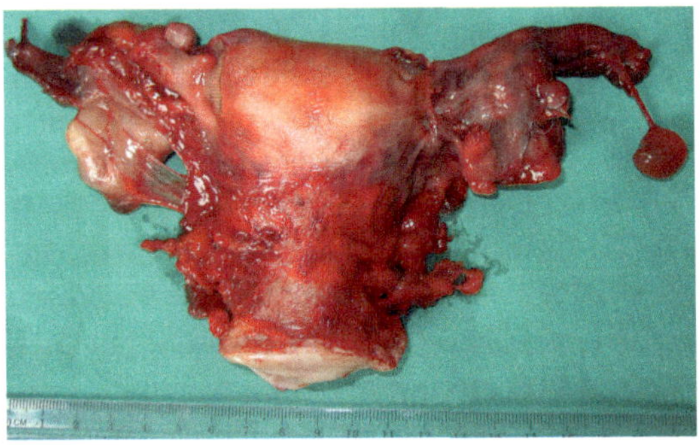

Fig. 18.218 Moderately differentiated squamous cell carcinoma of the cervix. Despite a delay of 15 months between histopathologic diagnosis and reevaluation and treatment, the tumor appears to be still limited to the cervix on the radical hysterectomy specimen (FIGO IB1)

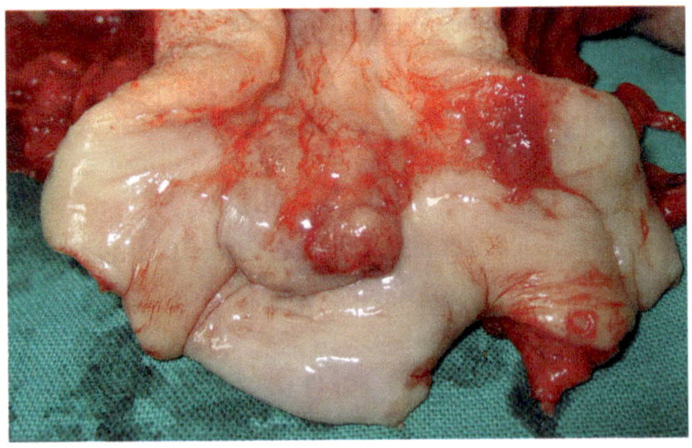

Fig. 18.220 Moderately differentiated squamous cell carcinoma of the cervix. The cervical portion of the radical hysterectomy specimen has been cut longitudinally at the 12 o'clock position. There appears to be only superficial invasion of the cervical tissue

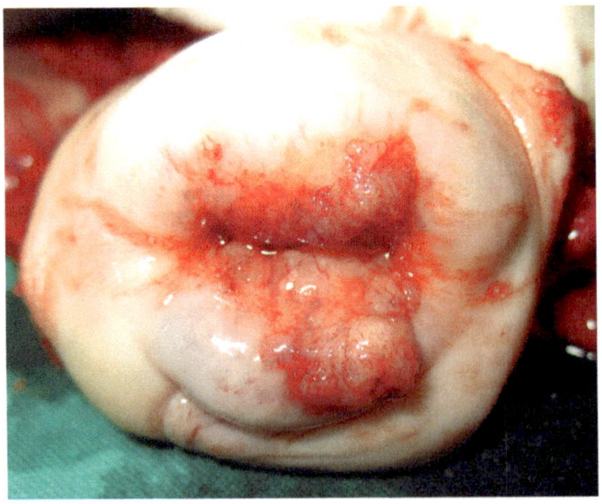

Fig. 18.219 Moderately differentiated squamous cell carcinoma of the cervix. On the surgical specimen, the cauliflower-like lesion seen earlier has collapsed and isha less pronounced. Macroscopically, the resection margins are free of disease

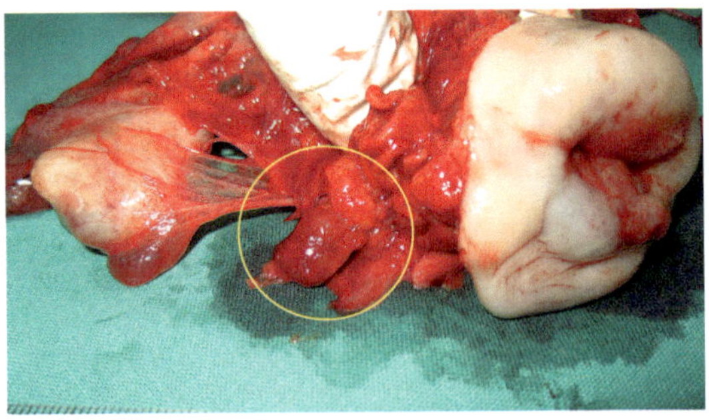

Fig. 18.221 Moderately differentiated squamous cell carcinoma of the cervix. There is a 2 x 3 cm lymph node within the right parametrium. Although no histopathological evaluation is available, parametrial lymph node involvement is possible

18.9.6 Hysterectomy for Suspected HSIL of the Cervix

A 38-year-old patient, P6, presents to META Referral Hospital, Mbeya, Tanzania, for cervical cancer screening. Her HIV status is found to be negative. On visual screening, a large acetowhite area is identified (VIA positive) (Fig. 18.222).

The subsequent colposcopy (Fig. 18.223) shows a slightly raised opaque lesion consistent with major change (grade 2 lesion) encompassing most of the two ventral quadrants of the cervix. The squamocolumnar junction is not visible (T3). The dorsal quadrants are partly involved with small areas of de-epithelization.

- Adequate colposcopy
- Squamocolumnar junction not visible
- T3
- Abnormal colposcopic findings: ventral two quadrants, opaque acetowhite (grade 2); dorsal two quadrants, partly involved with areas of de-epithelization (cannot rule out invasive disease)
  Fig. 18.223

At the time, no biopsy is performed due to limited resources and the very long processing time for surgical specimens of several weeks to several months. The lesion seems to be too large for cryotherapy. In addition, early invasive disease cannot be ruled out. Eventually, the patient opts for hysterectomy. Vaginal hysterectomy is performed (Fig. 18.224), and the patient is discharged on postoperative day 4.

A Pap smear obtained prior to hysterectomy (Figs. 18.225 and 18.226) shows high-grade squamous intraepithelial neoplasia (HSIL). There is no cytological evidence of invasive disease.

Histopathological results of the hysterectomy specimen are not available.

Commentary
Without histopathological evaluation, early invasive cancer cannot be ruled out. Paradoxically, treatment through hysterectomy had been available, whereas histopathology resources were highly limited. If this had not been the case, this kind of clinical management would be considered overtreatment. Also, according to Schockaert et al. (2008), the incidence of subsequent high-grade vaginal intraepithelial neoplasia (VAIN 2+) is as high as 7.4%.

When hysterectomy is performed without preoperative histopathologic evaluation, simple hysterectomy might be considered undertreatment if invasive disease is present and the criteria for FIGO stage IA1 cancer are not met.

Therefore, the above management option must be considered suboptimal and is only justifiable because of special circumstances.

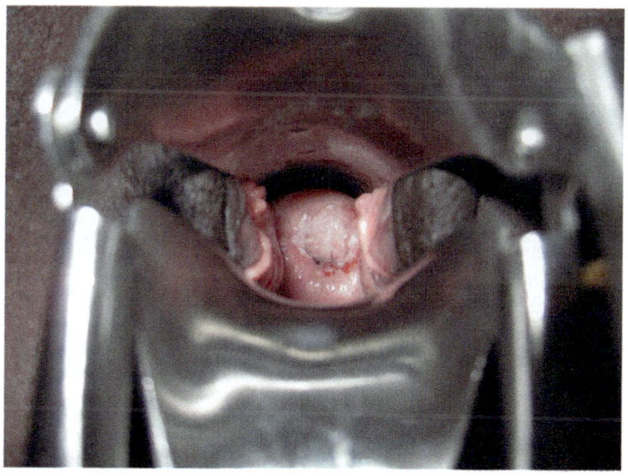

Fig. 18.222 A large acetowhite area is present encompassing most of the ventral quadrants of the cervix (VIA positive)

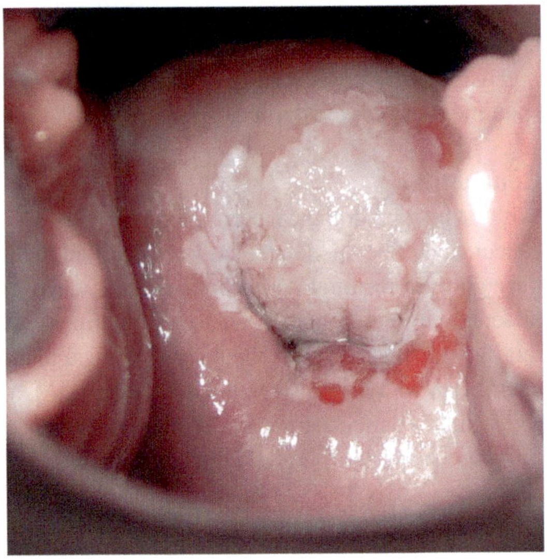

Fig. 18.223 The squamocolumnar junction is not visible (T3). There is a large irregular, opaque, and slightly raised lesion (grade 2) with circumscribed areas of de-epithelization posteriorly, so early invasive disease cannot be ruled out

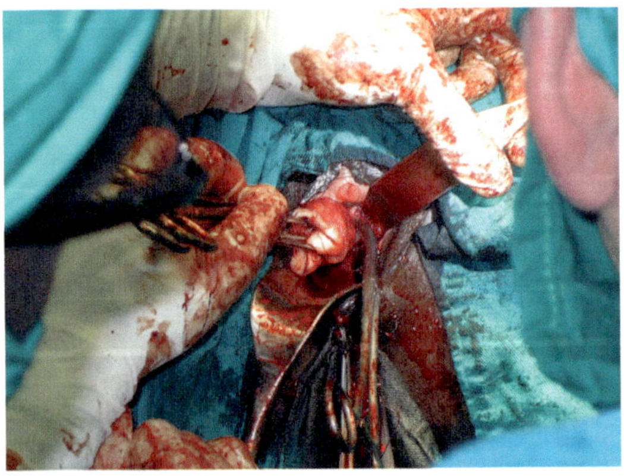

Fig. 18.224 Vaginal hysterectomy is performed for suspected HSIL+ disease without histopathological confirmation

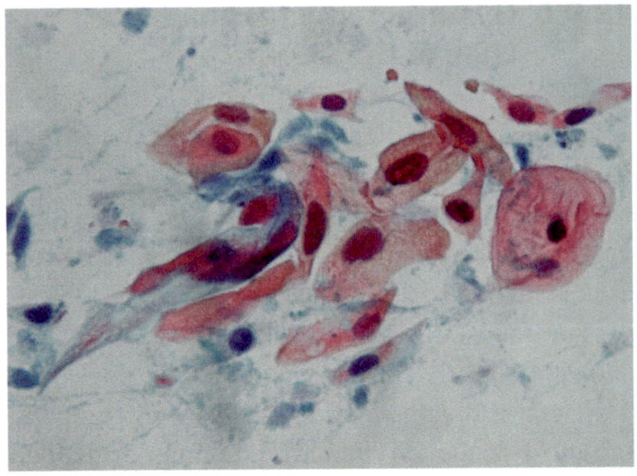

Fig. 18.225 Pap smear with HSIL. With the exception of the small intermediate squamous cell on the left, the nuclei are enlarged, dark (hyperchromatic), and polymorphous

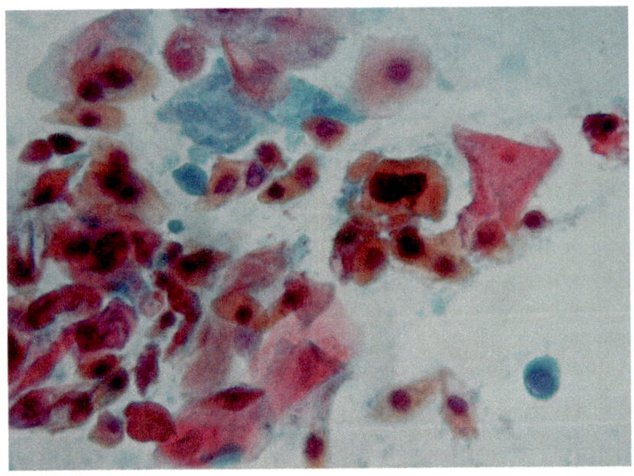

Fig. 18.226 Pap smear with HSIL. The nuclear morphology and the orange-colored stain of some of the abnormal cells suggest keratinization. Tumor diathesis is absent

18.9.7 HSIL of the Cervix and VIN in a 24-Year-Old HIV-Positive Patient

A 24-year-old nulliparous patient has been on medication for HIV infection for 2 years. She has tried to become pregnant, so far without success.

She now presents to META Referral Hospital, Mbeya, Tanzania, for cervical screening. She is found to be VIA positive (Fig. 18.227). Subsequently, colposcopy is performed (Figs. 18.228 and 18.229). The squamocolumnar junction is not visible. In all four quadrants, dense acetowhite areas with raised borders are seen with pronounced irregular mosaic especially of the left ventral and the left dorsal quadrants. According to colposcopic criteria, there is no evidence of invasive disease.

Despite the colposcopic diagnosis of HSIL disease, Pap smear is normal.

- Adequate colposcopy
- Squamocolumnar junction not visible
- T3
- Abnormal colposcopic findings: opaque acetowhite areas involving all four quadrants with irregular mosaic (major change, grade 2)
  Figs. 18.228 and 18.229

In addition to the diagnosis of grade 2 lesions (major change) of the cervix, patchy depigmentation of the vulva can be seen (Fig. 18.230). On closer inspection, there are several areas of leukoplakia and flat wart-like changes on the small labia as well as close to the clitoris (Fig. 18.231). The most likely clinical diagnosis is vulvar intraepithelial neoplasia (VIN).

Due to the large cervical area involved, cryotherapy is not feasible, so LEEP is performed under spinal anesthesia for removal of the cervical lesions (Fig. 18.232).

Commentary

Although no histopathology results are available, the colposcopic findings are typical for both HSIL (CIN3) disease of the cervix and VIN. Surprisingly, the Pap smear taken from this large lesion had been negative, i.e., most likely false negative. This is not surprising as the sensitivity of routine cytology for the detection of HSIL is less than 50%: 43.5% according to a study by Petry et al. (2003).

LEEP surgery had been done under spinal anesthesia. Although loop resections of the cervix can be performed under local anesthesia, it may be advisable to use spinal anesthesia if extensive cervical resections are required as in the case presented here, in order to reduce the patient's discomfort.

The treatment of vulvar intraepithelial disease, especially when it is located close to the clitoris, is a major challenge, when no CO_2 laser equipment is available. Topical imiquimod, which is also effective in VIN disease (van Seters et al. 2008; Terlou et al. 2011), is expensive and usually unavailable. Therefore, the vulvar lesion had neither been biopsied nor treated to avoid mutilation and scarring.

Not treating vulvar intraepithelial disease is suboptimal as there is an approximate 2.3% likelihood of developing invasive disease within a median duration of 109 months with a range of 12–327 months (Wallbillich et al. 2012). In a cohort of immunocompromised patients with HIV infection, the likelihood of progressive disease will be higher.

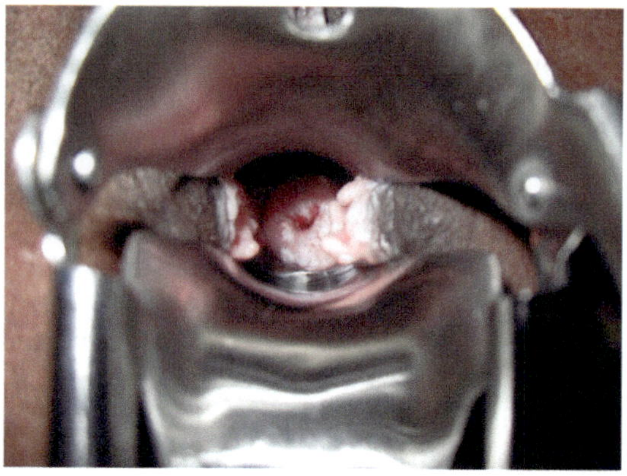

Fig. 18.227 A 24-year-old patient with HIV infection: visual inspection (VIA) of the cervix gives a positive result

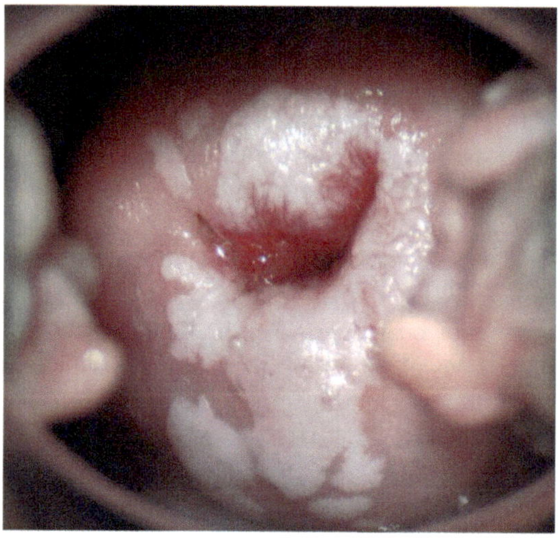

Fig. 18.228 On colposcopic exam, dense acetowhite areas with raised borders are seen in all four quadrants

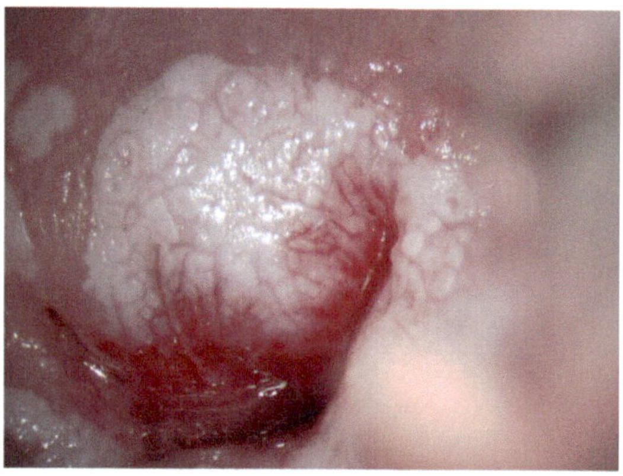

Fig. 18.229 The dense acetowhite lesion has an irregular mosaic pattern

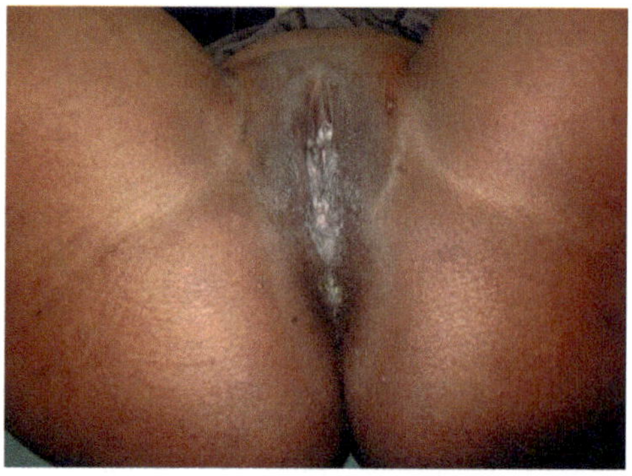

Fig. 18.230 There is a patchy depigmentation of the vulva suspicious for vulva intraepithelial neoplasia (VIN) in addition to cervical neoplasia

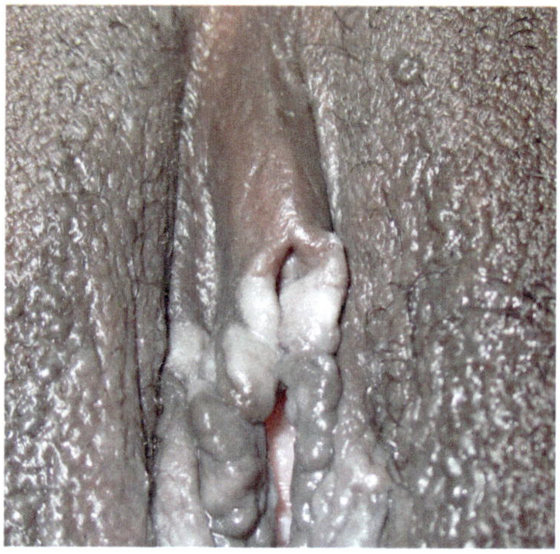

Fig. 18.231 On colposcopic exam, there are patchy areas of leukoplakia as well as flat wart-like changes on the small labia and close to the clitoris corroborating a clinical diagnosis of VIN

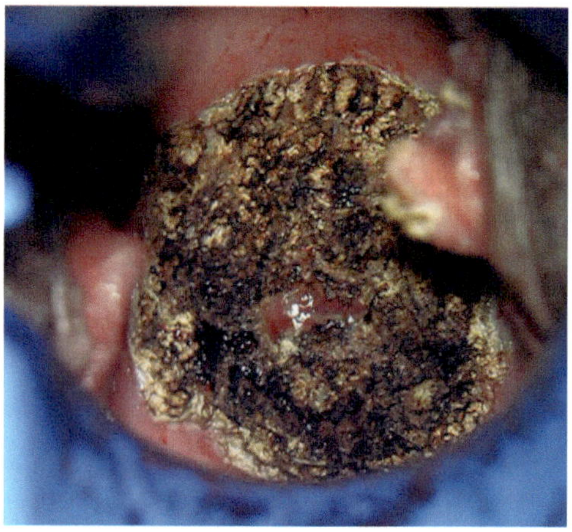

Fig. 18.232 Colposcopic aspect of the cervix immediately after removal of acetowhite lesions by loop resection and subsequent thermocoagulation

18.9.8 HSIL of the Cervix Not Eligible for Cryosurgery

A 37-year-old Tanzanian patient, P2, presents for cervical screening at Mbeya Referral Hospital. Previously, she has tested HIV positive. However, no further details on this infection are known.

On VIA exam she is found to be positive (Fig. 18.233). Colposcopic exam reveals an acetowhite area adjacent to the squamocolumnar junction encompassing most of the left dorsal and part of the right dorsal quadrants (Figs. 18.234 and 18.235). Especially on the left side, the abnormal epithelium is extending far into the periphery, so the patient is not eligible for treatment with the cryotherapy probe.

LEEP is performed under spinal anesthesia (Fig. 18.236). The patient is discharged from the hospital on the second postoperative day.

- Adequate colposcopy
- Squamocolumnar junction visible
- T1
- Abnormal colposcopic findings: dorsal two quadrants with opaque acetowhite changes (major change, grade 2) Fig. 18.234

A Pap smear obtained prior to LEEP (Figs. 18.237 and 18.238) is suspicious for a high-grade squamous intraepithelial lesion (HSIL).

Commentary
Histological confirmation of HSIL by tissue biopsy had not been performed due to limited access to a qualified pathologist.

Cryotherapy treatment is the treatment of choice within a VIA-based screening program. By comparison, LEEP is more expensive, needs a more complex set of instruments, and constitutes a surgical procedure that needs to be done by a medical doctor. In the scenario presented here, the cryo-tip would not have been large enough to cover the entire left dorsal quadrant where the grade 2 lesion is most pronounced. Therefore, LEEP had been chosen over cryotherapy.

LEEP is an outpatient procedure. However, as in the case presented here, the personal and family situation of the individual patient has to be taken into account and short hospitalization might be required. Also, cervical wound healing is going to be delayed in HIV patients (Pfaendler et al. 2015).

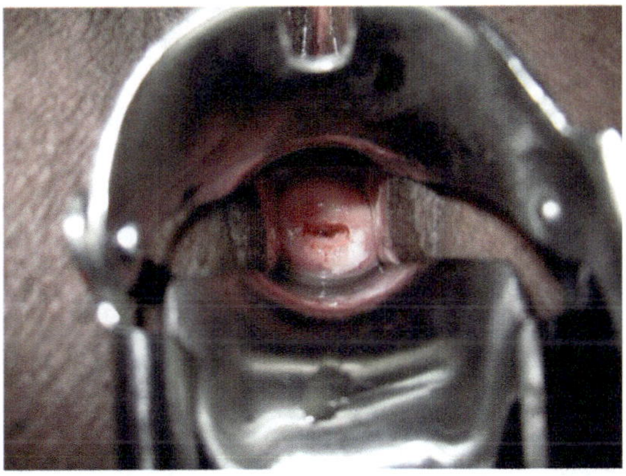

Fig. 18.233 A 37-year-old Tanzanian patient presenting to the screening clinic is found to be VIA positive

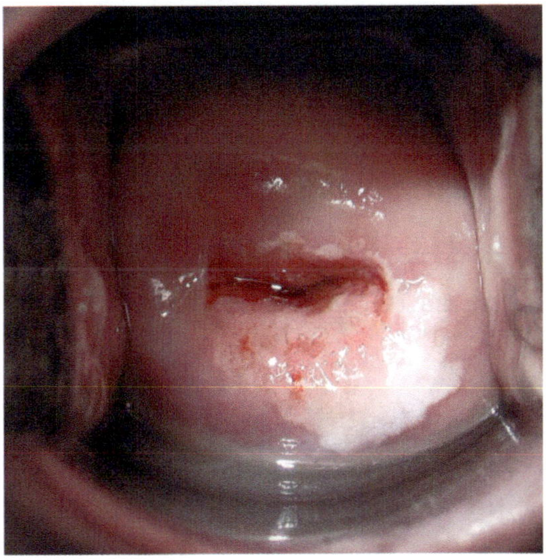

Fig. 18.234 On colposcopy, acetowhite changes of the dorsal two quadrants are noted with the opaque acetowhite lesion extending into the periphery of the left dorsal quadrant

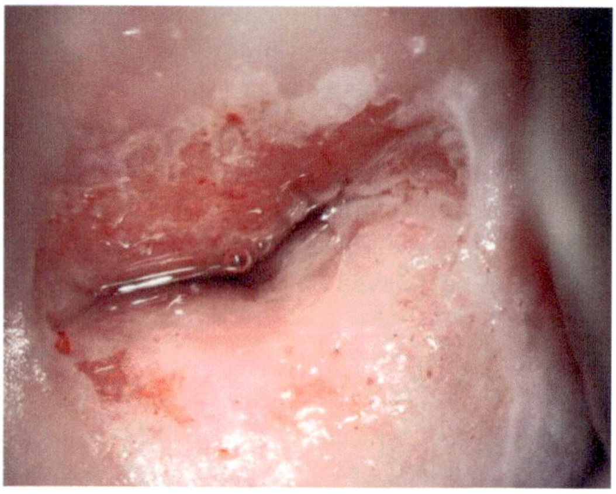

Fig. 18.235 A small band of acetowhite epithelium is visible ventrally

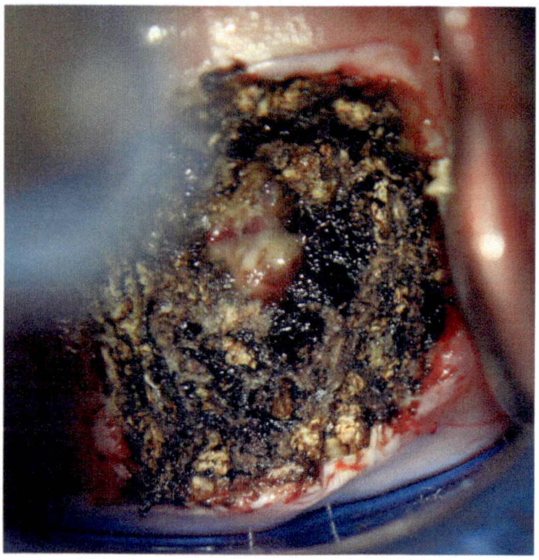

Fig. 18.236 Cervix immediately following ablative treatment via LEEP

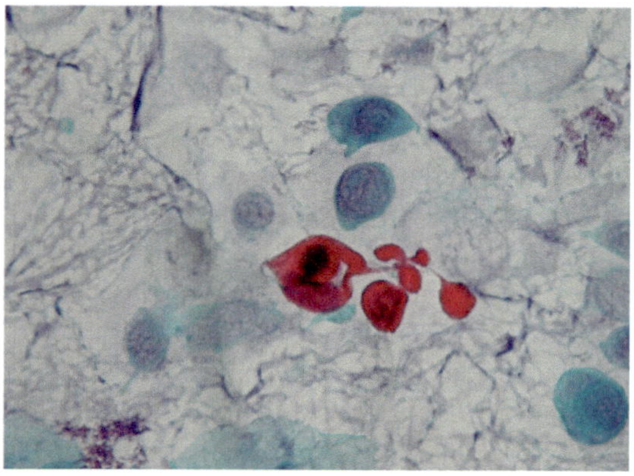

Fig. 18.237 Pap smear suspicious for HSIL (CIN3): several atypical squamous cells with large nuclei are seen including an eosinophilic cell with a dense nucleus indicating atypical keratinization

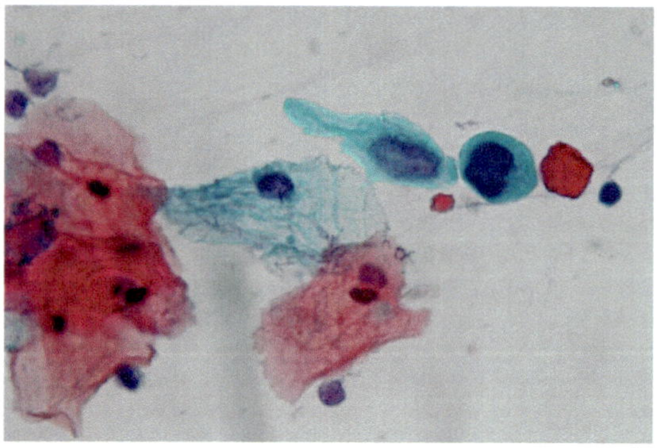

Fig. 18.238 Pap smear suspicious for HSIL (CIN3): two cells with enlarged nuclei are located next to a group of normal superficial and intermediate squamous cells

18.9.9 FIGO Stage IIIB Squamous Cell Carcinoma of the Cervix

A 51-year-old Tanzanian patient presents to META Referral Hospital, Mbeya, with significant vaginal bleeding. On speculum exam (Fig. 18.239) and subsequent colposcopy (Fig. 18.240), the posterior valve of the instrument rapidly fills with blood from a friable tumor encompassing the entire aspect of the cervix. The pelvic exam reveals a 6 cm cervical tumor which involves both parametria and extends toward the pelvic sidewall. The tumor also involves the anterior vagina down to the lower one third of the vaginal wall. A Pap test obtained at the time of the clinical exam is suspicious for keratinizing squamous cell carcinoma (Fig. 18.241).

Eighteen months prior, the patient tested HIV positive and was subsequently screened for cervical cancer. She was found to be VIA positive with involvement of more than 75% of the cervix. A Pap test showed HSIL. Three months later, biopsies were performed revealing squamous cell carcinoma of the cervix. At that time, FIGO stage IIIB disease was suspected and the patient was referred for primary chemoradiation at Ocean Road Hospital located in the Tanzanian capital Dar es Salaam.

Commentary

It remains unclear why this patient did not receive the recommended chemoradiation treatment at an earlier point of time. However, the distance from Mbeya to Dar es Salaam, where the only cancer hospital is located, is more than 800 km, which is expensive for an average Tanzanian citizen.

Furthermore, there are other inconsistencies within the patient's clinical history. Disease progression from high-grade intraepithelial neoplasia to advanced-stage squamous cell carcinoma within 3 months is highly unlikely, even in the HIV-positive patient. Possibly, early-stage invasive disease had been overlooked by both VIA exam and Pap smear. In this case, significant progression of disease within a 3-month period is possible as demonstrated by Kantelhardt et al. (2014) on a group of Ethiopian women with cervical cancer. During an average treatment delay of 3.8 months, the proportion of patients with stage IIIB/IVA disease went up from 33.5% to 63.9%.

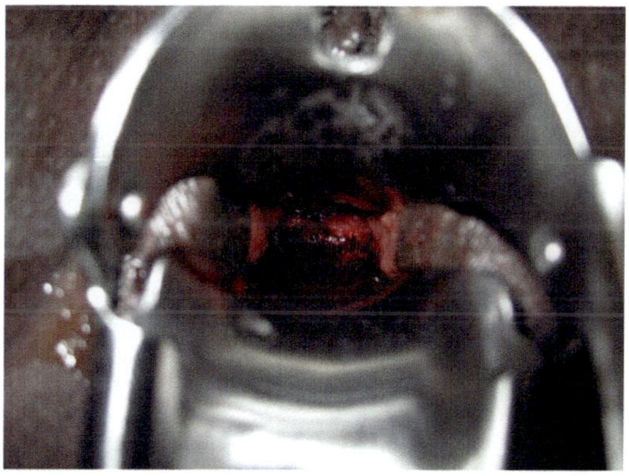

Fig. 18.239 FIGO stage IIIB squamous cell carcinoma of the cervix in a 51-year-old Tanzanian patient: the posterior part of the speculum rapidly fills with blood from the friable cervical tumor

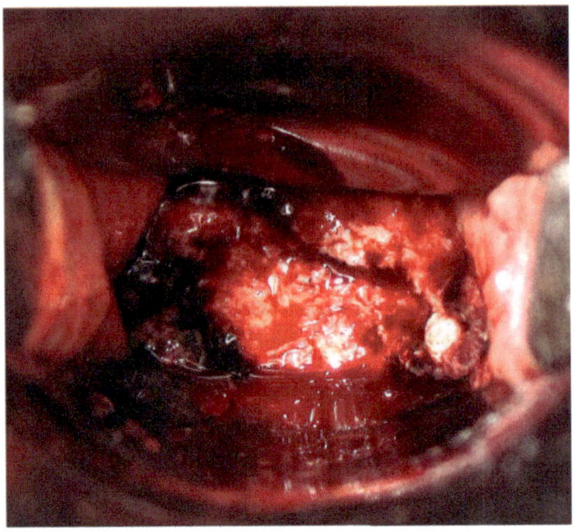

Fig. 18.240 FIGO stage IIIB squamous cell carcinoma of the cervix: tumor tissue, which is bleeding on touch, has replaced the cervix

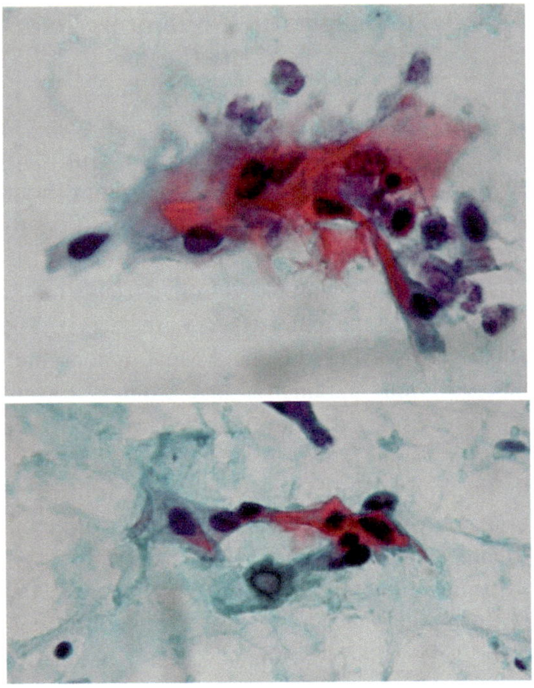

Fig. 18.241 Pap smear suspicious for keratinizing squamous cell carcinoma of the cervix: eosinophilic cells exhibit marked nuclear polymorphism with several dark nuclei

18.9.10 Operable FIGO Stage IIB Cancer of the Cervix

A 61-year-old patient presents to META Referral Hospital, Mbeya, Tanzania, for treatment of biopsy-proven squamous cell carcinoma of the cervix. Her HIV status is negative. On speculum exam and colposcopy, there is abnormal tissue growth close to the cervical os with coarse irregular punctation that bleeds upon touch (Figs. 18.242 and 18.243).

On transvaginal and rectal exams, the uterus is partially mobile. The tumor invades the left parametrial tissue. However, the left pelvic sidewall does not appear to be involved, so FIGO stage IIB disease is suspected.

As it is highly unlikely that the patient will receive chemoradiation in a timely manner, exploratory laparotomy is performed to evaluate operability. Radical hysterectomy and bilateral salpingo-oophorectomy are performed. The cervix is significantly enlarged with involvement of the left parametrium (Fig. 18.244). Macroscopically, resection margins are free of disease. A 1 cm firm lymph node is removed from the left external iliac vessels.

A preoperative Pap smear is suspicious for keratinizing squamous cell carcinoma (Figs. 18.245 and 18.246).

The immediate postoperative course is unremarkable. No histopathological exam of the specimen is available.

Commentary

The treatment of choice for clinical stage IIB disease is primary radiation therapy consisting of brachy- and teletherapy. However, at the time this patient needed to be treated, she would not have had access to an appropriate cancer treatment facility providing radiation therapy in a timely manner. Therefore, the decision had been made to explore the uterus surgically and to make an intraoperative decision on resectability. Although radical removal of the uterus had been possible, the patient might have benefitted from adjuvant chemoradiation, which again had not been available at the time.

Only one enlarged lymph node had been removed, as systematic pelvic and paraaortic lymph node dissection in the case of macroscopically normal tissue would not have benefitted the patient in the absence of a subsequent histopathological evaluation as well as the absence of an adjuvant treatment facility.

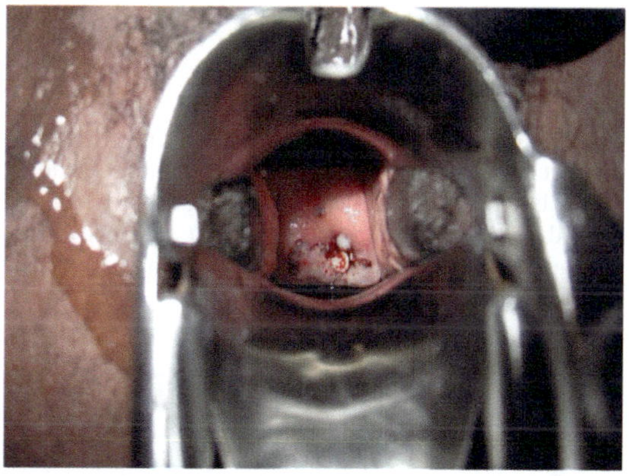

Fig. 18.242 Biopsy-proven squamous cell carcinoma of the cervix: Close to the cervical os as well as around the dorsal aspect of the cervix, abnormal tissue growth can be seen

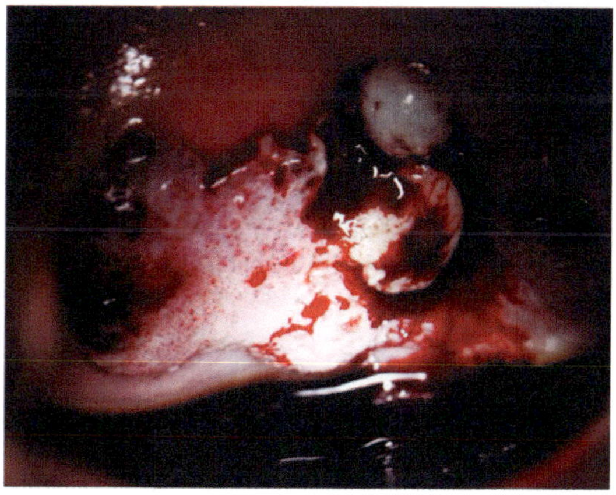

Fig. 18.243 Colposcopy of biopsy-proven squamous cell carcinoma of the cervix: the tumor tissue shows irregular and coarse punctation and is vulnerable

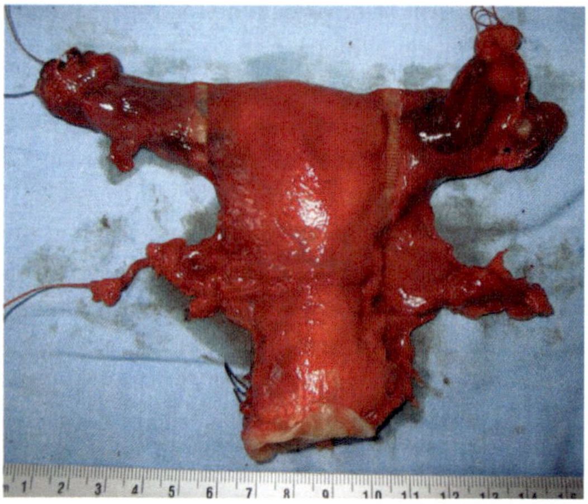

Fig. 18.244 (Clinically staged) FIGO stage IIB squamous cell carcinoma of the cervix: a radical hysterectomy and a bilateral salpingo-oophorectomy have been performed. The caudal aspect of the left parametrium is enlarged asymmetrically consistent with parametrial invasion

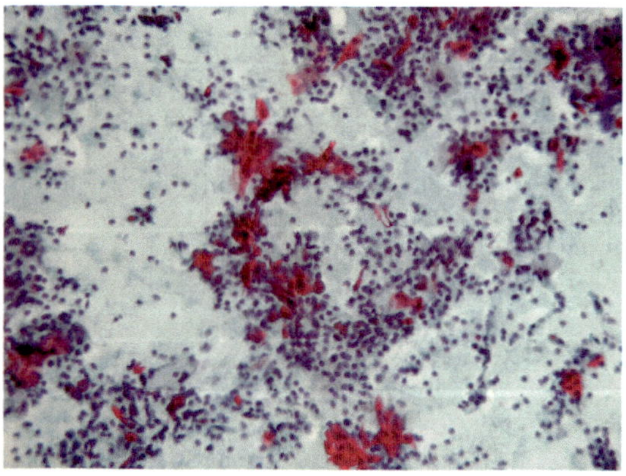

Fig. 18.245 Pap smear suspicious for keratinizing squamous cell carcinoma: the tumor cells are surrounded by marked tumor diathesis consisting predominantly of white blood cells and a hazy background of proteinaceous precipitates

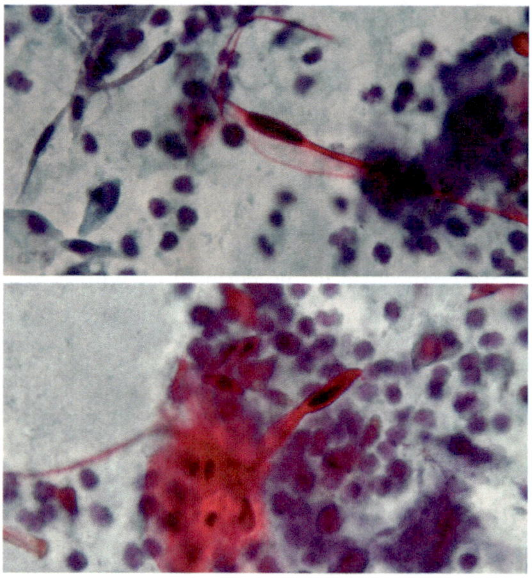

Fig. 18.246 Pap smear suspicious for keratinizing squamous cell carcinoma: keratinized spindle cells

18.9.11 Large Cervical Condyloma in an HIV-Positive Patient

A 35-year-old patient, P3, from the Southern Highlands of Tanzania has been found to be HIV positive 2 months prior. She is not yet on antiretroviral therapy. She has been screened at a peripheral health facility and diagnosed as VIA positive. On colposcopy (Figs. 18.247 and 18.248), a large condyloma is visible with multiple satellite lesions encompassing almost the entire cervix with coarse acetowhite epithelium reaching into the cervical canal. The squamocolumnar junction is not visible (T3). Surprisingly, no condyloma of the vagina and/or vulva are present.

- Adequate colposcopy
- Squamocolumnar junction not visible
- T3
- Abnormal colposcopic findings: large condyloma encompassing the dorsal two quadrants with satellite lesions on the ventral two quadrants, coarse acetowhite epithelium around and within the cervical canal (major change, grade 2)
  Figs. 18.247 and 18.248

A LEEP resection is performed under spinal anesthesia with complete removal of the abnormal tissue.

Commentary

Cervical condyloma does not necessarily represent a precancerous lesion as it may be caused by HPV 6 and/or HPV 11, the so-called "low-risk" HPV types not associated with the development of cancer of the cervix. However, a large cervical condyloma might also be associated with HSIL.

Cryotherapy would not have been possible due to the extent of the lesion.

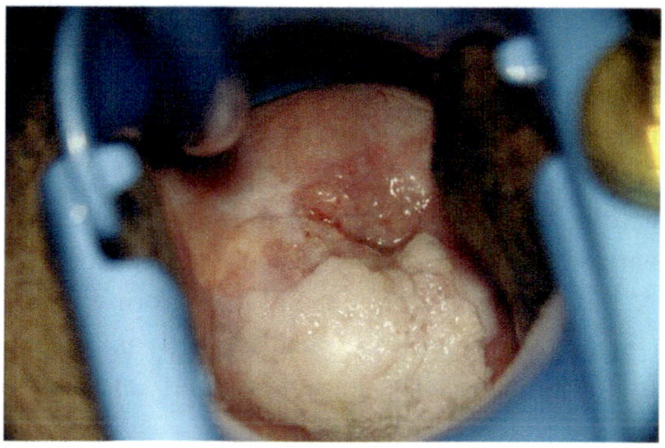

Fig. 18.247 Large cervical condyloma in a 35-year-old HIV-positive patient

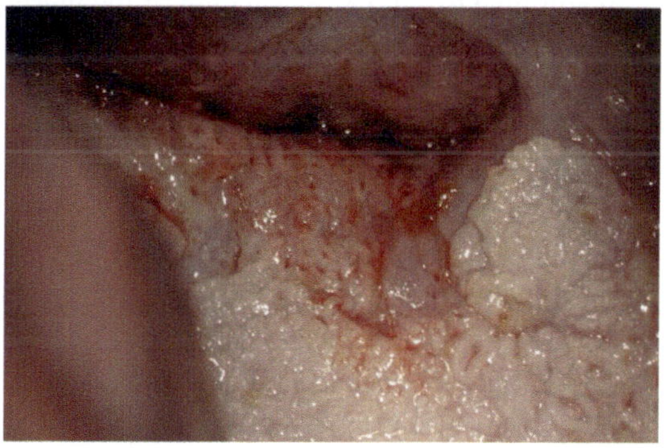

Fig. 18.248 Typical exophytic condyloma acuminatum of the cervix dorsally with coarse acetowhite epithelium reaching into the cervical canal

18.9.12 Choriocarcinoma Mimicking Carcinoma of the Cervix

A 47-year-old HIV-negative patient, P7, is admitted to a remote local hospital in the Southern Highlands of Tanzania. She is in hypovolemic shock with a hemoglobin of 3.1 g/dl. The patient is bleeding from the vagina. Gynecological examination shows an 8 cm mass protruding from the cervix (Fig. 18.249). There appears to be no parametrial or vaginal involvement. On ultrasound exam, there is no hydronephrosis. At this time, a clinical diagnosis of stage IB2 carcinoma of the cervix is made with a differential diagnosis of "myoma in statu nascendi." A Pap smear is taken from the tumor surface (Figs. 18.250 and 18.251) as well as several tumor biopsies. The patient is then referred to META Referral Hospital, Mbeya.

At META Referral Hospital, a comprehensive patient's history is obtained and the patient reexamined. On several previous occasions, she has been admitted to META: evacuation of the uterus has been attempted twice due to spontaneous abortion and continuous bleeding. Two months prior, a cervical biopsy from a bluish nodule located at the cervix has been obtained. At that time, the ß-HCG test of the urine had been positive. Therefore, choriocarcinoma was suspected. The patient had left the hospital untreated on her own accord before the diagnosis could be established.

At the time of readmission at META, biopsy results are not back yet. On reexamination a bluish nodule in the vagina close to the vulva is identified (Fig. 18.252), which had been overlooked at the previous exam, thus further confirming the diagnosis of choriocarcinoma. A chest X-ray shows multiple pulmonary metastases (Fig. 18.253).

As there is continuous and potentially life-threatening bleeding from the vagina, exploratory laparotomy is performed and the uterus removed. The tumor has perforated the anterior uterine wall and is infiltrating the peritoneum of the bladder. Another metastatic nodule is identified on the anterior aspect of the sigmoid colon (Fig. 18.254).

Eventually, a histopathological diagnosis of choriocarcinoma is obtained (Figs. 18.255, 18.256, and 18.257).

Subsequently, treatment with combination therapy of methotrexate, actinomycin C, and cyclophosphamide is initiated. The patient suffers from significant side effects such as oral and genital ulceration. However, there is evidence of a response to therapy as the nodule close to the vulva is regressing. Due to the side effects, the patient is given methotrexate only for the second course of chemotherapy. During this course of chemotherapy, the patient dies unexpectedly. The cause of death remains unclear.

Commentary

Sub-Saharan African countries are chronically short of trained pathologists (Adesina et al. 2013). Thus, histopathology is either not available or subject to long delays.

A Pap smear had been obtained. Reporting of the result had been delayed, so it did not contribute to patient management. However, as Kadivar and Hosseini (2007) point out, cytological features of choriocarcinoma are not characteristic enough to differentiate GTN from poorly differentiated squamous cell carcinoma. Even immunocytochemistry—if available—would not be helpful as some squamous cell carcinomas are positive for ß-HCG, and the presence of cytokeratin staining does not reliably rule out GTN.

As pointed out earlier, a clinical diagnosis of invasive cervical carcinoma is feasible in most cases. However, there are pitfalls as in this case of advanced choriocarcinoma protruding from the cervix. Initially, the correct clinical diagnosis had been made. However, the patient did not return for treatment. On readmission to the peripheral hospital due to hypovolemic shock, the patient did not adequately relate her history. Nevertheless, the correct diagnosis would have been made if the vaginal metastasis located close to the vulva had not been overlooked.

It is helpful to keep in mind that advanced gestational trophoblastic neoplasia (GTN) within the vagina is a possibility. In Africa, choriocarcinoma occurs three times more frequently than in Western Europe (Fig. 18.258).

According to the FIGO staging system (Fig. 18.259), the patient had stage III disease.

GTN is classified according to a risk score which also helps to select treatment (Fig. 18.260). In this case known risk factors are age > 40 years (1); antecedent abortion (1); interval from pregnancy about 2 months (0); largest tumor size 8 cm

(2); lung metastases (0); number of metastases 5–8 (2); and no previously failed chemotherapy (0). The resulting stage/risk score is reported as III:6.

However, the risk score and possibly also the stage may be underestimating the disease, because some key diagnostic elements are missing: liver and/or brain metastases, which occur frequently in advanced choriocarcinoma, had not been ruled out. In addition, serum β-HCG levels are not available.

Communication with the patient and her family had been difficult and she did not adhere to the doctors' recommendations possibly out of fear and a lack of understanding of the treatment rationale.

Although a multiple agent chemotherapy regimen had been initiated with a demonstrable clinical response, the patient died during a second course of chemotherapy consisting of methotrexate only. Ultimately, the cause of death remains unclear.

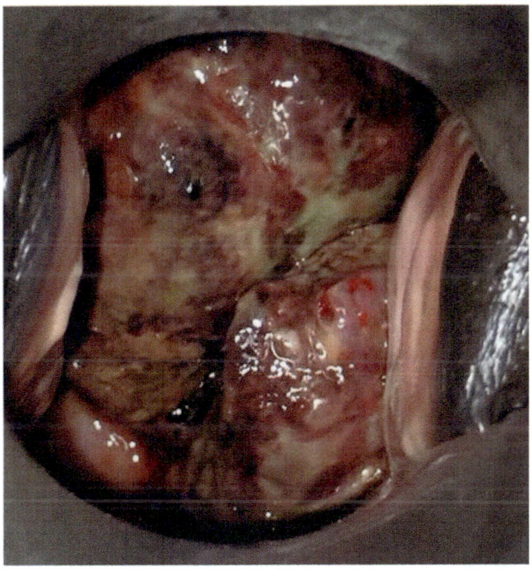

Fig. 18.249 Advanced choriocarcinoma misdiagnosed as carcinoma of the cervix. An 8 cm mass is protruding from the cervix

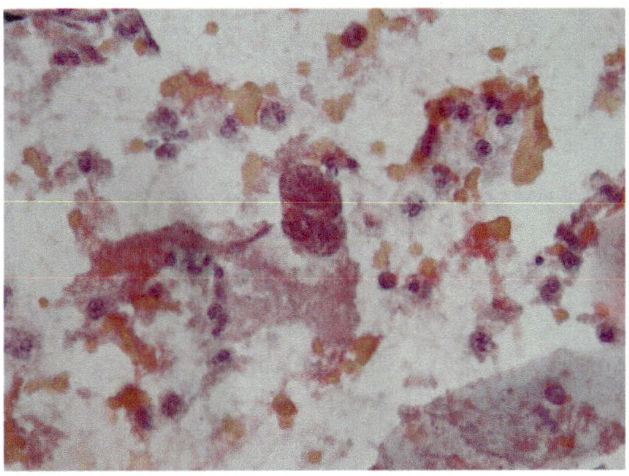

Fig. 18.250 Pap smear of advanced choriocarcinoma protruding from the cervix. The background of the sample with red and white blood cells as well as cell debris is typical for so-called tumor diathesis. In the center of the photograph are two multinucleated cells with coarse chromatin

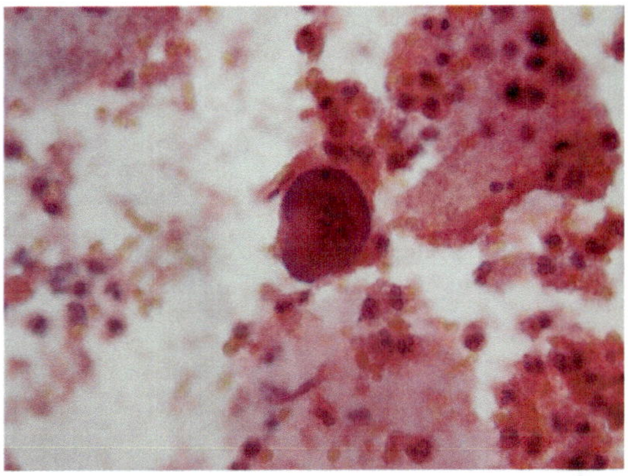

Fig. 18.251 Pap smear of advanced choriocarcinoma protruding from the cervix. Again, there is tumor diathesis. A bizarre multinucleated cell is seen which exhibits abundant cytoplasm

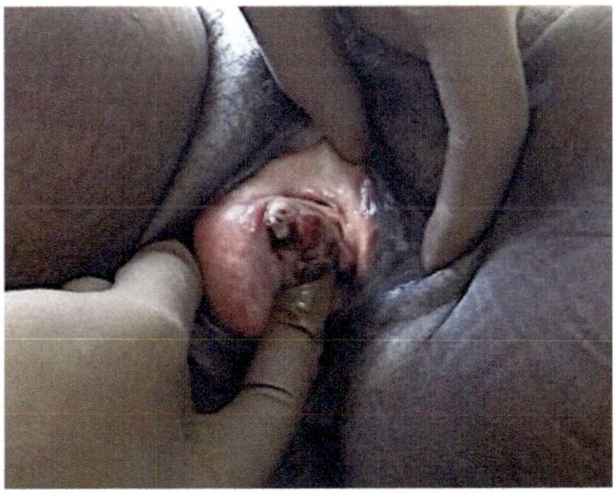

Fig. 18.252 Advanced choriocarcinoma with vaginal metastasis. A vaginal nodule close to the vulva is seen, a finding which is characteristic for GTN but would be highly unusual for squamous cell carcinoma of the cervix

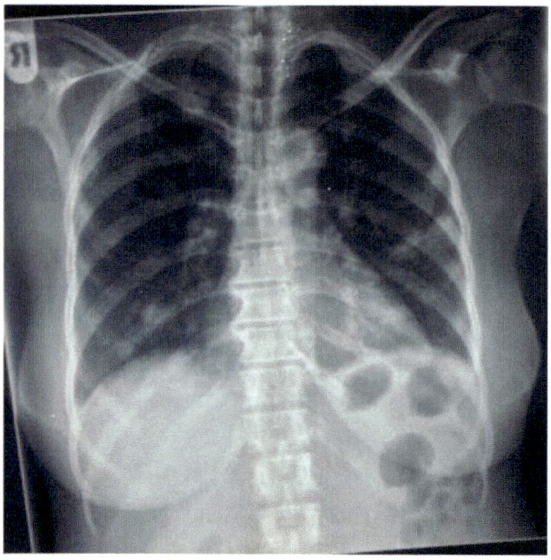

Fig. 18.253 Multiple pulmonary metastases from advanced choriocarcinoma

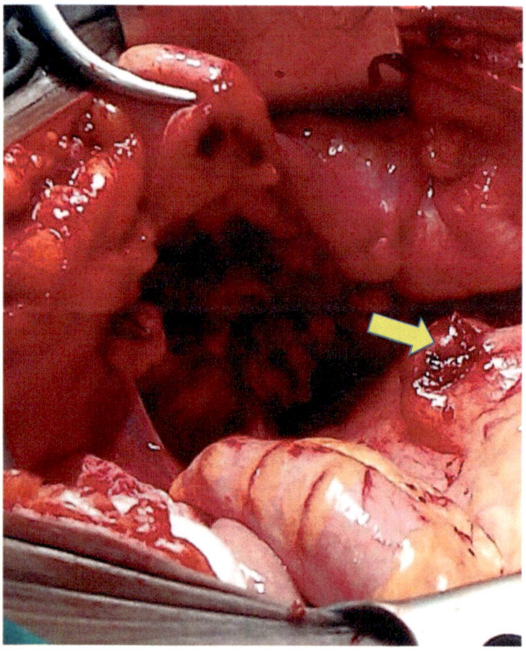

Fig. 18.254 Hemorrhagic nodule located at the anterior aspect of the sigmoid colon, which represents a metastasis of choriocarcinoma

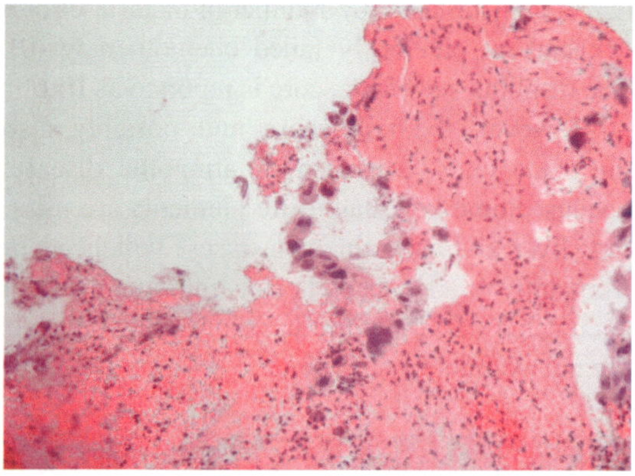

Fig. 18.255 Choriocarcinoma of the cervix

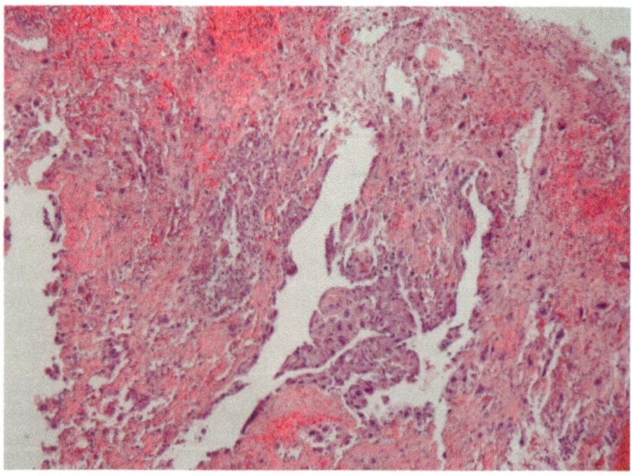

Fig. 18.256 Choriocarcinoma of the cervix

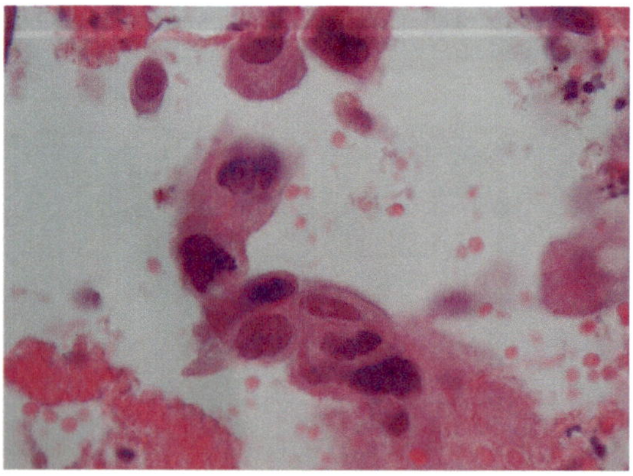

Fig. 18.257 Choriocarcinoma of the cervix

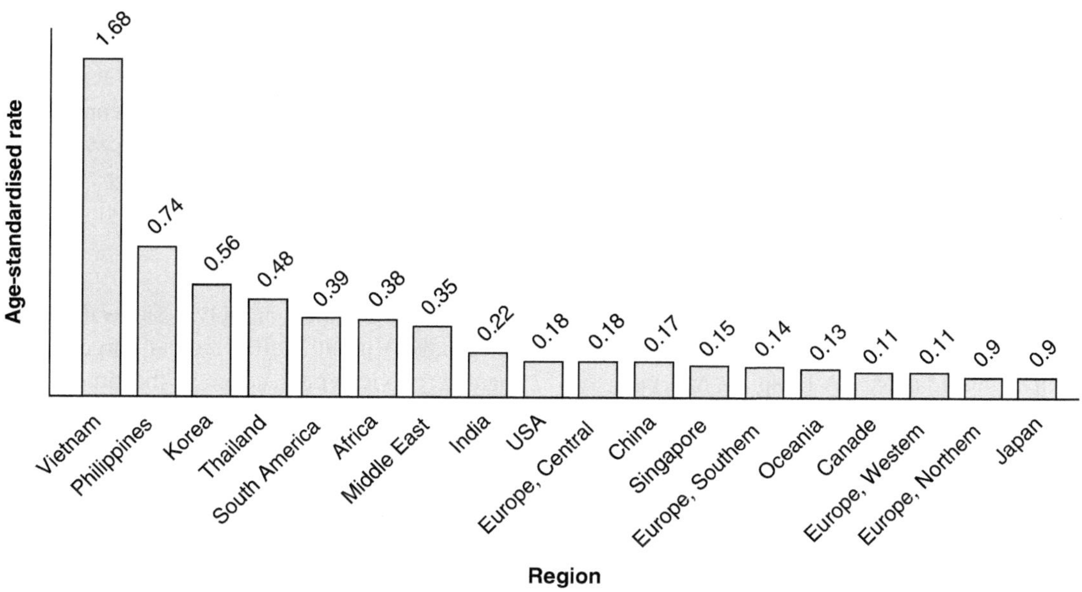

Fig. 18.258 Choriocarcinoma: age-standardized incidence rate per 100,000 women in various regions of the world (Altieri et al. 2003)

FIGO Stage	Description
I	Gestational trophoblastic tumors strictly confined to the uterine corpus
II	Gestational trophoblastic tumors extending to the adnexae or to the vagina, but limited to the genital structures
III	Gestational trophoblastic tumors extending to the lungs, with or without genital tract involvement
IV	All other metastatic sites

Fig. 18.259 FIGO staging of gestational trophoblastic neoplasia (GTN) (Ngan et al. 2015)

FICO/WHO risk factor scoring with FIGO staging	0	1	2	4
Age	<40	>40	–	–
Antecedent pregnancy	Mole	Abortion	Term	
Interval from index pregnancy, months	<4	4–6	7–12	>12
Pretreatment hCG mIU/mL	$<10^3$	$>10^3$-10^4	$>10^4$-10^5	$>10^5$
Largest tumor size including uterus, cm	–	3–4	≥5	–
Site of metastases including uterus	lung	Spleen, kidney	Gastrointestinal tract	Brain, liver
Number of metastases identified	–	1–4	5–8	>8
Previous failed chemotherapy	–	–	Single drug	Two or more drung

Fig. 18.260 FIGO/WHO prognostic scoring system for gestational trophoblastic neoplasia (GTN) (Ngan et al. 2015)

18.9.13 Radical Hysterectomy and Pelvic Lymph Node Dissection for FIGO Stage IB2 Carcinoma of the Cervix

A 39-year-old patient is a nurse at a regional district hospital of Mbeya, Tanzania. She tests HIV positive. After experiencing postcoital bleeding, she presents to her local hospital. Cervical biopsy is performed and reveals moderately differentiated squamous cell carcinoma. The patient is then evaluated at META Hospital, Mbeya.

On speculum exam, there is a bleeding mass of soft tissue which appears to have replaced the entire cervix (Fig. 18.261). Colposcopy exam after application of 5% acetic acid reveals a cauliflower-like growth pattern (Fig. 18.262). When using the 15-fold colposcopic magnification as well as the green filter (Fig. 18.263), atypical tumor vessels are visible. The tumor is approximately 5 cm in diameter. There is no clinical evidence of vaginal or parametrial invasion, so the diagnosis of cervical carcinoma FIGO stage IB2 is established.

Subsequently, a Piver class III radical hysterectomy is performed with bilateral salpingo-oophorectomy (Fig. 18.264). Macroscopically, the cancer growth is limited to the ventral aspect of the cervix and has been removed with a wide resection margin (Fig. 18.265). Pelvic lymph nodes are also removed (Fig. 18.266). The obturator lymph nodes are enlarged. Histologically all nodes are free of cancer. On histologic exam the lymph nodes are cancer-free.

Initially, the patient does well postoperatively and resumes work as a nurse. Three months later, however, she presents with a bilateral pelvic mass with a diameter of about 5 cm. Ultrasound-guided fine needle aspiration biopsy is positive for squamous cell carcinoma. Subsequently, she is referred to Ocean Road Cancer Institute in Dar es Salaam for radiation treatment in combination with chemotherapy.

Commentary

Massive lymph node or pelvic sidewall recurrence only 3 months after radical surgery with negative pelvic lymph nodes at the time of the initial surgery is quite unusual, even when taking into account that the patient tested HIV positive. A 1991 study from the University of Michigan showed a 5-year survival of 93% of patients with negative nodes at the time of surgery for stage IB squamous cell carcinoma of the cervix (Hopkins and Morley 1991a, b).

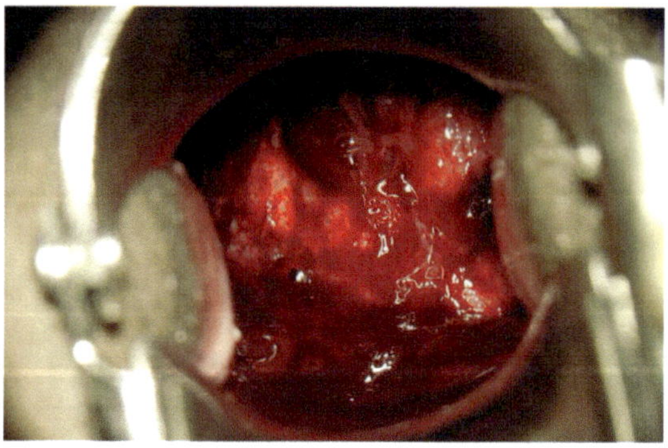

Fig. 18.261 A 39-year-old patient with squamous cell carcinoma of the cervix. On speculum exam, the cervix cannot be visualized. Instead, a friable tumor mass is seen

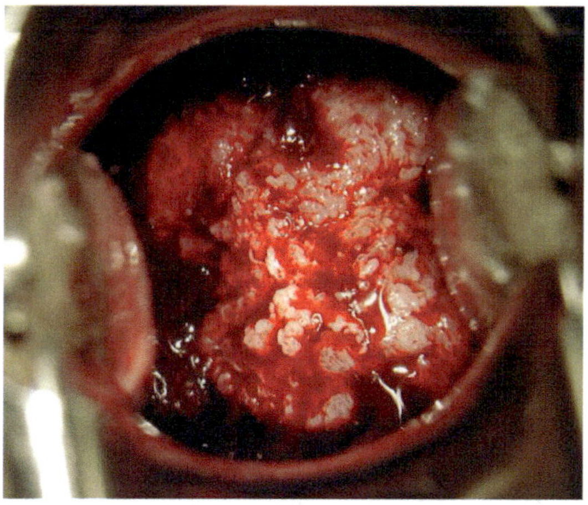

Fig. 18.262 A 39-year-old patient with squamous cell carcinoma of the cervix. After the application of 5% acetic acid solution, the tumor growth appears to be cauliflower-like

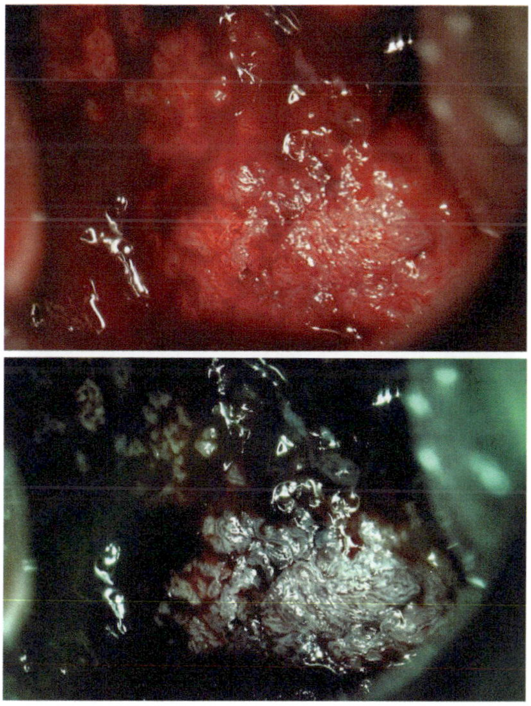

Fig. 18.263 A 39-year-old patient with squamous cell carcinoma of the cervix. Atypical vessels are visible when using the green filter

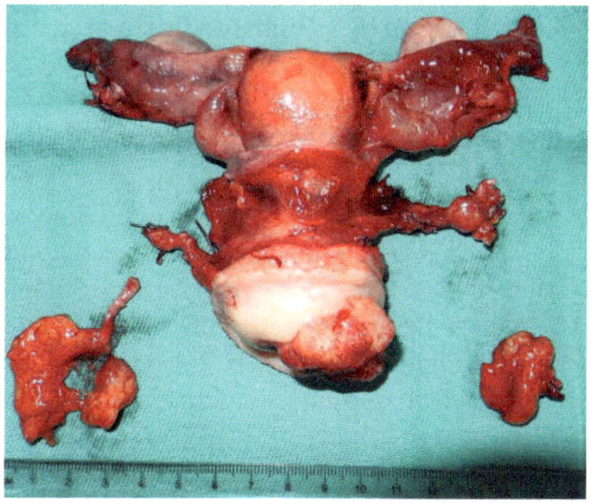

Fig. 18.264 A 39-year-old patient with squamous cell carcinoma of the cervix. The specimen encompasses the uterus with parametria including the uterine arteries, upper vaginal cuff, ovaries, and fallopian tubes. In addition, bilateral pelvic lymph nodes have been removed

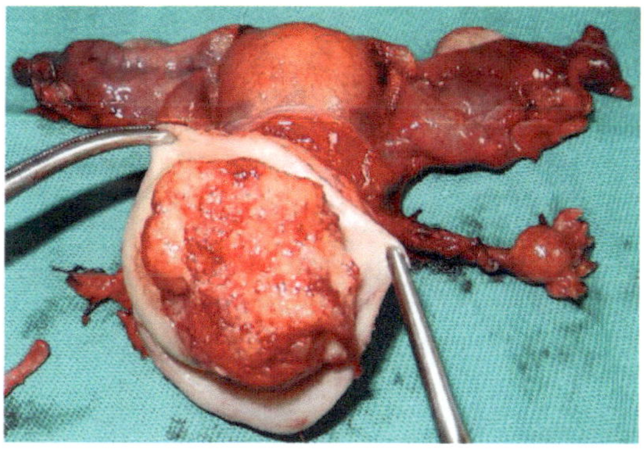

Fig. 18.265 A 39-year-old patient with squamous cell carcinoma of the cervix. The tumor is exophytic and located at the ventral aspect of the cervix

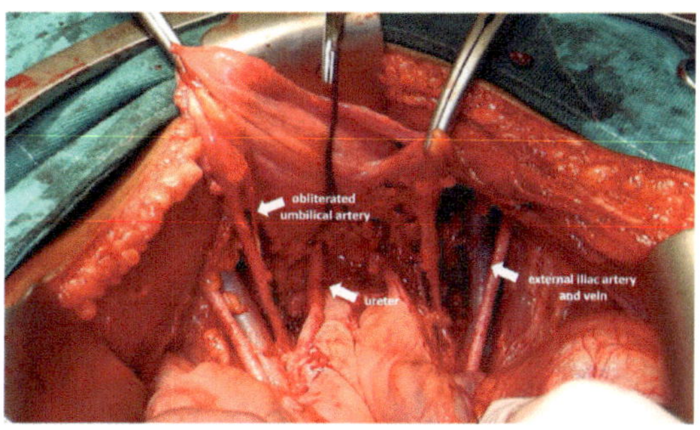

Fig. 18.266 After completion of the radical hysterectomy with bilateral pelvic lymphonodectomy, the retroperitoneal structures are clearly visible

18.9.14 Large VIA-Positive Lesion Treated by Loop Resection

One year prior, a 41-year-old patient, P2, underwent cervical screening at META hospital in Mbeya, Tanzania, and was found to be VIA negative. As she was HIV positive, repeat exam was scheduled after 1 year. Now the visual inspection is positive with opaque acetowhite lesions within all four quadrants of the cervix. In addition, there are superficial tissue abrasions close to the cervical canal (rag sign).

- Adequate colposcopy
- Squamocolumnar junction not visible
- T3
- Abnormal colposcopic findings: opaque acetowhite patches in all four quadrants of the cervix, rag sign (major change, grade 2)
  Fig. 18.267

As the lesion is too extensive for cryotherapy, a LEEP resection is performed (Fig. 18.268). Multiple tissue fragments are removed with a total resection volume of 2 cm^3 (Fig. 18.269).

The histological exam reveals benign nonkeratinized squamous epithelium as well as multiple normal endocervical glands. There is no evidence of neoplasia.

Two months after the surgery, the cervix has healed completely and is found to be VIA negative. The patient is scheduled for yearly Pap smears.

Commentary

Colposcopically, the cervical lesion is classified as a major change and HSIL is suspected. However, the histologic exam of the specimen is inconsistent with any grade of dysplasia. According to a meta-analysis by Fokom-Domgue et al. (2015), pooled specificity of VIA was 87.4% (77.1– 93.4%), so a considerable number of patients will be overtreated when using visual inspection alone for treatment decision.

Sometimes p16 immunostaining is helpful in order to identify small volume lesions. The p16 biomarker can also be useful when there is a discrepancy between colposcopic and cytopathological evaluation and histopathology (Galgano et al. 2010) as in the case presented here. However, p16 immunostaining is not available in low-resource environments such as southern Tanzania.

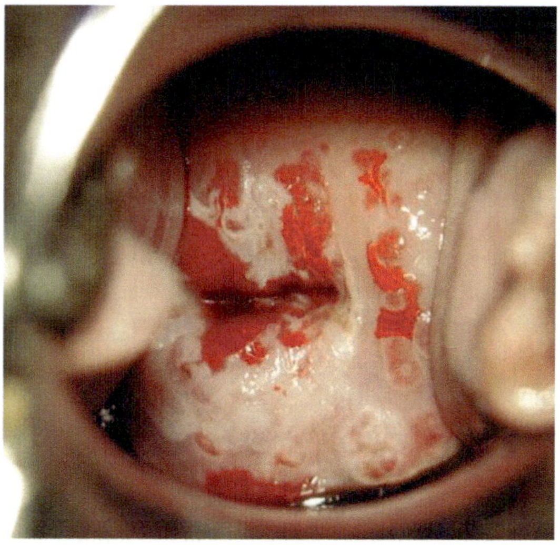

Fig. 18.267 Major change with multiple opaque acetowhite areas as well as abrasion close to the cervical canal (rag sign)

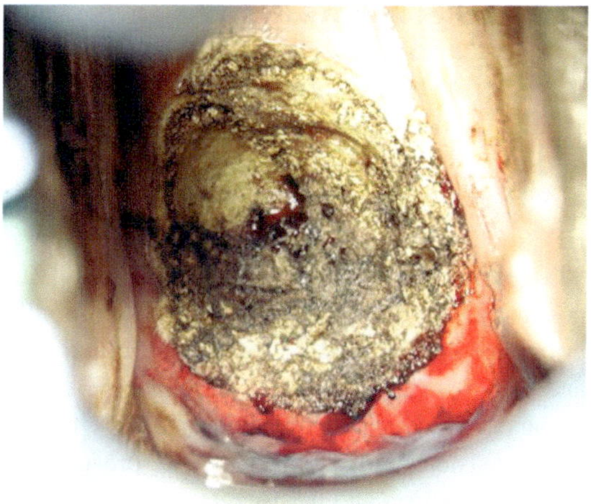

Fig. 18.268 Cervix after loop resection and coagulation for a VIA-positive lesion

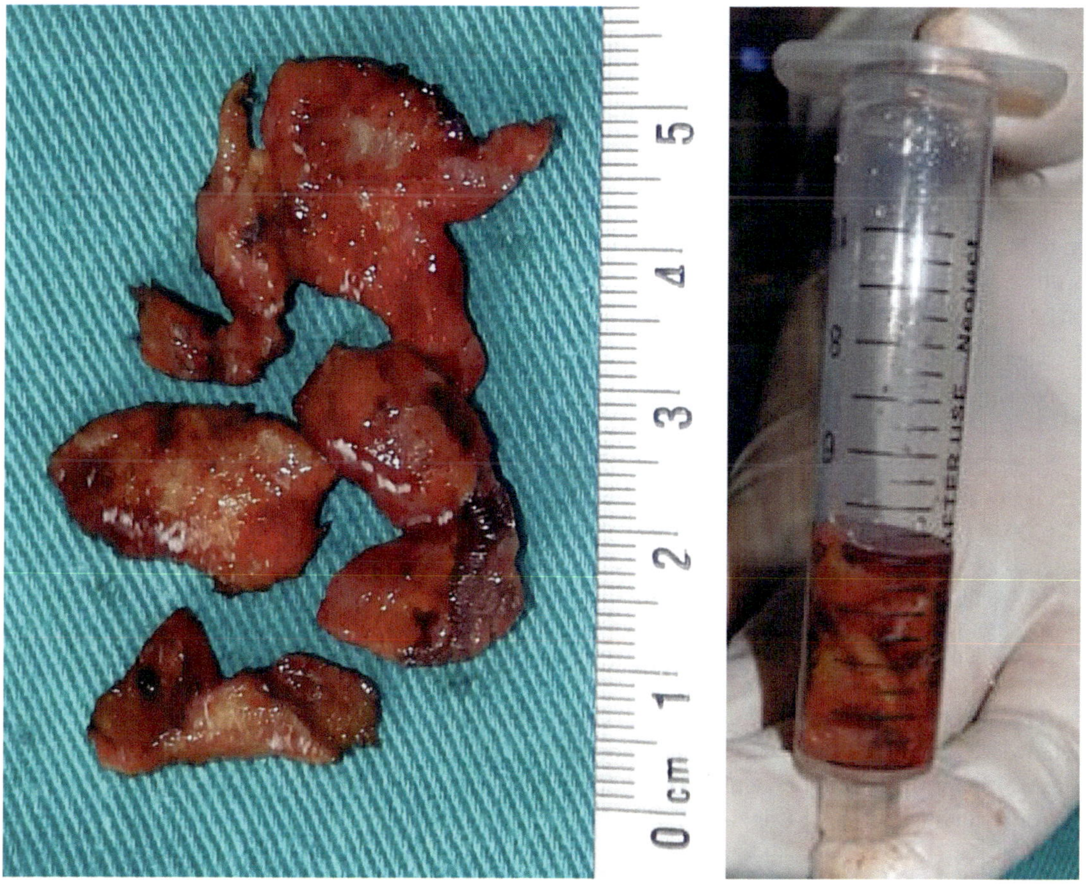

Fig. 18.269 The resected cervical tissue is fragmented as a small electrosurgical loop has been used requiring multiple passes. A tissue volume of 2 cm^3 determined using Archimedes' principle has been removed

18.9.15 Recurrent CIN3 and Condylomata Acuminata of the Vulva in a 51-Year-Old HIV-Positive Patient

A 51-year-old patient, P10, has been receiving HIV medication since 2012. Her CD4 count is 383 cell/µl. Eleven months prior, she was VIA positive and underwent cryotherapy. Four months prior, she complained of lower abdominal pain and mucopurulent vaginal discharge. A Pap smear was taken and revealed HSIL. A biopsy was consistent with CIN3. Now she presents for repeat evaluation and treatment.

On clinical inspection she has several pigmented warty lesions around the vulva and the anus (Fig. 18.270). On higher magnification (Fig. 18.271) these lesions are typical condyloma acuminata.

There is copious white discharge (Fig. 18.272). After application of the acetic acid, the cervical canal is flush with the surface of the upper vagina (Fig. 18.273). There is a small opaque and slightly raised acetowhite lesion at the 6 to 9 o'clock position close to the cervical opening (Fig. 18.274). The squamocolumnar junction is not visible. Lugol's test is partially positive with multiple yellow patches (Fig. 18.275) consistent with cervicitis.

- Adequate colposcopy
- Squamocolumnar junction not visible
- T3
- Abnormal colposcopic findings: small opaque and slightly raised densely acetowhite lesion at the 6 to 9 o'clock position close to the cervical canal (major change, grade 2)
  Figs. 18.273 and 18.274

The abnormal tissue around the cervical os is removed by several passes with a small electrosurgical loop followed by coagulation including the surrounding partially Lugol-negative tissue (Fig. 18.276). The resection volume is small (0.6 cm^3) (Fig. 18.277).

The vulvar condylomata are coagulated using the monopolar needle (Figs. 18.278 and 18.279).

Commentary

Condylomata acuminata frequently occur in HIV-positive patients. According to a study by Conley et al. (2002) the prevalence was 5.6% compared to 1% in HIV-negative patients.

Conley et al. also showed that HIV infection increases the risk of vulvar intraepithelial neoplasia. Thus, if there is any doubt regarding the diagnosis of vulvar or perianal condyloma, colposcopically guided biopsy is indicated.

The treatment of choice for condylomata acuminata is topical application of podofilox, podophyllin, or imiquimod. Surgical removal consists of tangential excision, curettage, or—as in the case presented here—electrocautery. Ideally, genital warts are removed by CO_2 laser vaporization to avoid scarring.

Both the quadrivalent Gardasil® (Ali et al. 2013) and the nonavalent Gardasil 9® vaccines are highly effective as condyloma prophylaxis because they include HPV types 6 and 11.

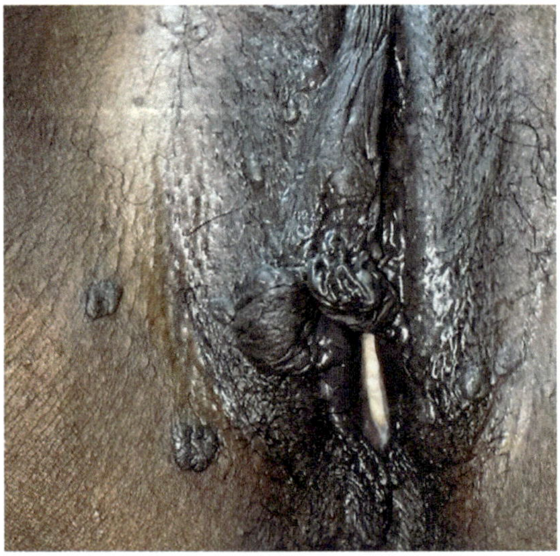

Fig. 18.270 Condylomata acuminata. Several pigmented warty lesions of the vulva

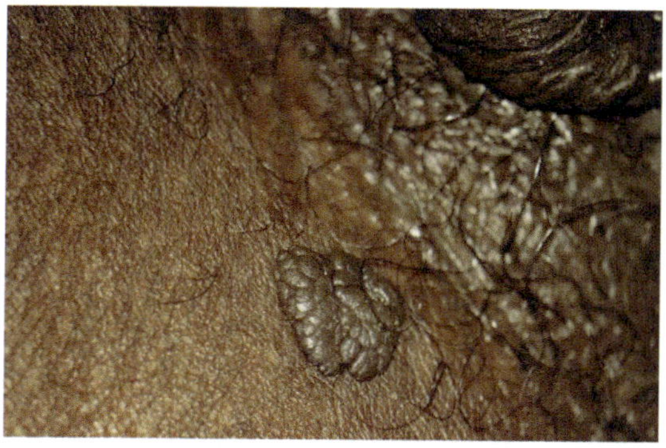

Fig. 18.271 Round papillary wart consistent with condyloma acuminata

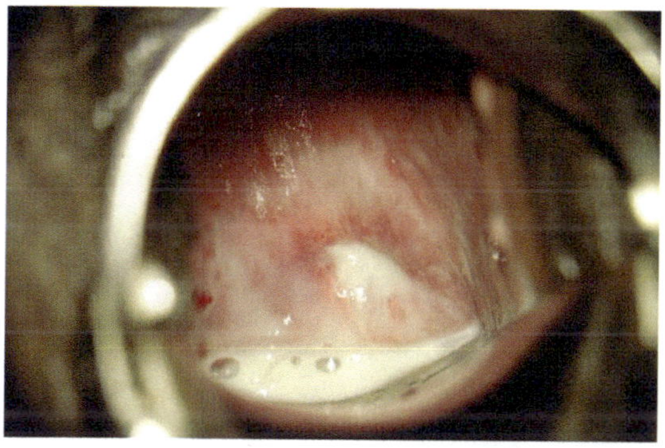

Fig. 18.272 Copious white frothy discharge

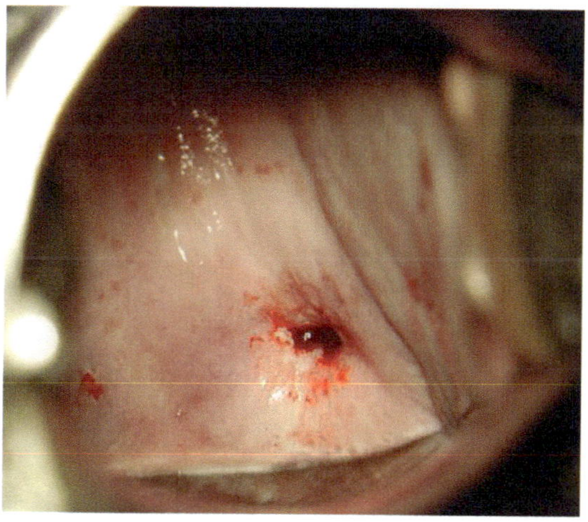

Fig. 18.273 The opening of the cervical canal is almost flush with the surface of the upper vagina

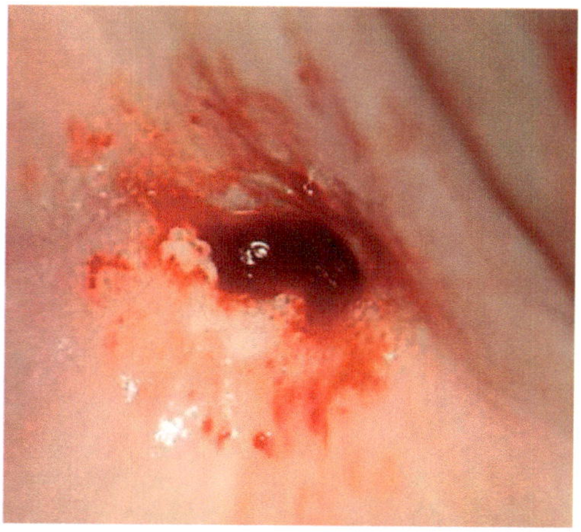

Fig. 18.274 Small opaque and slightly raised densely acetowhite lesion at the 6 to 9 o'clock position

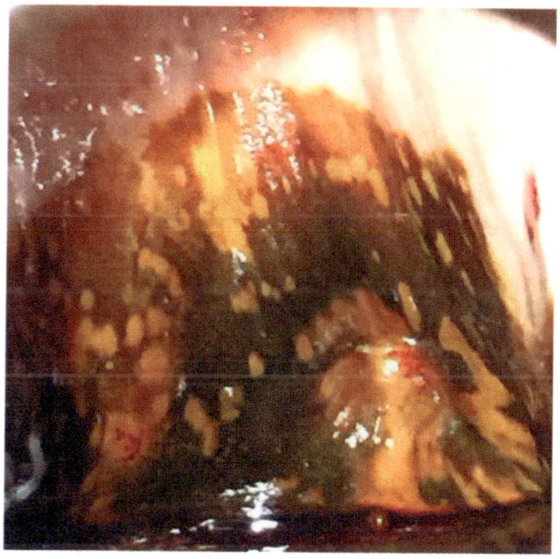

Fig. 18.275 Lugol's test shows partial staining of cervix and vagina with unstained yellowish patches consistent with cervicitis

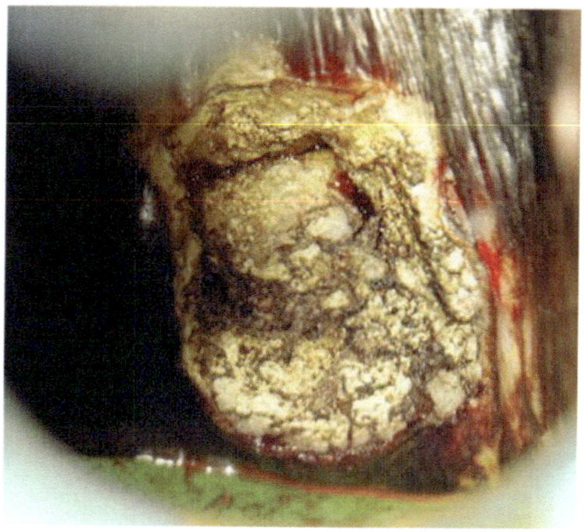

Fig. 18.276 Cervix and upper vagina after LOOP resection of the cervix and the surrounding tissue

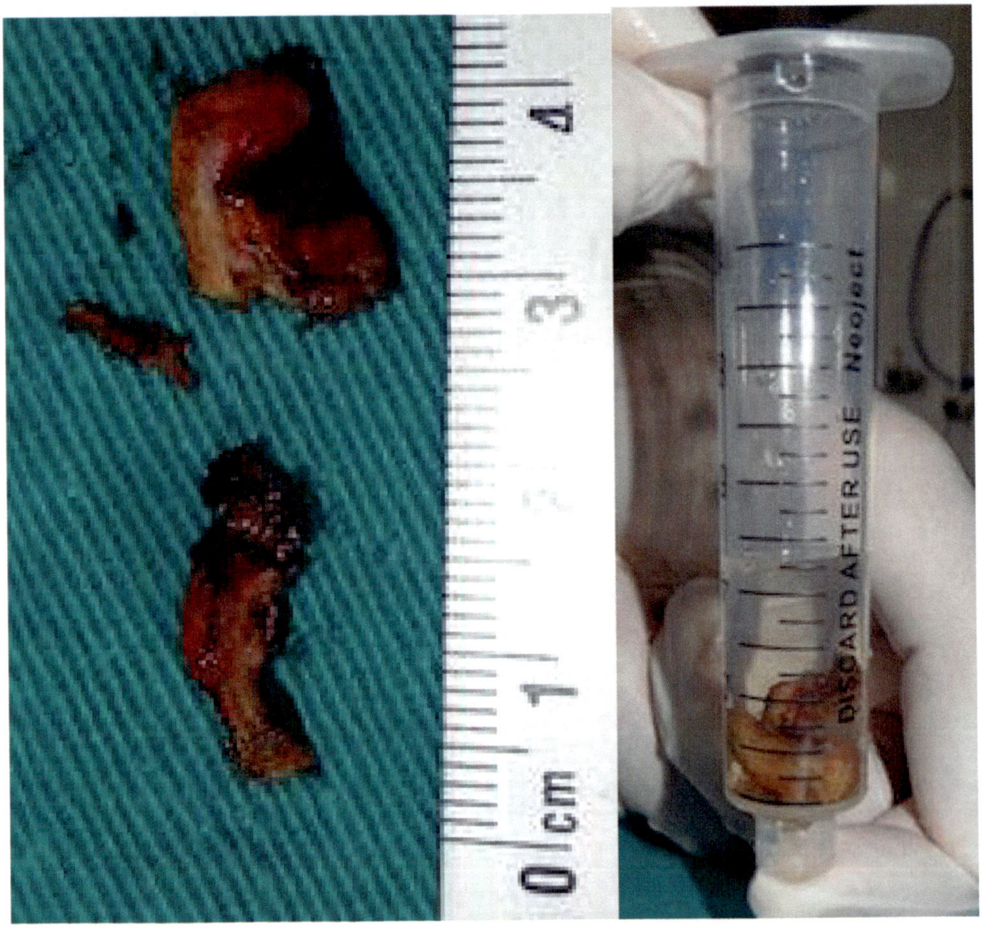

Fig. 18.277 Archimedes' principle is used to estimate the resection volume: 0.6 cm^3

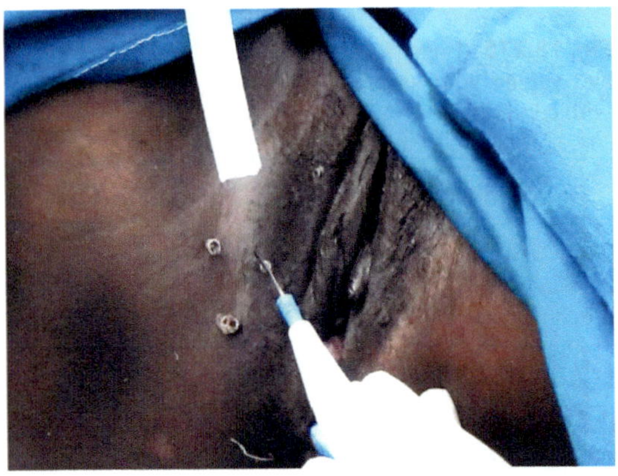

Fig. 18.278 With the tip of the electrosurgical scalpel (needle), the warts are coagulated

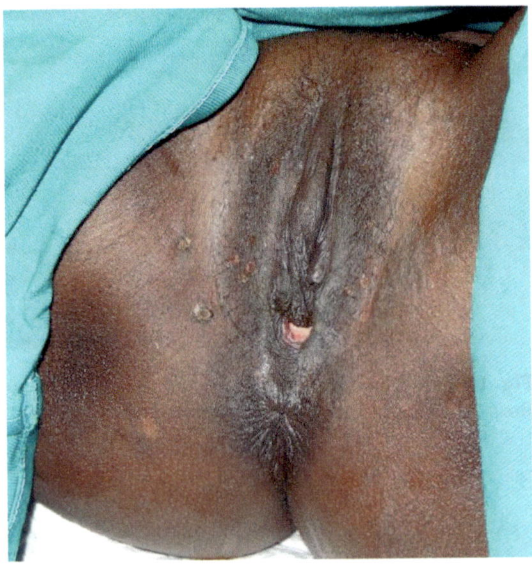

Fig. 18.279 Vulva after cauterization of condylomata acuminata

18.9.16 FIGO Stage IB1 Carcinoma of the Cervix Treated by Radical Hysterectomy and Bilateral Pelvic Lymph Node Dissection

A 35-year-old patient, P5, presented to META Hospital, Mbeya, Tanzania, complaining of post-coital bleeding. Cervical biopsies revealed well-differentiated squamous cell carcinoma of the cervix. Kidneys were normal on ultrasound. The HIV test was negative.

On colposcopic exam (Fig. 18.280) the cervix is distorted with a defect at the 6 o'clock position and significant bleeding from the cervical os and the irregular cervical surface. After the application of 5% acetic acid (Fig. 18.281), ulceration of the central aspect of the cervix can be seen as well as some opaque acetowhite changes in the periphery. On vaginal and rectal palpation, there is a 4 cm cervical mass that appears to be limited to the cervix without parametrial or vaginal involvement. The uterus is firm and enlarged as in a 12-week gestation. Clinical stage IB1 disease is suspected.

Radical hysterectomy, bilateral salpingo-oophorectomy, and bilateral pelvic lymph node dissection are performed (Fig. 18.282). Macroscopically, the tumor is resected completely (Fig. 18.283). Lymph nodes are enlarged but soft.

No histological evaluation is available at this point.

Commentary

Despite the fact that radical surgery for carcinoma of the cervix is rarely performed in Tanzania due to the lack of crucial resources, this patient has been treated according to international standards including the removal of regional lymph nodes. However, this example shows that the lack of a sufficient capacity for histopathologic evaluation in most countries of Sub-Saharan Africa (Adesina et al. 2013) leads to suboptimal management of cancer patients. If one or more lymph nodes had been found to be positive in this patient, adjuvant treatment by chemoradiation would have been indicated.

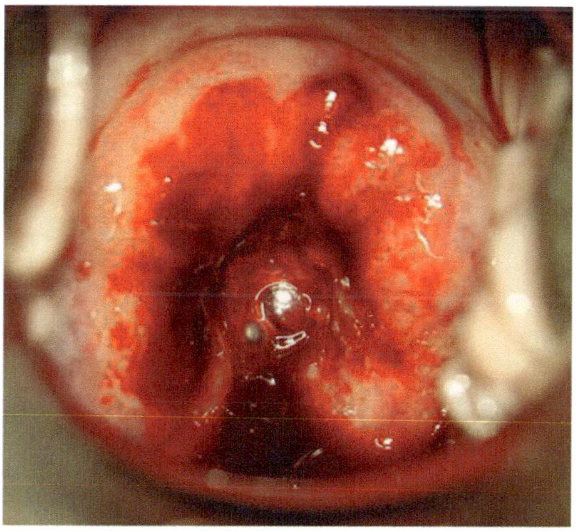

Fig. 18.280 FIGO stage IB squamous cell carcinoma of the cervix. The cervix is distorted with a defect at the 6 o'clock position with significant bleeding

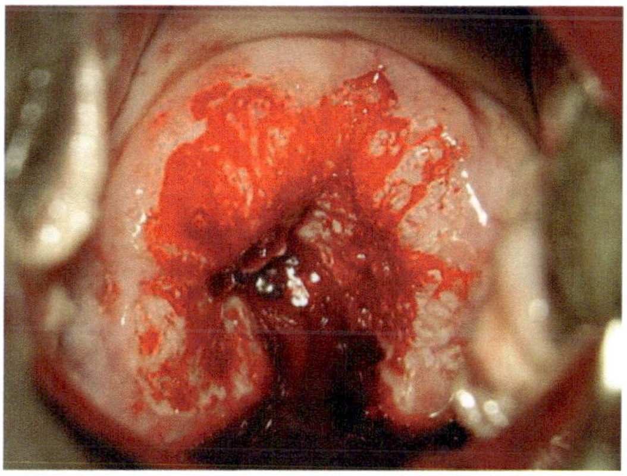

Fig. 18.281 FIGO stage IB squamous cell carcinoma of the cervix. After the application of 5% acetic acid, ulceration of the central aspect of the cervix is more pronounced with some acetowhite staining in the periphery

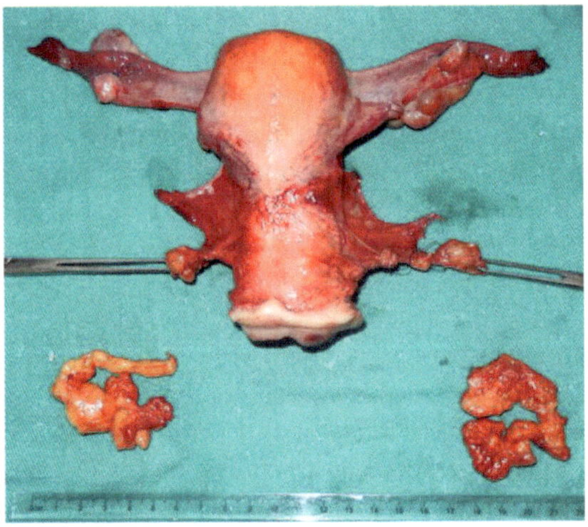

Fig. 18.282 FIGO stage IB squamous cell carcinoma of the cervix removed by Piver type III radical hysterectomy, bilateral salpingo-oophorectomy, as well as bilateral pelvic lymph node dissection

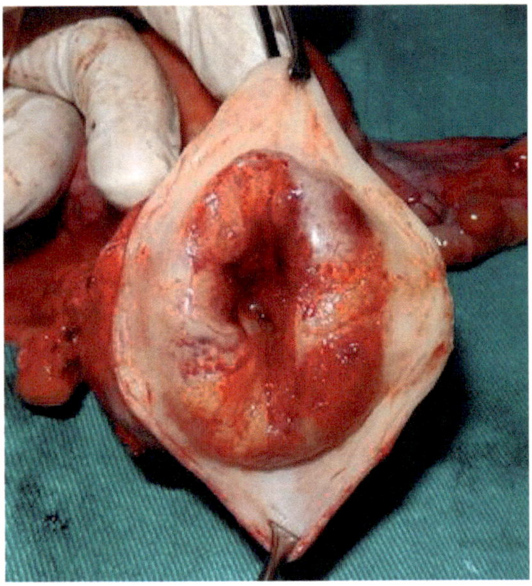

Fig. 18.283 The cancer growth is limited to the cervix without vaginal cuff involvement

18.9.17 Myoma in Statu Nascendi 1

A 36-year-old patient, P2, presented to META Hospital in Mbeya, Tanzania, with heavy vaginal bleeding during the past 2 weeks. She is HIV positive with pronounced facial lipodystrophy due to her HIV medication. Her CD4 count is 800 cell/μl.

On speculum exam, a large firm mass is seen protruding into the vagina. There is no acetowhite reaction (Fig. 18.284) and no Lugol staining either (Fig. 18.285).

On vaginal palpation, a 4–5 cm smooth and firm tumor is seen protruding from the cervix. The entire circumference of the cervix can be palpated.

Treatment includes removal of the fibroid by gentle rotation around its pedicle until it comes off (Figs. 18.286 and 18.287). Usually, no additional measures for hemostasis are required. However, the surgeon should be prepared for immediate hysterectomy, preferably through the vaginal route, if uncontrollable bleeding occurs.

Commentary

If a pedunculated fibroid becomes necrotic, confusion with cancer is possible. However, in the case presented here, the smooth tumor surface that does not react to acetic acid or Lugol solution as well as the fact that the cervical circumference can be palpated leads to the correct diagnosis.

An ultrasound study from the United States by Baird et al. (2003) has shown that uterine fibroid tumors develop in most women before menopause. However, in black women, these fibroids develop at earlier ages. This is possibly due to a higher prevalence of estrogen receptor alpha polymorphism in black women (Al-Hendy and Salama 2006).

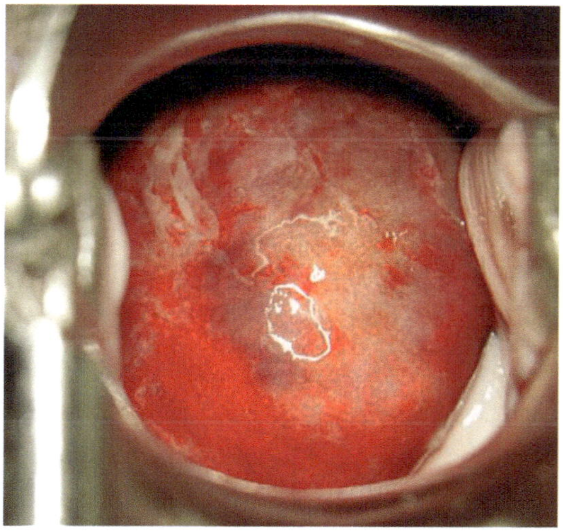

Fig. 18.284 Myoma in statu nascendi. On speculum exam, a large mass is seen protruding into the vagina. The cervix is not visible. The tumor does not react to the 5% acetic acid solution

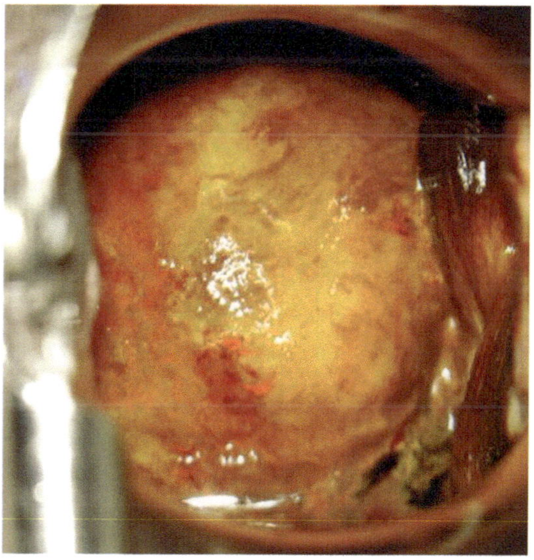

Fig. 18.285 Myoma in statu nascendi that is entirely Lugol negative

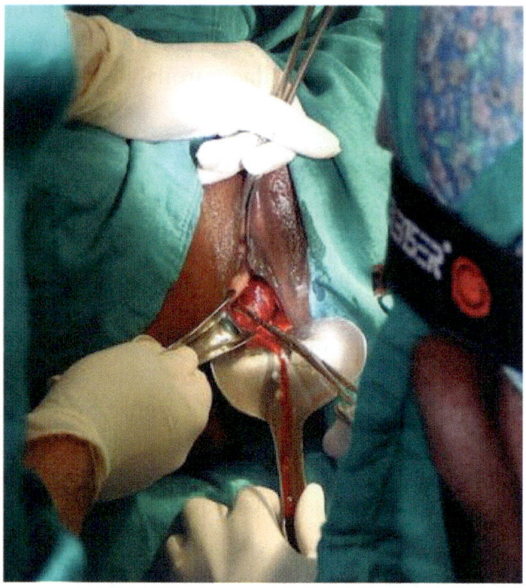

Fig. 18.286 Myoma in statu nascendi. The tumor is firmly grasped by bullet forceps and rotated slowly and gently until the pedicle comes off

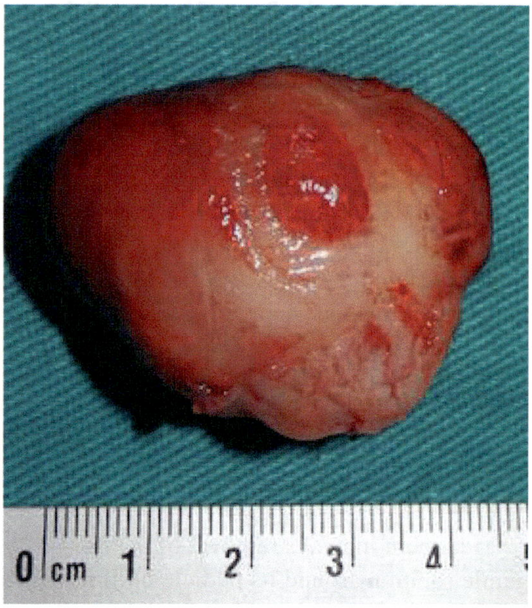

Fig. 18.287 Myoma in statu nascendi after removal

18.9.18 Myoma in Statu Nascendi 2

A 38-year-old patient, G3 P3, is HIV negative. She presents to META Hospital, Mbeya, Tanzania, complaining of vaginal bleeding. The patient herself suspects prolapse of the uterus.

On speculum exam a 3 x 3 cm mass can be seen protruding from the cervical os and which is attached through a narrow stalk out of the uterus. The surface of the tumor is slightly uneven (Fig. 18.288). However, on colposcopic inspection there is no ulceration and no suspicion of cancer (Fig. 18.289).

The diagnosis of a myoma in statu nascendi is made and the fibroid tumor is removed by gently rotating it around its stalk (Fig. 18.290) with curettage of the uterus to remove any residual tissue that may interfere with contraction of the uterus and thus with hemostasis.

Commentary

The surface of the fibroid tumor is not entirely smooth. Together with vaginal bleeding, this might be confused with carcinoma. However, vaginal palpation will clarify the diagnosis as the cervical circumference can be identified. Sometimes the stalk can also be palpated.

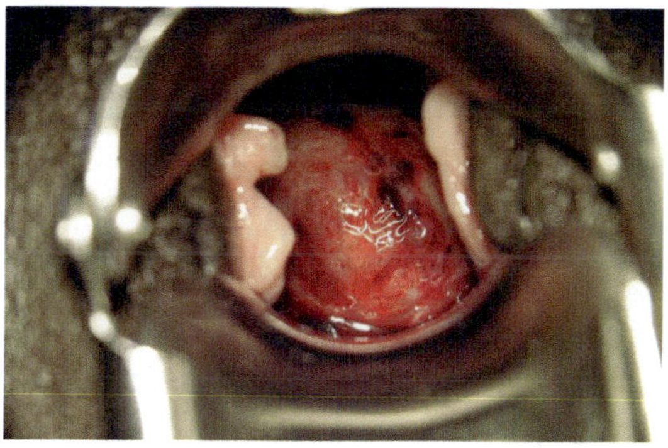

Fig. 18.288 Myoma in statu nascendi. A tumor is protruding from the cervix. However, this is not the cervix itself but rather a fibroid tumor attached to a pedicle protruding from the cervix

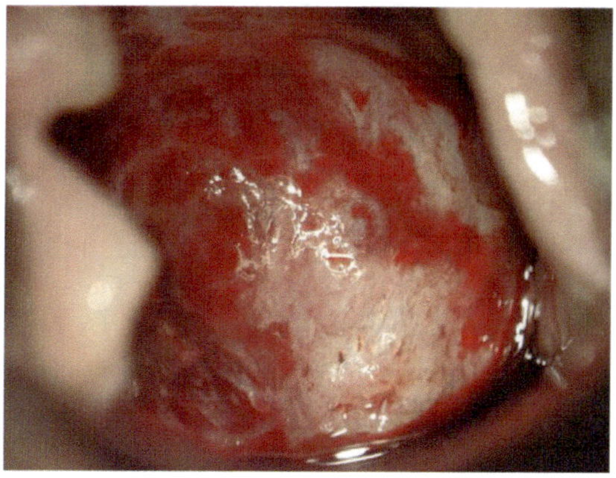

Fig. 18.289 Myoma in statu nascendi. The surface of the fibroid tumor is not entirely smooth and there is bleeding. In some cases, differential diagnosis to carcinoma can be difficult

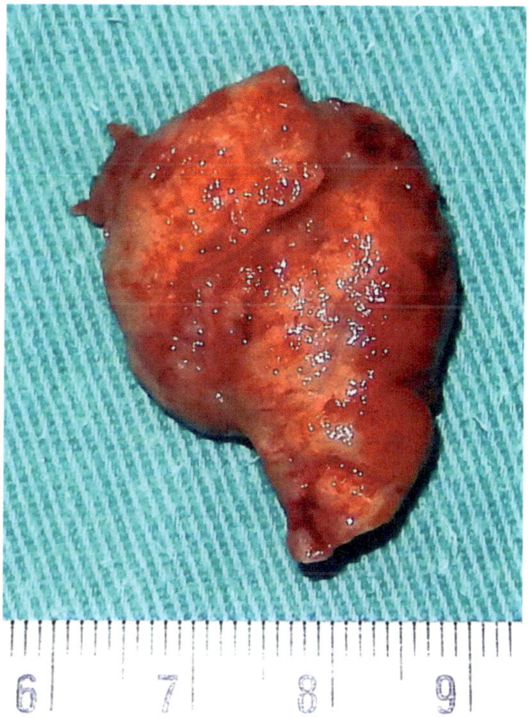

Fig. 18.290 Myoma in statu nascendi. In the lower half of the picture, the tumor tapers toward the former attachment of the pedicle

18.9.19 VIA+/VILI+ Patient Treated by LEEP

A 23-year-old patient, P1, is HIV negative. She presents to META Hospital, Mbeya, for screening. She does not have any complaints.

Before the application of acetic acid, the cervix looks normal (Fig. 18.291). After the acetic acid has been applied, the cervix is VIA positive. On colposcopic inspection, there is opaque acetowhite staining at the 12 o'clock position close to the squamocolumnar junction (major change). In addition, there are several less prominent and less opaque acetowhite regions with sharp borders, both ventrally and dorsally (minor change) (Figs. 18.292 and 18.293).

- Adequate colposcopy
- Squamocolumnar junction partially visible
- T3
- Abnormal colposcopic findings: ventral two quadrants with opaque acetowhite and ridge sign (grade 2); ventral and dorsal quadrants with transparent acetowhite staining and sharp borders (grade 1) Figs. 18.292 and 18.293

The cervix is VILI positive with iodine-negative/yellowish areas close to the squamocolumnar junction with sharp delineation (Fig. 18.294).

As the abnormal tissue area exceeds more than about 75% of the cervical surface, loop resection is performed instead of cryotherapy to remove all Lugol-negative tissue (Fig. 18.295). A small loop is used for the entire procedure, so multiple fragments are removed (Fig. 18.296). A histological report is not available due to the lack of local resources.

Commentary

Although no histological report is available, the likelihood of HSIL is very high as the colposcopic evaluation is consistent with a ridge sign, i.e., an opaque acetowhite ridge at the squamocolumnar junction. Scheungraber et al. (2009) demonstrated that a ridge sign is a highly specific marker for the presence of high-grade dysplasia. Furthermore, it is associated with HPV 16 infection and young age.

The patient was 23 years old when she presented for screening. Furthermore, she does not belong to a particular risk group as her HIV status is negative. The target population for screening is usually 30 years or older. The Tanzanian government, has defined a target population of 30–50 years of age (The United Republic of Tanzania Ministry of Health and Welfare Service 2011). However, patients who present for screening outside this age range should not be denied service. This is especially true for older patients whose risk for cervical cancer increases over time.

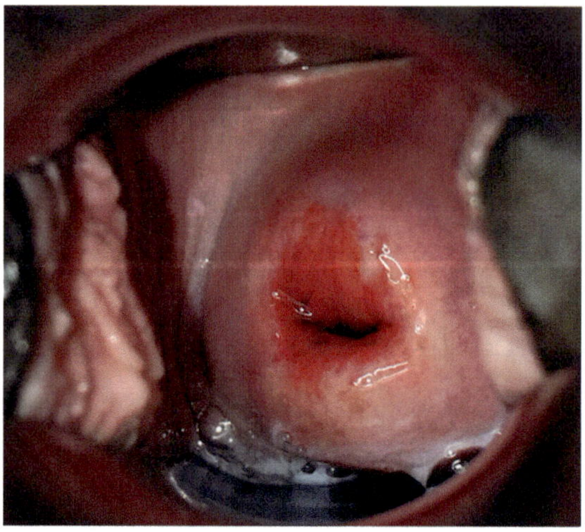

Fig. 18.291 Normal-appearing cervix prior to application of acetic acid

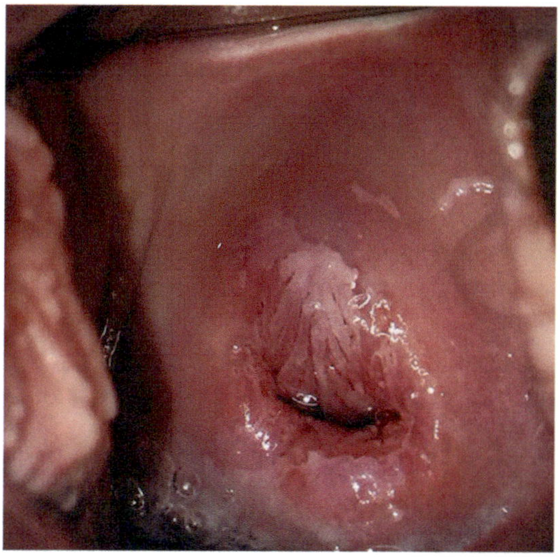

Fig. 18.292 After application of acetic acid, the cervix is VIA positive. Colposcopically, both major (anterior/ventral cervix) and minor changes (posterior/dorsal cervix) are seen

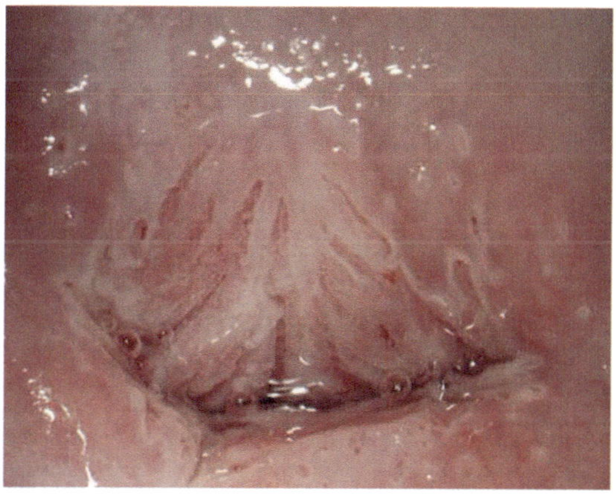

Fig. 18.293 Colposcopy reveals a typical ridge sign (major change)

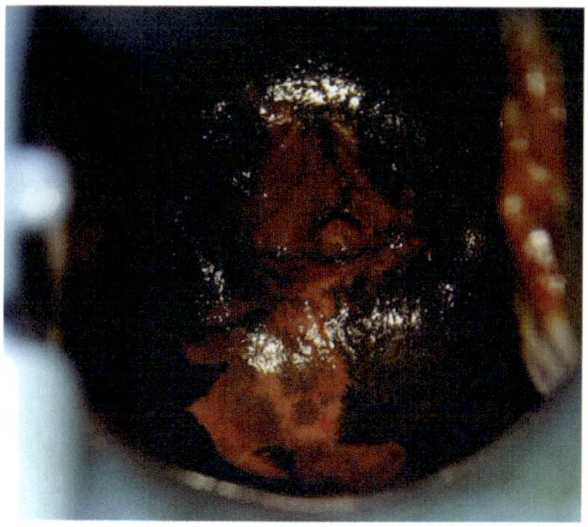

Fig. 18.294 Cervix after applying Lugol's solution: VILI +

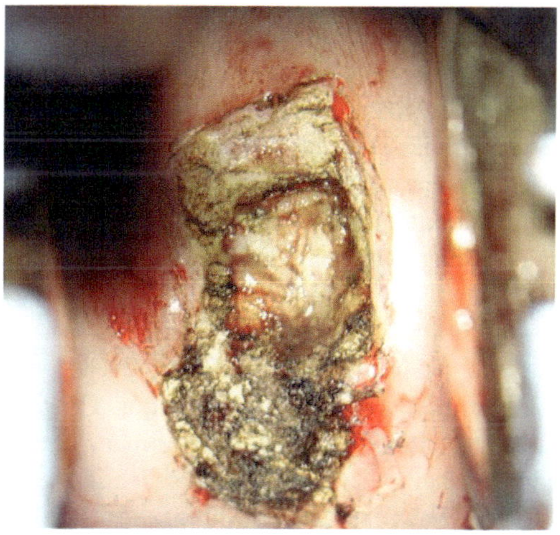

Fig. 18.295 Cervix immediately after LEEP

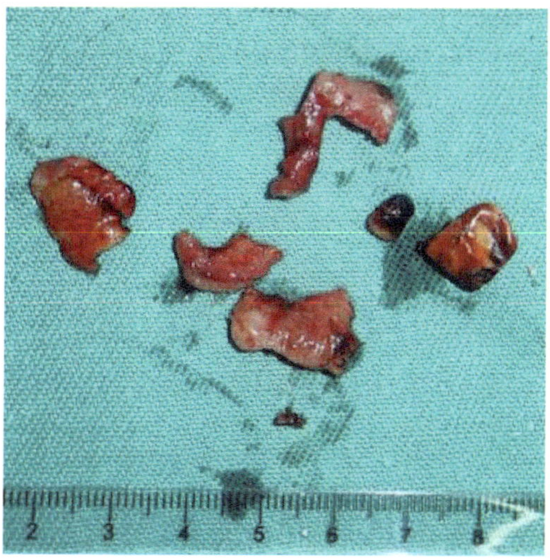

Fig. 18.296 LEEP. Multiple fragments have been removed using a small loop

18.9.20 Advanced Cervical Cancer with Urinary Fistula Formation

The patient presents to META Referral Hospital, Mbeya, Tanzania, with foul-smelling watery discharge. She does not know her own age and is estimated to be about 75 years old. Her HIV status is unknown.

On gynecological exam, no cervix can be identified. Instead, there is a large friable mass encompassing the entire anterior vaginal wall including the lower one third (Fig. 18.297). The patient smells of urine. On closer inspection, a bladder fistula is seen with a large part of the bladder mucosa visible (Fig. 18.298). On palpation, there is a nodular mass involving the left pelvic sidewall and partial involvement of the right side. Biopsies are taken which show poorly differentiated squamous cell carcinoma (FIGO stage IVA).

The patient is referred to palliative care as she would not be eligible for treatment at a cancer center according to present Tanzanian guidelines.

Commentary

The prognosis for patients with FIGO stage IVA carcinoma of the cervix is poor. However, treatment options exist such as primary chemoradiation therapy or primary and secondary exenteration (Waggoner 2003; Marnitz et al. 2006). However, especially the ultraradical surgery option with its high complication rate and the necessity of sophisticated and expensive perioperative as well as postoperative management is presently not feasible in many countries.

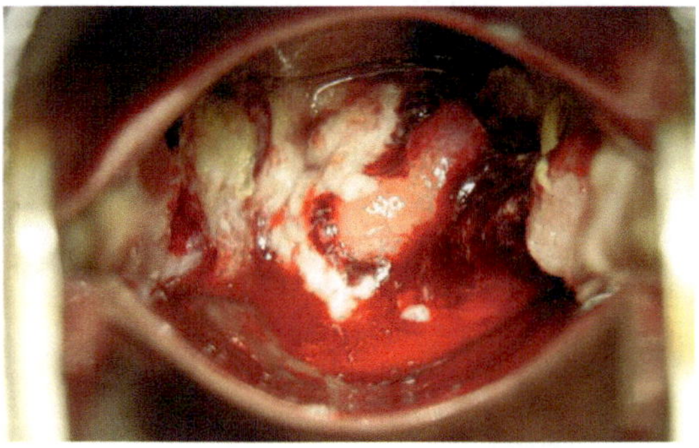

Fig. 18.297 Poorly differentiated squamous cell carcinoma of the cervix FIGO stage IVA. A large area of friable and necrotic tumor tissue is seen which has destroyed the cervix and part of the vagina

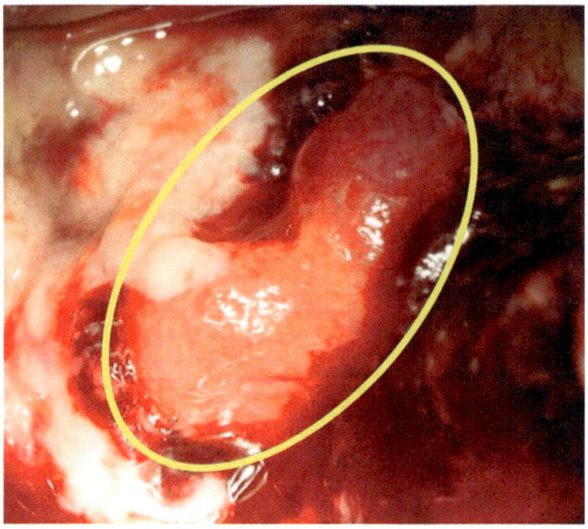

Fig. 18.298 Poorly differentiated squamous cell carcinoma of the cervix FIGO stage IVA. On closer inspection, a urinary fistula is identified exposing a large area of bladder mucosa

18.9.21 Cervical Carcinoma Without Ulceration or Exophytic Growth Pattern

A 31-year-old patient, P3, has presented 7 months ago to META Referral Hospital, Mbeya, Tanzania, with watery discharge and vaginal bleeding. For the past 3 years, she has been trying to conceive. A cervical biopsy is taken and shows well-differentiated squamous cell carcinoma.

For the previous 12 months, the patient has been on HIV treatment with a CD4 count of 210 cells/μl.

She now presents for further evaluation and treatment. On speculum exam there is significant bleeding through the cervical canal. The surface of the cervix is irregular. However, there is no tissue defect and no exophytic growth pattern (Fig. 18.299). After the application of 5% acetic acid, there is acetowhite staining which is partially opaque and partially transparent (Fig. 18.300). With higher magnification an irregular surface at the 3 and 9 o'clock position can be seen (Fig. 18.301).

On palpation, the cervix are felt to be of normal size without parametrial and/or vaginal infiltration. FIGO stage is determined as IB1.

The patient has remarried recently and would like to become pregnant again. She and her husband are counseled that radical hysterectomy would be advisable and the patient is scheduled for surgery.

Nevertheless, 6 months later she is pregnant in her 23rd week of gestation.

Commentary

Most invasive cervical carcinomas present either with tissue defects (ulceration) or an exophytic growth pattern. In this regard the macroscopic and colposcopic appearance of the cervix was unusual. However, vaginal bleeding and the irregular surface of the ectocervix had been suspicious for cancer. Possibly a major part of the invasive disease is located within the endocervix.

Despite efforts to explain the situation to the patient as well as her husband and despite the doctors' advice that radical surgery would be necessary, the patient had become pregnant again. Although there are reports that treatment delay for cervical cancer due to pregnancy might be acceptable (Amant et al. 2014), this is only true for lymph node-negative disease, i.e., the pelvic lymph nodes would have to be removed laparoscopically for histopathologic examination.

With histologically proven FIGO stage IB1 cancer of the cervix, delivery should be by cesarean section in order to avoid uncontrollable cervical bleeding. At that time operability needs to be reevaluated.

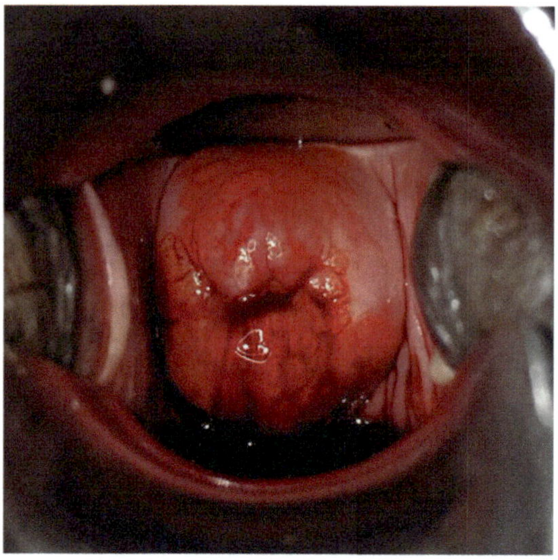

Fig. 18.299 FIGO stage IB1 squamous cell carcinoma of the cervix with bleeding and irregular cervical surface. However, there is no ulceration and no exophytic growth pattern

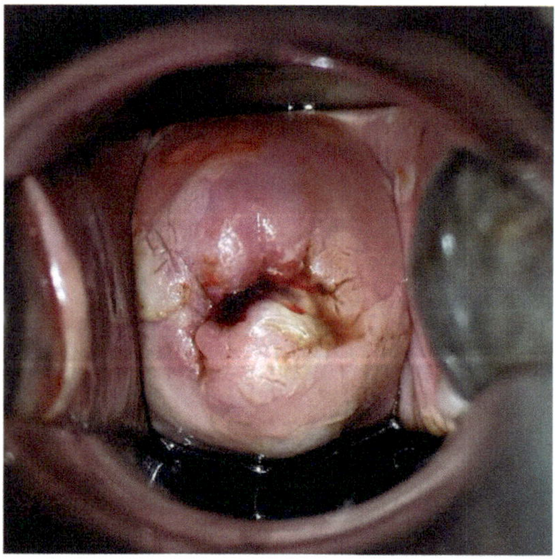

Fig. 18.300 FIGO stage IB1 squamous cell carcinoma of the cervix. There is acetowhite staining which is partially transparent and partially opaque

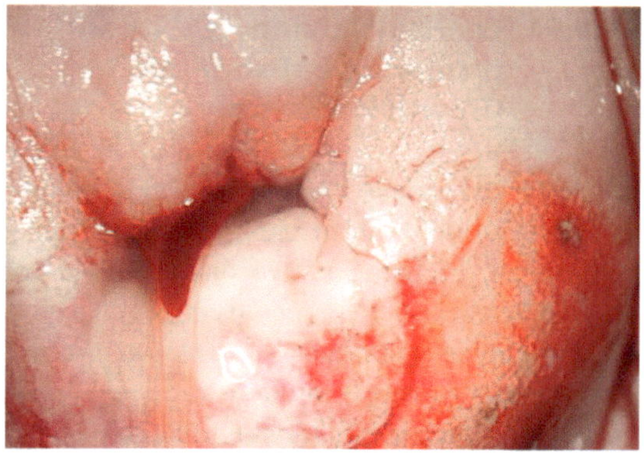

Fig. 18.301 The surface epithelium at the 3 and 9 o'clock position is highly irregular

References

ACOG (2016) Practice Bulletin No. 168: cervical cancer screening and prevention. Obstet Gynecol 128(4):e111–e130

Adesina A, Chumba D, Nelson AM, Orem J, Roberts DJ, Wabinga H et al (2013) Improvement of pathology in sub-Saharan Africa. Lancet Oncol 14(4):e152–e157. https://doi.org/10.1016/S1470-2045(12)70598-3

Al-Hendy A, Salama SA (2006) Ethnic distribution of estrogen receptor-α polymorphism is associated with a higher prevalence of uterine leiomyomas in black Americans. Fertil Steril 86(3):686–693. https://doi.org/10.1016/j.fertnstert.2006.01.052

Ali H, Donovan B, Wand H, Read TR, Regan DG, Grulich AE et al (2013) Genital warts in young Australians five years into national human papillomavirus vaccination programme: national surveillance data. BMJ 346:f2032. https://doi.org/10.1136/bmj.f2032

Altieri A, Franceschi S, Ferlay J, Smith J, La Vecchia C (2003) Epidemiology and aetiology of gestational trophoblastic diseases. Lancet Oncol 4(11):670–678

Amant F, Halaska MJ, Fumagalli M, Dahl Steffensen K, Lok C, Van Calsteren K et al (2014) Gynecologic cancers in pregnancy: guidelines of a second international consensus meeting. Int J Gynecol Cancer 24(3):394–403. https://doi.org/10.1097/IGC.0000000000000062

Baird DD, Dunson DB, Hill MC, Cousins D, Schectman JM (2003) High cumulative incidence of uterine leiomyoma in black and white women: ultrasound evidence. Am J Obstet Gynecol 188(1):100–107. https://doi.org/10.1067/mob.2003.99

Benedet JL, Wilson PS, Matisic JP (1992) Epidermal thickness measurements in vaginal intraepithelial neoplasia. A basis for optimal CO2 laser vaporization. J Reprod Med 37(9):809–812

Benedet JL, Odicino F, Maisonneuve P, Beller U, Creasman WT, Heintz AP et al (2003) Carcinoma of the cervix uteri. Int J Gynaecol Obstet 83(Suppl 1):41–78

Bhatla N, Aoki D, Sharma DN, Sankaranarayanan R. (2018) Cancer of the cervix uteri. Int J Gynaecol Obstet.143 Suppl.3:22–36

Borghi C, Bogani G, Ditto A, Martinelli F, Signorelli M, Chiappa V et al (2018) Invasive Paget disease of the vulva. Official journal of the International Gynecological Cancer Society. Int J Gynecol Cancer. 28(1):176–82

Bornstein J, Bentley J, Bosze P, Girardi F, Haefner H, Menton M et al (2012a) 2011 colposcopic terminology of the International Federation for Cervical Pathology and Colposcopy. Obstet Gynecol 120(1):166–172. https://doi.org/10.1097/AOG.0b013e318254f90c

Bornstein J, Sideri M, Tatti S, Walker P, Prendiville W, Haefner HK, Nomenclature Committee of International Federation for Cervical Pathology and Colposcopy (2012b) 2011 terminology of the vulva of the International Federation for Cervical Pathology and Colposcopy. J Low Genit Tract Dis 16(3):290–295. https://doi.org/10.1097/LGT.0b013e31825934c7

Brook I (2008) Microbiology and management of soft tissue and muscle infections. Int J Surg 6(4):328–338. https://doi.org/10.1016/j.ijsu.2007.07.001

Buckley CH, Fox H (1988) Epithelial tumours of the vulva. In: Ridley CM (ed) The vulva. Livingstone, Edinburg, p 287

Castellano Megias VM, Ibarrola de Andres C, Martinez Parra D, Lara Lara I, Perez Palacios C, Conde Zurita JM (2002) Cytology of extramammary Paget's disease of the vulva. A case report. Acta Cytol 46(6):1153–1157

Cohain JS, Buxbaum RE, Mankuta D (2017) Spontaneous first trimester miscarriage rates per woman among parous women with 1 or more pregnancies of 24 weeks or more. BMC Pregnancy Childbirth 17(1):437–437. https://doi.org/10.1186/s12884-017-1620-1

Condon JR, Rumbold AR, Thorn JC, O'Brien MM, Davy MJ, Zardawi I (2009) A cluster of vulvar cancer and vulvar intraepithelial neoplasia in young Australian indigenous women. Cancer Causes Control 20(1):67–74. https://doi.org/10.1007/s10552-008-9218-6

Conley LJ, Ellerbrock TV, Bush TJ, Chiasson MA, Sawo D, Wright TC (2002) HIV-1 infection and risk of vulvovaginal and perianal condylomata acuminata and intraepithelial neoplasia: a prospective cohort study. Lancet 359(9301):108–113. https://doi.org/10.1016/S0140-6736(02)07368-3

Costa S, Negri G, Sideri M, Santini D, Martinelli G, Venturoli S et al (2007) Human papillomavirus (HPV) test and PAP smear as predictors of outcome in conservatively treated adenocarcinoma in situ (AIS) of the uterine cervix. Gynecol Oncol 106(1):170–176

Das N, Naik R, Jackson S, De Barros Lopes A, Monaghan JM, Godfrey KA, Hatem MH (2005) Recurrent smear abnormalities where repeat loop treatment is not possible: is hysterectomy the answer? Gynecol Oncol 97(3):751–754. https://doi.org/10.1016/j.ygyno.2005.01.003

de Araujo Souza PS, Villa LL (2003). Genetic susceptibility to infection with human papillomavirus and development of cervical cancer in women in Brazil. Mutat Res 544:375–83

Delgado G, Bundy BN, Fowler WC, Stehman FB, Sevin B, Creasman WT et al (1989) A prospective surgical pathological study of stage I squamous carcinoma of the cervix: a Gynecologic Oncology Group study. Gynecol Oncol 35(3):314–320. https://doi.org/10.1016/0090-8258(89)90070-X

Duggan B, Muderspach LI, Roman LD, Curtin JP, d'Ablaing G III, Morrow CP (1993) Cervical cancer in pregnancy: reporting on planned delay in therapy. Obstet Gynecol 82(4 Pt 1):598–602

Fanning J, Lambert HC, Hale TM, Morris PC, Schuerch C (1999) Page's disease of the vulva: prevalence of associated vulvar adenocarcinoma, invasive Paget's disease, and recurrence after surgical excision. Am J Obstet Gynecol 180(1 Pt 1):24–27

Fokom-Domgue J, Combescure C, Fokom-Defo V, Tebeu PM, Vassilakos P, Kengne AP, Petignat P (2015)

Performance of alternative strategies for primary cervical cancer screening in sub-Saharan Africa: systematic review and meta-analysis of diagnostic test accuracy studies. BMJ 351:h3084. https://doi.org/10.1136/bmj.h3084

Galgano MT, Castle PE, Atkins KA, Brix WK, Nassau SR, Stoler MH (2010) Using biomarkers as objective standards in the diagnosis of cervical biopsies. Am J Surg Pathol 34(8):1077–1087. https://doi.org/10.1097/PAS.0b013e3181e8b2c4

Grote HJ, Nguyen HV, Leick AG, Bocking A (2004) Identification of progressive cervical epithelial cell abnormalities using DNA image cytometry. Cancer 102(6):373–379. https://doi.org/10.1002/cncr.20644

Gu M, Ghafari S, Lin F (2005) Pap smears of patients with extramammary Paget's disease of the vulva. Diagn Cytopathol 32(6):353–357. https://doi.org/10.1002/dc.20260

Haidopoulos D, Rodolakis A, Stefanidis K, Blachos G, Sotiropoulou M, Diakomanolis E (2002) Behcet's disease: part of the differential diagnosis of the ulcerative vulva. Clin Exp Obstet Gynecol 29(3):219–221

Hampl M, Deckers-Figiel S, Hampl JA, Rein D, Bender HG (2008) New aspects of vulvar cancer: changes in localization and age of onset. Gynecol Oncol 109(3):340–345. https://doi.org/10.1016/j.ygyno.2008.01.041

Hertel H, Köhler C, Grund D, Hillemanns P, Possover M, Michels W, Schneider A (2006) Radical vaginal trachelectomy (RVT) combined with laparoscopic pelvic lymphadenectomy: prospective multicenter study of 100 patients with early cervical cancer. Gynecol Oncol 103(2):506–511

Hilal Z, Rezniczek GA, Alici F, Kumpernatz A, Dogan A, Alieva L, Tempfer CB (2018) Loop electrosurgical excision procedure (LEEP) with or without intraoperative colposcopy: a randomized trial. Am J Obstet Gynecol 219(4):377.e1–377.e7. https://doi.org/10.1016/j.ajog.2018.07.023

Hopkins MP, Morley GW (1991a) A comparison of adenocarcinoma and squamous cell carcinoma of the cervix. Obstet Gynecol 77(6):912–917

Hopkins MP, Morley GW (1991b) Stage IB squamous cell cancer of the cervix: clinicopathologic features related to survival. Am J Obstet Gynecol 164(6 Pt 1):1520–1527

Jeng CJ, Shen J, Huang SH (2006) Partial trachelectomy: a new treatment choice for persistent or recurrent high grade cervical intraepithelial neoplasia. Gynecol Oncol 100(2):231–232. https://doi.org/10.1016/j.ygyno.2005.09.039

Kadivar M, Hosseini A (2007) Cytological findings of intrauterine and cervical choriocarcinoma. Cytopathology 19(1):61–62. https://doi.org/10.1111/j.1365-2303.2006.00421.x

Kantelhardt EJ, Moelle U, Begoihn M, Addissie A, Trocchi P, Yonas B et al (2014) Cervical cancer in Ethiopia: survival of 1,059 patients who received oncologic therapy. Oncologist 19(7):727–734. https://doi.org/10.1634/theoncologist.2013-0326

Kyrgiou M, Koliopoulos G, Martin-Hirsch P, Arbyn M, Prendiville W, Paraskevaidis E (2006) Obstetric outcomes after conservative treatment for intraepithelial or early invasive cervical lesions: systematic review and meta-analysis. Lancet 367(9509):489–498. https://doi.org/10.1016/S0140-6736(06)68181-6

Lellé RJ (2007) HPV-Test nicht sinnvoll bei zytologischem Dysplasieverdacht - Korrelation von Zervixzytologie, Histologie und HPV-Status. Frauenarzt 48(4):356–359

Lellé RJ, Maier E, Eltze E, Böcker W (2000) Das villoglanduläre Karzinom: eine seltene Sonderform zervikaler Adenokarzinome mit günstiger Prognose. Geburtsh Frauenheilk 60:349–436

Marnitz S, Köhler C, Müller M, Behrens K, Hasenbein K, Schneider A (2006) Indications for primary and secondary exenterations in patients with cervical cancer. Gynecol Oncol 103(3):1023–1030. https://doi.org/10.1016/j.ygyno.2006.06.027

Martin-Hirsch PL, Paraskevaidis E, Kitchener H (2000) Surgery for cervical intraepithelial neoplasia. Cochrane Database Syst Rev 2:CD001318

Mayrand MH, Duarte-Franco E, Rodrigues I, Walter SD, Hanley J, Ferenczy A et al (2007) Human papillomavirus DNA versus Papanicolaou screening tests for cervical cancer. N Engl J Med 357(16):1579–1588. https://doi.org/10.1056/NEJMoa071430

Mitsuhashi A, Sekiya S (2000) Loop electrosurgical excision procedure (LEEP) during first trimester of pregnancy. Int J Gynaecol Obstet 71(3):237–239

Moreno-Arias GA, Conill C, Sola-Casas MA, Mascaro-Galy JM, Grimalt R (2003) Radiotherapy for in situ extramammary Paget disease of the vulva. J Dermatolog Treat 14(2):119–123

Moschella F, Cordova A (2000) Innervated island flaps in morphofunctional vulvar reconstruction. Plast Reconstr Surg 105(5):1649–1657

Murzaku EC, Penn LA, Hale CS, Pomeranz MK, Polsky D (2014) Vulvar nevi, melanosis, and melanoma: an epidemiologic, clinical, and histopathologic review. J Am Acad Dermatol 71(6):1241–1249. https://doi.org/10.1016/j.jaad.2014.08.019

Nauth HF (2002) Gynäkologische Zytodiagnostik. Thieme Verlag (Stuttgart)

Negri G, Rigo B, Vittadello F, Mian C, Egarter-Vigl E (2007) Abnormal cervicovaginal cytology with negative human papillomavirus testing. Cancer 111(5):280–284

Ngan HYS, Seckl MJ, Berkowitz RS, Xiang Y, Golfier F, Sekharan PK, Lurain JR (2015) Update on the diagnosis and management of gestational trophoblastic disease. Int J Gynecol Obstet 131(S2):S123–S126. https://doi.org/10.1016/j.ijgo.2015.06.008

Nwanodi O, Choi C, Khulpateea N (2008) Cervicovaginal cytology and diagnosis of ovarian or peritoneal cancer: case report and literature review. Arch Gynecol Obstet 277(2):171–174. https://doi.org/10.1007/s00404-007-0428-z

Ortoft G, Henriksen T, Hansen E, Petersen L (2010) After conisation of the cervix, the perinatal mortality as a result of preterm delivery increases in subsequent pregnancy. BJOG 117(3):258–267. https://doi.org/10.1111/j.1471-0528.2009.02438.x

Pecorelli S (2009) Revised FIGO staging for carcinoma of the vulva, cervix, and endometrium. Int J Gynaecol Obstet 105(2):103–104

Petry KU, Scheffel D, Bode U, Gabrysiak T, Kochel H, Kupsch E et al (1994) Cellular immunodeficiency enhances the progression of human papillomavirus-associated cervical lesions. Int J Cancer 57(6):836–840

Petry KU, Kochel H, Bode U, Schedel I, Niesert S, Glaubitz M et al (1996) Human papillomavirus is associated with the frequent detection of warty and basaloid high-grade neoplasia of the vulva and cervical neoplasia among immunocompromised women. Gynecol Oncol 60(1):30–34

Petry KU, Menton S, Menton M, van Loenen-Frosch F, de Carvalho Gomes H, Holz B et al (2003) Inclusion of HPV testing in routine cervical cancer screening for women above 29 years in Germany: results for 8466 patients. Br J Cancer 88(10):1570–1577

Pfaendler KS, Sahasrabuddhe VV, Katundu K, Mwanahamuntu MH, Kapambwe S, Vermund SH, Parham GP (2015) Factors associated with post-cryotherapy wound healing among HIV-infected women in a low-resource sub-Saharan African setting. Gynecol Oncol 137:69. https://doi.org/10.1016/j.ygyno.2015.01.165

Pinto KR, Lu DW, Rader JS, Davila RM (2004) Double cervix with bilateral and synchronous HSIL associated with different high-risk HPV types. A case report. Acta Cytol 48(2):273–277

Piver MS, Rutledge F, Smith JP (1974) Five classes of extended hysterectomy for women with cervical cancer. Obstet Gynecol 44(2):265–272

Reich O, Pickel H, Lahousen M, Tamussino K, Winter R (2001) Cervical intraepithelial neoplasia III: long-term outcome after cold-knife conization with clear margins. Obstet Gynecol 97(3):428–430

Rome RM, England PG (2000) Management of vaginal intraepithelial neoplasia: a series of 132 cases with long-term follow-up. Int J Gynecol Cancer 10(5):382–390

Schaefer K, Peters D, Aulmann S, Sohn C, Eichbaum MH (2012) Value and feasibility of LLETZ procedures for pregnant women with suspected high-grade squamous intraepithelial lesions and microinvasive cervical cancer. Int J Gynaecol Obstet 118(2):141–144. https://doi.org/10.1016/j.ijgo.2012.02.019

Scheungraber C, Koenig U, Fechtel B, Kuehne-Heid R, Duerst M, Schneider A (2009) The colposcopic feature ridge sign is associated with the presence of cervical intraepithelial neoplasia 2/3 and human papillomavirus 16 in young women. J Low Genit Tract Dis 13(1):13–16. https://doi.org/10.1097/LGT.0b013e318180438a

Schockaert S, Poppe W, Arbyn M, Verguts T, Verguts J (2008) Incidence of vaginal intraepithelial neoplasia after hysterectomy for cervical intraepithelial neoplasia: a retrospective study. Am J Obstet Gynecol 199(2):113 e1–5. https://doi.org/10.1016/j.ajog.2008.02.026

Shimada M, Kigawa J, Nishimura R, Yamaguchi S, Kuzuya K, Nakanishi T et al (2006) Ovarian metastasis in carcinoma of the uterine cervix. Gynecol Oncol 101(2):234–237. https://doi.org/10.1016/j.ygyno.2005.10.004

Sidor J, Diallo-Danebrock R, Eltze E, Lellé RJ (2006) Challenging the concept of microinvasive carcinoma of the vulva: report of a case with regional lymph node recurrence and review of the literature. BMC Cancer 6:157

Snast I, Sharon E, Kaftory R, Noyman Y, Oren-Shabtai M, Lapidoth M et al (2020) Nonsurgical treatments for extramammary Paget disease: a systematic review and meta-analysis. Dermatology 236(6):493–499. https://doi.org/10.1159/000506832

Staender S, Reinhardt HW, Luger TA (2006) Topische Cannaboidagonisten. Eine effektive neue Möglichkeit zur Behandlung von chronischem Pruritus. Hautarzt 57(9):801–807

Terlou A, van Seters M, Ewing PC, Aaronson NK, Gundy CM, Heijmans-Antonissen C et al (2011) Treatment of vulvar intraepithelial neoplasia with topical imiquimod: seven years median follow-up of a randomized clinical trial. Gynecol Oncol 121(1):157–162. https://doi.org/10.1016/j.ygyno.2010.12.340

The United Republic of Tanzania Ministry of Health and Welfare Service (2011) Tanzania service delivery guidelines for cervical cancer prevention and control

Utsugi K, Shimizu Y, Akiyama F, Hasumi K (2002) Villoglandular papillary adenocarcinoma of the uterine cervix with bulky lymph node metastases. Eur J Obstet Gynecol Reprod Biol 105(2):186–188

van den Einden LC, Grefte JM, van der Avoort IA, Vedder JE, van Kempen LC, Massuger LF, De Hullu JA (2012) Cytology of the vulva: feasibility and preliminary results of a new brush. Br J Cancer 106(2):269–273. https://doi.org/10.1038/bjc.2011.533

van Seters M, van Beurden M, ten Kate FJ, Beckmann I, Ewing PC, Eijkemans MJ et al (2008) Treatment of vulvar intraepithelial neoplasia with topical imiquimod. N Engl J Med 358(14):1465–1473. https://doi.org/10.1056/NEJMoa072685

Waggoner SE (2003) Cervical cancer. Lancet 361(9376):2217–2225. https://doi.org/10.1016/S0140-6736(03)13778-6

Wallbillich JJ, Rhodes HE, Milbourne AM, Munsell MF, Frumovitz M, Brown J et al (2012) Vulvar intraepithelial neoplasia (VIN 2/3): comparing clinical outcomes and evaluating risk factors for recurrence. Gynecol Oncol 127(2):312–315. https://doi.org/10.1016/j.ygyno.2012.07.118

WHO Classification of Tumours Editorial Board (2020) Female genital tumours. IARC Press, Lyon

Wright VC (1999) Colposcopy of adenocarcinoma in situ and adenocarcinoma of the uterine cervix: differentiation from other cervical lesions. J Low Genit Tract Dis 3(2):83–97

Zong L, Wang W, He Y, Cheng N, Xiang Y (2019) Carcinoma of the lower female genital tract in patients with genitourinary malformations: a clinicopathologic analysis of 36 cases. J Cancer 10(13):3054–3061. https://doi.org/10.7150/jca.30486

GPSR Compliance

The European Union's (EU) General Product Safety Regulation (GPSR) is a set of rules that requires consumer products to be safe and our obligations to ensure this.

If you have any concerns about our products, you can contact us on ProductSafety@springernature.com

In case Publisher is established outside the EU, the EU authorized representative is:

Springer Nature Customer Service Center GmbH
Europaplatz 3
69115 Heidelberg, Germany

Batch number: 09321893

Printed by Printforce, the Netherlands